Deciphering PROCEDURAL CODING 2018

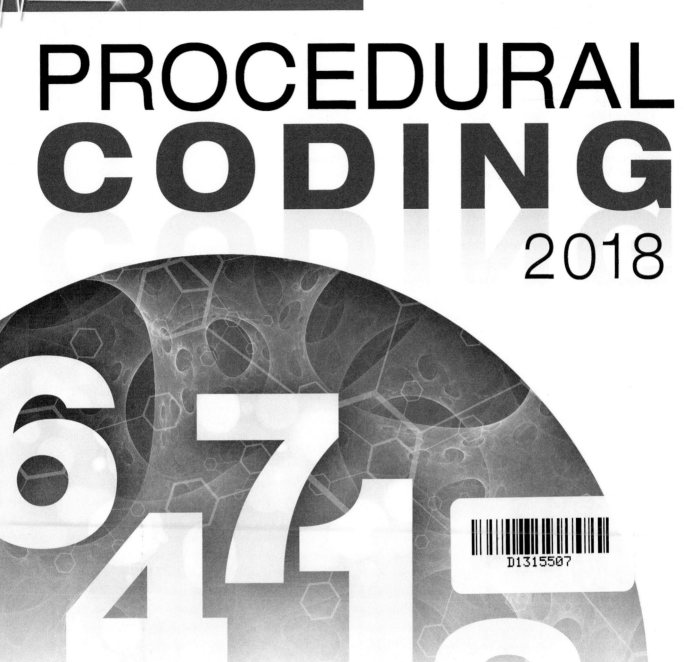

Ruth A. Berger • Sharon Y. McBride

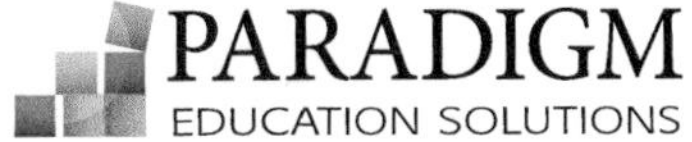

St. Paul

Division President: Linda Hein
Vice President, Content Management: Christine Hurney
Managing Editor: Carley Fruzzetti
Developmental Editor: Stephanie Schempp
Director of Production: Timothy W. Larson
Production Editor: Carrie Rogers
Senior Design and Production Specialist: Jaana Bykonich
Copy Editor: Deb Brant
Proofreader: Lori Ryan
Indexer: Terry Casey
Illustrators: A.D.A.M., a business unit of Ebix, Inc.; S4Carlisle Publishing Services
Vice President, Digital Solutions: Chuck Bratton
Digital Projects Manager: Tom Modl
Digital Solutions Manager: Gerry Yumul
Digital Production Manager: Aaron Esnough
Vice President, Sales and Marketing: Scott Burns
Director of Marketing: Lara McLellan

ISBN 978-0-76388-437-6 (print)
ISBN 978-0-76388-439-0 (ebook)

875 Montreal Way
St. Paul, MN 55102
Email: CustomerService@ParadigmEducation.com
Website: ParadigmEducation.com

Printed in the United States of America

28 27 26 25 24 23 22 21 20 19 1 2 3 4 5 6 7 8 9 10

Brief Contents

Contents

Chapter 5 Using the Health Record to Report Codes 125

Unit 2 Procedure Coding 149

Chapter 6 Evaluation and Management Services Coding 151

Preface

Deciphering Procedural Coding 2018 provides students with an up-to-date, accurate, and accessible introduction to Current Procedural Terminology (CPT®) coding. This textbook is designed to give students entering the field a firm foundation in all of the essential knowledge areas, including CPT®, Healthcare Common Procedure Coding System (HCPCS), modifiers, abstracting codes from electronic health records (EHRs), coding evaluation and management (E/M) services, anesthesia, surgical procedures, radiology procedures, pathology and laboratory procedures, medicine, reimbursement, and compliance.

This text is designed for students taking a course in CPT® coding, for those enrolled in a certified, accredited associate degree program, and for students planning to take a professional coding certification exam. To get the best benefit from this text, students should already have taken and passed a course in medical terminology.

This book also provides students with the opportunity to begin exploring Paradigm's live, web-based electronic health record application, the EHR Navigator. Developed by modeling the best features of many industry EHR systems, the EHR Navigator offers students hands-on practice and the freedom to explore this increasingly important technology at their own pace.

Chapter Features: A Visual Walk-Through

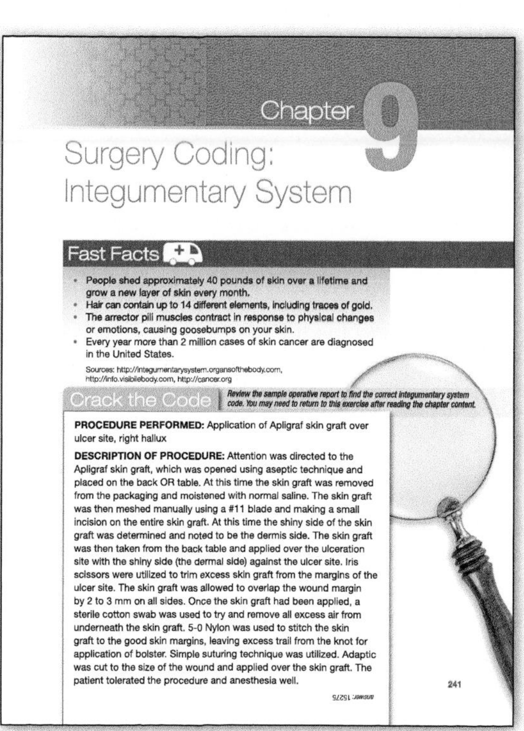

Chapter 9

Surgery Coding: Integumentary System

Fast Facts

- People shed approximately 40 pounds of skin over a lifetime and grow a new layer of skin every month.
- Hair can contain up to 14 different elements, including traces of gold.
- The arrector pili muscles contract in response to physical changes or emotions, causing goosebumps on your skin.
- Every year more than 2 million cases of skin cancer are diagnosed in the United States.

Sources: http://integumentarysystem.organsofthebody.com, http://info.visibilebody.com, http://cancer.org

Crack the Code *Review the sample operative report to find the correct integumentary system code. You may need to return to this exercise after reading the chapter content.*

PROCEDURE PERFORMED: Application of Apligraf skin graft over ulcer site, right hallux

DESCRIPTION OF PROCEDURE: Attention was directed to the Apligraf skin graft, which was opened using aseptic technique and placed on the back OR table. At this time the skin graft was removed from the packaging and moistened with normal saline. The skin graft was then meshed manually using a #11 blade and making a small incision on the entire skin graft. At this time the shiny side of the skin graft was determined and noted to be the dermis side. The skin graft was then taken from the back table and applied over the ulceration site with the shiny side (the dermal side) against the ulcer site. Iris scissors were utilized to trim excess skin graft from the margins of the ulcer site. The skin graft was allowed to overlap the wound margin by 2 to 3 mm on all sides. Once the skin graft had been applied, a sterile cotton swab was used to try and remove all excess air from underneath the skin graft. 5-0 Nylon was used to stitch the skin graft to the good skin margins, leaving excess trail from the knot for application of bolster. Simple suturing technique was utilized. Adaptic was cut to the size of the wound and applied over the skin graft. The patient tolerated the procedure and anesthesia well.

answer: 15275

241

Each chapter contains several engaging in-text and margin features to aid student learning. These features challenge students to think critically, expand their knowledge through online research, and test their mastery of chapter content. Designed to aid students of all learning styles, these features also highlight the importance of professionalism and soft skills.

Appealing one-page chapter openers immediately draw students into the chapter topics by piquing their interest with fun facts and a coding exercise.

1 **Learning Objectives** establish a clear set of goals for each chapter.

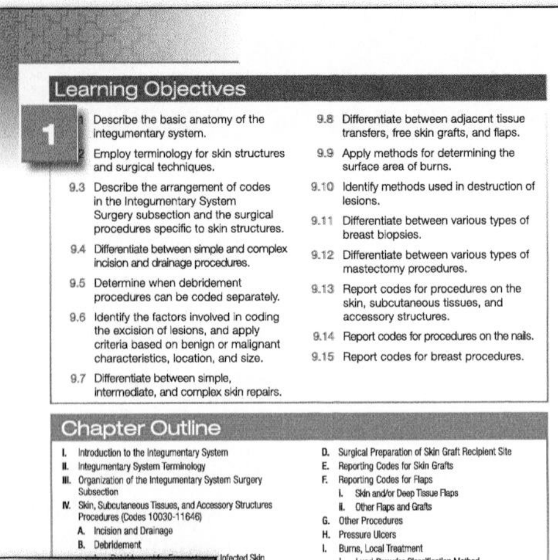

Learning Objectives

Describe the basic anatomy of the integumentary system.

Employ terminology for skin structures and surgical techniques.

9.3 Describe the arrangement of codes in the Integumentary System Surgery subsection and the surgical procedures specific to skin structures.

9.4 Differentiate between simple and complex incision and drainage procedures.

9.5 Determine when debridement procedures can be coded separately.

9.6 Identify the factors involved in coding the excision of lesions, and apply criteria based on benign or malignant characteristics, location, and size.

9.7 Differentiate between simple, intermediate, and complex skin repairs.

9.8 Differentiate between adjacent tissue transfers, free skin grafts, and flaps.

9.9 Apply methods for determining the surface area of burns.

9.10 Identify methods used in destruction of lesions.

9.11 Differentiate between various types of breast biopsies.

9.12 Differentiate between various types of mastectomy procedures.

9.13 Report codes for procedures on the skin, subcutaneous tissues, and accessory structures.

9.14 Report codes for procedures on the nails.

9.15 Report codes for breast procedures.

Chapter Outline

I. Introduction to the Integumentary System
II. Integumentary System Terminology
III. Organization of the Integumentary System Surgery Subsection
IV. Skin, Subcutaneous Tissues, and Accessory Structures Procedures (Codes 10030-11646)
A. Incision and Drainage
B. Debridement
... Infected Skin
... Tissue Infection
... teristics of Lesions
...)
...70-11772)
...-11983)
...2001-16036)
...rmediate,
...ngement

D. Surgical Preparation of Skin Graft Recipient Site
E. Reporting Codes for Skin Grafts
F. Reporting Codes for Flaps
i. Skin and/or Deep Tissue Flaps
ii. Other Flaps and Grafts
G. Other Procedures
H. Pressure Ulcers
I. Burns, Local Treatment
i. Lund-Browder Classification Method of Burn Estimating
ii. Escharotomy
IX. Destruction Codes (17000-17999)
A. Destruction, Benign or Premalignant Lesions
B. Destruction, Malignant Lesions, Any Method
X. Breast Procedures (Codes 19000-19499)
A. Incision
B. Excision
i. Types of Breast Biopsies
ii. Coding for Breast Biopsies
C. Introduction
D. Mastectomy Procedures
E. Repair and/or Reconstruction, Other Procedures
XI. Chapter Summary

Chapter 9 Surgery Coding: Integumentary System

2 **Key terms** are set in bold and defined in the Glossary.

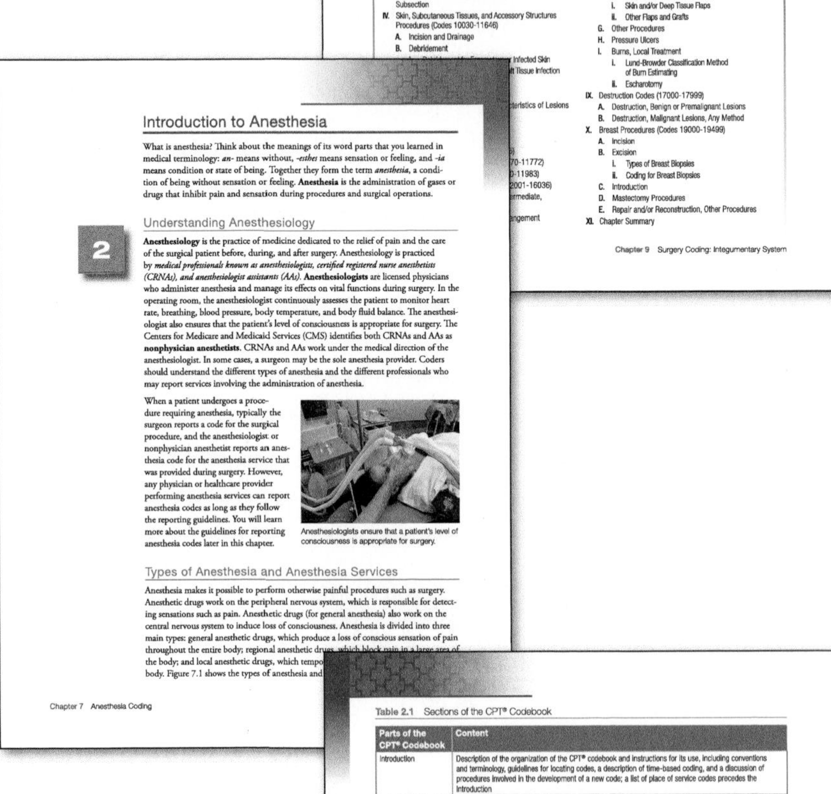

Introduction to Anesthesia

What is anesthesia? Think about the meanings of its word parts that you learned in medical terminology: *an-* means without, *-esthes* means sensation or feeling, and *-ia* means condition or state of being. Together they form the term *anesthesia*, a condition of being without sensation or feeling. **Anesthesia** is the administration of gases or drugs that inhibit pain and sensation during procedures and surgical operations.

Understanding Anesthesiology

Anesthesiology is the practice of medicine dedicated to the relief of pain and the care of the surgical patient before, during, and after surgery. Anesthesiology is practiced by *medical professionals known as anesthesiologists, certified registered nurse anesthetists (CRNAs), and anesthesiologist assistants (AAs).* **Anesthesiologists** are licensed physicians who administer anesthesia and manage its effects on vital functions during surgery. In the operating room, the anesthesiologist continuously assesses the patient to monitor heart rate, breathing, blood pressure, body temperature, and body fluid balance. The anesthesiologist also ensures that the patient's level of consciousness is appropriate for surgery. The Centers for Medicare and Medicaid Services (CMS) identifies both CRNAs and AAs as **nonphysician anesthetists**. CRNAs and AAs work under the medical direction of the anesthesiologist. In some cases, a surgeon may be the sole anesthesia provider. Coders should understand the different types of anesthesia and the different professionals who may report services involving the administration of anesthesia.

When a patient undergoes a procedure requiring anesthesia, typically the surgeon reports a code for the surgical procedure, and the anesthesiologist or nonphysician anesthetist reports an anesthesia code for the anesthesia service that was provided during surgery. However, any physician or healthcare provider performing anesthesia services can report anesthesia codes as long as they follow the reporting guidelines. You will learn more about the guidelines for reporting anesthesia codes later in this chapter.

Anesthesiologists ensure that a patient's level of consciousness is appropriate for surgery.

Types of Anesthesia and Anesthesia Services

Anesthesia makes it possible to perform otherwise painful procedures such as surgery. Anesthetic drugs work on the peripheral nervous system, which is responsible for detecting sensations such as pain. Anesthetic drugs (for general anesthesia) also work on the central nervous system to induce loss of consciousness. Anesthesia is divided into three main types: general anesthetic drugs, which produce a loss of conscious sensation of pain throughout the entire body; regional anesthetic dr... the body; and local anesthetic drugs, which tempo... body. Figure 7.1 shows the types of anesthesia and...

Chapter 7 Anesthesia Coding

Table 2.1 Sections of the CPT® Codebook

Parts of the CPT® Codebook	Content
Introduction	Description of the organization of the CPT® codebook and instructions for its use, including conventions and terminology, guidelines for locating codes, a description of time-based coding, and a discussion of procedures involved in the development of a new code; a list of place of service codes precedes the Introduction
Category I codes	A listing of 5-digit numeric codes (organized in numeric order unless otherwise stated in the codebook) that represents procedures and services that have been approved by the Food and Drug Administration (FDA)
Category II codes	A listing of 5-digit alphanumeric supplemental tracking codes, all ending with the letter F, that are used to report quality measurements to identify whether a facility is compliant with HIPAA regulations
Category III codes	A listing of 5-digit alphanumeric temporary codes for emerging technologies, services, and procedures. Category III codes end in the letter T.
Appendixes	Expanded definitions of modifiers, clinical examples, and other content associated with code selection and reporting. See Table 2.4 on page 51 for a full description of the appendixes.
Index	A comprehensive listing of code descriptions in alphabetic order according to procedure, anatomical site, condition, eponym, synonym, or abbreviation

The Introduction Section of the CPT® Codebook

The **Introduction** is located at the beginning of the CPT® codebook. Typically, the introduction includes a brief history of CPT®, standards for using the CPT® codebook, a description of the content of the codebook, and information regarding code format. The information provided in the Introduction is specific to a particular CPT® codebook publication, which can vary. Always read the Introduction before you start using the codebook to assign codes.

CPT® Code Set Categories

CPT® codes are divided into 3 categories: I, II, and III. Each category represents a specific type of code used to identify services and procedures. No code numbers are alike, and each code has its own unique meaning. As you learn more about the categories of CPT® codes, keep in mind that even if a medical provider has a particular specialty, he or she may perform services or procedures whose codes are located in any section of the CPT® codebook, as long as they are within the scope of practice.

Category I Codes

RED FLAG

Some Category I codes are not listed in numeric sequence in the CPT® codebook. In the codebook, a number symbol (#) is placed in front of a code number to identify that the code is out of numeric order.

Category I codes are the first and largest set of codes in the CPT® codebook. They represent procedures or services that are performed by physicians and other qualified healthcare providers with some regularity and are approved by the FDA. The codes are used to report the services and procedures to insurance payers to request payment. These services or procedures may take place in a hospital, a physician office, or an outpatient facility, such as a diagnostic imaging center. Outpatient services provided in a hospital are also reported with CPT® codes.

Category I codes are 5-digit numeric codes. They appear in the CPT® codebook in numeric order, except for the Evaluation and Management (E/M) section, which

40 Chapter 2 Getting to Know CPT®

3 **Red Flag** margin alerts identify subjects requiring special attention when coding.

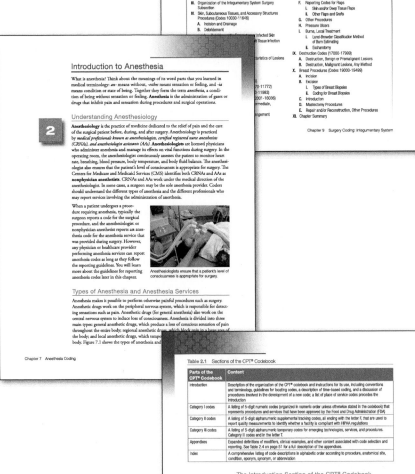

4 **Coding Clicks** margin features speak to today's digitally savvy students and integrate Internet resources and online learning opportunities.

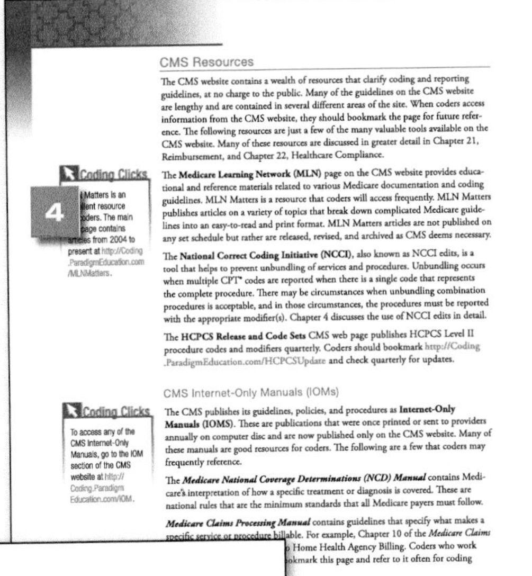

CMS Resources

The CMS website contains a wealth of resources that clarify coding and reporting guidelines, at no charge to the public. Many of the guidelines on the CMS website are lengthy and are contained in several different areas of the site. When coders access information from the CMS website, they should bookmark the page for future reference. The following resources are just a few of the many valuable tools available on the CMS website. Many of these resources are discussed in greater detail in Chapter 21, Reimbursement, and Chapter 22, Healthcare Compliance.

Coding Clicks: ...Matters is an ...ent resource ...oders. The main ...page contains ...articles from 2004 to present at http://Coding.ParadigmEducation.com/MLNMatters.

The **Medicare Learning Network (MLN)** page on the CMS website provides educational and reference materials related to various Medicare documentation and coding guidelines. MLN Matters is a resource that coders will access frequently. MLN Matters publishes articles on a variety of topics that break down complicated Medicare guidelines into an easy-to-read and print format. MLN Matters articles are not published on any set schedule but rather are released, revised, and archived as CMS deems necessary.

The **National Correct Coding Initiative (NCCI)**, also known as NCCI edits, is a tool that helps to prevent unbundling of services and procedures. Unbundling occurs when multiple CPT® codes are reported when there is a single code that represents the complete procedure. There may be circumstances when unbundling combination procedures is acceptable, and in those circumstances, the procedures must be reported with the appropriate modifier(s). Chapter 4 discusses the use of NCCI edits in detail.

The **HCPCS Release and Code Sets** CMS web page publishes HCPCS Level II procedure codes and modifiers quarterly. Coders should bookmark http://Coding.ParadigmEducation.com/HCPCSUpdate and check quarterly for updates.

CMS Internet-Only Manuals (IOMs)

Coding Clicks: To access any of the CMS Internet-Only Manuals, go to the IOM section of the CMS website at http://Coding.ParadigmEducation.com/IOM.

The CMS publishes its guidelines, policies, and procedures as **Internet-Only Manuals (IOMS)**. These are publications that were once printed or sent to providers annually on computer disc and are now published only on the CMS website. Many of these manuals are good resources for coders. The following are a few that coders may frequently reference.

The ***Medicare National Coverage Determinations (NCD) Manual*** contains Medicare's interpretation of how a specific treatment or diagnosis is covered. These are national rules that are the minimum standards that all Medicare payers must follow.

Medicare Claims Processing Manual contains guidelines that specify what makes a specific service or procedure billable. For example, Chapter 10 of the *Medicare Claims* ... Home Health Agency Billing. Coders who work ... bookmark this page and refer to it often for coding ...

...*anual* contains guidance for CMS contractors who are ...er records and reimbursements for compliance with ...s book discusses coding compliance in detail.

Chapter 2 Getting to Know CPT®

5 **Index Insider** margin features guide students on how to best navigate the CPT® codebook's Index.

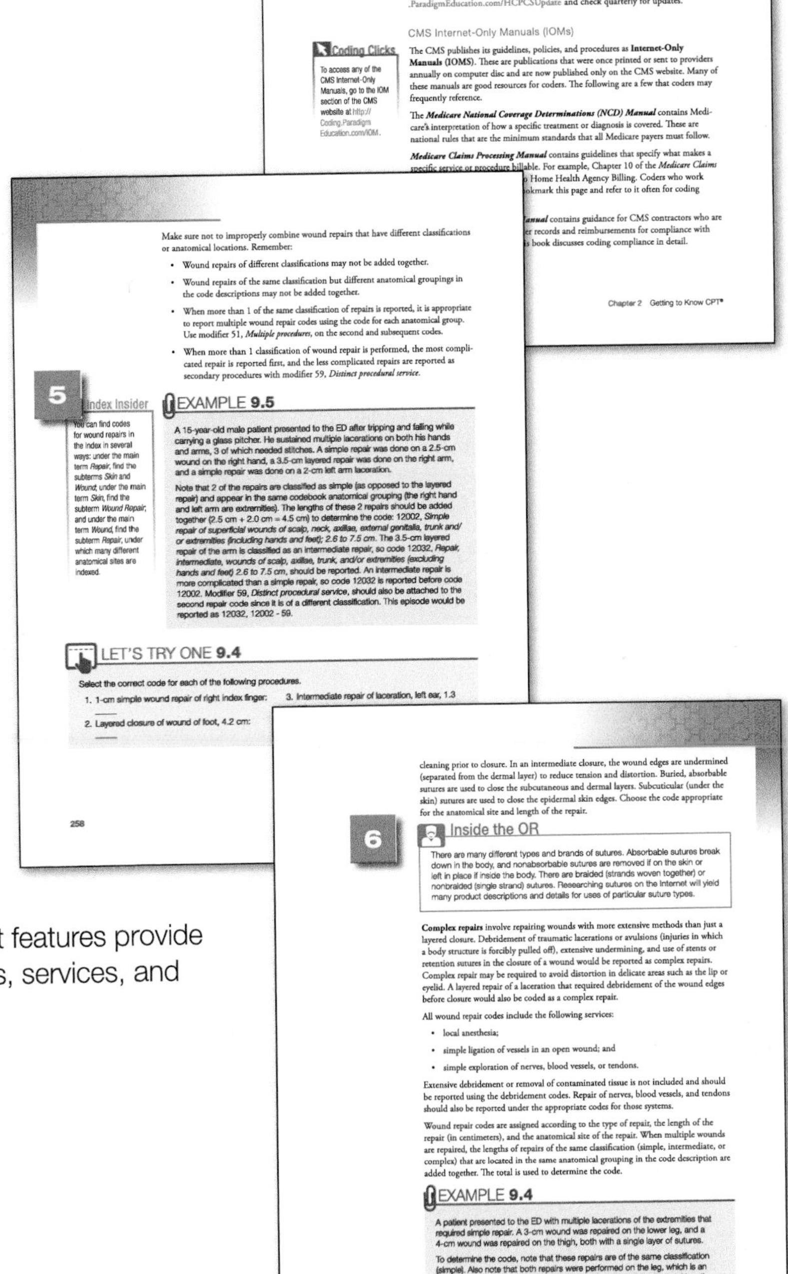

Make sure not to improperly combine wound repairs that have different classifications or anatomical locations. Remember:

- Wound repairs of different classifications may not be added together.
- Wound repairs of the same classification but different anatomical groupings in the code descriptions may not be added together.
- When more than 1 of the same classification of repairs is reported, it is appropriate to report multiple wound repair codes using the code for each anatomical group. Use modifier 51, *Multiple procedures*, on the second and subsequent codes.
- When more than 1 classification of wound repair is performed, the most complicated repair is reported first, and the less complicated repairs are reported as secondary procedures with modifier 59, *Distinct procedural service*.

Index Insider: You can find codes for wound repairs in the Index in several ways: under the main term *Repair*, find the subterms *Skin* and *Wound*; under the main term *Skin*, find the subterm *Wound Repair*; and under the main term *Wound*, find the subterm *Repair*, under which many different anatomical sites are indexed.

EXAMPLE **9.5**

A 15-year-old male patient presented to the ED after tripping and falling while carrying a glass pitcher. He sustained multiple lacerations on both his hands and arms, 3 of which needed stitches. A simple repair was done on a 2.5-cm wound on the right hand, a 3.5-cm layered repair was done on the right arm, and a simple repair was done on a 2-cm left arm laceration.

Note that 2 of the repairs are classified as simple (as opposed to the layered repair) and appear in the same codebook anatomical grouping (the right hand and left arm are extremities). The lengths of these 2 repairs should be added together (2.5 cm + 2.0 cm = 4.5 cm) to determine the code: 12002, *Simple repair of superficial wounds of scalp, neck, axillae, external genitalia, trunk and/or extremities (including hands and feet); 2.6 to 7.5 cm*. The 3.5-cm layered repair of the arm is classified as an intermediate repair, so code 12032, *Repair, intermediate, wounds of scalp, axillae, trunk, and/or extremities (excluding hands and feet) 2.6 to 7.5 cm*, should be reported. An intermediate repair is more complicated than a simple repair, so code 12032 is reported before code 12002. Modifier 59, *Distinct procedural service*, should also be attached to the second repair code since it is of a different classification. This episode would be reported as 12032, 12002 - 59.

LET'S TRY ONE **9.4**

Select the correct code for each of the following procedures.

1. 1-cm simple wound repair of right index finger: ___
2. Layered closure of wound of foot, 4.2 cm: ___
3. Intermediate repair of laceration, left ear, 1.3 ...

258

cleaning prior to closure. In an intermediate closure, the wound edges are undermined (separated from the dermal layer) to reduce tension and distortion. Buried, absorbable sutures are used to close the subcutaneous and dermal layers. Subcuticular (under the skin) sutures are used to close the epidermal skin edges. Choose the code appropriate for the anatomical site and length of the repair.

Inside the OR

There are many different types and brands of sutures. Absorbable sutures break down in the body, and nonabsorbable sutures are removed if on the skin or left in place if inside the body. There are braided (strands woven together) or nonbraided (single strand) sutures. Researching sutures on the Internet will yield many product descriptions and details for uses of particular suture types.

Complex repairs involve repairing wounds with more extensive methods than just a layered closure. Debridement of traumatic lacerations or avulsions (injuries in which a body structure is forcibly pulled off), extensive undermining, and use of stents or retention sutures in the closure of a wound would be reported as complex repairs. Complex repair may be required to avoid distortion in delicate areas such as the lip or eyelid. A layered repair of a laceration that required debridement of the wound edges before closure would also be coded as a complex repair.

All wound repair codes include the following services:

- local anesthesia;
- simple ligation of vessels in an open wound; and
- simple exploration of nerves, blood vessels, or tendons.

Extensive debridement or removal of contaminated tissue is not included and should be reported using the debridement codes. Repair of nerves, blood vessels, and tendons should also be reported under the appropriate codes for those systems.

Wound repair codes are assigned according to the type of repair, the length of the repair (in centimeters), and the anatomical site of the repair. When multiple wounds are repaired, the lengths of repairs of the same classification (simple, intermediate, or complex) that are located in the same anatomical grouping in the code description are added together. The total is used to determine the code.

EXAMPLE **9.4**

A patient presented to the ED with multiple lacerations of the extremities that required simple repair. A 3-cm wound was repaired on the lower leg, and a 4-cm wound was repaired on the thigh, both with a single layer of sutures.

To determine the code, note that these repairs are of the same classification (simple). Also note that both repairs were performed on the leg, which is an extremity. Therefore, you can add their lengths to determine the total length you will use to choose the code (3 cm + 4 cm = 7 cm). The combination of this documentation indicates code 12002, *Simple repair of superficial wounds of scalp, neck, axillae, external genitalia, trunk and/or extremities (including hands and feet); 2.6 cm to 7.5 cm*.

Chapter 9 Surgery Coding: Integumentary System 257

6 **Inside the OR** margin and in-text features provide insight into how specific surgeries, services, and procedures are performed.

7 **A&P Review** margin features present tips that relate anatomy and physiology to coding.

A **sialolithotomy** (codes 42330 through 42340) is an incisional treatment for a **salivary duct stone**, which is a concretion that blocks the passage of saliva to the oral cavity. A biopsy of a salivary gland is reported by the technique used to collect the specimen, code 42400 for a needle biopsy and code 42405 for an incisional biopsy.

A **sialography** is an x-ray image of the salivary glands. Dye may be injected to enhance the image, delivered through a small catheter that is inserted into the associated salivary duct. In this case, report code 42550, ***Injection procedure for sialography***. For radiological supervision and interpretation of the sialography, separately report radiology code 70390, ***Sialography, radiological supervision and interpretation***. Chapter 18 discusses the Radiology section of the CPT® codebook in detail.

LET'S TRY ONE **13.5**

Choose the correct code for the following procedure.

A patient with facial paralyses on the left side underwent bilateral parotid duct diversions to control drooling. The physician performed a Wilke type procedure, which involved an intraoral incision of the overlying parotid duct. The ducts were diverted and sutured to the mucosa so that the saliva into the duct was rerouted.

What is the correct code for this procedure? _____

Pharynx, Adenoids, and Tonsils (Codes 42700-42999)

7 A&P Review

The adenoids and tonsils are a part of the lymphatic system. Adenoids, also known as the *pharyngeal tonsils*, are located in the back of the throat (pharynx) and up into the nasal cavity. Tonsils are located on the sides of the throat.

Surgical procedures of the pharynx, adenoids, and tonsils are categorized as incision, excision and destruction, repair, and other procedures. Incision and drainage codes 42700 through 42725 are selected based on the location of the abscess (peritonsillar, retropharyngeal, or parapharyngeal) and the approach (intraoral or external). Biopsy codes are selected based on the location of the lesion in the pharynx: oropharynx, if posterior to the mouth, and nasopharynx, if near the opening to the nasal cavity. When a laryngoscope is used to view the interior of the larynx for the collection of a biopsy, report the appropriate laryngoscopy biopsy code from the Respiratory System Surgery subsection of the CPT® codebook. The respiratory system is discussed in Chapter 11.

Excisions of Adenoids and Tonsils

Tonsils and adenoids defend the body against bacteria and viruses that enter through the mouth or nose. Sometimes tonsils and adenoids become infected. **Tonsillectomy** is removal of the tonsils, a viable treatment for chronic tonsillitis or for cancer of the tonsils. **Adenoidectomy** is the surgical removal of the **adenoids** (also known as the *pharyngeal tonsils*, located at the back of the throat). Chronic nasopharyngitis is a condition that is effectively treated by an adenoidectomy. A tonsillectomy and adenoidectomy may be performed during the same surgical session or independently. Codes are selected based on the age of the patient and if the tonsils and adenoids are removed during the same surgical session. Selection of adenoidectomy codes 42830 through 42836 requires the identification of the procedure as primary or secondary. A secondary adenoidectomy is performed when the primary excised tissue has grown back.

376 Chapter 13 Surgery Coding: Digestive System

8 **Coding for CMS** margin and in-text features notify students of considerations and guidelines related to Medicare and Medicaid requirements.

Table 21.1 Government Health Insurance Plans

Program	Government Level (Federal or State)	Descriptic
Maternal and Child Health Program	Joint federal and state	Provides func ers, women, needs, and th
Medicaid	Joint federal and state	Helps individu pay for healt government, from state to
Medicare	Federal	For people w with end-stag coverage: • Part A care i health • Part B outpat • Part C plan offered by a private company that contracts with Medicare to provide all Part A and Part B benefits. Most Medicare Advantage plans offer prescription drug coverage; • **Part D (prescription drug coverage)**—prescription drug insurance coverage provided by private companies.
Medicare/Medicaid, often referred to as Medi/Medi	Joint federal and state	Individuals who are enrolled in both Medicare and Medicaid programs
TRICARE	Federal	Healthcare program for active duty members of the military and their families, as well as activated National Guard and Reserve personnel, retired military personnel, and surviving family members of deceased veterans
CHAMPVA (Civilian Health and Medical Program of the Department of Veterans Affairs)	Federal	Healthcare program provided by the US Department of Veterans Affairs for the families of veterans permanently disabled or killed in the line of duty who are not eligible for TRICARE; CHAMPVA for Life (CFL) is an extension of CHAMPVA benefits to those 65 years and older

Coding Clicks

Find the MAC for your jurisdiction using the interactive CMS map at http://Coding.ParadigmEducation.com/CMSMap.

Coding for CMS 8

Medicare uses a network of contractors called Medicare Administrative Contractors (MACs) to process Medicare claims, enroll healthcare providers in the Medicare program, and educate providers on Medicare billing requirements. Contractors designated as "A/B MACs" process Medicare Part A and Part B claims for defined geographic areas called *jurisdictions*. As Medicare sets national coverage standards on specific services, procedures, supplies, and diagnoses, MACs are tasked with applying these national coverage determinations (NCDs) to their local jurisdictions. These local rules are called *local coverage determinations (LCDs)*. An LCD may be more restrictive than an NCD. Coders must become familiar with the LCD that applies to the jurisdiction of the patient's Medicare plan. Documentation that does not meet the LCD requirements will affect coverage of services.

Chapter 21 Reimbursement

9 **Learn Your Way** in-text features provide students tips for mastering textbook content based on their learning styles.

9 Learn Your Way

Reflective learners prefer concrete experience and reflective observation, and they choose to watch rather than do. If you are a reflective learner, observing a real-life skin graft procedure will appeal to you. The accompanying links show how skin grafts are performed. The first link is an animated video meant for patients who will receive skin grafts. The second link is a video of a real split-thickness skin graft surgery and is graphic in nature. Viewer discretion is advised.

http://Coding.ParadigmEducation.com/SkinGraft1

http://Coding.ParadigmEducation.com/SkinGraft2

Surgical Preparation of Skin Graft Recipient Site

Surgical preparation of the recipient site is a procedure in which nonviable tissue is removed by excision. The surgeon prepares the recipient's tissue to receive a graft by excising skin, subcutaneous tissue, scars, burn eschar (pieces of dead tissue), and lesions to provide a healthy tissue bed for the new skin. Codes 15002 through 15005 are used to report surgical preparation of a recipient site. Modifier 51, ***Multiple procedures***, is not used with codes 15002 through 15005, as the guidelines state that they are to be coded in addition to the graft procedure. There are 2 criteria for code selection:

- the anatomical location with respect to the groupings given in the codes: 15002 and 15003 for trunk, arms, and legs; and 15004 and 15005 for face scalp, eyelids, mouth, neck, ears, orbits, genitalia, hands, feet, fingers, and toes;
- the size of the site, given in percentage of body area for infants and children younger than 10 years of age, and in square centimeters for adults.

If multiple recipient sites are prepared, the surface area of all wounds in the same anatomical grouping in the code description can be added together.

Reporting Codes for Skin Grafts

Codes for skin grafts are determined by the type of graft (autograft, split thickness, skin substitute, etc.), the anatomical site, and the surface area. Read the operative note carefully to obtain this information. The area of the graft is measured in square centimeters, and the codes have minimum baseline measurements ranging from 10 sq cm to 100 sq cm. Add-on codes are used to report additional surface area. Pay special attention to the code descriptions, which group anatomical areas similarly to those in the wound repair codes. Skin grafts are coded to the recipient site (where the graft is placed). The donor site (where the graft was taken from) does not affect code assignment.

262 Chapter 9 Surgery Coding: Integumentary System

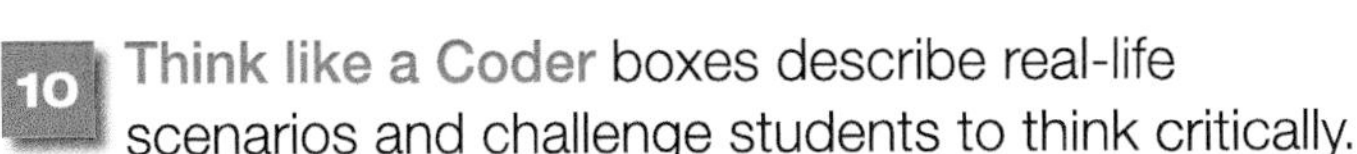

10 **Think like a Coder** boxes describe real-life scenarios and challenge students to think critically.

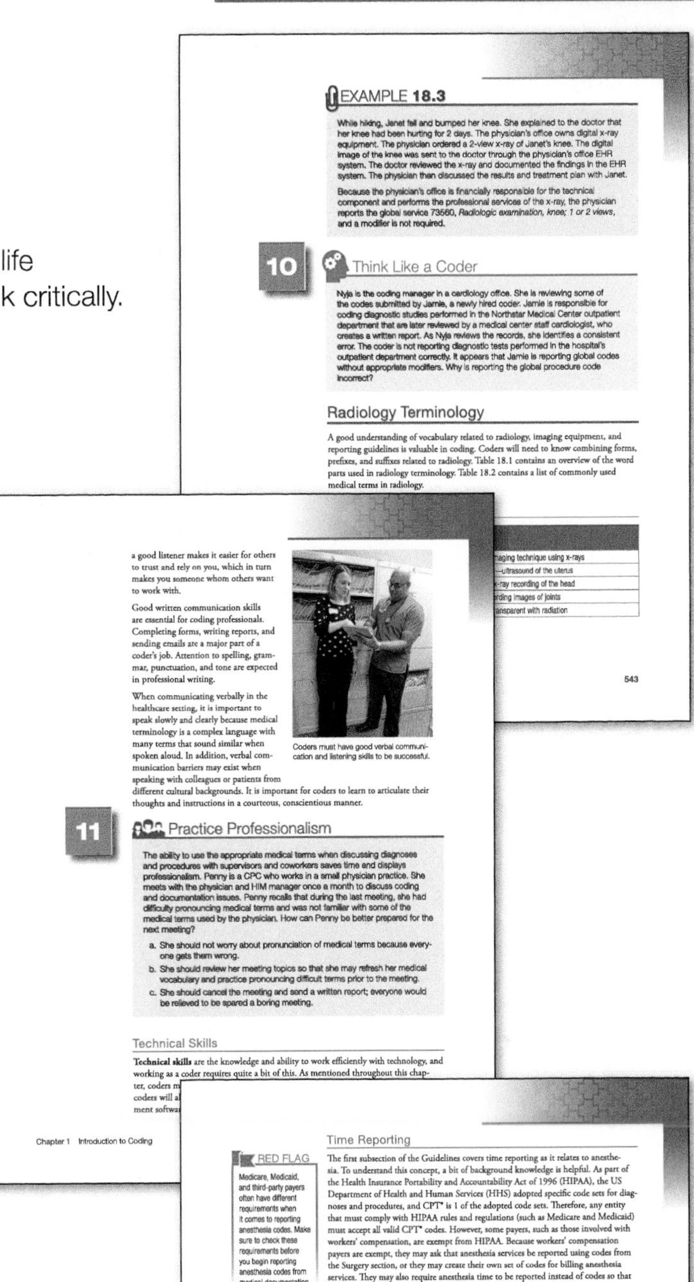

EXAMPLE 18.3

While hiking, Janet fell and bumped her knee. She explained to the doctor that her knee had been hurting for 2 days. The physician's office owns digital x-ray equipment. The physician ordered a 2-view x-ray of Janet's knee. The digital image of the knee was sent to the doctor through the physician's office EHR system. The doctor reviewed the x-ray and documented the findings in the EHR system. The physician then discussed the results and treatment plan with Janet.

Because the physician's office is financially responsible for the technical component and performs the professional services of the x-ray, the physician reports the global service 73560, *Radiologic examination, knee; 1 or 2 views*, and a modifier is not required.

10 Think Like a Coder

Nyla is the coding manager in a cardiology office. She is reviewing some of the codes submitted by Jamie, a newly hired coder. Jamie is responsible for coding diagnostic studies performed in the Northstar Medical Center outpatient department that are later reviewed by a medical center staff cardiologist, who creates a written report. As Nyla reviews the records, she identifies a consistent error. The coder is not reporting diagnostic tests performed in the hospital's outpatient department correctly. It appears that Jamie is reporting global codes without appropriate modifiers. Why is reporting the global procedure code incorrect?

Radiology Terminology

A good understanding of vocabulary related to radiology, imaging equipment, and reporting guidelines is valuable in coding. Coders will need to know combining forms, prefixes, and suffixes related to radiology. Table 18.1 contains an overview of the word parts used in radiology terminology. Table 18.2 contains a list of commonly used medical terms in radiology.

543

a good listener makes it easier for others to trust and rely on you, which in turn makes you someone whom others want to work with.

Good written communication skills are essential for coding professionals. Completing forms, writing reports, and sending emails are a major part of a coder's job. Attention to spelling, grammar, punctuation, and tone are expected in professional writing.

When communicating verbally in the healthcare setting, it is important to speak slowly and clearly because medical terminology is a complex language with many terms that sound similar when spoken aloud. In addition, verbal communication barriers may exist when speaking with colleagues or patients from different cultural backgrounds. It is important for coders to learn to articulate their thoughts and instructions in a courteous, conscientious manner.

Coders must have good verbal communication and listening skills to be successful.

11 Practice Professionalism

The ability to use the appropriate medical terms when discussing diagnoses and procedures with supervisors and coworkers saves time and displays professionalism. Penny is a CPC who works in a small physician practice. She meets with the physician and HIM manager once a month to discuss coding and documentation issues. Penny recalls that during the last meeting, she had difficulty pronouncing medical terms and was not familiar with some of the medical terms used by the physician. How can Penny be better prepared for the next meeting?

a. She should not worry about pronunciation of medical terms because everyone gets them wrong.
b. She should review her meeting topics so that she may refresh her medical vocabulary and practice pronouncing difficult terms prior to the meeting.
c. She should cancel the meeting and send a written report; everyone would be relieved to be spared a boring meeting.

Technical Skills

Technical skills are the knowledge and ability to work efficiently with technology, and working as a coder requires quite a bit of this. As mentioned throughout this chapter, coders m... coders will a... ment softwa...

Chapter 1 Introduction to Coding

11 **Practice Professionalism** integrates soft skills, advising students on the importance of preparing for the workplace.

Time Reporting

The first subsection of the Guidelines covers time reporting as it relates to anesthesia. To understand this concept, a bit of background knowledge is helpful. As part of the Health Insurance Portability and Accountability Act of 1996 (HIPAA), the US Department of Health and Human Services (HHS) adopted specific code sets for diagnoses and procedures, and CPT® is 1 of the adopted code sets. Therefore, any entity that must comply with HIPAA rules and regulations (such as Medicare and Medicaid) must accept all valid CPT® codes. However, some payers, such as those involved with workers' compensation, are exempt from HIPAA. Because workers' compensation payers are exempt, they may ask that anesthesia services be reported using codes from the Surgery section, or they may create their own set of codes for billing anesthesia services. They may also require anesthesia time to be reported instead of codes so that fees can be calculated based on that time. Although a coding professional may not be required to calculate fees for billing purposes, it is helpful to understand how fees based on anesthesia time are determined.

RED FLAG

Medicare, Medicaid, and third-party payers often have different requirements when it comes to reporting anesthesia codes. Make sure to check these requirements before you begin reporting anesthesia codes from medical documentation.

Anesthesia fees are based on the complexity of the surgical procedure and the period of time during which anesthesia services are provided. **Anesthesia time** starts when the anesthesiologist begins to prepare the patient to receive services and ends when the anesthesiologist is no longer in personal attendance, at which point the patient may be placed in postoperative care. When multiple surgical procedures are performed during a single anesthesia session, the anesthesia code reported should represent the most complex procedure, and the time for all procedures should be combined. The **American Society of Anesthesiologists (ASA)** annually publishes a relative-value guide that contains the base values for anesthesia codes, physical status modifiers, and qualifying circumstances codes. A higher base value indicates a more complex procedure. Anesthesia time is calculated in units, with each payer determining the number of minutes in each time unit. Base units, time units, and modifying factors are added together and multiplied by a dollar amount (conversion factor; set by the anesthesia provider) to calculate the anesthesia fees.

12 EXAMPLE 7.2

A 76-year-old female underwent a vaginal hysterectomy under general anesthesia. The anesthesia code for this procedure is 00944, *Anesthesia for vaginal procedures (including biopsy of labia, vagina, cervix or endometrium); vaginal hysterectomy*, with a base unit of 6 (according to the ASA's relative-value guide). The anesthesia time for the hysterectomy was 60 minutes, and the patient is a Medicare beneficiary, so 4 time units are reported (Medicare and Medicaid use 15-minute units). Because the patient is 76 years old, qualifying circumstances code 99100, *Anesthesia for a patient of extreme age, younger than 1 year and older than 70*, is also reported, which is a modifying factor for calculating fees. The anesthesia provider has set the conversion factor at $100. Therefore, the anesthesia fee is calculated using the following formula: 6 base units + 4 time units + 1 modifying factor x $100 = $1100.

Chapter 7 Anesthesia Coding 203

12 **Examples** offer realistic patient scenarios and show students how to select the correct code based on the performed procedure.

13 **Concepts Checkpoint** activities encourage students to stop periodically to test their learning within each chapter. The answers to the chapter Concepts Checkpoint questions are located in the Appendix.

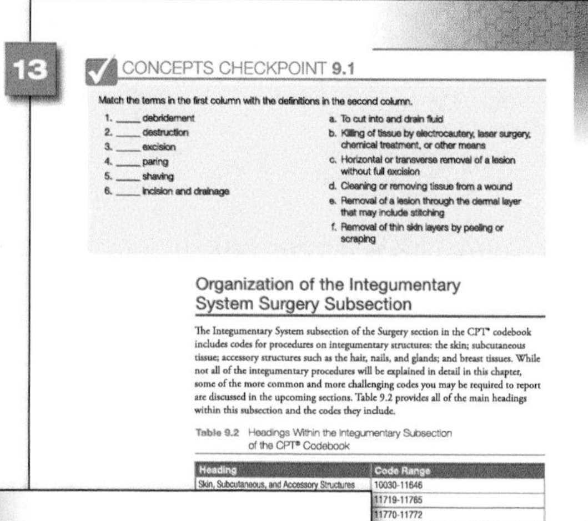

13

CONCEPTS CHECKPOINT **9.1**

Match the terms in the first column with the definitions in the second column.

1. _____ debridement
2. _____ destruction
3. _____ excision
4. _____ paring
5. _____ shaving
6. _____ incision and drainage

a. To cut into and drain fluid
b. Killing of tissue by electrocautery, laser surgery, chemical treatment, or other means
c. Horizontal or transverse removal of a lesion without full excision
d. Cleaning or removing tissue from a wound
e. Removal of a lesion through the dermal layer that may include stitching
f. Removal of thin skin layers by peeling or scraping

Organization of the Integumentary System Surgery Subsection

The Integumentary System subsection of the Surgery section in the CPT® codebook includes codes for procedures on integumentary structures: the skin; subcutaneous tissue; accessory structures such as the hair, nails, and glands; and breast tissues. While not all of the integumentary procedures will be explained in detail in this chapter, some of the more common and more challenging codes you may be required to report are discussed in the upcoming sections. Table 9.2 provides all of the main headings within this subsection and the codes they include.

Table 9.2 Headings Within the Integumentary Subsection of the CPT® Codebook

Heading	Code Range
Skin, Subcutaneous, and Accessory Structures	10030-11646
	11719-11765
	11770-11772
	11900-11983
	12001-16036
	17000-17999
	19000-19499

245

14 **Let's Try One** activities provide coding practice based on the concepts learned in the text. The answers to the chapter Let's Try One activities are located in the Appendix.

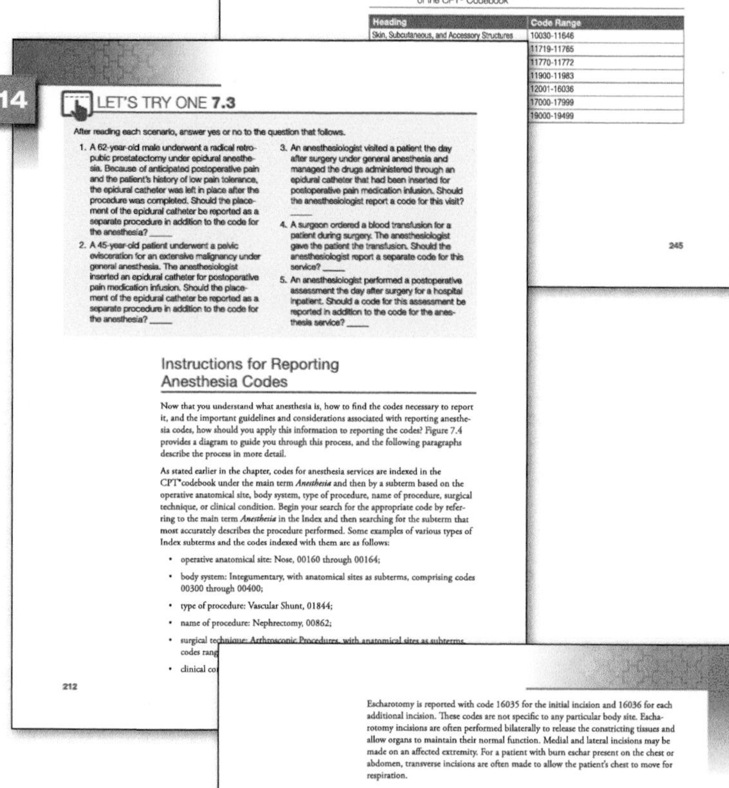

14

LET'S TRY ONE **7.3**

After reading each scenario, answer yes or no to the question that follows.

1. A 62-year-old male underwent a radical retropubic prostatectomy under epidural anesthesia. Because of anticipated postoperative pain and the patient's history of low pain tolerance, the epidural catheter was left in place after the procedure was completed. Should the placement of the epidural catheter be reported as a separate procedure in addition to the code for the anesthesia? _____
2. A 45-year-old patient underwent a pelvic evisceration for an extensive malignancy under general anesthesia. The anesthesiologist inserted an epidural catheter for postoperative pain medication infusion. Should the placement of the epidural catheter be reported as a separate procedure in addition to the code for the anesthesia? _____
3. An anesthesiologist visited a patient the day after surgery under general anesthesia and managed the drugs administered through an epidural catheter that had been inserted for postoperative pain medication infusion. Should the anesthesiologist report a code for this visit? _____
4. A surgeon ordered a blood transfusion for a patient during surgery. The anesthesiologist gave the patient the transfusion. Should the anesthesiologist report a separate code for this service? _____
5. An anesthesiologist performed a postoperative assessment the day after surgery for a hospital inpatient. Should a code for this assessment be reported in addition to the code for the anesthesia service? _____

Instructions for Reporting Anesthesia Codes

Now that you understand what anesthesia is, how to find the codes necessary to report it, and the important guidelines and considerations associated with reporting anesthesia codes, how should you apply this information to reporting the codes? Figure 7.4 provides a diagram to guide you through this process, and the following paragraphs describe the process in more detail.

As stated earlier in the chapter, codes for anesthesia services are indexed in the CPT®codebook under the main term *Anesthesia* and then by a subterm based on the operative anatomical site, body system, type of procedure, name of procedure, surgical technique, or clinical condition. Begin your search for the appropriate code by referring to the main term *Anesthesia* in the Index and then searching for the subterm that most accurately describes the procedure performed. Some examples of various types of Index subterms and the codes indexed with them are as follows:

- operative anatomical site: Nose, 00160 through 00164;
- body system: Integumentary, with anatomical sites as subterms, comprising codes 00300 through 00400;
- type of procedure: Vascular Shunt, 01844;
- name of procedure: Nephrectomy, 00862;
- surgical technique: Arthroscopic Procedures, with anatomical sites as subterms, codes rang
- clinical co

212

15 **Tables** organize and summarize information covered in the chapter and serve as a study aid.

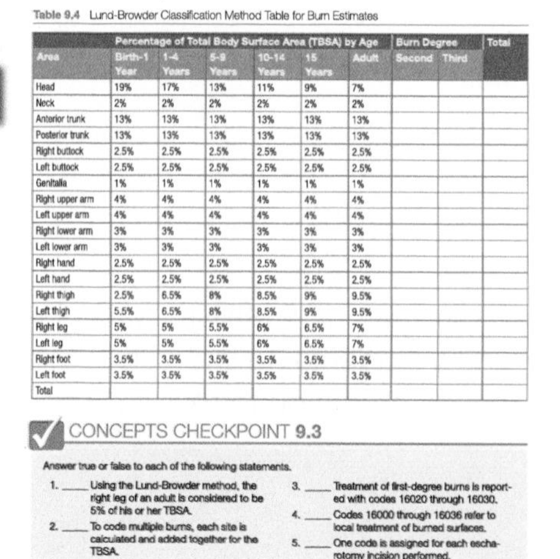

15

Escharotomy is reported with code 16035 for the initial incision and 16036 for each additional incision. These codes are not specific to any particular body site. Escharotomy incisions are often performed bilaterally to release the constricting tissues and allow organs to maintain their normal function. Medial and lateral incisions may be made on an affected extremity. For a patient with burn eschar present on the chest or abdomen, transverse incisions are often made to allow the patient's chest to move for respiration.

Table 9.4 Lund-Browder Classification Method Table for Burn Estimates

	Percentage of Total Body Surface Area (TBSA) by Age						Burn Degree		Total
Area	Birth-1 Year	1-4 Years	5-9 Years	10-14 Years	15 Years	Adult	Second	Third	
Head	19%	17%	13%	11%	9%	7%			
Neck	2%	2%	2%	2%	2%	2%			
Anterior trunk	13%	13%	13%	13%	13%	13%			
Posterior trunk	13%	13%	13%	13%	13%	13%			
Right buttock	2.5%	2.5%	2.5%	2.5%	2.5%	2.5%			
Left buttock	2.5%	2.5%	2.5%	2.5%	2.5%	2.5%			
Genitalia	1%	1%	1%	1%	1%	1%			
Right upper arm	4%	4%	4%	4%	4%	4%			
Left upper arm	4%	4%	4%	4%	4%	4%			
Right lower arm	3%	3%	3%	3%	3%	3%			
Left lower arm	3%	3%	3%	3%	3%	3%			
Right hand	2.5%	2.5%	2.5%	2.5%	2.5%	2.5%			
Left hand	2.5%	2.5%	2.5%	2.5%	2.5%	2.5%			
Right thigh	2.5%	6.5%	8%	8.5%	9%	9.5%			
Left thigh	5.5%	6.5%	8%	8.5%	9%	9.5%			
Right leg	5%	5%	5.5%	6%	6.5%	7%			
Left leg	5%	5%	5.5%	6%	6.5%	7%			
Right foot	3.5%	3.5%	3.5%	3.5%	3.5%	3.5%			
Left foot	3.5%	3.5%	3.5%	3.5%	3.5%	3.5%			
Total									

CONCEPTS CHECKPOINT **9.3**

Answer true or false to each of the following statements.

1. _____ Using the Lund-Browder method, the right leg of an adult is considered to be 5% of his or her TBSA.
2. _____ To code multiple burns, each site is calculated and added together for the TBSA.
3. _____ Treatment of first-degree burns is reported with codes 16020 through 16030.
4. _____ Codes 16000 through 16036 refer to local treatment of burned surfaces.
5. _____ One code is assigned for each escharotomy incision performed.

Chapter 9 Surgery Coding: Integumentary System 267

16 **Body system illustrations** help students make the connection between anatomy and physiology and coding.

17 **BioDigital** links direct students to interact with the BioDigital Human, offering them hands-on practice exploring different body systems.

18 Eye-catching **photographs** reinforce the text and help students to visualize coding concepts and real-world patient interactions.

19 **Images** of the EHR Navigator interface illustrate the key components of an EHR system as described in the chapter content.

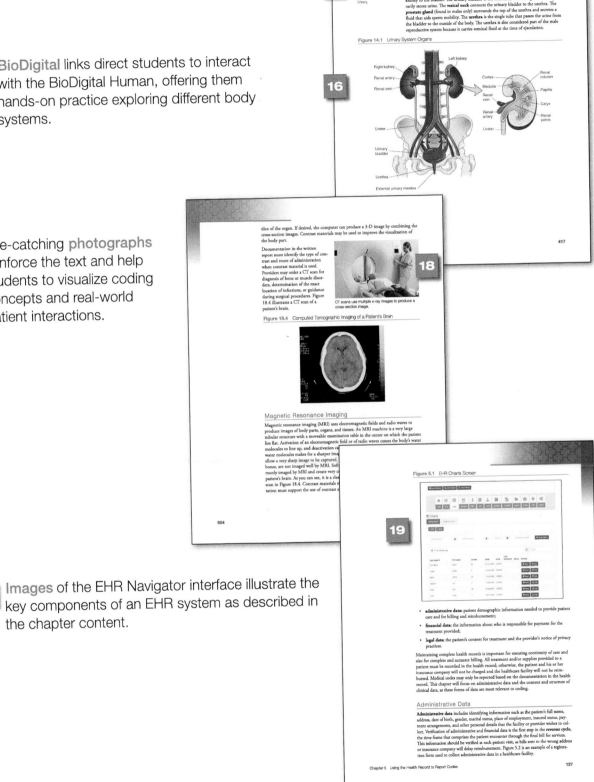

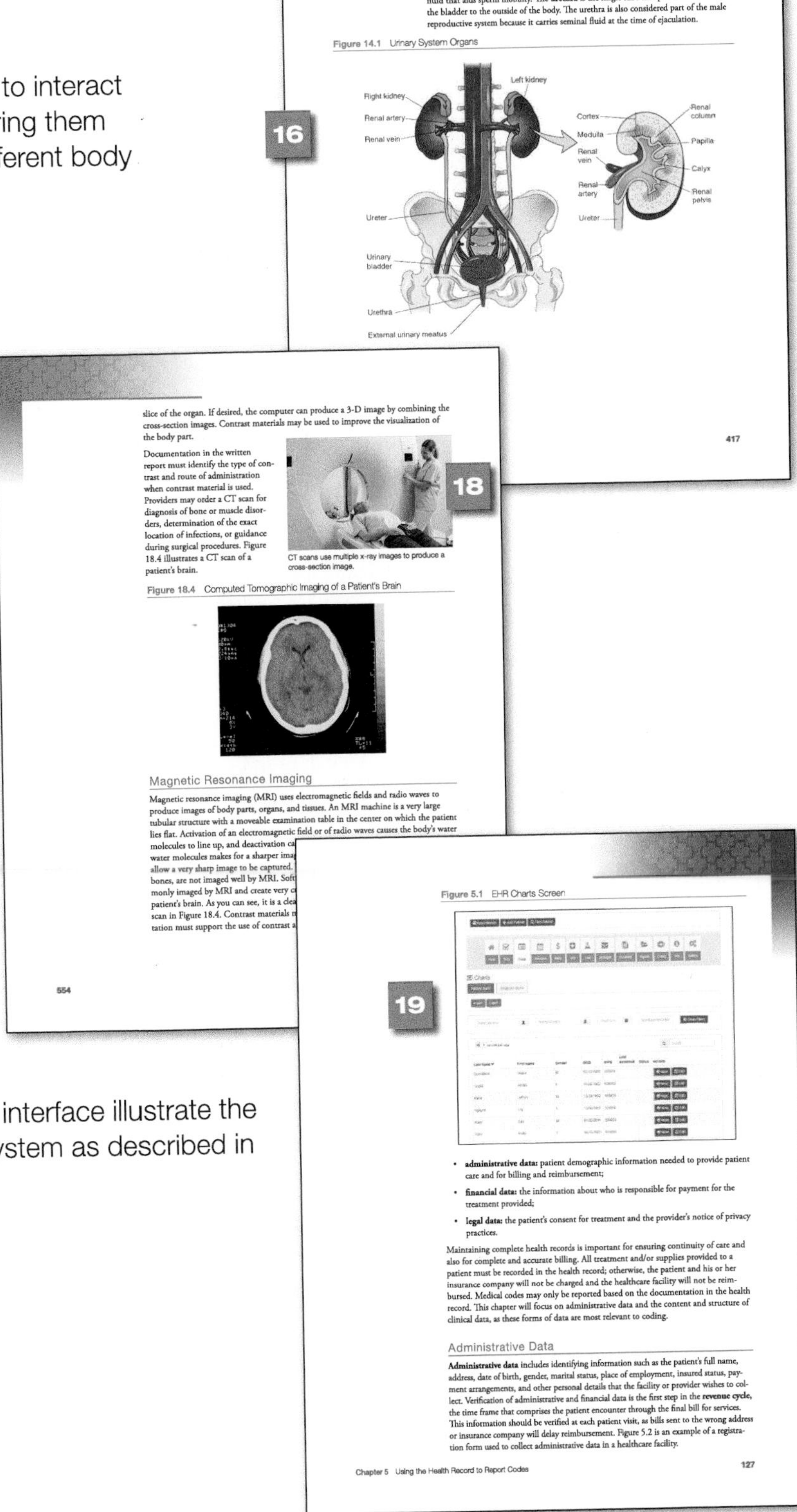

17

3-D
To explore the urinary system in the BioDigital Human, go to: http://Coding.ParadigmEducation.com/BioDigital_Urinary.

Introduction to the Urinary System

The **urinary system** removes waste from the body, regulates fluid volume, and maintains electrolyte balance in the body's fluids. Organs involved in this system are the kidneys, bladder, ureters, and urethra. The **kidneys** are a pair of bean-shaped organs located behind the peritoneum on each side of the vertebral column, as shown in Figure 14.1. In the kidney, the **renal pelvis** is the interior reservoir that collects urine. The **ureters** are the 2 tubes (1 connected to each kidney) that carry the urine from the kidney to the bladder. The urinary **bladder** is the muscular, hollow organ that temporarily stores urine. The **vesical neck** connects the urinary bladder to the urethra. The **prostate gland** (found in males only) surrounds the top of the urethra and secretes a fluid that aids sperm mobility. The **urethra** is the single tube that passes the urine from the bladder to the outside of the body. The urethra is also considered part of the male reproductive system because it carries seminal fluid at the time of ejaculation.

Figure 14.1 Urinary System Organs

16

417

slice of the organ. If desired, the computer can produce a 3-D image by combining the cross-section images. Contrast materials may be used to improve the visualization of the body part.

Documentation in the written report must identify the type of contrast and route of administration when contrast material is used. Providers may order a CT scan for diagnosis of bone or muscle disorders, determination of the exact location of infections, or guidance during surgical procedures. Figure 18.4 illustrates a CT scan of a patient's brain.

18

CT scans use multiple x-ray images to produce a cross-section image.

Figure 18.4 Computed Tomographic Imaging of a Patient's Brain

Magnetic Resonance Imaging

Magnetic resonance imaging (MRI) uses electromagnetic fields and radio waves to produce images of body parts, organs, and tissues. An MRI machine is a very large tubular structure with a moveable examination table in the center on which the patient lies flat. Activation of an electromagnetic field or of radio waves causes the body's water molecules to line up, and deactivation ca[…] water molecules makes for a sharper ima[…] allow a very sharp image to be captured. […] bones, are not imaged well by MRI. Soft[…] monly imaged by MRI and create very c[…] patient's brain. As you can see, it is a clea[…] scan in Figure 18.4. Contrast materials m[…] tation must support the use of contrast a[…]

554

Figure 5.1 EHR Charts Screen

19

- **administrative data:** patient demographic information needed to provide patient care and for billing and reimbursement;
- **financial data:** the information about who is responsible for payment for the treatment provided;
- **legal data:** the patient's consent for treatment and the provider's notice of privacy practices.

Maintaining complete health records is important for ensuring continuity of care and also for complete and accurate billing. All treatment and/or supplies provided to a patient must be recorded in the health record; otherwise, the patient and his or her insurance company will not be charged and the healthcare facility will not be reimbursed. Medical codes may only be reported based on the documentation in the health record. This chapter will focus on administrative data and the content and structure of clinical data, as these forms of data are most relevant to coding.

Administrative Data

Administrative data includes identifying information such as the patient's full name, address, date of birth, gender, marital status, place of employment, insured status, payment arrangements, and other personal details that the facility or provider wishes to collect. Verification of administrative and financial data is the first step in the **revenue cycle,** the time frame that comprises the patient encounter through the final bill for services. This information should be verified at each patient visit, as bills sent to the wrong address or insurance company will delay reimbursement. Figure 5.2 is an example of a registration form used to collect administrative data in a healthcare facility.

Chapter 5 Using the Health Record to Report Codes 127

20 Clear and colorful **diagrams** and **charts** help students better understand crucial concepts.

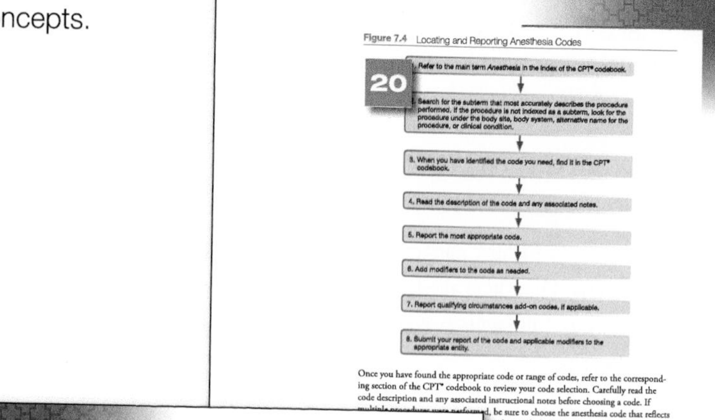

Figure 7.4 Locating and Reporting Anesthesia Codes
20
1. Refer to the main term Anesthesia in the Index of the CPT® codebook.
2. Search for the subterm that most accurately describes the procedure performed. If the procedure is not indexed as a subterm, look for the procedure under the body site, body system, alternative name for the procedure, or clinical condition.
3. When you have identified the code you need, find it in the CPT® codebook.
4. Read the description of the code and any associated notes.
5. Report the most appropriate code.
6. Add modifiers to the code as needed.
7. Report qualifying circumstances add-on codes, if applicable.
8. Submit your report of the code and applicable modifiers to the appropriate entity.

21 Examples of **healthcare forms** provide additional detail and visual reinforcement of chapter topics.

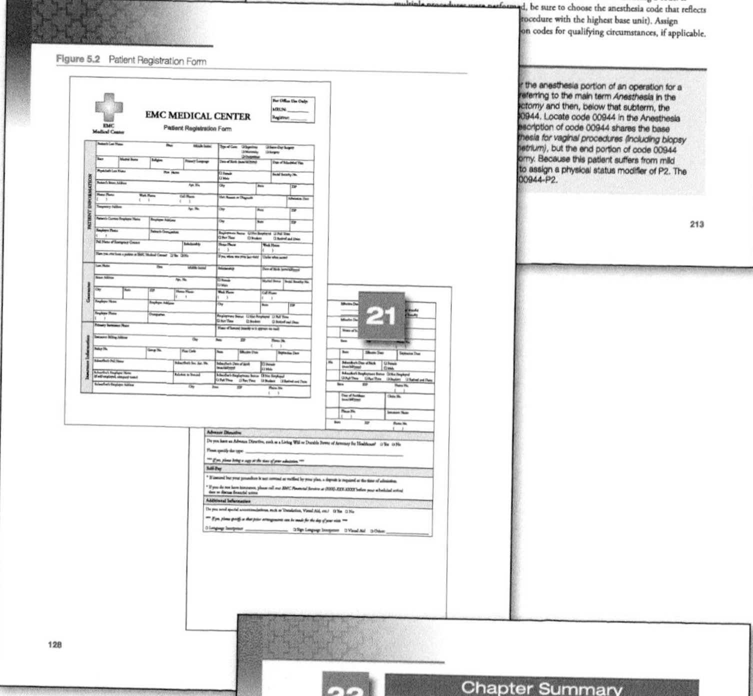

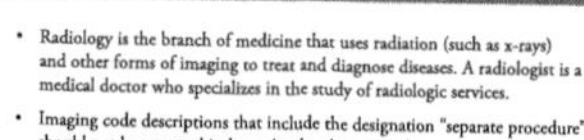

22 **Chapter Summary** lists deliver an overview of the key points of each chapter.

23 Students are directed to the Navigator+ to complete coding review activities, which test recall and comprehension of major chapter concepts, coding practice questions, designed to give students hands-on practice with coding scenarios, and case studies for more advanced practice.

22

Chapter Summary

- Radiology is the branch of medicine that uses radiation (such as x-rays) and other forms of imaging to treat and diagnose diseases. A radiologist is a medical doctor who specializes in the study of radiologic services.
- Imaging code descriptions that include the designation "separate procedure" should not be reported independently when carried out as an integral part of the procedure.
- When a contrast material is used in a diagnostic study, the phrase "with contrast" is included in the order for the study and in the written details of the procedure.
- Radiology codes are considered global services, which means that the services include a technical component and a professional component. When only the technical component of a radiology service is performed, append HCPCS modifier TC to the CPT® code. To report only the professional component, append CPT® modifier 26 to the CPT® code.
- A computed tomography scan (CT scan), sometimes referred to as a *CAT scan*, is an imaging technique that processes multiple x-rays to produce cross-section images of soft tissues and bones.
- Magnetic resonance imaging (MRI) is a technique that uses electromagnetic fields and radio waves to produce images of body parts, organs, and tissue.
- Ultrasound, also referred to as *ultrasonography*, is an imaging procedure that uses high-frequency sound waves to capture images or real-time video of internal organs.
- A fluoroscopy is an x-ray technique that captures continuous images in real time.
- Mammograms can be performed for screening or diagnostic purposes.
- Bone and joint studies identify abnormalities of bones and joints.
- Radiation oncology is a medical specialty that uses high-energy ionizing radiation to treat malignant and benign tumors.
- Nuclear medicine is the clinical discipline that uses radioactive substances to diagnose and treat diseases with chemical or pharmaceutical compounds.

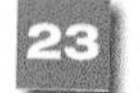

23 **Navigator+**

Access interactive chapter review exercises, practice activities, flash cards, and study games.

578 Chapter 18 Radiology Coding

Components

In addition to the many helpful features illustrated on the previous pages, *Deciphering Procedural Coding 2018* includes electronic resources designed to enhance student comprehension and assist students of all learning styles in preparing for a successful career in CPT ® coding.

Digital Textbook Content Delivery

For students who prefer studying digitally, this text is available in an electronic format. The digital content is web-based and always available. It can be accessed for offline use via an iOS app, available for free on iTunes.

Navigator

Navigator+

Navigator+ is a learning management system that contains the *Deciphering Procedural Coding 2018* end-of-chapter activities, case studies, web projects, and assessments, as well as flashcards, quizzes, and other interactive learning opportunities designed to reinforce textbook concepts and learning objectives. Through the Navigator+ site at http://Coding.ParadigmEducation.com/Navigator, instructors can set up a *Deciphering Procedural Coding* course. The Navigator+ site requires students to log in using the enrollment key provided by their instructor and the passcode provided with this textbook.

For instructors using their own learning management system, Navigator+ allows LTI connectivity, so instructors have the ability to export digital course content into their school's LMS (Blackboard, Canvas, D2L, or Common Cartridge). This means student work is instantly captured and reported, while grades are seamlessly updated into the school's LMS. Instructors can create, delete, modify, and schedule assignments.

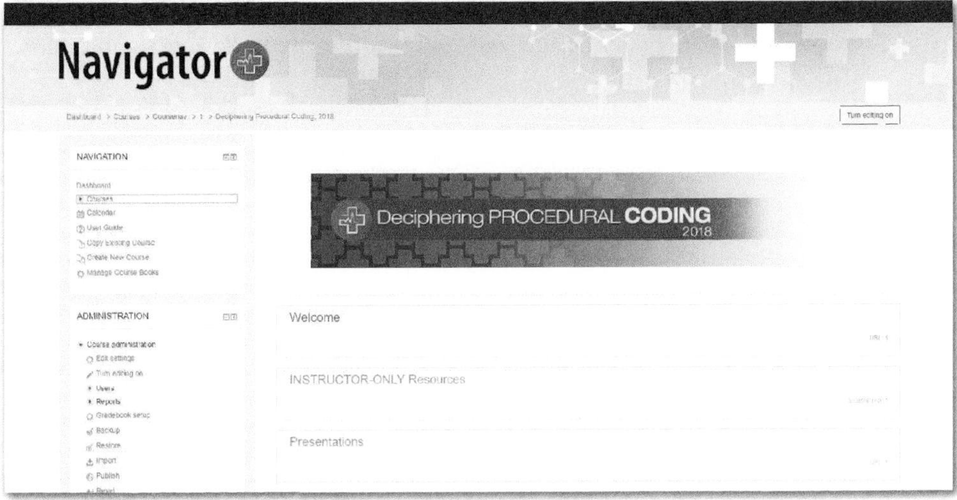

EHRNAVIGATOR

EHR Navigator

Access to EHR Navigator is included with this textbook. The EHR Navigator is a live software program from Paradigm Education Solutions that replicates professional practice and prepares students for today's workplace.

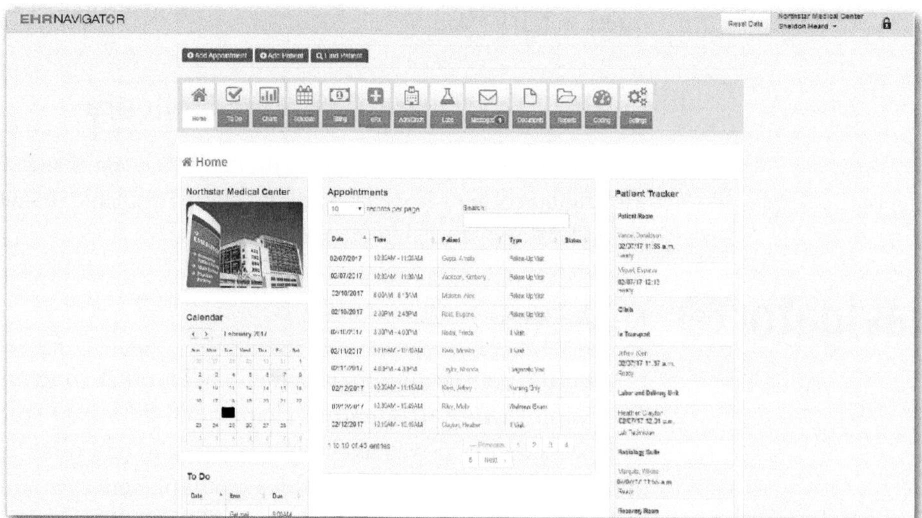

The EHR Navigator provides students with experience using a realistic patient record to code.

Instructor eResources

The Instructor eResources for *Deciphering Procedural Coding 2018*, provides instructors with helpful tools for planning and delivering their courses and assessing student learning. In addition to course planning tools and syllabus models, the Instructor eResources provide chapter-specific teaching hints and answers for all end-of-chapter activities. The Instructor Resources also offer PowerPoint® presentations and ready-to-use chapter quizzes and exams.

About the Authors

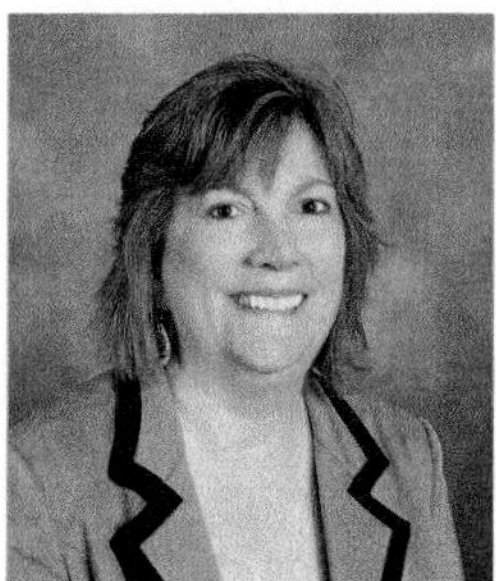
Ruth Berger

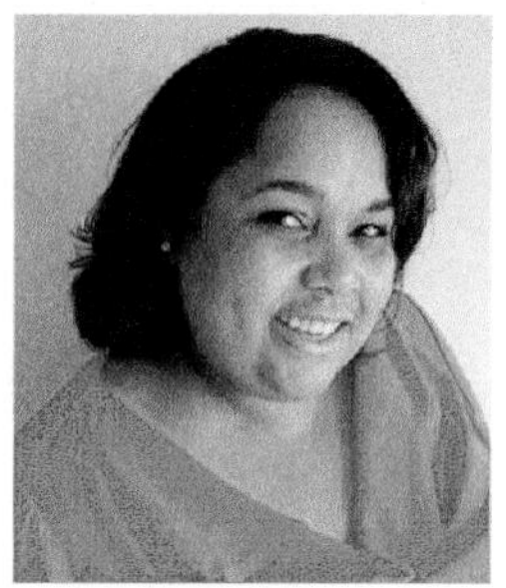
Sharon McBride

Ruth Berger is the HIT Program Coordinator at Rasmussen College in Brooklyn Park, Minnesota. She holds the American Health Information Management Association (AHIMA) certification of Registered Health Information Administrator (RHIA). Ruth has a master's degree in career and technical education from the University of Wisconsin—Stout, a bachelor's degree in healthcare management from Southern Illinois University, and an associate of applied science in medical records from the College of Lake County. She formerly taught in Illinois, Wisconsin, and Florida. Ruth brings decades of accredited HIM experience to her current teaching role in an associate degree program. She has previously worked in acute care as a manager of coding and compliance, been the assistant director of an HIM department, and held many other roles in HIM. Ruth has served on numerous committees and advisory boards in her career.

Sharon McBride is a Certified Professional Coder (CPC) and a Certified Professional Compliance Officer (CPCO) through the AAPC. Sharon is the Educational Coordinator for her local AAPC chapter. She works as a medical record auditor for a hospital management network and occasionally teaches medical coding certification preparation courses. Sharon also holds a master's degree in professional studies, with a concentration in training and development from the University of Memphis. She attained her bachelor's degree in organizational leadership, with a concentration on healthcare administration from Union University in Jackson, Tennessee. During her 20 years in healthcare administration, Sharon has held positions as a medical coder, insurance specialist, and practice administrator. As a consultant, she worked with physicians and practice managers to implement electronic health record (EHR) and practice management systems. As a physician's office compliance officer, she created compliance programs, conducted medical record audits, and provided education to physicians based on her audit findings. Sharon's passion to help others led her to pursue a career in education at Anthem Career College. While with Anthem, she taught all medical billing and coding modules, created coding specialty short course curricula, and held the position of program chair.

Acknowledgments

The quality of this body of work is a testament to the feedback we have received from the many contributors and reviewers who participated in the creation of *Deciphering Procedural Coding 2018*.

Reviewers

We would like to thank the following reviewers for offering valuable comments and suggestions on the content of this textbook:

Telma O'Neal, MEd, RHIA, CPAR
Virgina College

LaShunda Blanding Smith, PhD, RHIA, CPC, CHC, CHDA, CHTS-IM/TR/PW
National American University

A special thanks to Dr. McPartland for his review of all of the clinical material in the text.

Shawn McPartland, MD, JD,
Health Career Institute

Writers and Testers

Christine Bushaw, RHIT, MEd; Shelina Hardwick-Moses, MBA, MSHCA, CPhT, PhTR; Lynette Hessling, MSHI, RHIA, CHTS-PW, CHTS-TR

An additional special acknowledgment of gratitude goes out to the members of the Paradigm Education Solutions Health Information Technology Advisory Board for sharing their thoughts and advice throughout the development of this text.

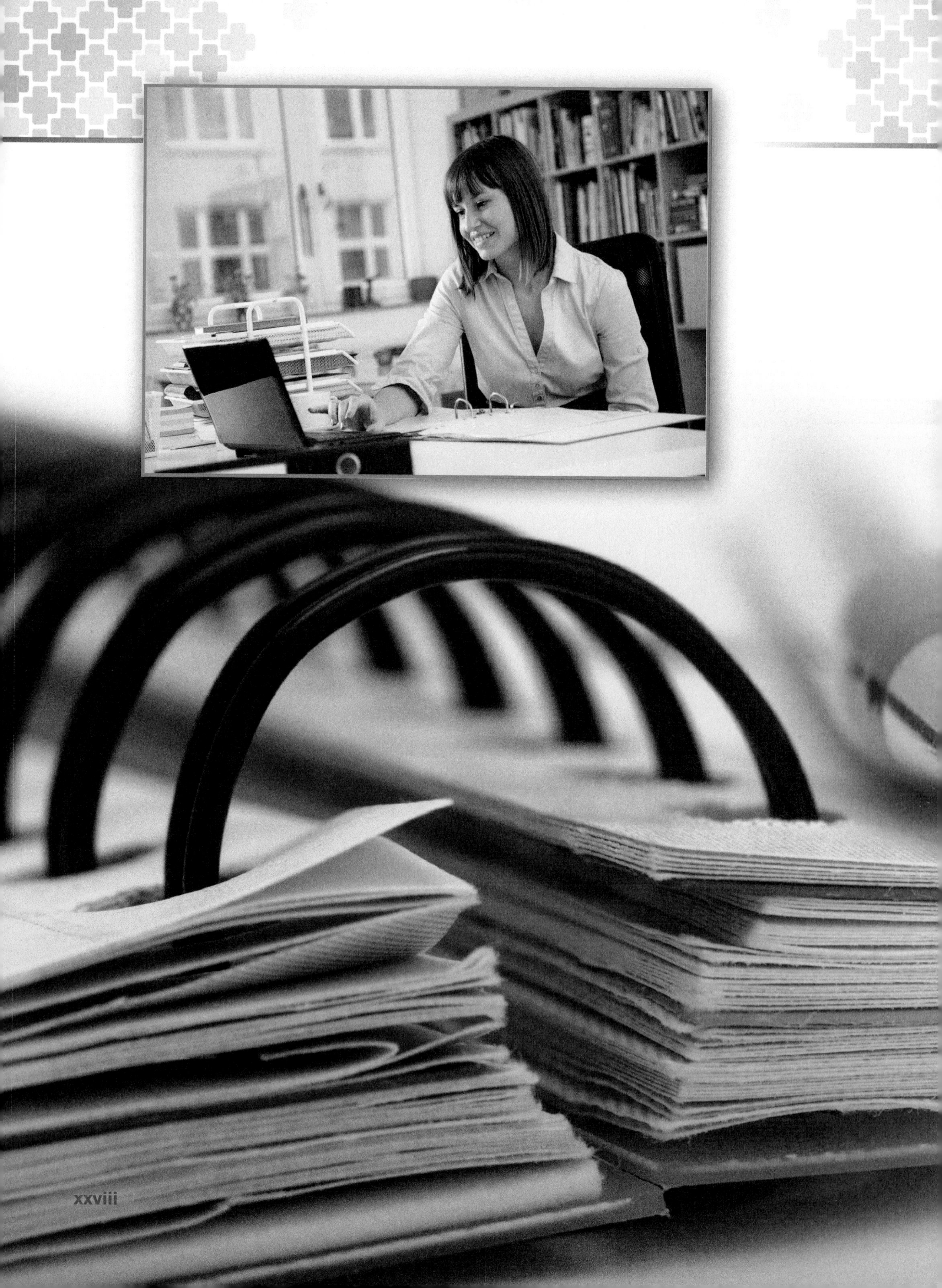

Unit 1

Introduction to Coding

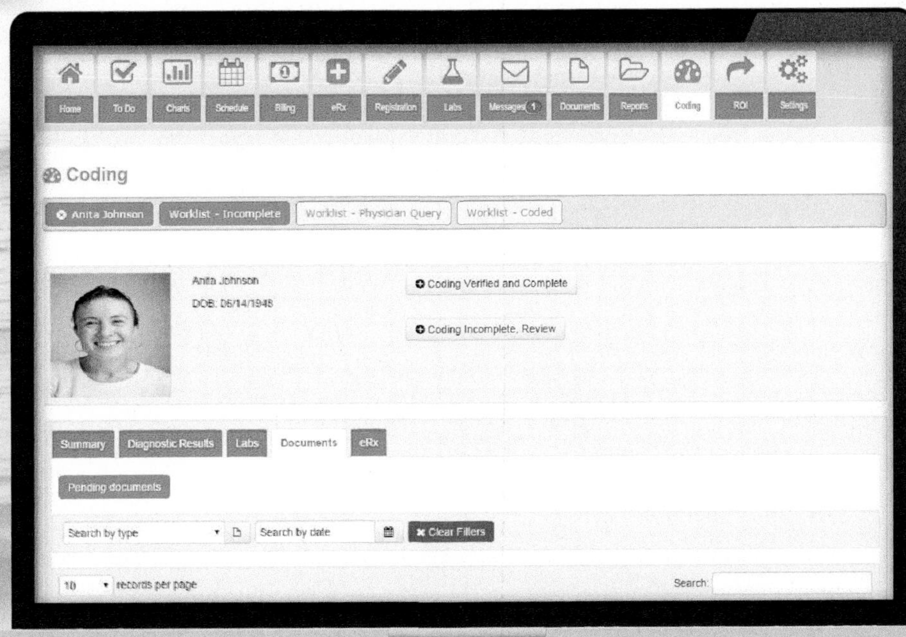

Chapter 1

Introduction to Coding

Fast Facts

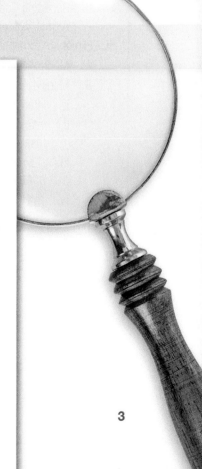

- According to the Bureau of Labor Statistics, jobs in the healthcare industry are predicted to increase 18% between 2016 and 2026, adding about 2.3 million new jobs.
- Medical coding jobs are projected to grow by more than 13% through 2026.
- Seventy percent of US adults seek care, information, or support from a doctor or other healthcare professional.
- The most common reason to see a doctor is for skin-related disorders, such as cysts, acne, and dermatitis.

Sources: http://bls.gov, http://pewinternet.org

Crack the Code

You may need to return to this exercise after reading the chapter content.

Morgan is a coding student who is excited to learn how medical codes are used in the healthcare industry. She is a recent high school graduate who decided to take a medical coding training certification program at the local community college. Upon completion of the coding program, Morgan will have expertise in physician-based settings such as physician offices, group practices, multispecialty clinics, and specialty centers. She will also be recognized as an expert in health information documentation, data integrity, and quality. Upon completion of the coding program, what American Health Information Management Association (AHIMA) coding certification examination will she qualify to take?

answer: The certified coding associate (CCA®) coding certification exam and registered health information technician (RHIT®) exam (if the college program is accredited through the Commission on Accreditation for Health Informatics and Information Management Education (CAHIIM)).

Learning Objectives

1.1 Define medical coding and the purpose for using medical codes.

1.2 Discuss how the health record is used to identify services and procedures that can be reported using medical codes.

1.3 Explore the benefits and challenges associated with the transition from paper records to electronic health records (EHRs).

1.4 Define medical nomenclatures and classification systems.

1.5 Explain the coder's relationship with health information management (HIM) and the billing cycle.

1.6 Identify certification requirements for coders.

1.7 Discuss essential skills for medical coders.

1.8 Describe common careers for medical coders.

1.9 Discuss healthcare providers and their significance to medical coding.

1.10 Discuss how coding ethics and compliance plans decrease fraud and abuse.

Chapter Outline

- **I.** What Is Medical Coding and Why Do We Use It?
- **II.** Coding and the Health Record
  - **A.** Electronic Health Records
  - **B.** Reporting Codes From the Health Record: A Brief Overview
- **III.** Exploring Nomenclatures and Classification Systems
  - **A.** Medical Nomenclatures
  - **B.** Medical Classification Systems
    - **i.** International Classification of Diseases
    - **ii.** International Classification of Functioning, Disability, and Health
    - **iii.** *Diagnostic and Statistical Manual of Mental Disorders*
    - **iv.** The Healthcare Common Procedure Coding (HCPCS) System
    - **v.** Current Dental Terminology (CDT)
- **IV.** The Role of Coding in Health Information Management
  - **A.** HIM in Hospitals Versus Physician Offices
  - **B.** HIM and the Revenue Cycle
- **V.** Required Education and Credentials for Medical Coders
  - **A.** The AAPC Medical Coding Organization
  - **B.** American Health Information Management Association (AHIMA)
- **VI.** Essential Skills for Medical Coders
  - **A.** Professionalism
  - **B.** Communication Skills
  - **C.** Technical Skills
  - **D.** Critical Thinking Skills
- **VII.** Career Opportunities in Coding
  - **A.** Coding Manager
  - **B.** Medical Coding Specialist
  - **C.** Medical Coding Auditor
- **VIII.** Healthcare Providers
  - **A.** Healthcare Practitioners
  - **B.** Nonphysician Practitioners
  - **C.** Allied Health Professionals
- **IX.** Coding Ethics
- **X.** Chapter Summary

What Is Medical Coding and Why Do We Use It?

Medical coding is the process of assigning standardized alphanumeric identifiers to the diagnoses and procedures documented in a health record. A **diagnosis** is a statement or conclusion that describes a patient's illness, disease, or health problem. A **procedure** is an activity performed on an individual to improve health, treat disease or injury, or identify a diagnosis. A **health record** is legal documentation in the form of a physical or electronic file in which doctors, nurses, and other healthcare professionals detail the diagnoses and procedures they provide to a particular patient. Health records also contain pertinent administrative and financial data about each patient.

When healthcare professionals document diagnoses and procedures in a health record, they do not always do so in a uniform way. For example, 2 physicians might describe the same procedure in different terms, as shown in Figure 1.1. Assigning standardized alphanumeric codes to this medical data makes it easier to immediately interpret, share, compare, classify, and manipulate the data for reimbursement, research, and planning.

Figure 1.1 How Different Medical Notes Can Result in the Same Code

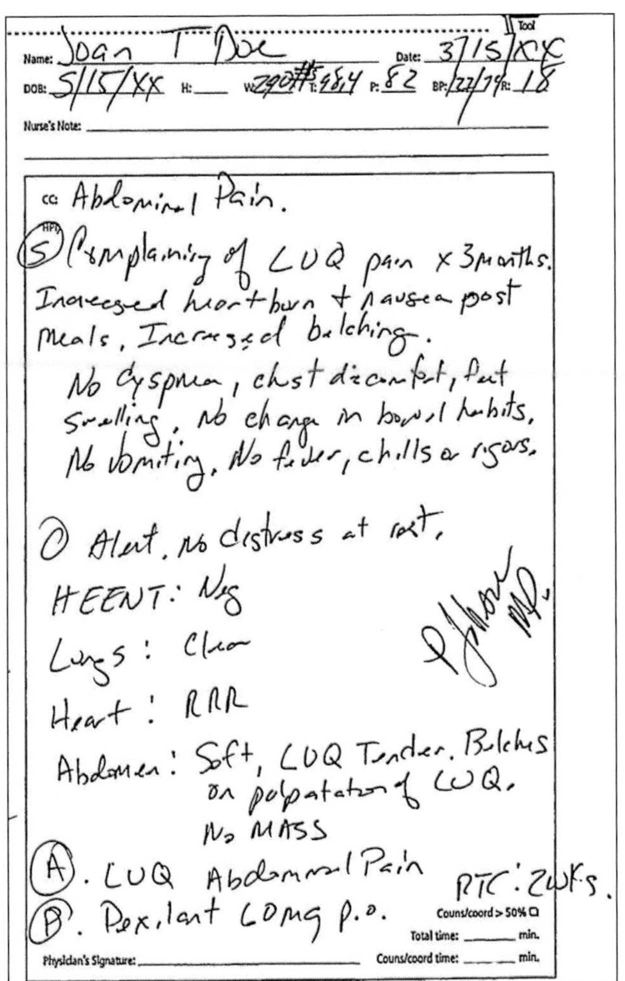
Name: Joan T Doe Date: 3/15/XX
DOB: 5/15/XX H: ___ W: 290# T: 98.4 P: 82 BP: 122/74 R: 18
Nurse's Note:

CC: Abdominal Pain.
HPI (S) Complaining of LUQ pain x 3 months. Increased heartburn + nausea post meals. Increased belching.
No dyspnea, chest discomfort, foot swelling. No change in bowel habits. No vomiting. No fever, chills or rigors.

(O) Alert. No distress at rest.
HEENT: Neg
Lungs: Clear
Heart: RRR
Abdomen: Soft, LUQ Tender. Belches on palpation of LUQ. No MASS

(A). LUQ Abdominal Pain
(P). Dexilant 60mg p.o. RTC: 2wks.

Couns/coord > 50% ☐
Total time: ______ min.
Physician's Signature: ______ Couns/coord time: ______ min.

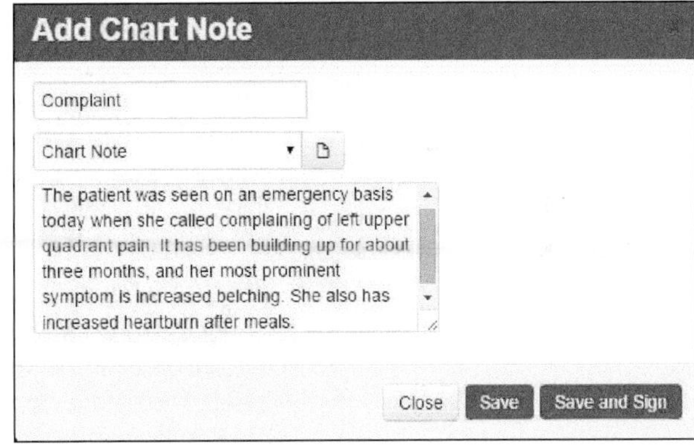

Learn Your Way

Students learn and process information in many different ways. Dr. Richard Felder, Hoechst Celanese Professor of Chemical Engineering at North Carolina State University, and Dr. Linda K. Silverman, an educational psychologist, developed the Felder-Silverman model of learning styles. They created a questionnaire called "The Index of Learning Styles" based on this model that measures students' preferences in 4 dimensions: reflecting versus acting, reasoning logically versus intuitively, experiencing new information verbally versus visually, and tackling assignments step by step versus as a big picture. Most people tend to prefer certain stages of the learning process over others, allowing different learning styles to be categorized based on these tendencies. The index identifies the following types of learners:

- Active versus reflective learners. Active learners retain knowledge best by doing something physical with the information, such as presenting it or discussing it with others. Reflective learners prefer thinking about the information quietly by themselves first.
- Sensing versus intuitive learners. Sensing learners like facts, solving problems, and memorization. Intuitive learners do better with making connections, abstracting information, and solving formulas.
- Visual versus verbal learners. Visual learners learn best when they see information in pictures, diagrams, flow charts, videos, etc. Verbal learners prefer words for explanations—written or spoken.
- Sequential versus global learners. Sequential learners understand best when given step-by-step, logical, linear instructions. Global learners seek to understand the big picture first so they can understand the purpose and order of the pieces and steps.

According to the Felder-Silverman model, people who learn by thinking out a process before acting are considered reflective learners. As a reflective learner, you find it easiest to master a concept when you understand how it applies to everyday life. You may be interested to know that medicine is just 1 of the many industries that rely on codes to keep track of data and predict trends. For example, retail stores use codes to manage inventory and track supply and demand. Notice the codes that appear on the cash register screen as your items are scanned. These codes provide many different forms of data to help the store conduct its business efficiently.

To take the self-scoring questionnaire about your preferences according to the Felder-Silverman model, visit http://Coding.ParadigmEducation.com/LearningStyles.

Coded data is used by healthcare providers to seek reimbursement from the government, private insurance companies, and other third-party payers. A **third-party payer** is an entity other than the patient that is financially responsible for payment of the medical bill. Patients who pay for the entire visit themselves are referred to as **self-pay patients**. Third-party payers are so named because there are typically 3 parties involved in the care of the patient:

- party 1, the patient;
- party 2, the healthcare provider;
- party 3, the entity that pays the medical bill other than the patient.

Coded data is also used in public health management to monitor the incidence and prevalence of diseases as well as death rates. To monitor health trends, nations track **morbidity**, which consists of illness statistics, and **mortality**, which consists of death statistics. Coded information enables the storage and retrieval of diagnostic information for clinical, epidemiological, and quality-control purposes. The following are examples of how coded data can be used for planning and research purposes.

EXAMPLE 1.1

Hometown Hospital has experienced an increase in the number of patients seen in the cardiac care center over the past 3 months. To determine if the hospital needs to invest further in cardiac care services to meet the growing need, the hospital administrator gathers information. The administrator uses the hospital's computer system to collect all the recent cases that have cardiac diagnosis and procedure codes. This information shows how many patients were seen for cardiac-related conditions during this time and, more specifically, how each of these patients was diagnosed and treated.

EXAMPLE 1.2

Becky Johnson is the tumor registrar for Montgomery Hospital. Her job is to use coded diagnoses and procedures to identify patients who have been recently seen at Montgomery Hospital for cancer-related conditions and to enter information from their health records into a tumor registry database. The information in this database is used by the Centers for Disease Control and Prevention (CDC) to help predict public health issues and improve healthcare delivery in the United States.

Coding and the Health Record

A health record is a physical or electronic file containing confidential patient health information, such as a health history, prescriptions, lab results, x-rays, and other diagnostic reports. The health record is the main source from which medical coders **abstract**, or take away, the information they need to assign codes. Physicians, nurses, medical assistants, and allied health professionals are responsible for entering information into the health record. Accuracy is of the utmost importance when working with data in health records: incomplete or erroneous entries can lead to poor patient care, dangerous medication errors, and inaccurate coding and billing. The health record will be discussed in greater detail in Chapter 5.

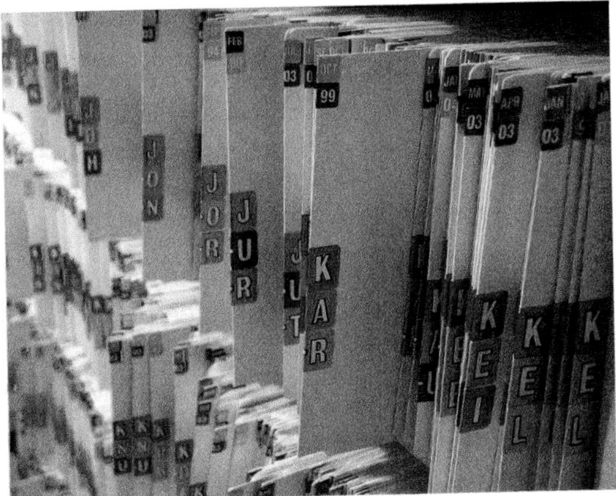

Health records contain confidential patient health information.

The steps in reporting codes from an operative report are generally the following:

1. Read the report and verify that the diagnosis and procedure listed at the top of the report are supported by the documentation of the procedure provided in the body of the report (sometimes called the *operative technique*).
2. After verifying that everything matches, the coder uses several resources, such as codebooks and coding databases, to locate the correct codes for both the diagnosis and the procedure.
3. If the documentation supports a different procedure or diagnosis than that listed by the physician, the coder should review the facility policies and procedures, which typically instruct the coder to query or ask for clarification from the provider.
4. If working in a physician practice, enter the code(s) into the patient's financial account in the **practice management system (PMS)**, which is the software used by physician practices to store, organize, bill, and reconcile patient financial accounts. You will learn more about these systems in Chapter 21.
5. After the medical codes have been entered into the PMS, prepare the account for billing.

This is only a brief overview of the process—Chapter 5 will provide a more in-depth look at the health record and how to use it to report codes.

CONCEPTS CHECKPOINT 1.1

Fill in the blanks in each of the following statements.

1. A ______________ is a statement or conclusion that describes a patient's illness, disease, or health problem.
2. A ______________ is an activity performed on a patient to improve health, treat disease or injury, or identify a diagnosis.
3. Coders are responsible for reading the operative report to verify that the procedural documentation in the body of the report ______________ the procedure and diagnoses at the top of the report.
4. ______________ is the process of assigning numbers and letters to the diagnoses and procedures documented in a medical patient record.
5. ______________ are physical or electronic files in which doctors, nurses, and other healthcare professionals document the diagnoses and procedures they provide to each patient.

Exploring Nomenclatures and Classification Systems

RED FLAG

The terms *nomenclature* and *classification system* are similar and related, but they may not be used interchangeably.

A **nomenclature** is a system of naming things. Science has many different kinds of nomenclatures, including the ones used to name medical conditions and procedures. In a nomenclature, every concept has its own unique name, but prefixes and suffixes may be reused consistently to convey specific meanings. For example, the removal of the appendix is called an *appendectomy*, and the removal of the spleen is called a *splenectomy*. These 2 distinct procedures have different names, but they also share the suffix *–ectomy* to convey that they are both removal procedures.

A **classification system** is used to organize like medical conditions, procedures, or concepts into categories and assign them codes that, when deciphered, describe each item in detail. Classification systems relate to nomenclatures in that a nomenclature is necessary for naming the various items so that they can be organized using a classification system. The following sections will describe several medical nomenclatures and classification systems, including the Current Procedural Terminology (CPT®) classification system.

Medical Nomenclatures

Coding Clicks

Access the SNOMED-CT nomenclature through the NLM website at http://Coding.ParadigmEducation.com/SNOMED. Although access is free, registration is required.

The **Systematized Nomenclature of Medicine (SNOMED)** is a nomenclature that contains the names of diseases, bacteria, anatomical sites, procedures, and other medical terms, as well as the corresponding medical codes. Originally developed by the American College of Pathologists and England's National Health Service, the nomenclature is now owned by a consortium of countries called the International Health Terminology Standards Development Organisation (IHTSDO). The National Library of Medicine (NLM) is the United States's member of the IHTSDO and distributes the nomenclature at no charge. EHR systems use SNOMED to index, store, and combine medical data.

Like any other language, medical terminology contains different words and phrases that mean the same thing. For example, Dr. Anderson may refer to a condition using the term *scrotal hernia*, while Dr. Xiang may call it an *inguinal hernia*, even though these terms refer to the exact same condition. Although these 2 phrases mean the same thing, in the language of SNOMED, they are 2 distinct terms. In the past, if Dr. Anderson and Dr. Xiang were treating the same patient but were using different computer systems, the computers would not understand that the 2 doctors were referring to the same condition. To solve this problem, in 2014, the ARRA began requiring the use of **SNOMED-CT** (in which CT stands for *clinical terminology*) when entering information into EHRs. SNOMED-CT is specially designed to improve the accuracy of information entered into EHR systems as well as improve communication between EHR systems, thereby improving the quality of care patients receive when they seek treatment from different medical providers. SNOMED is available to the public at no charge on the NLM website.

MEDCIN is another medical nomenclature previously used in EHR systems. It enabled EHRs to index, store, and combine medical data. Although MEDCIN is a comprehensive nomenclature system, it is a privately owned system, thus limiting its availability for use in research and development of new technology. Although MEDCIN can no longer be used in EHR systems, it is still used by some medical research companies and other private companies that use medical terminology in their computer systems as part of their daily operation.

Medical Classification Systems

Your first experience with a classification system may have been in your elementary school library, which probably used the Dewey Decimal Classification (DDC) to organize its books. The DDC assigns a call number to each book, and each part of the call number communicates a piece of information about the book. Using the DDC in the library allows students to look up books to check out and helps librarians to identify whether a specific book is checked out, when it is scheduled to return, and what bookshelf it belongs on. In the bigger picture, call numbers may also be used by the library committee to analyze what books are most popular, what categories of books need more resources, and what categories have become obsolete.

Medical classification systems are similar to the DDC. When medical terms are categorized, they are assigned individual codes. The categorization of the medical terms creates a standard classification system that makes it easier to access, store, and share medical data.

The **Health Insurance Portability and Accountability Act of 1996 (HIPAA)** contains 2 provisions: Title I protects health insurance coverage during a job loss or transition, and Title II mandates national standards for electronic healthcare transactions. Title II is also known as the Administrative Simplification provisions, which require specific classification and nomenclature systems be used when reporting diagnoses and procedures. HIPAA-designated code sets are the *International Classification of Diseases, 10th Revision* (ICD-10), CPT®, and the Healthcare Common Procedure Coding System, Level II (HCPCS). Although this book focuses on procedure coding, it is important for coders to have an understanding of other medical classification systems as well.

International Classification of Diseases

The **International Classification of Diseases (ICD)** is a statistical classification system maintained by the World Health Organization (WHO). The ICD classification system is a family made up of several smaller classification systems that identify a variety of conditions and procedures. The World Health Organization Family of International Classifications (WHO-FIC) includes 3 basic classifications:

- ICD-10, also known as ICD;
- International Classification of Functioning, Disability and Health (ICF); and
- International Classification of Health Interventions (ICHI).

The WHO-FIC also includes "derived" classifications that provide additional detail for a clinical specialty or a special population. These classifications currently treat oncology, mental and behavioral disorders, neurology, dentistry, and stomatology. Two of these classification systems will be discussed in this chapter: the *International Classification of Diseases for Oncology, 3rd Edition* (ICD-O-3), and ICF.

ICD uses alphanumeric codes. Each character in an ICD code represents a piece of information about a specific diagnosis, procedure, device, or medication.

The CDC, researchers, and governmental agencies use medical data collected from the reporting of ICD diagnosis codes to analyze morbidity and mortality statistics.

International Classification of Diseases, 9th Revision (ICD-9) **ICD-9** is a diagnosis and procedure classification system. Originally implemented in 1979, ICD-9 was replaced by ICD-10 in October 2015. ICD-9 codes were used to report patient illnesses, injuries, and other conditions that require medical care. ICD-9 procedure codes were reported by facilities for **inpatient procedures** (named using nomenclatures such as SNOMED), which are medical procedures performed in the hospital.

International Classification of Diseases, 10th Revision, Clinical Modification (ICD-10-CM) **ICD-10-CM** is the diagnosis classification system that replaced the ICD-9 diagnosis classification system on October 1, 2015. ICD-10-CM codes range in length from 3 to 7 digits and use both numbers and letters, allowing for more specific disease categorization than the ICD-9 codes provided. All US medical providers, and most other developed countries, use ICD-10-CM codes to report diseases, illnesses, injuries, and other conditions that require medical care.

Coding Clicks

The organization of the ICD-10-PCS is described in the Centers for Medicare and Medicaid report *Development of the ICD-10 Procedure Coding System*, found at http://Coding.ParadigmEducation.com/ICD-10.

International Classification of Diseases, 10th Revision, Procedural Coding System (ICD-10-PCS) **ICD-10-PCS** is a classification system used to report procedures performed in an inpatient setting. ICD-10-PCS codes replaced the ICD-9 procedure codes on October 1, 2015. Unlike the ICD-9 procedure codes, which categorized procedures predominantly based on the anatomical site at which they were performed, ICD-10-PCS codes are assigned based on the purpose of the procedure. Selecting a procedure based on the purpose allows a single procedure code to be reported for several different types of conditions. For example, the ICD-9 code 27.62, *Correction of cleft palate*, is selected and located based on the condition of the patient and anatomical site. When coding the same procedure with ICD-10-PCS, the code 0CQ20ZZ, *Repair Hard Palate, Open Approach*, is selected based on the purpose, anatomic site, and other key components of the procedure. This allows the ICD-10-PCS codes to be used for a variety of conditions, whereas the ICD-9 procedure code was reported only for a single condition. ICD-10-PCS codes are 7 characters in length, allowing for the reporting of more detailed information regarding the procedure.

International Classification of Diseases for Oncology, 3rd Edition (ICD-O-3) **ICD-O-3** is a **neoplasm** (tumor) classification system, and its codes are also referred to as **morphology codes**, meaning that they describe the form and structure of tumors. ICD-O-3 categorizes neoplasms by their anatomical site, **histology** (microscopic anatomy, also known as **morphology**), behavior, and **grading** (cell stage). ICD-O-3 codes are primarily used to collect data in **cancer registries**, which keep track of statistical information regarding cancer behaviors and characteristics and supply this information to physicians, hospitals, and researchers.

International Classification of Functioning, Disability, and Health

The **International Classification of Functioning, Disability, and Health (ICF)** is a classification system used to categorize the health and disability functionality of individuals and the general population. ICF codes fall into 3 primary categories: body functions and structure, activities and participation, and severity and environmental factors. ICF codes complement ICD codes to provide a complete picture of a patient's health condition and its effects on his or her quality of life. ICF codes are typically used internally by disability insurers to collect data about people who file claims.

Diagnostic and Statistical Manual of Mental Disorders

</> Coding for CMS

CMS does not allow the reporting of DSM for mental illnesses. These conditions must be reported using ICD codes instead.

The ***Diagnostic and Statistical Manual of Mental Disorders* (DSM)** is a standard classification system developed by the American Psychiatric Association and used by mental health professionals to categorize mental illnesses. DSM codes are derived from diagnoses in the ICD classification system. The sixth revision of DSM is in development and will resemble ICD-10-CM in code structure and diagnosis descriptions.

The Healthcare Common Procedure Coding (HCPCS) System

The **Healthcare Common Procedure Coding System (HCPCS)**, pronounced "hik-piks," is a list of procedures, medical supplies, medical equipment, services, and drugs. HCPCS codes are used to request reimbursement for services rendered by outpatient medical providers and dentists. **Outpatient providers** are not employees of a hospital, but they may bill for their professional services performed in the hospital or in the medical office. HCPCS codes are reported in conjunction with ICD-10-CM codes (the next section explains how they correlate). HCPCS, like ICD, is a family of smaller classification systems. In HCPCS, the different parts of this family are referred to by level.

Healthcare Common Procedure Coding System, Level I (CPT®) HCPCS Level I codes are best known as **Current Procedural Terminology (CPT®)** codes. The trademarked CPT® code set is developed, maintained, and published by the **American Medical Association (AMA)**. The codes are used to report medical services and procedures performed by outpatient providers. Hospitals also maintain a database of CPT® and HCPCS codes with associated fees set by the insurance payer. The database, called the *chargemaster*, enables the hospital to bill for outpatient services performed in the hospital, such as x-rays. The majority of the procedures and services reported on medical insurance claims are CPT® codes.

CPT® codes are reported in conjunction with ICD-10-CM codes: the ICD-10-CM code provides the medical problem (diagnosis), and the CPT® code covers how it was treated (procedure). For example, if a patient presents to his physician with pain in his left upper arm and the physician orders an x-ray of the left arm, the physician reports ICD-10-CM code M79.622, *Pain in left upper arm*, to explain why the patient was seen, and CPT® code 73060, *Radiologic examination; humerus, minimum of 2 views*, to report the procedure performed to diagnose it. Coding and reporting guidelines for CPT® codes are the main focus of this book.

Healthcare Common Procedure Coding System, Level II **HCPCS Level II** codes, also referred to as **National Codes**, are another nomenclature of procedures, services, drugs, and items. CMS maintains and distributes HCPCS Level II codes. The code set is updated quarterly based on input from healthcare providers, manufacturers of healthcare equipment, professional societies, and third-party payers. HCPCS Level II codes are used only in outpatient settings such as medical offices, diagnostic centers, and ancillary surgery centers to report services, products, drugs, and procedures not covered by CPT® codes. Codes listed in HCPCS Level II are typically not identified in the CPT® code set; however, in the rare case that both code sets contain the same procedure or service, CMS prioritizes the reporting of HCPCS Level II codes over CPT® codes when services are provided to Medicare patients. More information regarding HCPCS Level II codes is provided in Chapters 2 and 3.

Current Dental Terminology (CDT)

The Code on Dental Procedures and Nomenclatures, commonly referred to as **Current Dental Terminology (CDT)**, is the common language used when describing dental procedures. CDT is a classification system of dental procedure codes reported by dentists to request reimbursement. It is also considered a nomenclature. In 2000, CDT was named as a HIPAA standard code set. The CDT codes are maintained by the **American Dental Association (ADA)**. Although these codes are not part of the HCPCS family, they are included in the HCPCS Level II codebook. More information regarding CDT codes is provided in Chapter 3.

CONCEPTS CHECKPOINT **1.2**

Match the acronym to the correct definition.

1. _____ CDT
2. _____ CPT®
3. _____ DSM
4. _____ ICD-10-CM
5. _____ ICD-10-PCS
6. _____ ICD-9
7. _____ ICD-O-3

a. A neoplasm (tumor) classification system
b. A standard classification system used by mental health professionals to categorize mental illnesses
c. A medical procedural classification system used for reporting procedures performed in an inpatient setting
d. A diagnosis classification system implemented in the United States on October 1, 2015
e. Used for reporting medical services and procedures performed by outpatient providers
f. A diagnosis and procedure classification system no longer used in the United States
g. A list of dental procedures reported by dentists to request reimbursement

mainly by medical billers to apply charges based on medical codes. However, it is important to be aware of them and how they work, as this can affect how you do your job as a coder. For example, some codes are hard-coded into the chargemaster and thus do not need to be assigned by a coding professional.

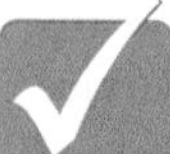

CONCEPTS CHECKPOINT 1.3

Fill in the blanks in each of the following statements.

1. The administrative, financial, and technological segments of medicine are all part of ______________.
2. Hospital coders are commonly referred to as ______________.
3. The ______________ consists of the steps necessary for a facility to receive reimbursement for services or procedures provided to a patient.
4. A ______________ is a comprehensive listing maintained by a hospital that contains all the services, procedures, and even medicines it provides, along with the price it charges for each item.
5. Coders in physician offices use ICD-10-CM to report diagnoses and _____ and _____ codes to report procedures and services.

Required Education and Credentials for Medical Coders

Medical facilities set the education requirements for the coders that they employ. Requirements span a spectrum from completion of a coding training program and a coding certification to degrees or certifications in HIM. Prior to selecting a coding training program or an HIM program, a student should research and investigate his or her desired career path. One way to do this is with the help of a **professional organization**—an association of people who have the same occupation. Members of these professional organizations have access to resources, professional training, certifications, and networking opportunities. Although there are many reputable professional associations within the HIM field, the 2 most recognized are the AAPC and AHIMA.

The AAPC Medical Coding Organization

Coding Clicks

Go to http://Coding.ParadigmEducation.com/AAPC and click the Continuing Education tab. Take a moment to explore the different ways you can obtain continuing education. Which methods are most appealing to you?

The **AAPC**, formerly the American Academy of Professional Coders but now known only by its initials, offers its members education and training programs, certifications, and networking and job opportunities. The AAPC administers certification examinations in medical coding for physician offices. Members who successfully pass the examination are awarded a **certified professional coder (CPC)** certificate. Completion of 80 hours of coding training and 1 year of on-the-job experience is required to take the CPC exam. Members who pass the coding exam but do not have the work experience are designated as apprentices until they attain the required work experience. The AAPC also administers certification exams for medical billing, medical auditing, compliance, and practice management, along with exams for a variety of medical specialties.

To maintain certifications obtained through the AAPC, coders are required to participate in continuing education. **Continuing education (CE)** typically comprises courses, webinars, workshops, and other offerings that allow professionals to stay up to date with changes and innovations in their field. Continuing education requirements for coders are based on the type of coding certification held.

American Health Information Management Association (AHIMA)

The **American Health Information Management Association (AHIMA)** is a membership organization that focuses on providing knowledge, resources, and tools to advance health information professional practices and standards for the delivery of quality health care. AHIMA provides training and networking opportunities, administers a number of certification exams, and awards credentials in the areas of HIM, coding, and data/documentation management. AHIMA offers certifications that verify expertise in various aspects of the HIM field. Only members of AHIMA are eligible to attain these credentials. Table 1.1 details the various AHIMA certifications and their requirements.

Table 1.1 AHIMA Certifications and Requirements

Credential Abbreviation	Credential Full Name	Educational Requirements	Focus	Biennial Continuing Education (CE) Hours Required
CCA	Certified coding associate	High school diploma or equivalent	Demonstrates coding competencies across all settings, including hospitals and physician practices.	20
CCS	Certified coding specialist	High school diploma or equivalent	Mastery-level professional skill in classifying medical data from patient records, generally in the hospital setting. Recognized as an expert in health information documentation, data integrity, and quality.	20
CCS-P	Certified coding specialist-physician-based	High school diploma or equivalent	Mastery-level coding practitioner with expertise in physician-based settings such as physician offices, group practices, multispecialty clinics, or specialty centers. Recognized as an expert in health information documentation, data integrity, and quality.	20
RHIT*	Registered health information technician	2-year associate's degree	Ensures quality of health records. Uses computer applications and systems. Applies skills in coding diagnoses and procedures for reimbursement and research.	20
RHIA*	Registered health information administrator	4-year bachelor's degree	Expertly manages patient health information. Possesses comprehensive knowledge of medical, administrative, ethical, and legal requirements and standards of healthcare delivery and privacy of protected patient information.	30

*RHIT and RHIA certifications are available only to the graduates of schools accredited by the Commission on Accreditation for Health Informatics and Information Management Education (CAHIIM), an independent accrediting organization that promotes and enforces accreditation standards for health information and health informatics education programs.

Source: http://ahima.org/certification

AHIMA coding credentials require the completion of coding training programs or real-world coding experience. Real-world experience is obtained from working either as a noncredentialed coder or a coder credentialed by another coding association. However, without a coding certification, this real-world experience is very difficult to obtain. AHIMA members may demonstrate coding competency by successfully passing 1 of several coding exams, listed here in order of increasing experience and proficiency:

- certified coding associate (CCA);
- certified coding specialist (CCS);
- certified coding specialist-physician-based (CCS-P).

The CCA is an entry-level coding certification for coders who have completed a coding training program but lack work experience. A coder with a CCA certification may work in physician offices or hospital coding departments; however, employers may expect them to attain CCS credentials within their first year of employment. The CCS certification is a high-level coding certification. CCS coders may work as inpatient coders or outpatient physician coders. The CCS certification tests members on their ability to analyze medical documentation for the purpose of identifying diagnoses and procedures and categorizing the severity of illnesses. The CCS-P certification demonstrates the coder's specialty knowledge of outpatient physician coding.

AHIMA members who meet specific postsecondary education requirements may take an examination that demonstrates their knowledge of medical coding and other key competencies of the HIM field. Successful candidates are awarded certification as a registered health information administrator (RHIA) or registered health information technician (RHIT).

RHIT and RHIA certifications are available only to the graduates of schools accredited by the **Commission on Accreditation for Health Informatics and Information Management Education (CAHIIM)**, an independent accrediting organization that promotes and enforces accreditation standards for health information and health informatics education programs. Students may take the RHIT or RHIA exam during the last semester of study or after all coursework has been completed. Students are encouraged to take the exam immediately after course completion.

It is essential for health information professionals to become lifelong learners and to remain current with all of the changes in the industry. To maintain certification, AHIMA-certified professionals are required to complete a certain number of hours of continuing education (CE) training in their chosen field every 2 years. Table 1.1 lists CE requirements for AHIMA certification programs. The number of CE hours required depends on the credential or certification.

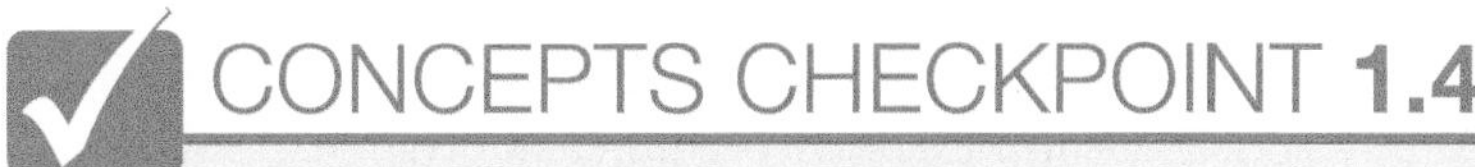

CONCEPTS CHECKPOINT **1.4**

Use the information in Table 1.1 to answer the following questions:

1. Which AHIMA certification requires the completion of a 2-year associate's degree? ______________
2. What are the CE requirements for each of the following certifications?
   a. CCA: ______________
   b. CCS: ______________
   c. RHIA: ______________
3. Which certifications have a minimum requirement of a high school diploma (or the equivalent)? ______________

Essential Skills for Medical Coders

Essential job skills that coders must acquire through training and education are the following:

- a comprehensive knowledge of medical terminology and anatomy;
- knowledge of governmental regulations that affect the healthcare industry;
- a facility with the use of coding reference books for CPT®, HCPCS Level II, and ICD-10 code sets, even though the majority of EHR systems have built-in encoders (coding databases that will be discussed in Chapter 5);
- up-to-date information about new developments in insurance plans, billing processes, and revenue systems;
- thorough familiarity with **medical compliance**, which is the process of meeting the regulations, recommendations, and standards of federal and state agencies that pay for medical services and procedures.

In addition to all of their knowledge related to healthcare processes and regulations, coders must also possess personal strengths of professionalism, communication skills, critical thinking skills, and technical skills.

Professionalism

A professional wardrobe is well fitting; not trendy; and free of wrinkles, holes, and stains.

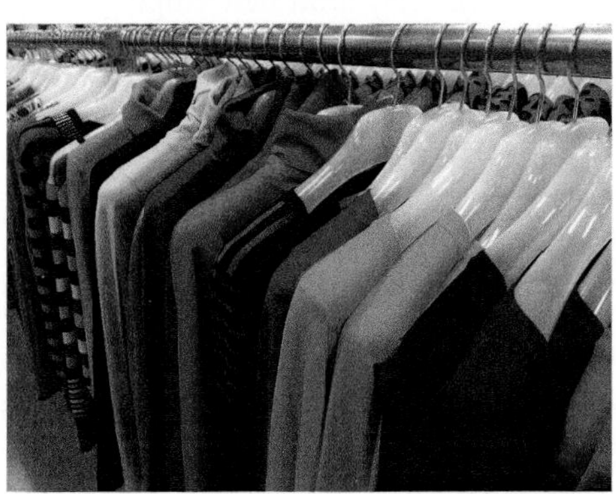

Professionalism refers to conducting oneself with responsibility, integrity, accountability, and excellence in the workplace. It also means communicating effectively and appropriately and maintaining a high level of productivity.

Professionalism begins with your appearance. A professional wardrobe is clean and free of wrinkles and defects, such as holes or stains, and fits well. The latest fashion trends are not always appropriate for work. Good personal hygiene practices such as styled hair, absence of body odors, and clean nails also exhibit professionalism. Lastly, most medical facilities have policies against excessive perfumes and colognes, so it is considerate to avoid wearing them while on the job.

As a professional, you will also be expected to demonstrate a strong work ethic. This includes being reliable and trustworthy, staying productive, maintaining a positive attitude, and showing a willingness to learn. Medical facilities rely on coders to complete all of their daily work on schedule. To meet this expectation, coders must attend work as scheduled and arrive on time. Even remote coders are required to work a specific number of hours per day, although they may have flexibility in choosing their hours. Unproductive coders create a backlog of uncoded records, which in turn delays billing and reimbursement for services and procedures and can jeopardize the financial stability of the medical facility. Show your employer that you are a professional by arriving on time and ready to work, with an open mind and a positive attitude.

Social Media in the Workplace

Social media is a general term that refers to websites and other online applications that allow large groups of people to share information for the purpose of developing social and personal contacts. Many social media websites and applications allow users to share information and images.

A survey conducted in 2014 by job search website CareerBuilder showed that 51% of employers who research an applicant's activity on social media decide not to offer employment after viewing posted content. In addition to the possible loss of job opportunities, inappropriate content may violate healthcare laws, offend coworkers and patients, or violate employment agreements. To decrease the probability that your social media activity negatively impacts your career, consider the following:

- Separate your personal social media accounts from your professional accounts.
- Avoid "friending" or "following" patients, clients, or coworkers.
- Remember that your deleted posts may still be accessible.
- Content shared on private personal social media pages can be exposed to members outside of the private page.
- Commenting about and/or posting images of a patient is unethical and violates HIPAA.
- Provocative comments and images may limit new employment offers or decrease opportunities for advancement with your current employer.

Communication Skills

Having strong **communication skills** means that you have the ability to convey information in a way that your audience can easily understand. Successful coders display a strong combination of listening, writing, and speaking skills.

Listening skills cannot be overemphasized. Coders interact daily with physicians and administrative staff, so they must learn to focus quickly and listen without formulating opinions, assumptions, or responses until the person has finished speaking. Being a good listener makes it easier for others to trust and rely on you, which in turn makes you someone whom others want to work with.

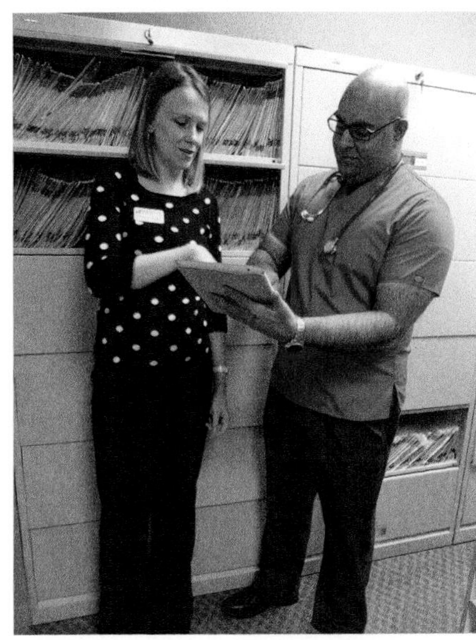

Coders must have good verbal communication and listening skills to be successful.

Good written communication skills are essential for coding professionals. Completing forms, writing reports, and sending emails are a major part of a coder's job. Attention to spelling, grammar, punctuation, and tone are expected in professional writing.

When communicating verbally in the healthcare setting, it is important to speak slowly and clearly because medical terminology is a complex language with many terms that sound similar when spoken aloud. In addition, verbal communication barriers may exist when speaking with colleagues or patients from different cultural backgrounds. It is important for coders to learn to articulate their thoughts and instructions in a courteous, conscientious manner.

Practice Professionalism

The ability to use the appropriate medical terms when discussing diagnoses and procedures with supervisors and coworkers saves time and displays professionalism. Penny is a CPC who works in a small physician practice. She meets with the physician and HIM manager once a month to discuss coding and documentation issues. Penny recalls that during the last meeting, she had difficulty pronouncing medical terms and was not familiar with some of the medical terms used by the physician. How can Penny be better prepared for the next meeting?

a. She should not worry about pronunciation of medical terms because everyone gets them wrong.
b. She should review her meeting topics so that she may refresh her medical vocabulary and practice pronouncing difficult terms prior to the meeting.
c. She should cancel the meeting and send a written report; everyone would be relieved to be spared a boring meeting.

Technical Skills

Technical skills are the knowledge and ability to work efficiently with technology, and working as a coder requires quite a bit of this. As mentioned throughout this chapter, coders must understand how to use EHRs and PMSs. In most medical settings, coders will also be required to use and understand word processing and data management software such as Microsoft Word and Excel. Coders also use email to send and receive messages daily. As the industry evolves, coders will be required to quickly learn and embrace new technologies that improve patient care, streamline workflow, share patient information, and increase reimbursement for medical services. These skills are especially important for remote coders, who depend on technology to communicate and complete daily tasks.

Critical Thinking Skills

Critical thinking skills include the ability to formulate ideas, solve problems, analyze situations, and think creatively. Medical facilities rely on coders to identify issues with daily operations that may affect the financial stability of the medical facility. For example, a medical coder might use his or her critical thinking skills to identify a pattern of claim rejections (instances in which an insurance company refused to reimburse the facility) related to the submission of a specific code. Identifying this pattern involves analyzing the data, researching policies and regulations related to the procedure code, and making a recommendation to management to correct the way the code is used. Coders can improve their critical thinking skills by accepting challenging work assignments, participating in activities that require creativity, and reading articles and books that offer new information and different perspectives. Professional organizations often offer journals or resources that can help coders stay on top of changes in the field.

Practice Professionalism

Destin is a CPC who works from home. Today he is having difficulty identifying a code to match the procedure documented in a patient's record. Although he has reviewed all of the relevant coding guidelines and references to better understand the procedure, he is still unable to find the information he needs. What should Destin do?

a. Destin should take the rest of the afternoon off. Once he has had a chance to clear his head, finding the solution to his problem will be much easier. He does not have any plans tomorrow, so he should be able to finish the rest of today's work then.
b. Destin should contact another coder from his company for assistance. Before he calls his colleague, he should make sure he has all the necessary reference materials readily available. When he talks to his colleague, he should clearly explain the problem, listen carefully to his colleague's response, answer any follow-up questions, and then express appreciation to his colleague for taking the time to help.
c. Destin should assign the code that he thinks is correct and move on. He has several records to code and cannot hold up an entire batch for 1 code.

Career Opportunities in Coding

Career opportunities for coding professionals are quite varied. When you are searching for employment, it is a good idea to review the qualifications and requirements for the position rather than dismissing a position based solely on the job title. For example, if you are looking specifically for a health record auditing position, you may find that a job posting for a physician documentation specialist requires many of the same professional skills and experiences. Searching for employment using only job titles could cause you to miss the perfect job opportunity. The following sections describe different coding-related positions.

Coding Manager

Coding managers are responsible for the daily operations of the coding department, which may include assigning coders their daily workloads, monitoring remote coders' productivity levels, distributing coding updates to the coding team, and working with managers of other departments to meet organizational goals. Coding managers may also be required to provide training to keep coders knowledgeable of coding and reporting guidelines. Coding managers need to have knowledge of human resources, medical billing and coding, and regulations that govern the healthcare industry. The minimum educational requirement for this position is typically an associate's degree in HIM in addition to a coding certification. RHIT or RHIA credentials may also be acceptable, depending on the policies of the individual medical facility.

Medical Coding Specialist

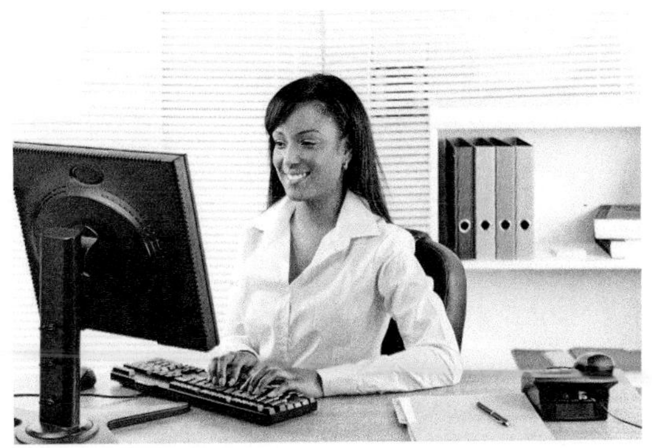

Coders translate medical information into medical codes. Strong computer skills are essential for this position.

Medical coding specialists (also known more commonly as *coders*) translate medical information into medical codes. They work closely with physicians, managers, and billing specialists to ensure that the codes selected are supported by health record documentation. A thorough understanding of ICD-10, CPT®, and HCPCS codes is a requirement for this position, as are strong computer and communication skills. An inquisitive nature is another useful quality, as much of a coding specialist's time will be spent searching for and assigning codes. In addition, a medical coding specialist must remain up to date on coding guidelines, government regulations, and compliance requirements. Coding certifications from AHIMA or AAPC are typically required for this position, which may be an entry-level position or a lifelong career.

Medical Coding Auditor

Coding Clicks

Want to explore more coding careers? Visit the Career and Student Center page of the AHIMA website at http://Coding.ParadigmEducation.com/AHIMACareers to find links to education and career planning resources.

Medical coding auditors review health records and patient claims to ensure that the documentation of medical services and procedures supports the claims submitted for reimbursement. They may also perform quality assurance (QA) audits. QA audits are performed on coded records to measure the accuracy of the medical coder. Coders must maintain a high coding accuracy rate, the exact level of which is set by the coding department at the facility. Coders who do not meet the coding accuracy requirement typically receive additional coding training and increased QA audits until they are able to consistently meet the company coding standards. This position requires knowledge of Medicare documentation guidelines, coding, and reporting guidelines for medical code sets, as well as state and federal regulations regarding the scope of practice for practitioners and allied health professionals. Good verbal and written communication skills are essential for this position, since auditors often need to educate the medical provider or coding team on audit findings. The minimum education required for this position is typically an associate's degree in HIM in addition to a coding certification. RHIT or RHIA credentials may be acceptable, depending on the policies of the individual medical facility.

Healthcare Providers

A **healthcare provider** is an individual who has completed the required education and is licensed to practice medicine, provide medical care, and/or perform procedures in a medical facility. This group includes medical doctors (MDs), doctors of osteopathy (DOs), physician assistants, certified nurse midwives, dentists, chiropractors, nurse practitioners, and psychologists, among others. Medical coders interact with healthcare providers on a daily basis.

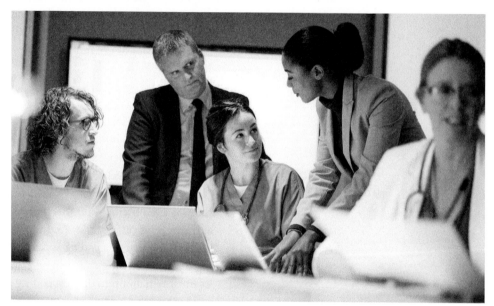

Medical coders often interact with a variety of healthcare professionals each day.

Healthcare Practitioners

A **healthcare practitioner** is another name for a person who practices medicine. The level of education required to become a healthcare practitioner depends on the licensing requirements for each position. For example, MDs and DOs must complete 4 years of undergraduate training, typically referred to as "premed" studies; 4 years of medical school; an internship; and a residency program. The **internship** allows medical students to practice medicine in a medical setting under the supervision of a teaching physician. Upon completion of an internship and after graduation, residency begins. **Residency**, which typically takes place in a hospital setting, allows graduates to apply their new knowledge and skills to a medical specialty of their choosing. During the internship and residency, there are rules that restrict the services that students can bill, so coders who work in university hospitals or for preceptors (teaching physicians) must have an understanding of these stages of practitioner education and any restrictions that come with them. After completion of residency, a medical doctor may choose to become board certified in a specific specialty. To maintain board certification and state licensure, the MD must participate in continuing education.

Nonphysician Practitioners

A **nonphysician practitioner (NPP)**, also referred to as a **midlevel**, is a medical provider who has completed undergraduate studies in a specific scope of patient care. Physician assistants (PAs) and nurse practitioners (NPs) are the most common types of NPPs. Becoming an NPP requires fewer years of education than becoming an MD. For example, registered nurses (RNs) usually take 1 of 3 education paths: a bachelor's degree in nursing, an associate's degree in nursing, or a diploma from an approved nursing program. To advance from an RN to an NP, an RN must complete additional academic training and acquire a specific amount of clinical experience. An NP has typically achieved the educational equivalent of a master's degree in nursing. NPs must be licensed to provide patient care. PAs must complete an accredited educational program that is the equivalent of a master's degree. All states require PAs to be licensed. Coding and reporting guidelines related to NPPs affect reimbursement, as there are certain services for which these healthcare professionals cannot bill, and coders must be aware of these guidelines. The reason for this restriction is predominantly based on the NPP's scope of knowledge, since they have not completed as much education as MDs.

Coding Clicks

Coding specialties are based on medical specialties. If you think you would like to tailor your career to a specific specialty (or are interested in learning more about the various specialties), you may want to review the specialties and subspecialties pages of the American Board of Medical Specialties' website at http://Coding.ParadigmEducation.com/ABMS.

Allied Health Professionals

Allied health professionals provide ancillary and support services to assist in the care of patients. They work as phlebotomists, physical therapists, respiratory therapists, occupational therapists, audiologists, radiographers, speech pathologists, optometrists, emergency medical technicians, medical laboratory scientists, and in a variety of other positions. Educational requirements for allied health professionals range from certification programs to doctoral degrees. State licensing requirements also vary. In addition, some allied health professionals, such as audiologists and optometrists, may request reimbursement for their services from insurance payers or work for physicians who pay them directly. Payment of allied health professionals is dependent on the insurance payer's billing guidelines. Allied health professionals that may bill insurance payers for their services must first meet state and insurance payer requirements.

CONCEPTS CHECKPOINT **1.5**

Provide a short answer to the following questions.

1. Coding managers are responsible for ______________.
2. Medical coding specialists must have a thorough understanding of ______________.

Coding Ethics

Just as **ethics** are a generally accepted standard of moral conduct, **coding ethics** are standards that medical coders are expected to follow as they perform their daily tasks. Because coders work with legally protected, confidential patient information, they must adhere to the highest ethical standards both at work and outside of work. AHIMA and AAPC have both drafted coding ethics guidelines that certified coders are required to follow. Certified coders and HIM professionals who violate their credentialing association's code of ethics may have their credentials revoked. Coders who violate state and federal regulations may face financial and/or criminal penalties.

In addition to maintaining certain ethical standards, coders must also remain in compliance with office policies and procedures and insurance payer documentation and reporting guidelines. The Office of the Inspector General of the US Department of Health and Human Services recommends that medical facilities adopt a **compliance plan**, which is an internal process that allows the medical facility to identify incidents that may result in the violation of federal or state regulations. The compliance plan also details how the facility will deal with violations. Coders should review and become familiar with the area of the compliance plan related to documentation and coding, which will explain what coders should do if they suspect fraud or abuse.

Fraud is intentionally submitting false information to benefit yourself or others. One example of fraud is **upcoding**, which happens when the provider bills for a higher level of services than what is supported by the documentation in the health record. If a physician documents fictional services for a patient he or she did not in fact see or treat and the coder codes the services so that the patient may be billed, the physician and the coder have both committed fraud. **Abuse** refers to incidents or practices (usually considered fraudulent) that are inconsistent with accepted sound medical business or fiscal practices. An example of abuse is suggesting to patients that additional services are needed when the services are not medically necessary. More information about governmental regulations, criminal penalties, and strategies to avoid participating in fraud and abuse is presented in Chapter 22.

Think Like a Coder

Penelope is a coding manager for a large coding company. During a meeting with the compliance department, she is notified that 2 of her coders have been upcoding. The compliance department says that they will work to reconcile any overpayment. What steps should Penelope take to resolve this issue? When Penelope returns to her office, she reviews the coding and documentation section of her company's compliance plan. The plan requires that she investigate to determine if the error is intentional or accidental.

When she conducts her investigation, Penelope determines that the coding errors were due to a lack of knowledge regarding a specific type of service. She follows the steps laid out in the compliance plan, discusses the errors with the coders, and schedules immediate coding training for those individuals. If the errors had been found to be intentional, Penelope would have followed the recommended reprimands outlined in the compliance plan.

CONCEPTS CHECKPOINT **1.6**

Fill in the blanks in each of the following statements.

1. Coding ethics are ______________ that medical coders are expected to follow as they perform their daily tasks.
2. ______________ is an internal process that allows the medical facility to identify incidents that may result in violation of federal or state regulations.
3. Fraud is ______________ submitting false information to benefit yourself or others.

Chapter Summary

- Medical coding is the process of assigning standardized alphanumeric identifiers to the diagnoses and procedures documented in a medical patient record.
- A diagnosis is a statement or conclusion that describes a patient's illness, disease, or health problem. A medical procedure is an activity performed on an individual to improve health, treat disease or injury, or identify a diagnosis.
- Health records are physical or electronic files in which doctors, nurses, and other healthcare professionals detail the diagnoses and procedures they provide to each patient. Health records also contain pertinent administrative and financial data about each patient.
- The health record is legal documentation of a patient's confidential health information, such as health history, diagnostic reports, and treatments provided.
- An electronic health record (EHR) can hold numerous years of health records, in addition to storing digital images of x-rays and other diagnostic images.
- A nomenclature is a system of naming things (diseases, body parts, procedures, etc.) so they can be organized.
- Classification systems organize like things into categories. The items are given codes that, when deciphered, describe the item in detail.
- A healthcare provider is an individual who is licensed to practice medicine and who provides medical care and/or performs procedures in a medical facility.
- The administrative, financial, and technological aspects of medicine are all part of health information managment (HIM). Coders, billers, managers, and health record technicians are considered HIM professionals.

- Medical facilities set the education requirements for the coders whom they employ. Requirements span from completion of a coding training program and a coding certification to degrees or certifications in HIM.
- Coders must have knowledge related to healthcare processes and regulations. Coders must also possess personal strengths of professionalism, communication skills, critical-thinking skills, and technical skills.
- Career opportunities for coding professionals are quite varied, such as coding managers, medical coding specialists, and medical coding auditors.
- Coding ethics are standards that medical coders are expected to follow as they perform their daily tasks. Coders must also remain in compliance with office policies and procedures and insurance payer documentation and reporting guidelines.

Navigator

Access interactive chapter review exercises, practice activities, flash cards, and study games.

Chapter 2

Getting to Know CPT®

Fast Facts

- Every year, the American Medical Association (AMA) updates and makes changes to the Current Procedural Terminology (CPT®) codes.
- In 2018, the AMA added 172 new CPT® codes, revised 60 codes, and deleted 82 codes.
- Code 99213, which describes an office or outpatient visit for the evaluation and management of an established patient, is the most billed CPT® code.
- In 2015, more than 2.8 billion codes were reported to Medicare for reimbursement.

Source: http://ama-assn.org, http://cms.gov

Crack the Code

Review the sample operative report to find the correct procedure code. You may need to return to this exercise after reading the chapter content.

DATE OF PROCEDURE: 5/15/2019

PROCEDURE PERFORMED: Arthrocentesis of left shoulder

SURGEON: Curtis Chaney, MD

ANESTHESIA: Local lidocaine

DESCRIPTION OF PROCEDURE: After administering a local anesthetic, the physician inserts a 22-gauge needle through the skin and into the left glenohumeral joint. The needle is inserted anteriorly, slightly inferior, and lateral to the coracoid process, aiming posteriorly toward the glenoid fossa. A small quantity of synovial fluid is removed. The needle is withdrawn and pressure is applied to stop any bleeding. The synovial fluid specimen is sent to a pathologist for analysis. The patient tolerated the procedure well without complications.

answer: 20610

Learning Objectives

2.1 Discuss the history of Current Procedural Terminology (CPT®) and the Healthcare Common Procedure Coding System (HCPCS) codes.

2.2 Explain the evolution of CPT® codes and HCPCS Level II codes.

2.3 Define the difference between CPT® codes and HCPCS Level II codes.

2.4 Describe the 3 levels of HCPCS codes.

2.5 Examine the relationship between CPT® and HIPAA.

2.6 Identify and discuss the organization of the CPT® codebook.

2.7 Define the different components of CPT® Categories.

2.8 Describe the content and uses of CPT® appendixes.

2.9 Understand how to locate main terms in the alphabetic Index.

2.10 Identify codebook conventions that assist in locating and assigning CPT® codes.

2.11 Define CPT® and HCPCS modifiers.

2.12 Describe how to use the CPT® codebook to locate and select procedure codes.

2.13 Discuss tools and resources used by coders.

Chapter Outline

- **I.** Current Procedural Terminology and the Healthcare Common Procedure Coding System
  - **A.** History and Evolution of CPT®
  - **B.** History and Evolution of HCPCS
    - **i.** HCPCS Level I Codes
    - **ii.** HCPCS Level II Codes
    - **iii.** HCPCS Level III Codes
  - **C.** CPT® and HIPAA
- **II.** Organization of the CPT® Codebook
  - **A.** Components of the CPT® Codebook
  - **B.** The Introduction Section of the CPT® Codebook
  - **C.** CPT® Code Set Categories
    - **i.** Category I Codes
    - **ii.** Category II Codes
    - **iii.** Category III Codes
  - **D.** Appendixes
  - **E.** Index
  - **F.** CPT® Codebook Conventions
    - **i.** Symbols
    - **ii.** The Cross-Reference *See*
  - **G.** Modifiers
  - **H.** Place of Service Codes
  - **I.** Locating and Selecting Codes Using the CPT® Codebook
- **III.** Tools and Resources
  - **A.** AMA Resources
  - **B.** CMS Resources
    - **i.** CMS Internet-Only Manuals (IOMs)
  - **C.** Digital Resources
- **IV.** Chapter Summary

Current Procedural Terminology and the Healthcare Common Procedure Coding System

As described in Chapter 1, the **Healthcare Common Procedure Coding System (HCPCS)** comprises 2 levels: Level I, **Current Procedural Terminology (CPT®)**, Fourth Edition; and HCPCS Level II, also referred to as **National Codes**. Together the 2 levels constitute the standards used to report medical, surgical, and diagnostic procedures as well as products and drugs.

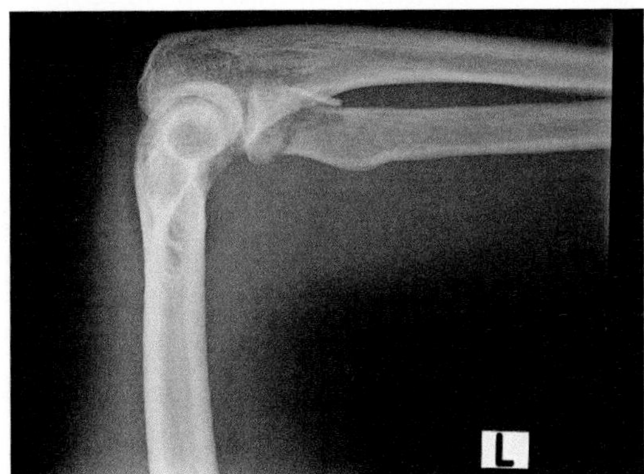

X-rays are 1 of the procedures located in the CPT® codebook.

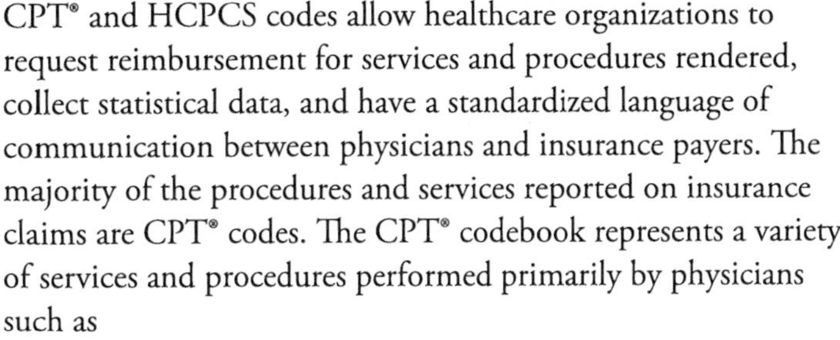

CPT® and HCPCS codes allow healthcare organizations to request reimbursement for services and procedures rendered, collect statistical data, and have a standardized language of communication between physicians and insurance payers. The majority of the procedures and services reported on insurance claims are CPT® codes. The CPT® codebook represents a variety of services and procedures performed primarily by physicians such as

- office visits;
- x-rays and other diagnostic imaging procedures;
- surgeries;
- laboratory tests; and
- hospital visits.

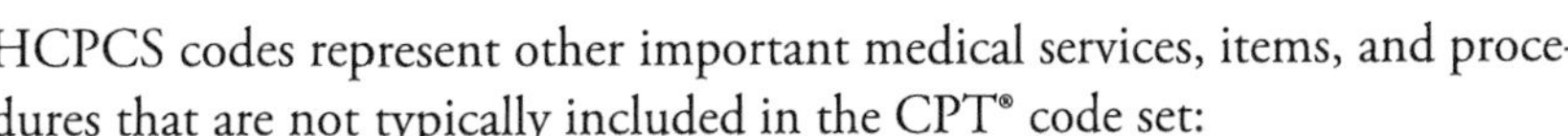

HCPCS codes represent other important medical services, items, and procedures that are not typically included in the CPT® code set:

- drugs;
- dental services;
- orthotics; and
- durable medical equipment.

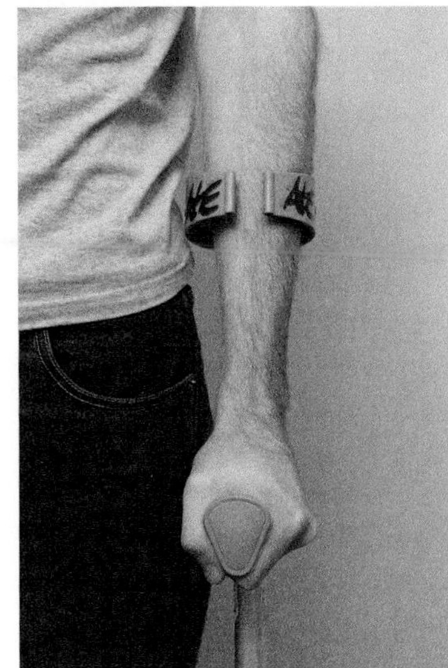

Codes for crutches and braces can be found in the HCPCS codebook.

CPT® and HCPCS codes may be reported independently of 1 another or together. Depending on the medical specialty you work with, you may never use HCPCS codes or you may use them frequently. For example, if you work for an orthopedic specialist, you may use CPT® codes to report surgeries and x-rays and HCPCS codes to report durable medical equipment, such as crutches and braces. If you work for a cardiovascular surgeon, you might report the CPT® codes for surgeries only and no HCPCS codes.

History and Evolution of CPT®

CPT® codes are developed, revised, and licensed for publication by the **American Medical Association (AMA)**, which holds the copyright for the CPT® codes. Since its inception in 1847, the AMA has worked to promote scientific advancements in medicine, improve public health, and enhance physician-patient relationships. It is now 1 of the most prominent medical associations in the United States. The AMA established the codes in 1966 to provide a uniform language to describe surgical, medical, and diagnostic services. Physicians and other healthcare providers finally had a reliable means of communicating with each other and insurance payers. The first publication used 4-digit codes that focused on surgical procedures and provided a limited range of codes for diagnostic tests. The publication of procedure codes with detailed standardized descriptions encouraged physicians to use the same descriptions when documenting procedures in health records. This standardized documentation allowed insurance payers to verify that the information in health records supported the codes submitted for reimbursement. The creation of CPT® also facilitated the collection of statistical information. Analysis of statistical data allowed the AMA to identify the need for additional codes and helped insurance payers create fee schedules that more accurately represented the services and procedures provided.

In 1970, the second edition of CPT® was published. It expanded the code sets to 5 characters and included more diagnostic and specialty code sections. Internal medicine codes were also introduced in the second edition. The third edition was published later in 1970, and in 1977, the fourth edition was released. With the fourth edition, the AMA enacted a system of periodic updates that kept pace with changes in procedures and the evolving medical community. CPT® is still in its fourth edition. Instead of revising the book's format, the AMA releases annual code updates that go into effect January 1 of each year. The AMA website updates the CPT® codes biannually.

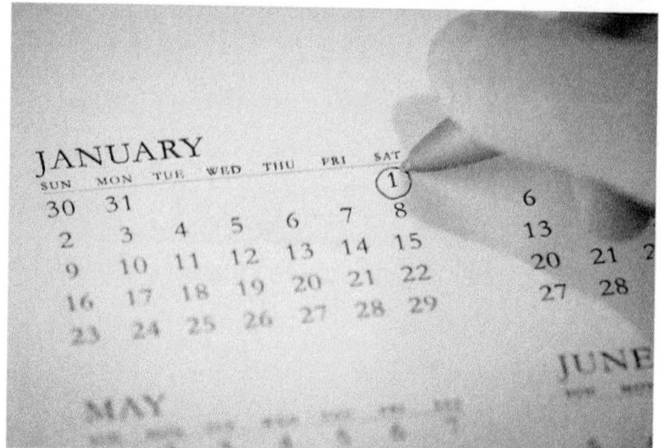

New CPT® codes go into effect January 1.

History and Evolution of HCPCS

HCPCS was established in 1978 by the Health Care Financing Administration (HCFA), now known as the **Centers for Medicare and Medicaid Services (CMS)**. At that time, HCPCS was called the HCFA Common Procedure Coding System. These codes were created to give Medicare and Medicaid providers a standardized code set that described services, procedures, drugs, and equipment not described by the CPT® codes. Initially, reporting HCPCS codes was voluntary, but during the 1980s, HCFA began to require the use of HCPCS codes when reporting services for Medicare and Medicaid patients. HCPCS Level II codes are distributed and maintained by CMS. CMS updates the code set quarterly. These updates are based on recommendations from healthcare providers, manufacturers of healthcare equipment, professional societies, and third-party payers.

In 1986, CMS adopted the CPT® coding system into the HCPCS coding family to allow for a more uniform coding system. The Omnibus Budget Reconciliation Act of 1987 then mandated the use of CPT® codes for reporting outpatient hospital surgical procedures to Medicare and Medicaid patients. Currently, in addition to the mandated use for governmental insurance, CPT® codes are used to report services and procedures to commercial payers (private insurance companies). The adoption of CPT® into the HCPCS system created different levels of procedure coding. To distinguish the different code sets in the HCPCS coding family, CMS divided them into 3 levels: HCPCS Levels I, II, and III.

HCPCS Level I Codes

HCPCS Level I codes are another name for CPT® codes. They are located in the CPT® codebook and not in the HCPCS codebook. HCPCS Level I/CPT® codes are used for reporting medical services and procedures performed by outpatient providers, who may then bill for their professional services. CPT® codes are rarely referred to as HCPCS Level I codes. However, CMS may use the name HCPCS Level I in coding and documentation guidelines published on its website. Figure 2.1 illustrates a HCPCS Level I/CPT®code.

Figure 2.1 Example of a HCPCS Level I/CPT® Code

77067	Screening mammography, bilateral (2-view study of each breast), including computer-aided detection (CAD) when performed

HCPCS Level II Codes

HCPCS Level II codes are referred to as National Codes. Level II codes are 5-character alphanumeric codes beginning with a letter and followed by 4 numbers. Descriptions of services, drugs, or products accompany each code. HCPCS Level II codes are used only in outpatient settings, such as medical offices, diagnostic centers, and ancillary surgery centers, to report services, products, drugs, and procedures not categorized by CPT® codes. Also included are codes that report dental services. Dental codes are HCPCS Level II codes that are maintained by the American Dental Association. CMS updates the HCPCS Level II codes quarterly based on input from healthcare providers, manufacturers of healthcare equipment, professional societies, and third-party payers. Figure 2.2 illustrates a HCPCS Level II code.

Figure 2.2 Example of a HCPCS Level II Code

J0120	Injection, tetracycline, up to 250 mg

Medicare requires the use of HCPCS codes whenever possible, while commercial payers prioritize CPT® codes. Because of this, there are some HCPCS and CPT® codes that represent the same procedure or service. For example, when a CPT® code and a HCPCS Level II code describe the same service or procedure, you would report the HCPCS Level II code for Medicare and the CPT® code for the commercial payer.

Coding for CMS

A 4-year-old received a flu shot. There are CPT® codes and HCPCS Level II codes for the influenza virus vaccine and its administration. If the patient has commercial medical insurance, you report the services with the CPT® codes: 90471, *Immunization administration (includes percutaneous, intradermal, subcutaneous, or intramuscular injections); 1 vaccine (single or combination vaccine/toxoid)*; and 90658, *Influenza virus vaccine, trivalent, split virus, when administered to individuals 3 years of age and older, for intramuscular use*. If the patient has Medicare, you report the services using HCPCS codes: G0008, *Administration of influenza virus vaccine,* and the appropriate HCPCS influenza code from code range Q2035 through Q2039.

HCPCS Level III Codes

HCPCS Level III codes became inactive in 2000. Level III codes were a separate code set approved by CMS and used by local and state agencies to report services not categorized by CPT® or HCPCS Level II codes. However, when HCPCS Level III codes were active, a coder would have the added responsibility of deciding which HCPCS level code set to report, based on the medical insurance payer. In 2000, the Health Insurance Portability and Accountability Act of 1996 (HIPAA) updated the Transaction and Code Sets Standards, designating CPT® and HCPCS Level II as the recognized code sets for reporting outpatient services and procedures. CMS incorporated useful services and procedures categorized in HCPCS Level III into Level II codes. Coders who work in medical collections departments may see a HCPCS Level III code on a Medicaid insurance claim form that was submitted prior to the compliance date in 2002. Because the code descriptions were maintained by local agencies, the coder may have to do extensive research to identify the service or procedure provided. Figure 2.3 illustrates a HCPCS Level III code.

Figure 2.3 Example of a HCPCS Level III Code

X5427 Extended Speech Therapy

CPT® and HIPAA

The **Health Insurance Portability and Accountability Act of 1996 (HIPAA)** is federal legislation enacted to provide continuing health coverage, reduce healthcare costs, and guarantee the security and privacy of health information. The Administrative Simplification provisions of the HIPAA final Privacy Rule published August 17, 2000, require the use of standardized code sets in electronic transactions. CPT® and HCPCS were designated as the standard code sets for reporting the following:

- physician services;
- physical and occupational therapy services;

- radiological procedures;
- clinical laboratory tests;
- other medical diagnostic procedures;
- hearing and vision services;
- transportation services, including by ambulance.

The final rule also named the *International Classification of Diseases, 9th Revision, Clinical Modification (ICD-9-CM), Volumes 1 and 2,* as the standard code set for reporting diagnosis codes; and the *International Classification of Diseases, 9th Revision, Procedure Coding System (ICD-9-PCS), Volume 3,* as the standard code set for reporting inpatient hospital procedures. As of October 1, 2015, CMS requires reporting ICD-10-CM codes for diagnoses and ICD-10-PCS codes for inpatient hospital procedures. More information regarding the ICD code sets is located in Chapter 1.

CONCEPTS CHECKPOINT **2.1**

Use information from the previous section to fill in the blanks.

1. When do new CPT® codes go into effect?

 ____

2. What association is responsible for developing, maintaining, and revising CPT® codes?

 ____

3. HCPCS stands for ______________.
4. HCPCS Level II codes are also known as ______________.
5. HCPCS Level I codes are better known as ______________.

Organization of the CPT® Codebook

To accurately assign CPT® codes, coders must have a working knowledge of the organization of the CPT® codebook, its parenthetic notes and symbols used to locate the most specific code, and coding and reporting guidelines.

Although the healthcare industry is increasingly providing medical documentation through the use of electronic health records (EHRs) that provide automatically generated lists of medical codes, knowledge of coding and reporting guidelines and the ability to locate and verify codes using the CPT® codebook remain essential to the financial stability of a medical practice. Because CPT® codes are used to request reimbursement for services and procedures, reporting incorrect codes may lead to delayed reimbursement, refund requests, or risk of adverse legal action. EHRs typically provide a drop-down menu that lists service and procedure codes. Drop-down menus do not have the space to include coding guidelines and do not provide the additional details needed to select the most accurate code. A thorough understanding of how to locate codes in the CPT® codebook to verify codes provided by EHR systems will increase coding accuracy. EHR systems in relation to coding will be explored in Chapter 5.

The following are some general tips for assigning medical codes using the CPT® codebook:

1. **Read thoroughly**. Whether you are reviewing the documentation in the medical record or the descriptions and notes in the codebook, there are many medical terms that have similar spellings and procedures that have various components. If you do not read thoroughly and double-check your work, you can easily assign the wrong code or miss an additional procedure that should also be coded.
2. **Know where to find the relevant guidelines in the CPT® codebook**. Guidelines provide instructions on how to code, document, and bill, among other topics. Although it is important to become familiar with the basic guidelines, you should never rely on your memory when assigning codes. Make it your mission as a coder to know how to quickly locate the appropriate coding guidelines to help you accurately assign a code.
3. **Know the scope of practice for your billing provider**. CPT® guidelines will define the type of medical provider that can perform specific services or procedures. If the procedure states "physician," do not report this code for the nurse practitioner. If the guidelines state "qualified health care professional," you may report this code for a non physician practitioner, such as a physician assistant. There will be several reminders of this and other guidelines throughout the chapters of this textbook.
4. **Make notes directly in your textbook and codebooks**. Highlight codes that are hard to locate or draw pictures to help you remember certain procedures. Write down any and all extra information that will help you accurately select and assign codes.

Highlighting codes in your textbook and codebook can help you remember certain procedures.

5. **Remember that if it is not written, it was not done**. Documentation is written, not spoken. Only assign codes for what is written in the health record—you cannot assign a code based on what the provider "always does" or if you "know what they mean."
6. **Watch for the criterion of medical necessity**. CMS states that "medical necessity of a service is the overarching criterion for payment in addition to the individual requirements of a CPT® code." Medical necessity is defined as the need for an item(s) or service(s) to be reasonable and necessary for the diagnosis or treatment of disease, injury, or defect. Medical necessity is something you will need to consider throughout your coding career. As you learn to code, keep this question in the back of your mind: Was the service or procedure medically necessary? For example, it is not medically necessary to do a foot x-ray for a patient who has been diagnosed with arm pain. If the answer to this question is ever no, the coder has a duty to discuss it with the provider or manager prior to submitting the claim.

Think Like a Coder

Samantha is a certified professional coder (CPC) who works for a family practitioner. While coding the health records for the previous day, Samantha discovers that several patients with urinalysis orders did not have their results documented. She thought that this was unusual, because the nurses typically entered results into the EHR system in a timely fashion. Without the results, Samantha cannot confirm that the tests were done. She discusses the situation with the laboratory nurse who indicates that he was training a new hire and did not have time to enter the results in the EHR system. He promises Samantha that the reports will be entered into the health records before the end of the workday. What should Samantha do?

a. Report the urinalysis codes on the nurse's assurances that the results would be posted in the health records by the end of the day.
b. Report the urinalysis codes for the patient she knows always get a urinalysis and place the others on hold.
c. Report urinalysis codes only for the records that have documented results and place all others on hold until the reports are in the records.
d. Place all records on hold and work on something else until the lab gets it together.

Components of the CPT® Codebook

Although the AMA owns, develops, and maintains CPT® codes, many different companies license the code set to publish CPT® codebooks. Some versions include glossaries, illustrations, and documentation guidelines, while others are more basic. You should select the version with which you are most comfortable. For the purpose of this textbook, we will review the elements that appear in the majority of CPT® codebooks, but you should note that the sections may appear in a different order than the 1 described here. This textbook follows the sequence of the AMA CPT® codebook.

The CPT® codebook categorizes procedures and services into lists that allow you to locate codes alphabetically or numerically: Within the main sections or tabular portion, codes are arranged in numeric sequence. In the Index, the descriptions of the codes are arranged in alphabetic sequence.

The codebook is divided into 6 parts: Introduction, Category I codes, Category II codes, Category III codes, the appendixes, and the Index. A brief description of each part is provided in Table 2.1. The Category I, II, and III portions of the codebook list the codes by number. The category portions also contain reporting guidelines, coding symbols, charts, figures, tables, examples, and several other tools to help you locate and assign the most accurate code. The Index lists the codes in alphabetic order by procedure, anatomical site, condition, **eponym** (a name based on or derived from the name of a person), or other designation.

Table 2.1 Sections of the CPT® Codebook

Parts of the CPT® Codebook	Content
Introduction	Description of the organization of the CPT® codebook and instructions for its use, including conventions and terminology, guidelines for locating codes, a description of time-based coding, and a discussion of procedures involved in the development of a new code; a list of place of service codes precedes the Introduction
Category I codes	A listing of 5-digit numeric codes (organized in numeric order unless otherwise stated in the codebook) that represents procedures and services that have been approved by the Food and Drug Administration (FDA)
Category II codes	A listing of 5-digit alphanumeric supplemental tracking codes, all ending with the letter F, that are used to report quality measurements to identify whether a facility is compliant with HIPAA regulations
Category III codes	A listing of 5-digit alphanumeric temporary codes for emerging technologies, services, and procedures. Category III codes end in the letter T.
Appendixes	Expanded definitions of modifiers, clinical examples, and other content associated with code selection and reporting. See Table 2.4 on page 51 for a full description of the appendixes.
Index	A comprehensive listing of code descriptions in alphabetic order according to procedure, anatomical site, condition, eponym, synonym, or abbreviation

The Introduction Section of the CPT® Codebook

The **Introduction** is located at the beginning of the CPT® codebook. Typically, the introduction includes a brief history of CPT®, standards for using the CPT® codebook, a description of the content of the codebook, and information regarding code format. The information provided in the Introduction is specific to a particular CPT® codebook publication, which can vary. Always read the Introduction before you start using the codebook to assign codes.

CPT® Code Set Categories

CPT® codes are divided into 3 categories: I, II, and III. Each category represents a specific type of code used to identify services and procedures. No code numbers are alike, and each code has its own unique meaning. As you learn more about the categories of CPT® codes, keep in mind that even if a medical provider has a particular specialty, he or she may perform services or procedures whose codes are located in any section of the CPT® codebook, as long as they are within the scope of practice.

Category I Codes

RED FLAG

Some Category I codes are not listed in numeric sequence in the CPT® codebook. In the codebook, a number symbol (#) is placed in front of a code number to identify that the code is out of numeric order.

Category I codes are the first and largest set of codes in the CPT® codebook. They represent procedures or services that are performed by physicians and other qualified healthcare providers with some regularity and are approved by the FDA. The codes are used to report the services and procedures to insurance payers to request payment. These services or procedures may take place in a hospital, a physician office, or an outpatient facility, such as a diagnostic imaging center. Outpatient services provided in a hospital are also reported with CPT® codes.

Category I codes are 5-digit numeric codes. They appear in the CPT® codebook in numeric order, except for the Evaluation and Management (E/M) section, which appears first in the codebook but covers codes 99201 through 99499. Because E/M codes are used to report the providers' assessment and supervision of medical conditions, they are the most frequently reported CPT® codes. Therefore, they are typically the first set of Category I codes listed in a CPT® codebook.

While a CPT® codebook's table of contents typically contains headings for Category II and Category III codes, it may not contain a heading for Category I. Instead, the Category I codes are divided into 6 **sections**, which typically appear in the order shown in Table 2.2.

Table 2.2 Category I Sections and Their CPT® Codes

Category I Section	CPT® Code Range(s)
Evaluation and Management	99201-99499
Anesthesia	00100-01999, 99100-99140
Surgery	10021-69990
Radiology	70010-79999
Pathology and Laboratory	80047-89398, 0001U-0017U
Medicine	90281-99199, 99500-99607

Category I sections are further divided into a hierarchy that this textbook refers to as subsections, headings, and categories:

- **Subsections** are titled based on procedures or anatomical sites. For example, 2 subsections of the Radiology section are Diagnostic Radiology and Diagnostic Ultrasound, and the Evaluation and Management section includes the subsections Consultation and Home Services. Surgery has subsections for the different body systems such as the Integumentary System and the Musculoskeletal System.
- **Headings** are the next order of division and can refer to a patient population, an anatomical site, or a type of procedure or service.
- **Categories** group the CPT® codes by a further level of specific topic related to the codes, often by the type of procedure performed.

Figure 2.4 illustrates how the Sections are divided.

Category I codes are designed to fully describe components and variations of basic services and procedures, and the use of both parent and indented codes helps to achieve this goal. The **parent code** is the first code listed in a group of related codes, as shown in Figure 2.5. The parent code contains a full description of the base procedure or service that is applicable to the codes indented below it. A parent code is sometimes referred to as a *stand-alone code.* The **base procedure** is the most basic procedure or service in the group of codes. An **indented code** listed below the parent code refers back to the base procedure or service and supplies additions to or variations of the base procedure. Look for the semicolon (;) in the description of the parent code—any information that appears before the semicolon is the base procedure. The description in an indented code replaces the description after the semicolon in the parent code for a unique coded procedure or service.

For example, in Figure 2.5, the base procedure in the parent code 55700 is *Biopsy, prostate* because it precedes the semicolon; what follows the semicolon completes the code for 55700, *Biopsy, prostate; needle or punch, single or multiple, any approach*. Likewise, code 55705 by virtue of the indentation has an implied relationship to the base procedure *Biopsy, prostate*, and the complete code 55705 is *Biopsy, prostate; incisional, any approach*. Notice how the part of the parent code description that comes before the semicolon is included in both code descriptions, even though the common portion of the code is not printed in its entirety in the CPT® codebook.

Figure 2.4 Divisions of the CPT® Codebook

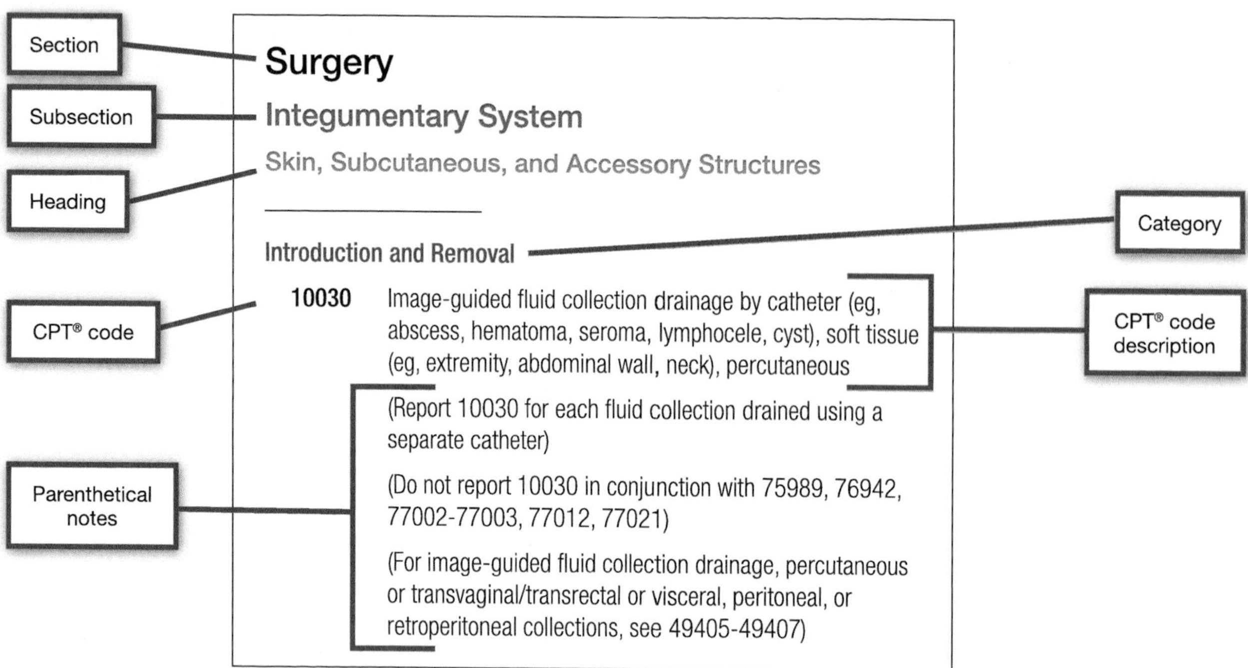

Figure 2.5 Example of Parent Codes and Indented Codes in the CPT® Codebook

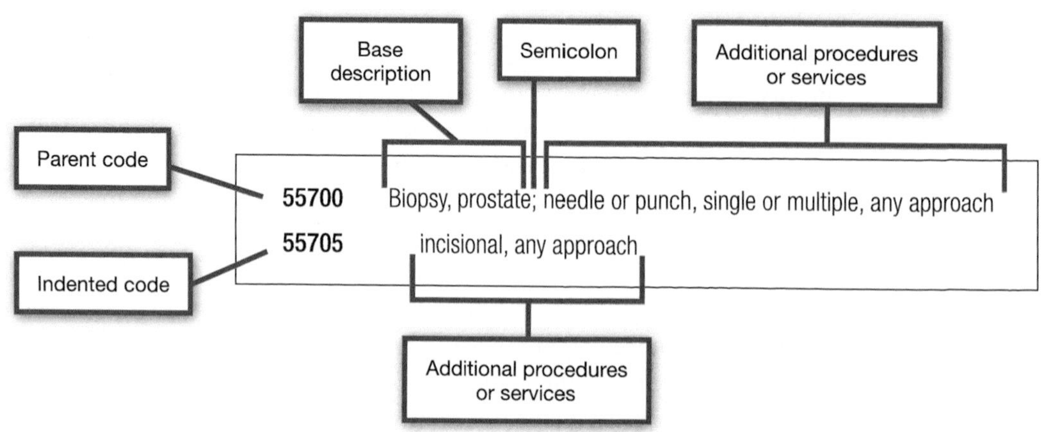

LET'S TRY ONE 2.1

Locate the following codes in the CPT® codebook and write down the procedure description.

1. 21215 ____________
2. 77078 ____________
3. 20612 ____________
4. 43236 ____________

CONCEPTS CHECKPOINT 2.2

Use information from the previous section to select the correct answers to the following questions.

1. What is the first listed code in a group of codes that fully describes the basic procedure or services but may not fully describe the procedure or service for which you are searching?
   a. the parent code
   b. an indented code
   c. the base procedure
   d. None of the answers are correct.
2. What is an eponym?
   a. a word opposite in meaning to a word in another language
   b. a name based on or derived from the name of a person
   c. a word or phrase that means exactly or nearly the same as another word or phrase in the same language
   d. All of the answers are correct.
3. Which category contains a listing of 5-digit numeric codes (organized in numeric order unless otherwise stated in the codebook) that represents procedures and services that have been approved by the FDA?
   a. Category I
   b. Category II
   c. Category III
   d. All of the answers are correct.
4. The _____ contains a comprehensive listing of procedures and services in alphabetic order according to procedure, anatomic site, condition, eponym, or other designation.
   a. Introduction
   b. appendixes
   c. Category I listing
   d. Index

Guidelines for Category I Codes Guidelines in the CPT® codebook are instructions from the AMA for how to accurately document and select services and procedures. Specific guidelines are located at the beginning of each Category I section. The guidelines include topics specific to each section and subsection. For example, the Anesthesia Guidelines include instructions on Time Reporting, Anesthesia Services, Supplied Materials, Separate or Multiple Procedures, Special Reports, Anesthesia Modifiers, and Qualifying Circumstances. These are instructions unique to Anesthesia codes—you will not find information on anesthesia modifiers or qualifying circumstances in the Guidelines for other sections.

Throughout the chapters in this book, we will discuss in detail the Guidelines related to each coding section. However, reading the explanations in this book is not a substitute for reviewing the Guidelines in the CPT® codebook. Always read the appropriate section Guidelines prior to coding for a specific specialty, and refer back to them as often as necessary.

In addition to the AMA Guidelines described above, this textbook may also refer to CMS guidelines, which provide further instructions for documentation of services and procedures. At times, AMA and CMS reporting guidelines do not match, and this textbook will point out when the 2 sets of guidelines are significantly different. Because CMS is the largest payer of medical services, it is important to learn the CMS guidelines that affect the medical facility where you work. CMS publishes a variety of coding and reporting guideline documents on its website. Prior to assigning a code for a Medicare beneficiary, you should always go the CMS website and search for guidelines for that specific service or procedure. Some CPT® codebooks reference CMS guidelines next to the affected codes; however, coders should get in the habit of consulting the CMS website quarterly for guideline updates.

</> Coding for CMS

CMS is the largest medical insurance payer in the United States. Most commercial payers base their reimbursement policies on CMS guidelines. All CMS policies and guidelines are published on the CMS.gov website. Medical providers may reference the CMS site for guidance on coding, billing, provider enrollment, and other information required to remain compliant with CMS policies. The Medicare.gov website contains enrollment, benefit, and other useful information for people eligible for Medicare and their family members and caregivers.

Unlisted Codes There may be circumstances when a physician performs a service or procedure that does not have a Category I code or a temporary code (found in Category III). Temporary codes are created to provide definitions for services or procedures that do not have a permanent Category I code. **Unlisted codes**, also referred to as *dummy codes*, are used to report the services or procedures that do not have a Category I or temporary code. Each CPT® section lists the associated unlisted code(s) for the common anatomical sites, procedures, or services. Note that these codes are to be used only when a code truly does not exist—not just when you cannot locate the appropriate code. If a CPT® code from a different section describes the procedure or service performed, then that code must be reported. Unlisted Category I codes are provided in the guidelines for each section and subsection. Unlisted codes are also listed in the alphabetic Index. Figure 2.6 illustrates unlisted codes in the CPT® codebook.

Figure 2.6 Examples of Unlisted Codes

19499	Unlisted procedure, breast
84999	Unlisted chemistry procedure
92499	Unlisted ophthalmological service or procedure

Because unlisted codes do not describe a specific service or procedure, third-party payers require a special report documenting the service or procedure performed to be submitted with the claim form. A **special report** is documentation that provides additional

Coding Clicks

Read more about how CPT® codes are developed, revised, and deleted at http://Coding.ParadigmEducation.com/Codes.

information about the service or procedure to the insurance payer, such as length of time spent, the extent and effort required, equipment used, and the medical necessity of the service or procedure. The special report may be in the form of operative reports, pathology reports, and/or progress notes that provide details of services rendered.

Data collected from the reporting of unlisted codes is used to identify the need for new CPT® codes.

The AMA constantly updates terms used in the CPT® codebook to reflect medical innovations. Healthcare professionals, medical associations, medical specialty societies, and other interested parties suggest changes and revisions to, as well as the inclusion of new terminology within, the CPT® codes. All proposed changes to a CPT® code are reviewed by the AMA CPT® Editorial Panel and the appropriate medical specialist society.

Think Like a Coder

Destin is a certified professional coder, and he has just started a new job at Regional Medical Center, coding for a family practice physician group. On his first day, he is given new coding books. The CPT® codebook is a different publication than the 1 he used with his previous employer and in school. What should Destin do to become familiar with the new codebook?

Time-Based Codes Although the majority of Category I codes describe a specific service or procedure, certain Category I codes may be applied based on the amount of face-to-face time the healthcare provider spends with the patient. This is called a **time-based code**. When a provider spends more than 50% of a visit counseling or coordinating care for the patient, the provider may select a time-based code from the E/M section. Certain other procedures and services, such as anesthesia, require the amount of time spent with the patient to be documented in the health record (and thus converted to a CPT® code). Time-based codes related to a particular procedure or service are located in the same section as that procedure or service. Selecting time-based codes requires a clear understanding of how time must be documented in the medical record and how the documentation of time is calculated.

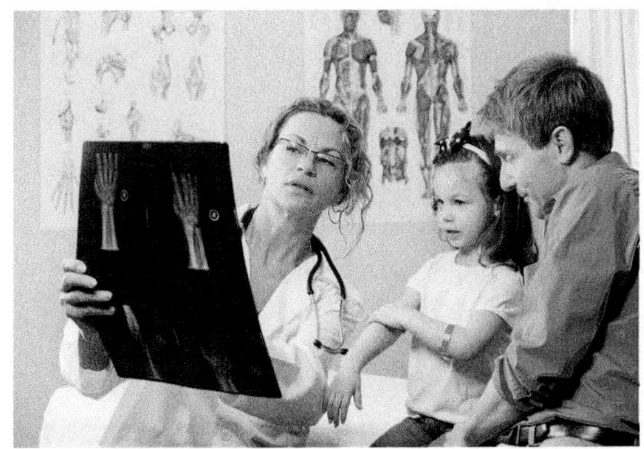

Only face-to-face time with a physician is included in time-based code calculations.

For example, a patient arrives at the physician's office at 8:00 a.m. and sits in the waiting room until he is brought back to the exam room at 8:30 a.m. The physician enters the exam room at 8:45 a.m. and spends 30 minutes in the exam room with the patient discussing the patient's lab results and answering the patient's questions. The physician discovers that a chest x-ray is not included in the record and is necessary to determine further treatment. The physician leaves the exam room at 9:15 a.m. He orders a chest x-ray on the patient. The patient is taken to have an x-ray at 9:30 a.m. After the x-ray, the patient returns to the exam room and waits 10 minutes alone for the physician to return to discuss the x-ray results. The physician returns to the room at 9:40 a.m. and spends 10 minutes reviewing the chest x-ray results and discussing treatment options with the patient. The patient leaves the clinic at 9:50 a.m.

The time the patient spends in the waiting room or alone in the exam room is not included in the time calculation. The time spent by the provider performing a procedure that can be reported with a separate CPT® code, such as the x-ray in the above example, is not included when calculating face-to-face time. Only the time the physician spent providing face-to-face services discussing the results of the lab test and treatment options is calculated for time-based coding. The calculation below identifies the physician's portion of the patient's visit that is factored into the time-based code.

30 minutes in the exam room with the patient providing counseling and coordination of care

\+ 10 minutes to review the chest x-ray results and discuss treatment options with the patient

40 minutes total time appropriate for selecting a time-based code

The guidelines for each section and subsection that contain time-based codes provide instructions regarding documentation requirements and how to accurately calculate time. For example, guidelines for time-based coding for office visits are different than those for critical care. This textbook will thoroughly review time-based coding associated with a specific code section.

CONCEPTS CHECKPOINT 2.3

Use information from the previous section to select the correct answers to the following questions.

1. Instructions from the AMA for how to accurately document and select services and procedures are called
   a. instructions.
   b. Guidelines.
   c. rationales.
   d. codes.
2. AMA Guidelines for specific Category I sections are located
   a. at the beginning of each specific Category I section and subsection.
   b. in the Index next to the code.
   c. at the end of each specific Category I section.
   d. at the beginning of each specific Category I section.
3. CMS guidelines are
   a. printed in all AMA CPT® codebooks.
   b. always the same as AMA coding and reporting guidelines.
   c. published on the CMS website.
   d. None of the answers are correct.
4. Which of the following is true regarding unlisted codes?
   a. Unlisted codes are used to report the services or procedures that do not have a Category I or temporary code.
   b. Unlisted codes are to be used only when a code truly does not exist for the documented procedure.
   c. Unlisted Category I codes are provided in the Guidelines for each section and subsection.
   d. All of the answers are correct.

LET'S TRY ONE 2.2

Select the correct unlisted code for the following procedures.

1. Unlisted preventive medicine service: _____
2. Unlisted procedure, casting or strapping: _____
3. Unlisted procedure, temporal bone, middle fossa approach: _____

LET'S TRY ONE **2.3**

Locate the guidelines for the Evaluation and Management (E/M) section to answer the following questions. Place an *X* by the areas that are not included in E/M Guidelines.

1. _____ Chief Complaint
2. _____ Classification of Evaluation and Management (E/M) Services
3. _____ Clinical Examples
4. _____ CPT® Surgical Package Definition
5. _____ Follow-Up Care for Therapeutic Surgical Procedures
6. _____ New and Established Patient
7. _____ Past History
8. _____ Separate Procedures
9. _____ Special Report
10. _____ System Review (Review of Systems)
11. _____ Time
12. _____ Unlisted Service

Category II Codes

Increasingly, the healthcare industry is looking for ways to measure the quality of care that patients receive. Category II codes are used for reporting performance measurements and tracking quality measures. The codes report details that took place during an office visit that are not described in a CPT® codebook. It is anticipated that the reporting of Category II codes will decrease some administrative burdens associated with reviewing, abstracting, and measuring quality of care. The reporting of Category II codes does not negate the reporting of Category I codes. Both codes may be reported together. However, Category II codes do not have any monetary value.

Coding Clicks

Providers may enroll in the PQRS incentive program by going to the PQRS section of the CMS website at http://Coding.ParadigmEducation.com/PQRS.

Reporting Category II codes is optional, unless the facility participates in the **Physician Quality Reporting System (PQRS)**, formerly known as the Physician Quality Reporting Initiative (PQRI). PQRS is a CMS program that provides incentive payments to physician practices with eligible providers who report Category II codes.

Category II codes are located immediately following the Category I codes. The subsection headings group the codes by performance-measure criteria: clinical components, diagnostic procedures and results, processes for patient safety, and services reflecting compliance with state or federal laws. Table 2.3 illustrates how CPT® Category II codes are arranged.

Category II codes are made up of 5 alphanumeric characters: the first 4 characters are numbers and the last character is always the letter *F*. Diseases or conditions related to the coded measure are referred to as *clinical topics*. Acronyms for a clinical topic are noted in parentheses following the code description. A superscripted number, attached to the parenthetical abbreviation, references the associated Category II Codes footnotes, which list the names and web addresses of the performance measure developers. Let's look at Category II code 0580F, *Multidisciplinary care plan developed or updated (ALS)*[8]. ALS is an abbreviation for *amyotrophic lateral sclerosis*. The superscripted number "8" references footnote 8 at the American Academy of Neurology website at http://Coding.ParadigmEducation.com/AAN.

Coding Clicks

To view the Category II clinical topics information, go to http://Coding.ParadigmEducation.com/ClinicalTopics.

Table 2.3 Category II Subsections and Code Ranges

Category II Subsections	Category II Code Range
Modifiers	1P-8P
Composite Codes	0001F -0015F
Patient Management	0500F-0584F
Patient History	1000F-1505F
Physical Examination	2000F-2060F
Diagnostic/Screening Processes or Results	3006F-3776F
Therapeutic, Preventive or Other Interventions	4000F-4563F
Follow-up or Other Outcomes	5005F-5250F
Patient Safety	6005F-6150F
Structural Measures	7010F-7025F
Nonmeasure Code Listing	9001F-9007F

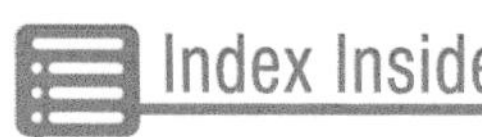

EXAMPLE **2.1**

If a patient is being treated for end stage renal disease (ESRD), the physician may need to create a care plan for hemodialysis, a process that filters waste from the body. Category II code 0505F, *Hemodialysis plan of care documented (ESRD, P-ESRD)*[1], indicates that the provider has set up a plan for the patient to have hemodialysis. The parenthetical abbreviation identifies the clinical topic as end stage renal disease and pediatric end stage renal disease. Superscripted number "1" references Category II footnote 1 at the website of the Physician Consortium for Performance Improvement (PCPI), http://physicianconsortium.org. Reporting the Category II code 0505F does not request payment for the hemodialysis plan of care that was part of the office visit. The office visit is reported by a Category I code that requests reimbursement, and the Category II code reports performance measurements.

Index Insider

The Index presents Category II codes under the main entry *Performance Measures*, organized by clinical topic.

LET'S TRY ONE **2.4**

Identify the following Category II codes in the subsections given.

1. Patient History—History obtained regarding new or changing moles (ML): _____
2. Therapeutic, Preventive, or Other Interventions—Anti-inflammatory/analgesic agent prescribed (OA): _____
3. Body Mass Index (BMI), documented (PV): _____

Category III Codes

Medical technologies are constantly changing with continuing experimentation. To address these medical advances, the AMA provides Category III codes, which are temporary codes used to report emerging technology, services, and procedures. Because they are still being developed, procedures and services covered by Category III codes are performed far less often than those covered by Category I codes. If you cannot locate a Category I code for a particular procedure or service, you should check the Category III codes before you decide to assign an unlisted code. If a Category III code exists for the procedure or service and you assign an unlisted code, the unlisted code would be considered inaccurate.

Category III codes are the third set of codes in the CPT® codebook, located immediately after the Category II codes. Category III codes are 5 alphanumeric characters in length: the first 4 characters are numbers, and the last character is always the letter *T*, as illustrated in Figure 2.7. These temporary codes are not divided into topical groupings as seen in other sections but rather are listed in numeric order.

Figure 2.7 Format of a Category III Code

0058T	Cryopreservation; reproductive tissue, ovarian Sunset January 2021

Reporting temporary codes allows CMS and the AMA to collect data regarding the usefulness and viability of these codes. If the data demonstrate widespread use and FDA approval, the AMA may convert a Category III code to a permanent Category I code by assigning the procedure or service a new, permanent 5-digit numeric code. The temporary code used to represent a procedure or service is archived for 5 years. After 5 years, if the procedure or services still do not warrant promotion to the Category I section of CPT®, it may be renewed by the governing committee for another 5 years, or it will automatically be removed from the CPT® codebook. The automatic removal is referred to as a *sunset date*. Not all temporary codes are converted to permanent codes; some may remain temporary for many years. There is no limit to the lifespan of a temporary code. Category III codes are also listed by service or procedure in the alphabetic Index. Category I codes contain parenthetical notes when a Category III code is available to assign.

Coding Clicks

For more information regarding CPT® code categories, go to http://Coding.ParadigmEducation.com/CodeCategories.

The AMA updates temporary codes biannually by adding, promoting, or archiving them as needed. Because these changes go into effect on January 1 of each year, it is important to always refer to the most recent edition of the codebook and review your office's coding and billing processes, EHR coding databases, and quick reference sheets when changes take place. New codebooks are available by October of the preceding year. Code updates, archives, and revisions are posted on the AMA website. Figure 2.8 illustrates a Category III code added in 2017.

Figure 2.8 Example of a Category III Code Added January 1, 2017

• 0487T	Biomechanical mapping, transvaginal, with report Sunset January 2023

CONCEPTS CHECKPOINT **2.4**

Use information from the previous sections to select the correct answers to the following questions.

1. Which of the following statements is *not* true of Category II codes?
   a. Category II codes are used for reporting performance measurements.
   b. Category II codes are the second set of codes in the CPT® codebook and are located immediately following the Category I codes.
   c. Reporting of Category II codes is optional, unless the facility participates in the Physician Quality Reporting System (PQRS).
   d. Category II codes have monetary value, the same as Category I codes.
2. PQRS stands for
   a. Physician Quality Reporting Services.
   b. Provider Quality Reporting System.
   c. Physician Quality Reporting System.
   d. Physician Quantitative Reporting System.
3. PQRS is a CMS program that provides incentive payments to physician practices with eligible providers who report Category II codes.
   a. True
   b. False

LET'S TRY ONE **2.5**

In your CPT® codebook, locate the beginning of the following sections, write down the first code listed, and briefly note the procedure or service described.

Example:

Pathology and Laboratory: 80047, Basic metabolic panel

Category I

1. Anesthesiology: ____________
2. Surgery: ____________
3. Radiology: ____________

Category II

4. Patient History: ____________
5. Diagnostic/Screening Processes or Results: ____________

Category III

6. What is the first listed code in Category III? ____________

RED FLAG

Remember that there are many different CPT® codebooks printed by different publishers. The codebook you use may include additional codebook conventions or have the alphabetic index in a different location than referenced in this textbook.

Appendixes

In most CPT® codebooks, the Category III codes are followed by the appendixes, which are sections of additional information to assist in the accurate reporting of CPT® codes (although the number and type of appendixes can vary by publisher). In the appendixes, you will find expanded definitions of modifiers, clinical examples, CPT® codes categorized by their special designations, and other content associated with code selection and reporting. Table 2.4 contains descriptions of Appendixes A through P, which appear in the CPT® codebook published by the AMA.

Table 2.4 Appendixes in the AMA CPT® Codebook

Appendix	Name	Description
A	Modifiers	CPT® and HCPCS modifiers and descriptions that may be added to 5-digit codes Modifiers are often used when assigning codes.
B	Summary of Additions, Deletions, and Revisions	A list of annual additions, deletions, and revisions Coders should review this section when they receive the updated codebook each year. Facilities may need to revise coding policies based on changes to codes that are reported often in their practices.
C	Clinical Examples	Clinical examples of services that correspond to various E/M codes
D	Summary of CPT® Add-on Codes	A list of add-on codes, which describe additional procedures or services that typically take place along with another procedure or service (reported with a primary code) Add-on codes are identified throughout the CPT® codebook with the + symbol.
E	Summary of CPT® Codes Exempt From Modifier 51	A list of CPT® codes that will not be used with modifier 51 Modifier 51 is reported when multiple surgeries are performed on the same day, during the same surgical session. Procedures that may not be reported with other procedures are exempt from being reported with modifier 51. Codes exempt from modifier 51 are identified throughout the CPT® codebook with the ⊘ symbol.
F	Summary of CPT® Codes Exempt From Modifier 63	A list of codes for procedures performed on infants less than 4 kg
G	Summary of CPT® Codes That Include Moderate (Conscious) Sedation	In 2017 the AMA discontinued the inclusion of moderate (conscious) sedation as a component of CPT® code sets and the bullseye symbol that identified these codes. Therefore, Appendix G no longer contains a list of any CPT® codes. When moderate sedation is administered by the same physician or qualified healthcare professional performing the therapeutic or diagnostic procedure, report the appropriate moderate sedation code(s) in addition to the CPT® code for the procedure. Chapter 20, Medicine Coding, contains additional information on how to accurately report the use of moderate sedation.
H	Alphabetical Clinical Topics Listing	The content of this appendix has been removed from the CPT® codebook and is now located on the AMA website.
I	Genetic Testing Code Modifiers	As a result of the creation of new molecular pathology codes in 2012, the AMA decided to remove this appendix in any future CPT® codebook publications. The AMA website provides additional background information regarding genetic testing and molecular pathology.
J	Electrodiagnostic Medicine Listing of Sensory, Motor, and Mixed Nerves	Nerves that apply to each sensory, motor, and mixed nerve conduction study listed under associated code range The family of nerves identified in this appendix is typically referenced when assigning codes for needle electromyogram (EMG). Each nerve represents 1 unit of study. Appendix J will be revisited in Chapter 20, where nerve studies are discussed in detail.
K	Product Pending FDA Approval	A summary of codes that are pending FDA approval and have been assigned a CPT® code In the main sections of the CPT® codebook, these codes are identified with the ⚡ symbol.
L	Vascular Families	A summary of the branches of vascular families when the starting point of intravascular catheterization is the aorta This appendix is frequently referred to when coding cardiovascular procedures.
M	Renumbered CPT® Codes—Citations Crosswalk	A list of deleted codes with descriptions and replacement codes
N	Summary of Resequenced CPT® Codes	A list of resequenced codes, which are codes that appear out of numeric sequence in the Category I, II, and III sections of the CPT® codebook In the codebook, a number symbol (#) is placed in front of a code number to identify that the code is out of numeric order.

O	Multianalyte Assays with Algorithmic Analyses	A limited set of administrative codes for multianalyte assays with algorithmic analyses (MAAA), which are procedures that utilize multiple results derived from assays of various types. MAAA tests are represented by a Category I CPT® code or an alphanumeric code that ends with "M," when a permanent Category I code has yet to be assigned.
P	CPT® Codes That May Be Used for Synchronous Telemedicine Services	Appendix P lists CPT® codes that may be reported with modifier 95, Synchronous Telemedicine Service rendered via a real-time interactive audio and video telecommunications system. Modifier 95 is reported with the appropriate CPT® code to certify that the Medicare beneficiary was in a Rural Health Clinic or a county outside of a Metropolitan Statistical Area during a telehealth service. Codes that meet the qualification of telehealth services are identified in the CPT® codebook by the star symbol. ★

Index

The **Index** is the last component of the CPT® codebook and is your starting point for locating a code for a service or procedure. It contains a comprehensive listing of codes in alphabetic order according to procedure, service, anatomical site, organ, condition, synonym, eponym, or abbreviation relevant to the code descriptor. It is formatted similarly to a dictionary, with guide words for the first and last entries on each page in the upper corners. You should always verify codes found in the Index by reviewing the full description of the code in the appropriate section of the CPT® codebook.

The Index does not contain detailed descriptions of procedures or services—only the main term and the modifying term(s) of the service or procedure. A **main term** is the primary component of a service or procedure. It may name the procedure or service, or an anatomical site, an organ, a related condition, an eponym, or an abbreviation. The main term typically appears in a larger font than the modifying terms and may also be printed in bold typeface. The following is an example of how main terms appear in the alphabetic Index.

RED FLAG

Do not confuse modifying terms with modifiers. Modifying terms appear in the CPT® Index under main terms. Modifiers are 2-character codes that are appended to a CPT® or HCPCS Level II code to add information or alter the code description.

Procedure: Electrocardiography

Service: Preventive Medicine

Organ or other anatomical site: Shoulder

Eponym: Clagett Procedure

Condition: Cleft Lip

Abbreviation: EEG

Modifying terms provide descriptions of codes associated with the main term. They are the indented terms listed below the main term. One main term may have up to 3 levels of indentations underneath it. The modifying term that is indented the farthest represents the most specific description available in the Index for that main term.

Figure 2.9 illustrates how modifying terms appear below a main term in the Index. If you were searching for the code for an excision of the epithelial layer of the cornea using a chelating agent, you may first locate the main term *Cornea* in the Index. Under *Cornea*, you would then locate the modifying term *Epithelium*, followed by the modifying term *Excision*, and, lastly, the modifying term *With Chelating Agent*. The codes for each indented modifying term are listed to the right of the term. When more than 1 code applies to the modifying term, a range of codes is provided. If 2 or more sequential codes apply, only the first and last codes in the sequence are listed, separated by a hyphen. Figure 2.9 illustrates how sequential codes appear in the Index. If several nonsequential codes apply, they are separated by commas. Figure 2.10 illustrates how nonsequential codes appear in the Index.

Figure 2.9 Example of Alphabetic Index Main Term and Modifying Terms

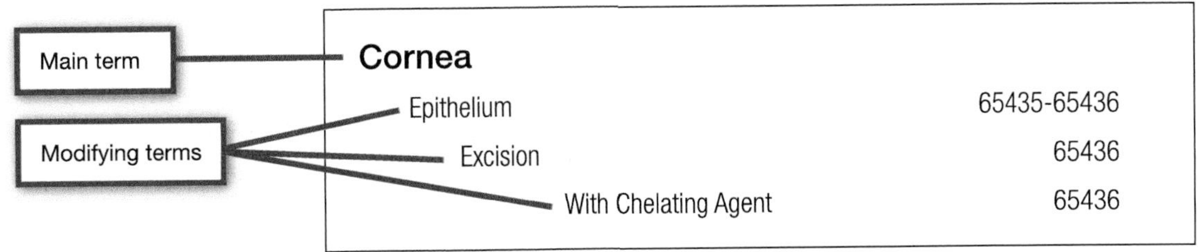

Figure 2.10 Example of Modifying Term That Lists Nonsequential Codes

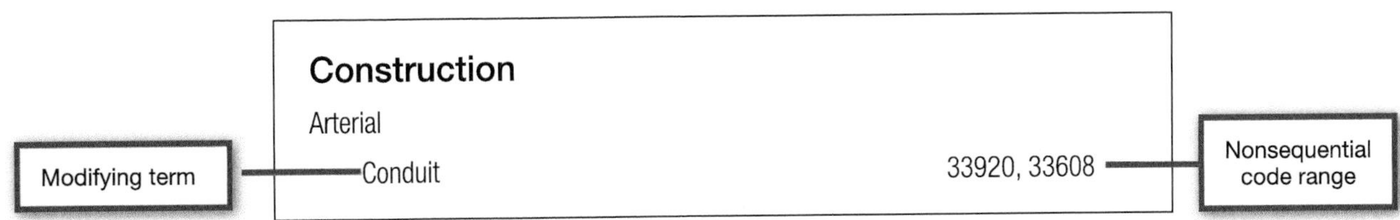

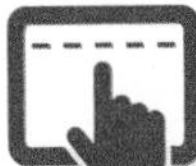

LET'S TRY ONE **2.6**

Using the Index, list the main term and modifying term for each procedure.

1. Aspiration of ganglion cyst:
   Main term: ______________
   Modifying term: ______________
2. Esophagogastroduodenoscopy, flexible, transoral; with biopsy:
   Main term: ______________
   Modifying term: ______________
3. Arteriovenous fistula abdomen repair:
   Main term: ______________
   Modifying term: ______________

CONCEPTS CHECKPOINT **2.5**

Use information from the previous sections to select the correct answers to the following questions.

1. Category III codes are
   a. temporary codes used to report emerging technology, services, and procedures.
   b. the third set of codes in the CPT® codebook, located immediately after the Category II codes.
   c. have 4 numbers and end with the letter "T."
   d. All of the answers are correct.
2. CPT® modifiers are
   a. located in Appendix A.
   b. located in the CPT® codebook Introduction.
   c. located in the guidelines of each section.
   d. located in Appendix A and in the CPT® codebook Introduction.
3. A summary of the branches of vascular families is located in
   a. Appendix A.
   b. Appendix G.
   c. Appendix L.
   d. Appendix O.
4. A list of CPT® codes that already includes moderate (conscious) sedation is located in
   a. Appendix A.
   b. Appendix G.
   c. Appendix L.
   d. Appendix O.

CPT® Codebook Conventions

Codebook conventions are words, symbols, punctuation, formatting, and abbreviations that are used to help locate and assign codes. CPT® uses a standard set of conventions in the codebook to help with code selection. These are typically defined in the introduction to the codebook. We will review the standard conventions set by the AMA, although you should be aware that some publishers may use additional conventions.

Symbols

Symbols are used to identify revised, new, and add-on codes, as well as code exemptions. They are placed in front of the CPT® code, and a quick reference of the symbol's meaning is typically included in the footer on that page of the codebook. Symbols appear only in the Category sections of the codebook, with the exception of the New or Revised Text symbol, ►◄, which also appears in the Guidelines to indicate coding guidelines that have been added or revised. Most codebooks also change the color of the added or revised text so that it is easily identifiable. Table 2.5 provides a comprehensive look at the symbols used within the AMA's CPT® codebook.

Table 2.5 Symbols Used in the CPT® Codebook

Symbol	Meaning	Description
★	CPT® codes that may be used for synchronous telemedicine services	Identifies codes that may be reported as telehealth services, when modifier 95, Synchronous telemedicine service rendered via a real-time interactive audio and video telecommunications system, is appended. Modifier 95 is reported with appropriate CPT® codes to certify that the beneficiary was physically located at a Rural Health Clinic or a county outside of a Metropolitan Statistical Area during the telehealth encounter. It also certifies that a physician has physically examined the vascular access site of dialysis patients with ESRD at least once per month. Appendix P of the CPT® codebook lists all telehealth services.
●	New code	New codes are added to the CPT® codebook annually and are preceded by a dot the first year they appear in the book.
►◄	New or revised text	The first year that new or revised text appears in the CPT® book, it is placed between 2 triangles. Some publishers also set the new or revised text in color so that the changes are more apparent. New or revised text may appear anywhere in the CPT® codebook.
▲	Description has been substantially altered from previous years	The first year after a code's description has been substantially altered from the previous years, an upward-pointing triangle is used to identify the affected code. This may happen, for example, when AMA updates out-of-date terminology.
#	Resequenced code	Resequenced codes appear out of numeric sequence in the CPT® codebook. This happens when a new code is needed in a section in which there are no unused numerals in sequence available. In these instances, an unused code from a different subsection is assigned for that service or procedure, and the new code is listed in the correct subsection with the # sign preceding it to indicate that it is out of numeric order. In the place where the new code would be listed if it had not been resequenced, a parenthetic note indicates that the code has been resequenced and explains where to find it.
+	Add-on code	Add-on codes describe procedures or services that typically take place with another procedure or service (represented by a primary code). Add-on code descriptions often include terminology such as "each additional" or "(List separately in addition to code for primary procedure)." Add-on codes typically appear below the codes to which they are assigned. Appendix D of the CPT® codebook lists all current add-on codes. Modifiers are added to CPT® codes to provide information regarding a change in the described procedure. Modifier 51 describes multiple procedures. Add-on codes and modifier 51 may not be reported together.

⊘	Code exempt from use with modifier 51	Modifier 51 is a CPT® modifier that is reported with surgical procedures when multiple surgeries are performed on the same day, during the same surgical session. Modifier 51 is reported with the additional procedures to reduce the payment for these services. When a code is exempt from the multiple procedure payment reduction, the ⊘ symbol is placed in front of the code. Add-on codes are exempt with modifier 51; however, the ⊘ code does not appear next to these codes. Appendix E contains a summary of CPT® codes exempt from modifier 51.
⚡	Pending FDA approval	When a CPT® code number is assigned to a procedure that is pending FDA approval, the ⚡ symbol precedes the code in the Category sections of the CPT® codebook. In rare instances, you may see the symbol with vaccines.
( )	Parenthetic note	Information inside parentheses is referred to as a *parenthetic note.* Parenthetic notes contain special information to help coders select and report the most accurate codes, such as deleted codes and restriction of code assignment. They are typically located below a code description or in the location where a code has been deleted. It is very important to read parenthetic notes prior to code selection.

The Cross-Reference *See*

The word *See* is used to indicate that you should cross-reference a different procedure or service to find what you are looking for. When you look for a code under the wrong main term, the word *See* is meant to guide you to the correct term. *See* may also appear after a modifying term to recommend that you look in a different location because that code may be more accurate.

LET'S TRY ONE **2.7**

Place the correct symbol next to the correct code.

⊘ ★ + # ▲

1. 17004 _____
2. 17250 _____
3. 22552 _____
4. 24071 _____
5. 31500 _____
6. 33369 _____
7. 99407 _____

Modifiers

Modifiers are 2-character codes that are sometimes added to CPT® codes or HCPCS Level II codes when the procedure, service, or item was altered from the code description. Modifiers supply payers with more information about services or procedures performed. CPT® modifiers comprise 2 numbers and are reported only with CPT® codes. Appendix A of the codebook contains full descriptions of CPT® modifiers.

HCPCS Level II modifiers comprise 2 alphanumeric or 2 alphabetic characters and are reported with both CPT® codes and HCPCS Level II codes. Full definitions of HCPCS modifiers are located in the HCPCS codebook. Some CPT® codebooks list the most commonly used HCPCS modifiers with brief descriptions. Chapter 4 is dedicated to CPT® and HCPCS Level II modifiers. Figure 2.11 illustrates a CPT® modifier, and Figure 2.12 shows a HCPCS modifier.

Figure 2.11 Example of a CPT® Modifier

81	Minimum Assistant Surgeon: Minimum surgical assistant services are identified by adding modifier 81 to the usual procedure number.

Figure 2.12 Example of a HCPCS Modifier

GA	Waiver of liability statement issued as required by payer policy, individual case

Place of Service Codes

Coding Clicks

Bookmark the Place of Service codes at http://Coding.ParadigmEducation.com/POS.

Place of service (POS) codes are 2-digit numeric codes developed by CMS that are used on the insurance claim form to identify the setting where a service or procedure takes place. Although outpatient providers report CPT® codes, services and procedures may take place in many different types of medical facilities. Some CPT® codes, such as those for evaluation and management services, are specific to the location where the service or procedure takes place. Coders typically do not assign POS codes unless they also have billing duties. Place of service codes are typically located in the front of the CPT® codebook, before the Introduction. If your CPT® codebook does not contain POS codes, bookmark the POS page on the CMS website. Table 2.6 contains the most common POS codes used in medical facilities.

Table 2.6 Most Common Place of Service Codes List

Place of Service Code(s)	Place of Service Name
01	Pharmacy
02	Telehealth
03	School
04	Homeless Shelter
09	Prison/Correctional Facility
10	Unassigned
11	Office
12	Home
13	Assisted Living Facility
18	Place of Employment–Worksite
20	Urgent Care Facility
21	Inpatient Hospital
22	On-Campus Outpatient Hospital
23	Emergency Department Hospital
24	Ambulatory Surgical Center
26	Military Treatment Facility
31	Skilled Nursing Facility
32	Nursing Facility
34	Hospice

Place of Service Code(s)	Place of Service Name
51	Inpatient Psychiatric Facility
52	Psychiatric Facility–Partial Hospitalization
53	Community Mental Health Center
54	Intermediate Care Facility/Mentally Retarded
55	Residential Substance Abuse Treatment Facility
56	Psychiatric Residential Treatment Center
57	Non residential Substance Abuse Treatment Facility
71	Public Health Clinic
72	Rural Health Clinic

CONCEPTS CHECKPOINT **2.6**

Use information from the previous sections to select the correct answers to the following questions.

1. A(n) _____ is the primary component of a service or procedure.
   a. main term
   b. modifying term
   c. eponym
   d. None of the answers are correct.
2. Codebook conventions are
   a. used to help locate and assign codes.
   b. words, symbols, punctuation, formatting, and abbreviations.
   c. large meetings regarding the codebook held once per year.
   d. None of the answers are correct.
3. The term *See*
   a. is not a code convention.
   b. is a code convention.
   c. indicates a cross-reference to a different code.
   d. never appears in the Index.
4. Modifiers
   a. supply payers with more information about services or procedures performed.
   b. may be numbers only, letters only, or a combination of numbers and letters.
   c. are used with CPT® and/or HCPCS Level II codes.
   d. None of the answers are correct.
5. _____ identify where a service or procedure takes place.
   a. Modifiers
   b. Category codes
   c. Place of service codes
   d. Codebook conventions

Locating and Selecting Codes Using the CPT® Codebook

Now that we have reviewed the contents of the CPT® codebook and the general rules and conventions that help you locate and understand codes, the next step is using the CPT® codebook to assign codes. The following are the necessary steps to accurately select a code using the CPT® codebook:

1. Review the health record to identify the procedure or service that needs to be coded. Operative reports typically list the name of the procedure performed at the top of the report. However, the documentation must support the listed procedure, so always review the complete report to confirm the procedure and

note any revisions or special circumstances. If the source document is unclear, you should always consult with the physician to verify the services performed. If the facility uses an EHR system, the coder may use the query (inquiry) feature, which allows the coder to submit questions and ask for further documentation directly from the healthcare provider.

2. Refer to the main term in the Index of the CPT® codebook.
3. Search for the modifying term(s) that most accurately describes the service or procedure performed. If the procedure is not indexed as a subterm, try the body site, the body system, or an alternative term.
4. Note the appropriate code range from the Index so that you have it on hand when referring to the category sections of the codebook.
5. Based on the code(s) you identified, refer to the appropriate section of the CPT® codebook.
6. Read any parenthetic notes and follow the instructions communicated by any symbols associated with a selected code.
7. Verify that the code description matches the procedure statement and documentation. If the facility uses an encoder (an online database discussed below), coders may read an electronic description of the service or procedure. If an encoder is not available, coders should reference medical terminology books, coding journals, and the Internet for detailed descriptions of procedures.
8. Assign the most appropriate code.
9. Assign a modifier(s) if necessary.
10. Report the code and/or modifier(s) to the appropriate entity.

Think Like a Coder

Christopher is a certified coding specialist working for a cardiologist who uses an EHR system. While reviewing the health records, Christopher discovers that some key components of a patient's procedure are not documented in the operative report. Because of this, he is unable to determine the most accurate CPT® code. What should Christopher do?

a. Guess and report the code he thinks is correct.
b. Query the physician for more information.
c. Ask his coworker what code he would report.

Coding Clicks

To learn more about how to join the AAPC or AHIMA, visit their websites:

- http://aapc.com
- http://ahima.org

Tools and Resources

Coders use a variety of tools and resources that help them to remain up to date with changes in coding, reporting guidelines, and the healthcare industry that affect their careers. The American Health Information Management Association (AHIMA) and AAPC publish professional journals dedicated to coding, compliance, documentation, and other topics related to health information management. These publications are available in print format or online to members at no additional charge. Members of these professional organizations also have access to professional training, certifications, and opportunities to network with others in the same field.

AMA Resources

In addition to developing, licensing, and publishing the CPT® code set, the AMA provides a selection of coding reference publications that may be purchased in printed format or online from the AMA website:

- *CPT® Assistant*, a monthly newsletter dedicated to addressing coding questions regarding specific services and procedures;
- *CPT® Changes: An Insider's View*, an annual publication released in November of the previous year that the changes take place. *CPT® Changes* contains detailed descriptions and rationales of why a CPT® code was added, revised, or deleted. The publication also includes new temporary codes;
- *Clinical Examples in Radiology*, a quarterly newsletter that provides clarification on a variety of clinical case examples that will assist coders in selecting radiology codes.

When a reference from 1 of these sources is specific to a CPT® code, the AMA's CPT® codebook lists the resource next to the code and uses the symbols illustrated in Figure 2.13.

Figure 2.13 AMA Source References in the CPT® Codebook

The symbols ➲ ➲ and ➲ appear after many codes throughout the AMA codebook and indicate that the AMA has published reference material regarding that particular code. Coders who have access to these resources may review the information for coding guidance.

➲ ➲ refers to an edition of *CPT® Assistant*

➲ refers to an edition of *Clinical Examples in Radiology*

Some encoders include access to these resources. Figure 2.14 illustrates how publication references appear in the AMA's CPT® codebook.

Figure 2.14 AMA Publication References in the CPT® Codebook

77073 Bone length studies (orthoroentgenogram, scanogram)

➲ ➲ *CPT® Assistant* Mar 07:7;

➲ *Clinical Examples in Radiology* Summer 07:12. Fall 08:10, Fall 10:6

CMS Resources

The CMS website contains a wealth of resources that clarify coding and reporting guidelines, at no charge to the public. Many of the guidelines on the CMS website are lengthy and are contained in several different areas of the site. When coders access information from the CMS website, they should bookmark the page for future reference. The following resources are just a few of the many valuable tools available on the CMS website. Many of these resources are discussed in greater detail in Chapter 21, Reimbursement, and Chapter 22, Healthcare Compliance.

> **Coding Clicks**
>
> MLN Matters is an excellent resource for coders. The main webpage contains articles from 2004 to present at http://Coding.ParadigmEducation.com/MLNMatters.

The **Medicare Learning Network (MLN)** page on the CMS website provides educational and reference materials related to various Medicare documentation and coding guidelines. MLN Matters is a resource that coders will access frequently. MLN Matters publishes articles on a variety of topics that break down complicated Medicare guidelines into an easy-to-read and print format. MLN Matters articles are not published on any set schedule but rather are released, revised, and archived as CMS deems necessary.

The **National Correct Coding Initiative (NCCI)**, also known as NCCI edits, is a tool that helps to prevent unbundling of services and procedures. Unbundling occurs when multiple CPT® codes are reported when there is a single code that represents the complete procedure. There may be circumstances when unbundling combination procedures is acceptable, and in those circumstances, the procedures must be reported with the appropriate modifier(s). Chapter 4 discusses the use of NCCI edits in detail.

The **HCPCS Release and Code Sets** CMS web page publishes HCPCS Level II procedure codes and modifiers quarterly. Coders should bookmark http://Coding.ParadigmEducation.com/HCPCSUpdate and check quarterly for updates.

CMS Internet-Only Manuals (IOMs)

> **Coding Clicks**
>
> To access any of the CMS Internet-Only Manuals, go to the IOM section of the CMS website at http://Coding.ParadigmEducation.com/IOM.

The CMS publishes its guidelines, policies, and procedures as **Internet-Only Manuals (IOMS)**. These are publications that were once printed or sent to providers annually on computer disc and are now published only on the CMS website. Many of these manuals are good resources for coders. The following are a few that coders may frequently reference.

The ***Medicare National Coverage Determinations (NCD) Manual*** contains Medicare's interpretation of how a specific treatment or diagnosis is covered. These are national rules that are the minimum standards that all Medicare payers must follow.

Medicare Claims Processing Manual contains guidelines that specify what makes a specific service or procedure billable. For example, Chapter 10 of the *Medicare Claims Processing Manual* is dedicated to Home Health Agency Billing. Coders who work for home health agencies will bookmark this page and refer to it often for coding guidance.

Medicare Program Integrity Manual contains guidance for CMS contractors who are responsible for reviewing provider records and reimbursements for compliance with CMS policies. Chapter 22 of this book discusses coding compliance in detail.

Local coverage determinations (LCDs) is an online CMS resource that details how Medicare Administrative Contractors (MACs) apply national coverage determinations (NCDs) to their assigned jurisdictions (regions). MACs are responsible for processing Medicare claims, enrolling healthcare providers into the Medicare program, and providing education and clarification regarding documentation and medical coverage.

Digital Resources

Encoders are online databases that allow coders to look up codes, review detailed descriptions of procedures, and review coding and reimbursement guidelines. EncoderPro and 3M are 2 of the most popular encoder programs. Most coders have access to encoder databases through subscriptions paid by their employers. Individuals may purchase subscriptions directly from the vendors' websites.

Computer-assisted coding (CAC) is an electronic tool used to analyze health records for keywords to recommend a diagnosis or procedure code. If the coder agrees with the recommended code, it is entered into the patient's financial record to prepare for billing. A CAC is a tool that increases coding accuracy and productivity. Coders who use CACs are required to review medical documentation to verify the recommended code. Many EHRs have CAC capabilities; however, the medical facility may choose not to activate it. Chapter 5 discusses encoders and CACs in more detail.

Practice Professionalism

Carter is a medical record auditor for the Central Physician Group. He has completed a medical record audit on Dr. Wilds, a physician who has been practicing medicine for only a few years. He is not familiar with many of the CMS guidelines that affect the group. Carter is scheduled to meet Dr. Wilds to discuss the audit findings. It is important that Carter conduct himself in a professional manner during the meeting. To do this, he must prepare for the meeting. He reviews the audit and his notes and visits the CMS website to print out various resources that support his findings to share with Dr. Wilds during the meeting. He arrives 15 minutes early to set up his computer and documents. He also brings his coding books, in the event that the physician wants to view the codes. When Dr. Wilds arrives, Carter greets him and begins to discuss the audit findings. He feels confident that he has all the resources needed to handle the physician's questions and knows that his preparation helps him to remain professional.

Chapter Summary

- Healthcare Common Procedure Coding System (HCPCS) is a group of codes used to describe medical, surgical, and diagnostic procedures as well as products and drugs.
- Current Procedural Terminology (CPT®), Fourth Edition, is a coding system that is used to assign 5-character codes to descriptions of medical, surgical, and diagnostic procedures.
- HCPCS Level I codes are CPT® codes.
- HCPCS Level II codes are referred to as National Codes. They are located in the HCPCS codebook.
- The Health Insurance Portability and Accountability Act of 1996 (HIPAA) Administrative Simplification section of the HIPAA final rule requires the use of CPT® and HCPCS codes to report procedures.
- To accurately assign CPT® codes, coders must have a working knowledge of the CPT® codebook organization, conventions, parenthetic notes, and symbols, as well as coding and reporting guidelines.
- Medical necessity of a service is the overarching criterion for payment in addition to the specific criteria of CPT® codes.
- The CPT® codebook categorizes procedures and services into lists that allow you to locate codes alphabetically or numerically.
- The codebook is divided into 6 parts: Introduction, Category I codes, Category II codes, Category III codes, the appendixes, and the Index.
- Category I codes are the first and largest set of codes in the CPT® codebook. They represent common procedures or services that are performed often and are approved by the FDA.
- Category II codes are optional codes used for reporting certain services and test results that support nationally established performance measures and that have an evidence base as contributing to quality patient care. The codes are not required for correct coding and may not be used as a substitute for Category I codes. These codes are intended to facilitate data collection about the quality of care.
- Category III codes are temporary codes used to report emerging technology, services, and procedures.
- The appendixes contain expanded definitions of modifiers, clinical examples, and other content associated with code selection and reporting.
- The Index lists the descriptions of procedures and services in alphabetic order by procedure, anatomical site, condition, eponym, or other designation.

- Guidelines in the CPT® codebook are instructions from the AMA for how to accurately document and select services and procedures. Specific guidelines are located at the beginning of each Category I section and subsection.
- Unlisted codes, also referred to as *dummy codes*, are used to report services or procedures not defined by any CPT® code.
- Time-based codes reflect face-to-face time the provider spends with the patient.
- Codebook conventions are words, symbols, punctuation, formatting, and abbreviations that are used to help locate and assign codes.
- Modifiers are 2-character codes that are sometimes added to CPT® or HCPCS Level II codes when the procedure, service, or item was altered from the code description.
- Place of service codes are 2-digit numeric codes used on the insurance claim form to identify where a service or procedure takes place.

Navigator

Access interactive chapter review exercises, practice activities, flash cards, and study games.

Chapter 3

HCPCS Coding

Fast Facts

- Many of the HCPCS codes are used to report products and drugs.
- In 2015, Medicare reimbursed for approximately 14 million influenza vaccines.
- More than 6.5 million Americans use a cane, walker, or crutches to assist their mobility.
- Cervical cancer is 1 of the easiest cancers to prevent with regular screening tests.

Sources: http://cms.gov, http://nih.gov, http://cancer.org

Crack the Code

Review the sample report to find the correct HCPCS code. You may need to return to this exercise after reading the chapter content.

HEARING CRITERIA: Puretone Audiometry. A patient fails the screening test if he or she does not respond to any 1 tone (frequency) at 20 dB hearing level in either ear.

SCREENING DATE: June 24, 2019

		FREQUENCY HZ		
		1000	2000	4000
Right Ear	HL 20	[XX] Pass [ ] Fail	[XX] Pass [ ] Fail	[XX] Pass [ ] Fail
Left Ear	HL 20	[ ] Pass [XX] Fail	[ ] Pass [XX] Fail	[XX] Pass [ ] Fail

REMARKS:

[ ] Within Normal Limits
[ ] Needs Rescreen (within two weeks)
[XX] Needs Referral

answer: V5008

Learning Objectives

3.1 Identify and discuss the organization of the HCPCS Level II code set.

3.2 Describe the components of HCPCS publications.

3.3 Define HCPCS Level II codebook sections.

3.4 Understand how to locate terms in the HCPCS Index.

3.5 Describe how to use the HCPCS tabular list to locate and assign HCPCS codes.

3.6 Identify the information included in the Table of Drugs and understand how to use it to locate codes.

3.7 Select HCPCS Level II codes to identify procedures, services, drugs, and equipment.

Chapter Outline

- **I.** The Healthcare Common Procedure Coding System Level II Code Set
  - **A.** Organization of HCPCS Code Set Publications
    - **i.** Guidance Components
    - **ii.** HCPCS Index
    - **iii.** Tabular List of HCPCS Level II National Codes
- **II.** HCPCS Level II National Codes Sections
  - **A.** Section A (Codes A0000–A9999): Transport Services Including Ambulance; Medical and Surgical Supplies; Administration, Miscellaneous, and Investigational Services
    - **i.** Transport Services Including Ambulance
    - **ii.** Medical and Surgical Supplies
    - **iii.** Administrative, Miscellaneous, and Investigational Services
  - **B.** Section B (Codes B4000–B9999): Enteral and Parenteral Therapy
  - **C.** Section C (Codes C1000–C9999): CMS Hospital Outpatient Payment System
  - **D.** Section D (Codes D0000–D9999): Dental Procedures
  - **E.** Section E (Codes E0100–E9999): Durable Medical Equipment (DME)
  - **F.** Section G (Codes G0000–G9999): Temporary Procedures and Professional Services
  - **G.** Section H (Codes H0001–H9999): Behavioral Health and/or Substance Abuse Treatment Services
  - **H.** Section J (Codes J0100–J9999): Drugs Administered Other Than Oral Method, Chemotherapy Drugs
    - **i.** Table of Drugs
  - **I.** Section K (Codes K0000–K9999): Temporary Durable Medical Equipment Regional Carriers
  - **J.** Section L (Codes L0100–L9900): Orthotics, Prosthetics
  - **K.** Section M (Codes M0000–M0301): Other Medical Services
  - **L.** Section P (Codes P0000–P9999): Pathology and Laboratory Services
  - **M.** Section Q (Codes Q0035–Q9999): Temporary Codes Assigned by CMS
  - **N.** Section R (Codes R0000–R9999): Diagnostic Radiology Services
  - **O.** Section S (Codes S0000–S9999): Temporary National Codes Established by Private Payers
  - **P.** Section T (Codes T1000–T9999): Temporary National Codes Established by Medicaid
  - **Q.** Section V (Codes V0000–V5364): Vision Services, Hearing Services
- **III.** Modifiers
- **IV.** Chapter Summary

The Healthcare Common Procedure Coding System Level II Code Set

Coding Clicks

Visit and bookmark the CMS's HCPCS Quarterly Update at http://Coding.ParadigmEducation.com/HCPCSUpdate. Because updates are posted quarterly, accessing the page is easier and more accurate than downloading the associated file.

As you learned in Chapter 2, the Healthcare Common Procedure Coding System (HCPCS) is used to report medical, surgical, and diagnostic procedures as well as products and drugs. There are 2 levels of HCPCS currently in use. The Level I codes are the CPT® codes developed by the American Medical Association (AMA) and published in the CPT® codebook. The Level II HCPCS codes are developed and released by the US governmental agency the Centers for Medicare and Medicaid Services (CMS). The codes are published on the CMS website as a collection of text and spreadsheet files. Updated quarterly, the code set consists of 4 basic files:

- *Alpha-Numeric HCPCS File*, a folder that consists of a text file that contains general information about the HCPCS database and the HCPCS code set in both text and spreadsheet formats;
- *Record Layout*, a text file that describes the organization of the codes;
- *Table of Drugs*, a PDF file that alphabetically lists drugs with their dosages, routes of administration, and codes;
- *Alpha-Numeric Index*, a PDF file that is a comprehensive alphabetic index to all of the codes.

The CMS updates HCPCS Level II codes in October for use in January of the following year. Changes to Medicare coverage policies associated with HCPCS Level II are published quarterly on the CMS website. Coders should periodically review HCPCS Level II updates on the CMS website for changes that may affect their medical practices.

Organization of HCPCS Code Set Publications

Although the Level II codes are developed by CMS and published on the CMS website, CMS does not publish a HCPCS codebook. HCPCS codebooks are published by independent publishing companies.

All HCPCS coding books contain the following components:

- a table of contents;
- a list of symbols and conventions;
- an introduction;
- HCPCS alphabetic index;
- Table of Drugs;
- the lists of HCPCS codes;
- a list of HCPCS modifiers.

Some features that can also be included are the following:

- HCPCS Updates: lists of new, revised, and deleted codes and modifiers as well as payment and payment status indicators for the current year;
- HCPCS Table of Drugs: the list of codes for generic drugs and biologicals with associated dosages and routes of administration;
- Chapter I of the National Correct Coding Initiative (NCCI) Policy Manual for Medicare Services: a discussion of general correct coding policies.

Guidance Components

HCPCS codebook publications offer helpful text features to navigate through the code set. Familiarity with your version will help you find and select the codes you need to report.

Table of Contents As with any introductory content in the HCPCS codebook, it is important to review the table of contents so that you are familiar with the format of the codebook and any additional resources. Additional resources could include an appendix, important notices, and URLs for accessing NCCI materials, CMS Internet-Only Manuals, and periodic updates.

Symbols and Conventions **Conventions** are abbreviations, symbols, and notes to help guide coders to the most accurate code. The CMS HCPCS Level II code set does not have a standard set of conventions to assist coders in location and reporting of codes. Publishers of HCPCS Level II codebooks develop their own set of conventions that work best with their publications, which typically mimic the conventions used in their CPT® codebooks. Because of the differences in conventions between publications, coders will need to review the conventions at the beginning of the HCPCS codebook they have chosen.

Introduction The HCPCS codebook Introduction section contains organizational and codebook conventions unique to that publication. Context and presentation of HCPCS Levels I, II, and III are described. Legends are provided to indicate the status of codes reflecting both CMS's and the publisher's updates.

HCPCS Level II Annual Code Updates Publishers may list HCPCS Level II annual updates to codes and payment and status indicators. Codes and modifiers are added, revised, and/or deleted by CMS annually. A **payment status indicator** is a letter *A* through *Y* that identifies Medicare's payment determination for procedures and items provided in ambulatory surgery centers (ASCs). For example, the payment status indicator E denotes that the associated procedure or item is not paid by Medicare when submitted on outpatient claims. Payment indicators help coders avoid submission of codes that will not be reimbursed and understand why specific HCPCS codes are not reimbursed. This payment status indicator letter is not a part of the HCPCS code. The publisher may place the payment indicator at the end of the HCPCS code description or somewhere near the code. Coding conventions signal whether the publisher includes payment status indicators and how to identify them. The complete list of status indicators and the definitions of each HCPCS code are published annually on the CMS website, in Addendum B of the Hospital Outpatient Prospective Payment System and Ambulatory Surgery Centers final rule.

HCPCS Table of Drugs Publishers may provide the Table of Drugs, a list of codes for generic drugs and biologicals with associated dosages and routes of administration. The Table of Drugs is discussed in this chapter.

National Correct Coding Initiative General Correct Coding Policies Publishers may include as an appendix the NCCI guidance on general correct coding policies located in Chapter I of the NCCI Policy Manual. The NCCI is discussed in detail in Chapter 4.

HCPCS Index

The HCPCS Index is a list of services, procedures, supplies, products, and drugs in alphabetic order. The associated HCPCS Level II code or codes are displayed next to the main term or subterm. When searching for a HCPCS Level II code, first look for the service, procedure, or item by the name in the code descriptor. Items that are not listed by name may be located by the type of item. If the service or procedure is related to a specific body part, search for the affected body system or body part by name. The example in Figure 3.1 will help you better understand how to search for main terms in the Index.

For example, a breast pump is listed in the Index under both main terms *Breast* and *Pump*. The main term represents several different types of products, and those products are listed below the main term, as shown in Figure 3.1.

> **Index Insider**
>
> There are many ways to find the same code. Open your HCPCS codebook, go to the Index, and look up *Breast pump* by going to the main entry "Pump." Did you find the same range of codes as those shown in Figure 3.1?

When more than 1 code is associated with the subterm, a range of codes is provided. A hyphen between the first code and the last code indicates a range of multiple sequential codes that are relevant. Relevant nonsequential codes are listed in a series divided by commas. The Index is meant only to help you locate codes—you should never report codes directly from the Index. Always verify codes in the tabular list prior to reporting them.

Figure 3.1 Example of a HCPCS Level II Index Entry

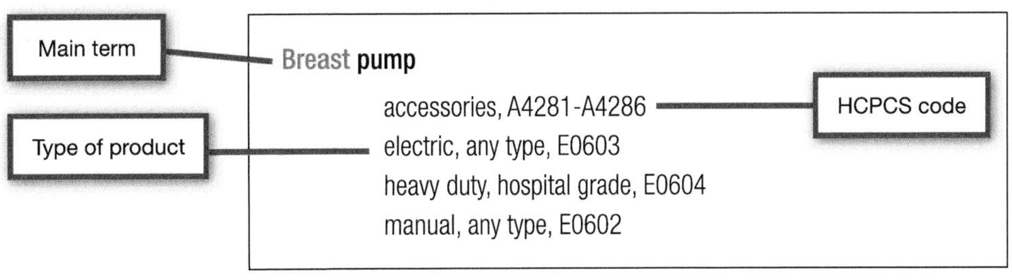

CONCEPTS CHECKPOINT 3.1

Place an *X* next to HCPCS coding book components that are contained in all publications.

a. _____ Chapter I of the National Correct Coding Initiative (NCCI) Policy Manual for Medicare Services

b. _____ HCPCS alphabetic index

c. _____ HCPCS Table of Drugs

d. _____ HCPCS Updates

e. _____ Introduction

f. _____ List of HCPCS modifiers

g. _____ List of symbols and conventions

h. _____ Lists of HCPCS codes

i. _____ Table of Contents

j. _____ Abbreviations

LET'S TRY ONE 3.1

Give the code, sequence of codes, or code range listed in the HCPCS Index for the following entries.

1. Blood, platelets, pheresis, leukocytes reduced: _____________
2. Cast, supplies: _____________
3. Collar, cervical, multiple post: _____________
4. Hand restoration: _____________
5. Nebulizer, pneumatic, administration set: _____________

Practice Professionalism

Always base your selection of HCPCS Level II codes on the documentation provided in the health record. Health record documentation will be discussed in detail in Chapter 5. Prior to assigning a code, review the documentation to ensure that the procedure, product, services, or drug matches the full description of the code. Take the following steps to select the appropriate HCPCS Level II code:

1. Review coding conventions located at the beginning of the HCPCS codebook.
2. Review the health record and identify the medical term(s) to be coded.
3. Locate the main term in the alphabetic index or go to the tabular list.
4. Locate the code in the tabular list.
5. In the tabular list, review all notes, symbols, abbreviations, and punctuation marks associated with the selected code.
6. Review the code description to ensure that the definition completely describes the services, products, drugs, or procedures documented in the health record.

Tabular List of HCPCS Level II National Codes

The **HCPCS Level II tabular list** is an alphanumeric list of HCPCS codes organized by sections. There are 17 sections for HCPCS Level II codes. Each section is represented by a letter, shown in Table 3.1, which begins each code within the section.

Some code sections are subdivided by type, anatomical site, product, or procedure. An example of code entries L1600 and L1610 is shown in Figure 3.2. The first character in the code, *L*, identifies them as belonging to the Orthotics section. The red heading, "Orthotic Devices: Lower Limb," identifies a grouping of codes, as does the subheading "Hip: Flexible." The section "Note" provides coders with further instruction on how to accurately assign codes in this section. The "Note" in section L1600 through L2999 instructs coders to add codes from the Additional Sections (located at the end of each subsection in Section L) if additional procedures from this subsection were performed. Code descriptions located at the right of each code provide its detailed definition. The figure callout notes the difference between the similar codes. Make sure to review the entire code description prior to selecting a code to ensure accurate code assignment.

Table 3.1 HCPCS Level II Tabular List Sections

Section	Code Range	Description
A	A0000–A9999	Transport services including ambulance; medical and surgical supplies; administration, miscellaneous, and investigational services
B	B4000–B9999	Enteral and parenteral therapy
C	C1000–C9999	CMS hospital outpatient payment system
D	D0000–D9999	Dental procedures
E	E0100–E9999	Durable medical equipment (DME)
G	G0000–G9999	Temporary procedures and professional services
H	H0001–H9999	Behavioral health and/or substance abuse treatment services
J	J0100–J9999	Drugs administered other than oral method, chemotherapy drugs
K	K0000–K9999	Temporary durable medical equipment regional carriers
L	L0100–L9900	Orthotics, prosthetics
M	M0000–M0301	Other medical services
P	P0000–P9999	Pathology and laboratory services
Q	Q0035–Q9999	Temporary codes assigned by CMS
R	R0000–R9999	Diagnostic radiology services
S	S0000–S9999	Temporary national codes established by private payers
T	T1000–T9999	Temporary national codes established by Medicaid
V	V0000–V5364	Vision services, hearing services

Figure 3.2 Example of the HCPCS Level II Tabular List

Orthotic Devices: Lower Limb

Note: The procedures in L1600-L2999 are considered as base or basic procedures and may be modified by listing procedures from the additional sections and adding them to the base procedure.

Hip: Flexible

L1600	Hip orthosis, abduction control of hip joints, flexible, frejka type with cover, prefabricated item that has been trimmed, bent, molded, assembled, or otherwise customized to fit a specific patient by an individual with expertise
L1610	Hip orthosis, abduction control of hip joints, flexible, (frejka cover only), prefabricated item that has been trimmed, bent, molded, assembled, or otherwise customized to fit a specific patient by an individual with expertise

Difference in code description

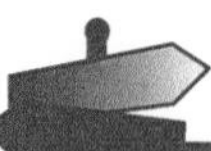

Learn Your Way

According to the Learning Styles Index, if you are an active learning type, you prefer to do technical tasks that are hands-on and practical. Look at Figure 3.2. Are there any terms in this code description for which you do not know the meaning? Use a medical dictionary to look up unfamiliar terms. This will help expand your knowledge and improve your coding skills. For all kinds of learners, hands-on action can help memory.

HCPCS Level II National Codes Section

Not all sections are used by all medical specialties. However, it is important that coders have an understanding of the content of each HCPCS Level II tabular list section.

Section A (Codes A0000–A9999): Transport Services Including Ambulance; Medical and Surgical Supplies; Administration, Miscellaneous, and Investigational Services

Section A of the HCPCS codebook contains codes for transport services, medical and surgical supplies, administration services, and investigational services. Miscellaneous services, procedures, and products are also categorized in this section.

Transport Services Including Ambulance

Ambulance services codes are reported using section A codes. Medicare limits reimbursement for ambulance services to:

- transportation of the beneficiary to an approved healthcare facility;
- transportation by ambulance that is medically necessary;

- transportation by an ambulance provider that meets all state and local regulations to operate as a medical transportation service.

The coder will review the health record associated with the medical transportation to identify medications administered, the patient's condition, miles traveled, and pertinent information required for coding accuracy. Prior to coding ambulance services, coders should review *Medicare Claims Processing Manual, Chapter 15 – Ambulance*, published on the CMS website. These CMS guidelines detail ambulance billing procedures, including health record documentation requirements. Individual commercial insurance payers have medical transportation polices that should also be reviewed.

Medical and Surgical Supplies

Section A contains codes for medical and surgical supplies that are separately reportable. Typically, the cost of these items is included in surgery or procedure fees. However, when nonroutine supplies are used, or regular supplies used exceed the typical amount for that specific procedure, then the supply may be billed. The health record must document the specific name of the supply, the medical necessity for the nonroutine or higher-than-normal quantity, and the number of supplies used. For example, if a patient has a wound that needs suturing, the surgical tray that contains the supplies needed to close the wound is included in the routine procedure. However, if the medical documentation states that the wound was very deep and required the use of 2 or more surgical trays during the in-office procedure, the coder should report the additional surgical trays with HCPCS Level II code A4550, *Surgical trays.* The insurance payer may require a special report to validate the use of additional supplies or nonroutine supplies.

Administrative, Miscellaneous, and Investigational Services

Codes listed in section A as administrative, miscellaneous, and investigational are used to report services and procedures that do not have a specific HCPCS code. These are considered catchall codes. For example, if a new medical supply is approved by the Food and Drug Administration (FDA) and provided to a patient or used during a procedure, it is billed with the appropriate miscellaneous, administrative, or investigational code. Section A codes may also include items and services such as exercise equipment and other items/services that are not included in Medicare benefits. An example is illustrated in Figure 3.3. Radiopharmaceutical diagnostic imaging agents and nonprescription drugs are also listed in the Administrative, Miscellaneous, and Investigational Services section.

Figure 3.3 Example of an Administrative, Miscellaneous, and Investigational Level II Code

A9270	non-covered item or service

Section B (Codes B4000–B9999): Enteral and Parenteral Therapy

Enteral and parenteral therapy is the process of providing a patient with nutrition to sustain life when he or she is unable to consume food orally. **Parenteral therapy** requires the insertion of a catheter into the basilic or cephalic vein in the arm and is threaded into the superior vena cava above the right atrium. A solution composed of nutrients tailored for the patient is administered through the catheter.

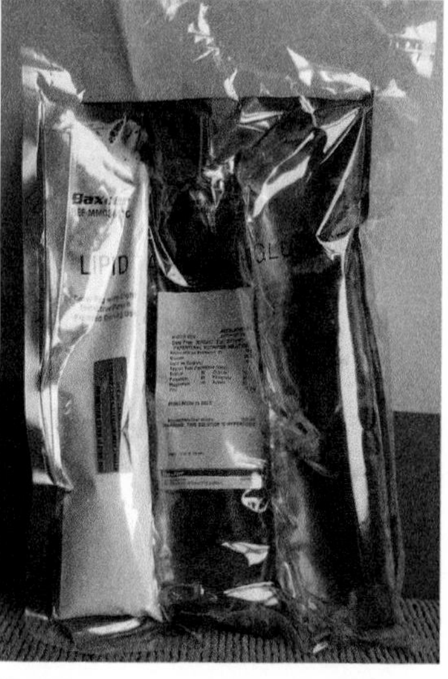

Premixed total parenteral nutrition solution can be used in the home healthcare setting.

Enteral nutrition therapy is the process of providing a patient with nutrition via a feeding tube. A feeding tube may be inserted through the nose or a surgical opening in the patient's stomach. The nasal feeding tube is referred to as *nasogastric*. The insertion of a feeding tube into the stomach is called a *jejunostomy* when the nutritional liquid is directed into the small intestine (the bowel) and a gastrostomy if directed into the stomach. The process of administering the nutrients is referred to as **infusion**. When the infusion is complete, the catheter or surgical opening (indicated by the suffix *-stomy*) is plugged until the next infusion. The initial procedure is performed in the hospital. Once the patient is healthy enough to return home and adequately trained on the infusion technique, the patient continues the treatments at home. Medical supplies, feeding solutions, and infusion services are reported with codes from section B of HCPCS Level II. Some codes in this section include the administration of the nutritional solution. If the code does not include the administration component of the services, an additional code is required to fully report the services. Figure 3.4 shows an example of a code for the infusion pump, and Figure 3.5 shows a code for the nutritional mix. If medication is administered via the feeding tube, an additional code to describe the specific drug is also reported.

Figure 3.4 Example of a Parenteral Therapy Pump Code

B9004	Parenteral nutrition infusion pump, portable

Figure 3.5 Example of a Parenteral Nutritional Mix Code

B4220	Parenteral nutrition supply kit; premix, per day

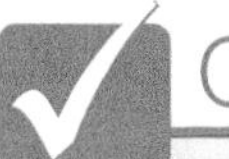

CONCEPTS CHECKPOINT 3.2

Use information from the previous sections to identify if the following statements are true or false.

1. _____ All sections of HCPCS Level II are used by all medical specialties.
2. _____ *Medicare Claims Processing Manual, Chapter 15 – Ambulance*, published on the CMS website, contains guidelines for reporting ambulance billing procedures.
3. _____ Medical supplies, feeding solutions, and infusion services are reported with codes from section B of HCPCS Level II.
4. _____ If medication is administered via a feeding tube, an additional code to describe the specific drug is also reported.
5. _____ The process of administering nutrients is referred to as *intravenous consumption*.

Section C (Codes C1000–C9999): CMS Hospital Outpatient Payment System

C codes are temporary codes established by CMS for the Hospital Outpatient Prospective Payment System and are valid only for Medicare on claims for hospital outpatient department services and procedures. When the temporary code is replaced by a permanent code, the C code is deleted and cross referenced to the permanent code. **Hospital Outpatient Prospective Payment System (OPPS)** is a reimbursement method used by CMS to reimburse hospitals or facilities for certain medical services that take place in the outpatient department. HCPCS C codes are reported for device categories; new technology procedures; and drugs, biologicals, and radiopharmaceuticals that do not have other HCPCS code assignments. Non-OPPS hospitals, critical access hospitals (CAHs), Indian health service hospitals (IHSs), hospitals located in American Samoa, Guam, Saipan, or the Virgin Islands, and Maryland-waiver hospitals may report these HCPCS C codes at their discretion.

LET'S TRY ONE 3.2

Use the HCPCS codebook to locate the correct HCPCS Level II code for the following services.

1. Ostomy pouch, closed; for use on barrier with locking flange, with filter (2 piece), 1: _____
2. Leg strap; foam or fabric, replacement only, 1 set: _____
3. Ketone test, specimen blood: _____
4. Humidifier water chamber: _____

Section D (Codes D0000–D9999): Dental Procedures

D codes are used to report dental procedures. They are developed and maintained by the American Dental Association. The dental industry refers to these codes as **Current Dental Terminology (CDT)**. Many CDT codes have counterparts in the CPT®codebook, and your HCPCS Level II codebook may provide cross-references to

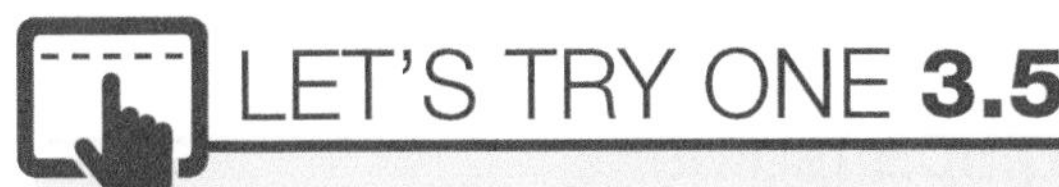

LET'S TRY ONE **3.5**

Use the HCPCS codebook to locate the correct HCPCS Level II code for the following services, procedures, and equipment.

1. Power wheelchair, group 3 heavy duty, single power option, sling/solid seat/back, patient weight 301 to 450 pounds: _____
2. Thoracic, rib belt, custom fabricated: _____
3. Ankle foot orthosis, posterior solid ankle, plastic, custom fabricated: _____
4. Infusion, albumin (human), 25%, 50 ml: _____
5. Fern test: _____

Section S (Codes S0000–S9999): Temporary National Codes Established by Private Payers

S codes are temporary codes that are used by commercial payers to report drugs, services, and supplies that do not have a HCPCS Level II code. These codes are designed to meet the needs of billing and claim processing policies unique to private insurers. Some S codes may be reported to state Medicaid programs.

Section T (Codes T1000–T9999): Temporary National Codes Established by Medicaid

RED FLAG

Do not confuse HCPCS Level II T codes with CPT® Category III temporary codes that have 4 digits preceding the T.

T codes are temporary codes that are established for Medicaid to report drugs, services, and supplies that do not have a HCPCS Level II code. Medicare does not recognize these codes, but some commercial payers may accept T codes.

Section V (Codes V0000–V5364): Vision Services, Hearing Services

Section V codes V0000 through V2799 are used to report vision-related supplies, including spectacles, lenses, contact lenses, prostheses, and intraocular lenses. HCPCS V codes are mostly reported by vision centers that specialize in providing patients with vision equipment, such a contact lenses and eyeglasses. Typically, eyeglasses and eye exams are not covered by Medicare. However, Medicare may cover some vision services if the vision problem is related to an underlying medical condition, such as glaucoma.

V codes in the range V5008 through V5364 are used to report hearing services, speech tests, equipment, and devices. Services related to prescribing, fitting, changing, or examining hearing aids are not covered by Medicare. There are some HCPCS Level II L codes that also report hearing devices or equipment.

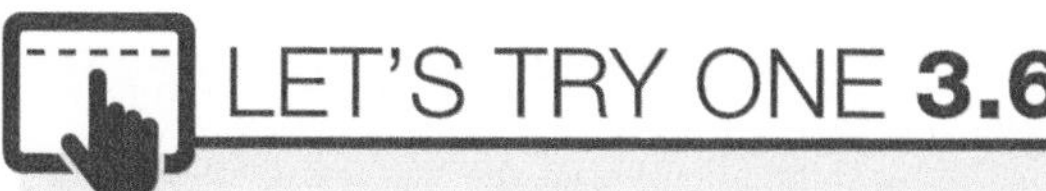

LET'S TRY ONE **3.6**

Use the HCPCS codebook to locate the correct HCPCS Level II code for the following services, procedures, and equipment.

1. Hearing assessment using audiometry for hearing aid evaluation and hearing loss measurement: _____
2. Iris supported intraocular lens: _____
3. Positioning seat for persons with special orthopedic needs: _____
4. Contact lens PMMA, bifocal, per lens: _____
5. Polishing/resurfacing of ocular prosthesis: _____

CONCEPTS CHECKPOINT **3.5**

Use the information from the previous section to identify if the following questions are true or false.

1. _____ A screening Papanicolaou smear is commonly referred to as a *Pap smear*.
2. _____ Medicare may cover some vision services if the vision problem is related to an underlying medical condition such as glaucoma.
3. _____ R codes are reported for equipment stored in the medical facility where the service is performed.
4. _____ There is a limit to the length of time a code will remain on temporary status.
5. _____ Written prescriptions for devices and items are required to order the orthotics.

Modifiers

Modifiers are the 2-character codes that are sometimes added to CPT® or HCPCS codes when the procedure, service, or item was altered from the code description. Modifiers supply payers with more information about services or procedures performed. Some modifiers increase payment, others decrease payment, and some are only informational and have no effect on reimbursement. Coders must review payer policy regarding acceptance of modifiers prior to reporting them. Incorrect usage of modifiers will result in delayed reimbursement. Chapter 4 discusses CPT® and HCPCS modifiers in detail.

Chapter Summary

- The Healthcare Common Procedure Coding System (HCPCS) is a coding system used to describe medical, surgical, and diagnostic procedures as well as products and drugs.
- HCPCS Level I codes are CPT® codes, developed and maintained by the AMA.
- HCPCS Level II codes are referred to as National Codes, developed and maintained by the CMS.
- The HCPCS Index is a list of services, procedures, supplies, products, and drugs in alphabetic order, which can be used to locate codes in the codebook tabular list.
- The HCPCS Level II tabular list presents the codes organized into sections, which are further subdivided by product and service categories.
- Section A codes are used to report transportation services, such as ambulances.
- Codes listed in section A that are categorized as administrative, miscellaneous, and investigational are used to report services and procedures that do not have a specific HCPCS code.
- Section B codes report the use of enteral and parenteral therapy.
- Section C codes are temporary codes for use with the outpatient prospective payment system.
- Dental procedures are reported with D codes. CMS puts a limit on reimbursement for dental procedures.
- Durable medical equipment (DME) is reported with E codes. Reporting of E codes sometimes requires the use of a Certificate of Medical Necessity (CMN).
- Section G codes report procedures and professional services. CMS requires the use of G codes to report services that are unique to the Medicare program.
- Section H codes are for behavioral and substance abuse treatment services.
- Section J codes report drugs administered other than through an oral method as well as chemotherapy drugs.
- The Table of Drugs can help coders with assignment of J codes.
- Section K codes are for temporary DME regional carriers.
- Orthotic and prosthetic services are found in the L code section. These include items like prosthetic limbs and orthopedic shoes.

- Section M codes are used for medical services not listed in other sections of the HCPCS Level II codebook.
- Section P codes are used for pathology and laboratory services, such as Pap smears.
- Section Q codes are temporary codes for miscellaneous services.
- Section R codes are used for diagnostic radiology services.
- Temporary national codes (non-Medicare or Medicaid) are reported with S codes.
- Section T codes are used by established state Medicaid agencies. T codes are temporary codes.
- Section V codes are used for vision services and hearing services, such as lenses, contact lenses, and speech tests.
- Modifiers are the 2-character codes that are sometimes added to CPT® or HCPCS codes when the procedure, service, or item was altered from the code description.

Navigator

Access interactive chapter review exercises, practice activities, flash cards, and study games.

Chapter 4

Principles of Coding and the Use of Modifiers

Fast Facts

- Many of the HCPCS and CPT® modifiers are related to various healthcare trends and growing areas of concern in the healthcare community.
- A shortage of more than 90,000 physicians is predicted in the United States by 2020. Modifier Q6, *Service furnished by a locum tenens physician*, is used when a substitute doctor provides care.
- In 2014, the CDC reported that nearly 2 million Americans either abused or were dependent on prescription opioid analgesics. Modifier HG is used for opioid addiction treatment programs.
- Nearly 93% of California mothers have breastfed their children. Modifier HD is used for programs for pregnant and nursing mothers.

Sources: http://www.bartonassociates.com, http://www.cdc.gov, http://calwic.org

Crack the Code

Review the sample operative report to find the correct procedure code and modifier. You may need to return to this exercise after reading the chapter content.

DATE OF PROCEDURE: 7/23/2019

SURGEON: Irene Watkins, MD

PROCEDURE PERFORMED: Closed treatment of left hip dislocation using the Stimson maneuver

INDICATIONS: Dislocation of left hip due to fall at home

ANESTHESIA: General

PROCEDURE: The patient is placed in the prone position with the lower limbs hanging from the end of the operative table. Pressure is placed on the sacrum for stabilization. The physician holds the knee and ankle flexed to 90 degrees and applies gentle downward pressure to the leg, just below the knee. The maneuver is unsuccessful. The physician repeats the Stimson maneuver with slightly stronger pressure. Due to the age of the patient and the amount of time the patient has been under anesthesia, the surgeon decides to discontinue the procedure. The patient is turned to the supine position and moved to recovery.

answer: 27252-53

Learning Objectives

4.1 Identify coding principles and pitfalls.
4.2 Understand the purpose of modifiers.
4.3 Use NCCI code sets to recognize appropriate usage of modifiers.
4.4 Differentiate between CPT® and HCPCS modifiers.
4.5 Increase knowledge of the reporting guidelines of CPT® modifiers.
4.6 Recognize CPT® symbols that prohibit modifier assignment.
4.7 Understand the reporting guidelines of selected HCPCS modifiers.

Chapter Outline

- **I.** Coding Principles and Guidelines
  - **A.** National Correct Coding Initiative (NCCI)
    - **i.** National Correct Coding Initiative (NCCI) Edits
    - **ii.** NCCI Edits Tables
    - **iii.** Medically Unlikely Edits Table
  - **B.** Medicare Physician Fee Schedule
- **II.** The Use of Modifiers
  - **A.** Modifiers and NCCI Edits
  - **B.** CPT® Modifiers
    - **i.** Modifier 22, *Increased Procedural Services*
    - **ii.** Modifier 23, *Unusual Anesthesia*
    - **iii.** Modifier 24, *Unrelated Evaluation and Management Service by the Same Physician or Other Qualified Health Care Professional During a Postoperative Period*
    - **iv.** Modifier 25, *Significant, Separately Identifiable Evaluation and Management Service by the Same Physician or Other Qualified Health Care Professional on the Same Day of the Procedure or Other Service*
    - **v.** Modifier 26, *Professional Component*
    - **vi.** Modifier 27, *Multiple Outpatient Hospital E/M Encounters on the Same Date*
    - **vii.** Modifier 32, *Mandated Services*
    - **viii.** Modifier 33, *Preventive Services*
    - **ix.** Modifier 47, *Anesthesia by Surgeon*
    - **x.** Modifier 50, *Bilateral Procedure*
    - **xi.** Modifier 51, *Multiple Procedures*
    - **xii.** Modifier 52, *Reduced Services*
    - **xiii.** Modifier 53, *Discontinued Procedure*
    - **xiv.** Modifier 54, *Surgical Care Only*
    - **xv.** Modifier 55, *Postoperative Management Only*
    - **xvi.** Modifier 56, *Preoperative Management Only*
    - **xvii.** Modifier 57, *Decision for Surgery*
    - **xviii.** Modifier 58, *Staged or Related Procedure or Service by the Same Physician or Other Qualified Health Care Professional During the Postoperative Period*
    - **xix.** Modifier 59, *Distinct Procedural Service*
    - **xx.** Modifier 62, *Two Surgeons*
    - **xxi.** Modifier 63, *Procedure Performed on Infants Less Than 4 kg*
    - **xxii.** Modifier 66, *Surgical Team*
    - **xxiii.** Modifier 73, *Discontinued Outpatient Hospital/Ambulatory Surgery Center (ASC) Procedure Prior to the Administration of Anesthesia*
    - **xxiv.** Modifier 74, *Discontinued Outpatient Hospital/Ambulatory Surgery Center (ASC) Procedure After Administration of Anesthesia*
    - **xxv.** Modifier 76, *Repeat Procedure or Service by Same Physician or Other Qualified Health Care Professional*
    - **xxvi.** Modifier 77, *Repeat Procedure by Another Physician or Other Qualified Health Care Professional*
    - **xxvii.** Modifier 78, *Unplanned Return to the Operating/Procedure Room by the Same Physician or Other Qualified Health Care Professional Following Initial Procedure for a Related Procedure During the Postoperative Period*
    - **xxviii.** Modifier 79, *Unrelated Procedure or Service by the Same Physician or Other Qualified Health Care Professional During the Postoperative Period*
    - **xxix.** Modifier 80, *Assistant Surgeon*
    - **xxx.** Modifier 81, *Minimum Assistant Surgeon*
    - **xxxi.** Modifier 82, *Assistant Surgeon (When Qualified Resident Surgeon Not Available)*
    - **xxxii.** Modifier 90, *Reference (Outside) Laboratory*
    - **xxxiii.** Modifier 91, *Repeat Clinical Diagnostic Laboratory Test*
    - **xxxiv.** Modifier 92, *Alternative Laboratory Platform Testing*
    - **xxxv.** Modifier 95, *Synchronous Telemedicine Service Rendered Via a Real-Time Interactive Audio and Video Telecommunications System*
    - **xxxvi.** Modifier 96, *Habilitative Services*
    - **xxxvii.** Modifier 97, *Rehabilitative Services*
    - **xxxviii.** Modifier 99, *Multiple Modifiers*
  - **C.** HCPCS Modifiers
    - **i.** Guidelines for Reporting Multiple HCPCS Modifiers
    - **ii.** Ambulance Services Modifiers
    - **iii.** Advance Beneficiary Notice of Noncoverage (ABN) Modifiers
    - **iv.** Modifier Q6, *Service Furnished by a Locum Tenens Physician*
    - **v.** Modifier TC, *Technical Component*
    - **vi.** Modifier 59, *Subset Modifiers*
    - **vii.** HCPCS Laterality Modifiers
- **III.** Chapter Summary

Coding Principles and Guidelines

CPT® and HCPCS Level II codes define medical and surgical procedures performed on patients. Some procedure codes are very specific, defining a single service such as CPT® code 93000, *Electrocardiogram, routine ECG with at least 12 leads; with interpretation and report*; other codes define procedures consisting of many services, such as CPT® code 58263, *Vaginal hysterectomy, for uterus 250 g or less; with removal of tube(s) and/or ovary(s), with repair of enterocele*. Because many procedures can be performed by different approaches, different methods, or in combination with other procedures, there are often multiple HCPCS/CPT® codes defining similar or related procedures.

CPT® and HCPCS Level II code descriptors usually do not explicitly describe all services included in a procedure. The CPT® codebook contains guidelines that indicate services inherent in a coded procedure or group of procedures, or defined as a package. As examples, postoperative care by the physician who performs a surgical procedure is always included in the surgical package; the anesthesia package of services includes certain preparation and monitoring services. Some pitfalls may arise out of these code characteristics, which experienced coders learn to avoid. These pitfalls include the following:

- downcoding, which is reporting a less extensive service or procedure than was performed;
- upcoding, which is reporting a comprehensive code when all of the procedures have not been performed;
- fragmenting a procedure into component parts;
- unbundling a bilateral procedure code into 2 unilateral procedure codes;
- unbundling services that are integral to a more comprehensive procedure.

The Centers for Medicare and Medicaid Services (CMS) has developed the National Correct Coding Initiative (NCCI) resources to help coders avoid these mistakes, which can delay the revenue cycle.

National Correct Coding Initiative (NCCI)

The **National Correct Coding Initiative (NCCI)** or CCI was first developed by CMS in 1996 to promote correct coding and to mitigate incorrect coding that leads to inappropriate payments for outpatient physician services. The NCCI tools help to prevent downcoding, upcoding, fragmenting, and unbundling of services and procedures. **Downcoding**, also referred to as *undercoding*, is reporting a code that represents a lower level of service or a less extensive procedure than what is supported by the documentation. **Upcoding**, also referred to as *overcoding*, is reporting a service or procedure that is more extensive than what the documentation supports. **Fragmenting**, commonly referred to as *unbundling*, is separately reporting services inherent in a procedure or group of procedures. **Unbundling** occurs when multiple CPT® codes are reported when there is a single code that represents the complete procedure. The single code that includes more than 1 procedure is called a **combination code**. There may be circumstances when unbundling a combination code is acceptable. When unbundling is acceptable, the separate procedure, which is typically the parent code, is reported with the appropriate modifier. There may also be circumstances when 2 services, 2 procedures, or some combination of these are reported for the same patient on the same date of service.

Coding Clicks

Coders should bookmark the *National Correct Coding Initiative Policy Manual for Medicare Services.* Follow the link to the NCCI Policy Manual on the CMS website, or visit http://Coding.ParadigmEducation.com/NCCI.

CMS publishes the *National Correct Coding Initiative Policy Manual for Medicare Services*. Located on the CMS NCCI web page, the manual explains why and how NCCI code combinations are determined. The manual also discusses in detail the proper use of selected modifiers when unbundling is allowed. NCCI identifies whether a selected combination can be reported together. The *NCCI Policy Manual for Medicare* is updated annually and takes effect January 1 of each year.

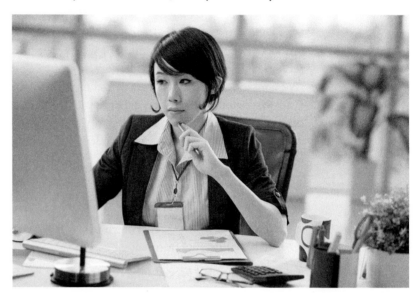

The NCCI tools provided online can help prevent downcoding, upcoding, fragmenting, and unbundling.

National Correct Coding Initiative (NCCI) Edits

CMS created NCCI Edits to help coders and physicians quickly identify code combinations. The NCCI Edits are Excel spreadsheets (tables) that list CPT® and HCPCS code combinations that in general should not be reported together. These inappropriate code combinations are referred to as an "edit."

The NCCI Edits also identify procedures that are mutually exclusive and may never be reported together. For example, a Pap smear screening code can never be reported with a prostate screening code. Women do not have prostates, and men do not receive Pap smear screens.

The NCCI Edits tables are available on the CMS and Medicaid websites. The tables are divided into 2 sections—2 for physicians and 2 for outpatient hospital services.

NCCI Edits Tables

To be confident that procedures reported together are accurate, a coder should reference the NCCI Edits tables published on the CMS or Medicaid website. The NCCI Edits tables contain both NCCI and Medically Unlikely Edits.

Coding Clicks

All coders should have the CMS NCCI Edits web page bookmarked on their computers. Go to the "NCCI Coding Edits" page on the CMS website at http://Coding.ParadigmEducation.com/NCCIEdits. At the bottom of the page, the "Related Links" list provides the downloadable Excel files.

Location of NCCI Edits Tables To access the NCCI Edits, the coder must go to the NCCI web page on CMS.gov to select the appropriate table. The links to the 2 hospital NCCI Edits tables and 2 physician NCCI Edits tables are located at the bottom of the web page as downloadable Excel files. Once you click the link and accept the license agreement terms, a zipped file will be downloaded to your computer. You can ignore the links provided for those familiar with the format of the data as previously released by the National Technical Information Service (NTIS), which is being phased out.

Format of NCCI Edits Tables Each table contains 6 columns—the first 2 are the code combinations—arranged in ascending numeric order based on column 1 codes. Figure 4.1 illustrates how the columns appear in the NCCI Edits table.

Figure 4.1 NCCI Edits Table

A	B	C	D	E	F
Column 1 / Column 2 Edits					
1	2	3	4	5	Modifier 0=not allowed 6
Column 1	Column 2	* = In existence prior to 1996	Effective Date	Deletion Date *=no data	1=allowed 9=not applicable
99215	G0101		19980401	19980401	9
99215	G0102		20000605	*	0
99215	G0104		19980401	19980401	9

The following list describes the content of each column of the NCCI Edits table:

- Column 1: primary code that is payable without a modifier;
- Column 2: secondary code that is not payable with the adjacent Column 1 code, unless a modifier is permitted and submitted;
- Column 3: indicates if the edit existed prior to 1996;
- Column 4: indicates the effective date of the edit (year, month, date);
- Column 5: indicates the deletion date of the edit (year, month, date);
- Column 6: identifies if use of modifier is permitted.

The coder will select the NCCI Edits table title with the appropriate code range for the first code value. For example, if you are looking for code combination 27524 and 51703 to report for a physician practice, open the *Practitioner PTP Edits v23.3 effective October 1, 2017* table appended with *The last row contains edit column 1 = 26010 and column 2 = 36909*. PTP refers to procedure to procedure edits. The column 1 numeric value gives the range; the column 2 value is incidental and does not have navigational value. Once the Excel file is open, the coder will see 6 columns that provide information on how to determine the appropriateness of the code combination.

Column 6 indicates whether it is acceptable to report codes in Columns 1 and 2 together: 0 indicates it is not allowed, 1 indicates it is allowed, and 9 indicates use of a modifier is not applicable. Table 4.1 shows the 3 indicators with their definitions.

Table 4.1 NCCI Edits Table Column 6 Modifier Indicator

Modifier Indicator	Definition
0 (Not Allowed)	There are no modifiers associated with NCCI that are allowed to be used with this code pair; there are no circumstances in which both procedures of the code pair should be paid for the same beneficiary on the same day by the same provider.
1 (Allowed)	The modifiers associated with NCCI are allowed with this code pair when appropriate.
9 (Not Applicable)	This indicator means that an NCCI edit does not apply to this code pair.

Source: "Modifier Indicator Table" from Medicare Learning Network, *How to Use the Medicare National Correct Coding Initiative (NCCI) Tools,* 2013, p. 6.

If the code pair combination is allowed (indicator 1), the modifier is placed on the code with the lowest relative value unit (RVU). The RVU is the value that CMS places on a specific service or procedure as determined by 3 components: physician work, practice expense, and malpractice risk. RVUs are discussed in Chapter 21. Modifiers should not be reported solely to bypass the reporting guideline restrictions of a procedure, but rather based on the medical necessity and documentation in the medical record.

Coding Clicks

CMS provides access to the MUE tables on its "Medically Unlikely Edits" web page at http://Coding.ParadigmEducation.com/MUE. Links to Practitioner Services, Facility Outpatient Services, and DME Supplier Services tables are at the bottom of the page.

Medically Unlikely Edits Table

Coders use Medically Unlikely Edits (MUEs) to identify the maximum number of a single procedure or service that may be reported on a single date of service. A single procedure or service rendered by the same provider is referred to as a *unit of service.* MUEs are listed in MUE tables for associated provider type. For example, a physician office will reference the Practitioner Services MUE table on CMS's "Medically Unlikely Edits" web page. Coders reference the MUE table before assigning modifier 50, *Bilateral procedure,* or modifier 51, *Multiple procedures.* Typically CMS does not list surgical MUEs with a maximum of 4 or more units, due to the concern of potential overcoding. The list of MUE also includes injectable medications or medical supplies that may exceed 4 units. The MUE table does not identify code combinations. To determine if a code combination is medically unlikely, refer to the appropriate NCCI Edits table. Medically Unlikely code combinations are indicated by the number "0" in Column 6 of the NCCI Edits table.

The MUE table is divided into 4 columns. As shown in Table 4.2, Column 1 lists CPT® or HCPCS codes in alphanumeric order. Column 2 identifies Practitioner Services MUE Values, which indicate the maximum units allowed for a single date of service. Column 3 identifies the MUE CMS Adjudication Indicator used for claim appeals. Column 4 identifies the rationale for the MUE.

Table 4.2 Medically Unlikely Edits Table Excerpt

Column 1 HCPCS/CPT® Code	Column 2 Practitioner Services MUE Values	Column 3 MUE Adjudication Indicator	Column 4 MUE Rationale
17110	1	2 Date of Service Edit: Policy	Code Descriptor / CPT® Instruction
17111	1	2 Date of Service Edit: Policy	Code Descriptor / CPT® Instruction
17250	4	3 Date of Service Edit: Clinical	Clinical: Data
17260	7	3 Date of Service Edit: Clinical	Clinical: Data

Source: CMS. Practitioner Services MUE Table – Effective 10/1/2016. CMS.gov. http://www.cms.gov/Medicare/Coding/NationalCorrectCodInitEd/MUE.html. Accessed November 25, 2016.

Medicare Physician Fee Schedule

The **Medicare Physician Fee Schedule (MPFS)** is a price list of services and procedures set by CMS. The MPFS lists the maximum amount that Medicare will pay a provider or vendor for a specific procedure or service. The MPFS is used by providers to determine coinsurance for Medicare beneficiaries and by insurance payers to set fees for services and procedures. The Physician Fee Schedule Look-Up Tool on the CMS Physician Fee Schedule web page lists detailed information related to the payment policy of services and procedures. Coders will reference the MPFS tool to look up the following types of information:

- RVU values for services and procedures;
- global days;
- whether applicable modifiers are allowed;
- whether a procedure allows for an assistant at surgery or a surgical team.

Coders should download the CMS Medicare Learning Network *How to Use the Searchable Medicare Physician Fee Schedule (MPFS)* booklet from the CMS website to use as a reference with the MPFS tool. Figure 4.2 illustrates a portion of the MPFS tool that identifies if selected modifiers are applicable. Figure 4.2 displays the headings that indicate the type of modifier associated with the code. The entire table is many more columns long. Only the portion pertaining to select common modifiers is illustrated in Figure 4.2. The arrows indicate that the table can be sorted. Table 4.3 provides brief definitions of the status indicators in Figure 4.2. Modifiers are described in detail in the CPT® modifier section of this chapter.

Figure 4.2 Medicare Physician Fee Schedule Searchable Tool Modifier Status Indicators

GLOBAL	MULT SURG	BILT SURG	ASST SURG	CO SURG	TEAM SURG

Coding Clicks

To learn how to use the searchable Medicare Physician Fee Schedule, coders should download the Medicare Learning Network resource *How to Use the Searchable Medicare Physician Fee Schedule* booklet at http://Coding.ParadigmEducation.com/MPFSBooklet. Access the CMS Physician Fee Schedule Search at http://Coding.ParadigmEducation.com/PhysicianFeeSchedule.

Table 4.3 Medicare Physician Fee Schedule Modifier Indicators

Indicator	Description
GLOBAL	Global Surgery Package Days
PREOP	Preoperative Percentage (CPT® modifier 56)
INTRAOP	Intraoperative Percentage (CPT® modifier 54)
POSTOP	Postoperative Percentage (CPT® modifier 55)
MULT SURG	Multiple Surgery Rules (CPT® modifier 51)
BILT SURG	Bilateral Surgery Rules (CPT® modifier 50)
ASST SURG	Assistant Surgery Rules (CPT® modifier 80)
CO SURG	Co-Surgeon Rules (CPT® modifier 62)
TEAM SUG	Team Surgeon Rules (CPT® modifier 66)

CONCEPTS CHECKPOINT 4.1

Indicate if the statement is true or false.

1. _____ The MUE table lists code combinations.
2. _____ Coders reference the MUE table to determine if they may assign modifier 50.
3. _____ The Practitioner Services MUE Values column indicates the minimum number of units to report.
4. _____ The Medicare Physician Fee Schedule (MPFS) is a price list of services and procedures set by CMS.

The Use of Modifiers

Modifiers are the 2-character codes that are sometimes added to 5-character CPT® or HCPCS codes when the procedure, service, or item was altered from the code description. Modifiers supply payers with more information about services or procedures performed. Some modifiers increase payment, others decrease payment, and some are only informational and have no effect on reimbursement. Although some modifiers are recognized by both Medicare and commercial payers, many are recognized only by 1 or the other. Coders must review payer policy regarding acceptance of modifiers prior to reporting them. Incorrect usage of modifiers will result in delayed reimbursement.

Modifiers and NCCI Edits

Coders reference NCCI Edits and the MPFS to determine if selected modifiers are allowed. NCCI Edits are relevant only to select CPT® and HCPCS Level II modifiers. Following is a list of CPT® modifiers associated with NCCI Edits. Detailed explanations of how to apply these modifiers are discussed in detail later in this chapter.

CPT® modifiers associated with NCCI Edits are the following:

- 24, *Unrelated Evaluation and Management Service, by the Same Physician or Other Qualified Health Care Professional, During a Postoperative Period*;
- 25, *Significant, Separately Identifiable Evaluation and Management Service by the Same Physician or Other Qualified Health Care Professional During a Postoperative Period*;
- 27, *Multiple Outpatient Hospital E/M Encounters on the Same Date*;
- 57, *Decision for Surgery*;
- 58, *Staged or Related Procedure or Service by the Same Physician or Other Qualified Health Care Professional During the Postoperative Period*;
- 59, *Distinct Procedural Service*;
- 78, *Unplanned Return to the Operating/Procedure Room by the Same Physician or Other Qualified Health Care Professional Following Initial Procedure for a Related Procedure During the Postoperative Period*;
- 79, *Unrelated Procedure or Service by the Same Physician or Other Qualified Health Care Professional During the Postoperative Period*;
- 91, *Repeat Clinical Diagnostic Laboratory Test.*

Below is a list of HCPCS modifiers associated with NCCI Edits. Detailed explanations of how to apply these modifiers are discussed in detail later in this chapter.

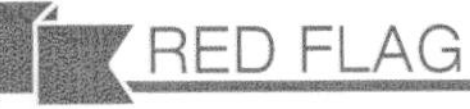

RED FLAG

The operative report includes details about the surgery performed. If the coder identifies details that indicate that the procedures should be billed separately, check the NCCI Edits first. Then decide which modifier should be reported.

HCPCS Level II modifiers associated with NCCI Edits are the following:

- Laterality modifiers;
- XE, *Separate encounter*;
- XS, *Separate structure*;
- XP, *Separate practitioner*;
- XU, *Unusual non-overlapping service.*

Encoder programs have NCCI Edits features that will help coders determine if the codes may be reported together. There are separate NCCI Edits for Medicaid. Medicaid edits are published quarterly on the Medicaid.gov website.

CONCEPTS CHECKPOINT **4.2**

Match the terms in the first column with the definitions in the second column.

1. _____ modifiers
2. _____ unbundling
3. _____ NCCI Edits

a. Two characters that are sometimes added to CPT® or HCPCS codes when the procedure, service, or item was altered from the code description

b. A tool that helps to prevent unbundling of services and procedures

c. The reporting of multiple CPT® codes when there is a single code that represents the complete procedure

CONCEPTS CHECKPOINT **4.3**

List 6 of the CPT® Surgery modifiers that are associated with NCCI edits.

1. _____
2. _____
3. _____
4. _____
5. _____
6. _____

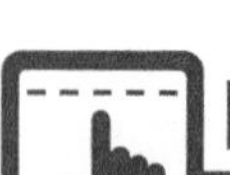

LET'S TRY ONE **4.1**

Using the NCCI Edits table below, write *yes* next to the code combinations that are allowed, write *no* next to the combinations that are not allowed, and place an *X* next the combinations that are not applicable.

1. _____ 45334 and 64550
2. _____ 45334 and 90772
3. _____ 45334 and 90783
4. _____ 45334 and 90784
5. _____ 45334 and 77001
6. _____ 45334 and 77002
7. _____ 45334 and 90760

Column 1	Column 2	* = In existence prior to 1996	Effective Date	Deletion Date * = no data	Modifier 0 = not allowed 1 = allowed 9 = not applicable
45334	64530		20090401	*	0
45334	64550		20090401	20090401	9
45334	69990		20000605	*	0
45334	76000		20091001	*	1
45334	76001		20091001	*	1
45334	77001		20110101	*	1
45334	77002		20110101	*	1
45334	90760		20060101	20081231	1
45334	90765		20060101	20081231	1
45334	90772		20060101	20081231	1
45334	90774		20060101	20081231	1
45334	90775		20060101	20081231	1
45334	90780		19960101	20041231	1
45334	90781		19960101	20041231	1
45334	90782		19960101	20041231	0
45334	90783		19960101	20041231	0
45334	90784		19960101	20041231	0

CPT® Modifiers

CPT® modifiers are 2-character numeric codes reported with CPT® codes to provide additional information to third-party payers. A coder might report a modifier if the service provided is different in some way from the CPT® code description, such as the service being greater than usually required. Adding a modifier may warrant an increase or decrease in payment, depending on the circumstances. Reporting the appropriate CPT® modifier with the code will notify the insurance payer that an adjustment in payment may be needed. Not all CPT® modifiers affect payment; some are informational only. A brief description of CPT® modifiers is located on the inside cover of most CPT® codebooks. A full description of each CPT® modifier is located in Appendix A of the CPT® codebook.

Modifier 22, *Increased Procedural Services*

Modifier 22 is used to describe services rendered that are substantially greater than what would normally be provided. Typically, the services include 2 or more of the following factors:

- unusually lengthy procedure;
- excessive blood loss relative to the procedure;
- presence of an excessively large surgical specimen;
- trauma extensive enough to complicate the procedure and not be billed as separate procedure codes;
- other pathologies, tumors, or malformations that directly interfere with the procedure but are not billed as separate procedure codes;
- services that are significantly more complex than comprised by the submitted CPT® or HCPCS code, with no recourse for reporting a second procedure code for the additional work.

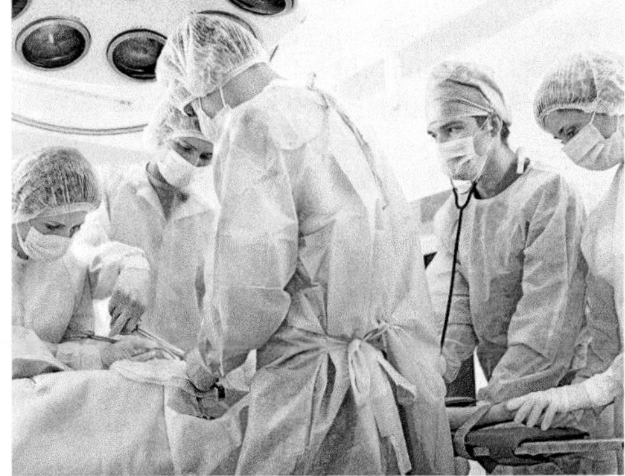

Modifier 22 may be used when there is excessive blood loss and a procedure is unusually lengthy or complicated. Documentation must support the reason for the increased procedural services.

Modifier 23, *Unusual Anesthesia*

This modifier is used to describe procedures that are usually performed without anesthesia or with local anesthesia (desensitizing a small body area) but due to special circumstances are performed with general anesthesia (induced state of unconsciousness) instead. Do not report this modifier with surgical codes. Only report modifier 23 with Anesthesia codes. Anesthesia will be described further in Chapter 7.

Modifier 24, *Unrelated E/M Service, Same Physician, During Postoperative Period*

Modifier 24 is used to indicate that the physician provided evaluation and management (E/M) care during the postoperative global period that was not related to the original procedure.

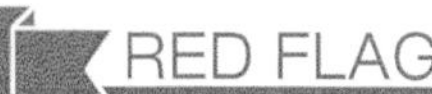

Coding Clicks

Coders must have a thorough knowledge of how the global period affects reimbursement. To read more about the global period, visit the Medical Learning Network at http://Coding.ParadigmEducation.com/MLNGlobalPeriod.

RED FLAG

The global period is the day before, day of, and days after a surgical procedure. The postoperative period is the days after a surgical procedure.

The **postoperative period** refers to the days after a procedure in which the physician is still managing the patient's corrected condition. The **global period** is a period of time in which follow-up visits after the original surgery may not be billed, unless services or procedures rendered are not part of the surgical package. The postoperative period is part of the global period. The difference is that the postoperative period begins the day after the procedure, and the global period begins the day before the procedure. The length of the global period is dependent on the procedure. Most diagnostic studies and some minor procedures have a 0-day global period, which means that the day of the procedure is the only day that is payable. E/M services on the same date of service as the minor surgical procedure are included in the payment for the procedure. Most minor surgeries have 10-day global periods, which is in fact 11 days—the day of the surgery plus 10 days of postoperative time. Major surgeries are usually 90 days, which is really 92 days—the day before the surgery, the day of the surgery, plus 90 days of postoperative time.

Add modifier 24 to the E/M procedure code under the following circumstances:

- An unrelated E/M service is performed by the same physician during the 0-, 10-, or 90-day global period.
- Documentation indicates the service was exclusively for treatment of the underlying condition and not for postoperative care.
- The same physician is managing immunosuppressant therapy or chemotherapy during the postoperative period of a transplant.
- The same physician provides unrelated critical care during the postoperative period.

EXAMPLE **4.1**

A 17-year-old male patient, who plays hockey for the local team, had treatment for a wrist fracture. This surgical procedure has 90 global days. The patient saw the same physician 45 days later with a sprained ankle; reporting of modifier 24 with the E/M code to evaluate and treat the sprained ankle is appropriate because the sprained ankle was not related to the wrist fracture. The code reported would be 99213, *Office or other outpatient visit for the evaluation and management of an established patient, which requires at least 2 of these 3 key components: An expanded problem focused history; An expanded problem focused examination; Medical decision making of low complexity,* with modifier 24, *Unrelated E/M service, same physician, during postoperative period*, appended.

Modifier 25, *Significant, Separately Identifiable E/M Service by the Same Physician on the Same Day of the Procedure or Other Service*

A physician may need to specify that on the day a procedure or service was performed, the patient's condition required a significant, separately identifiable E/M service above and beyond the other service provided or beyond the usual preoperative and postoperative care related to that procedure. Report both the primary service and the secondary E/M code. Append modifier 25 to the secondary E/M code. Modifier 25 is not used to report an E/M service that resulted in a decision to perform surgery. NCCI Edits will provide guidance when assigning this modifier.

EXAMPLE **4.2**

A 34-year-old established patient saw her gynecologist for her annual well-woman examination. The physician performed a comprehensive history and exam. In addition to the gynecological examination, a Papanicolaou (Pap) smear was collected. Preventative counseling on nutrition and reproductive health was provided. During the visit, the patient complained of foot pain, tenderness, and swelling. The physician found during the examination that the left foot was swollen. The patient was given a prescription for pain medication and scheduled to return in 2 weeks. The codes reported would be 99395, *Periodic comprehensive preventive medicine; age 18-39,* and 99212, *E/M established patients* (selected solely based only on services associated with the sprained foot). Modifier 25, *Significant, separately identifiable E/M service by the same physician on the same day of the procedure or other service* would be added to code 99212, so that 99395, 99212 - 25 was reported.

Modifier 26, *Professional Component*

Modifier 26, *Professional component,* is for certain procedures that require a combination of a physician or other qualified healthcare professional's services and a technical component. A global procedure is a procedure that clearly defines both the technical component and the professional component used to complete the procedure. In circumstances when only the technical component of services is rendered and the most accurate procedure code available is a global code, the global code would be reported with HCPCS Level II modifier TC, *Technical component.* In the same way, if a physician/provider supplies only the professional component, the global code would be reported with CPT® modifier 26, *Professional component.* For example, a patient has an x-ray performed in a physician's office. The physician looks at the x-ray film and writes a report. The physician reports the global code 71010, *Radiologic examination, chest; single view, frontal.* If the physician's office does not have x-ray equipment, the patient may go to an imaging center for the x-ray and bring the film back to the physician. Because code 71010 is a global code and the only code available that describes a single frontal view chest x-ray, both facilities report the same code. However, a modifier is added to the code to inform the insurance payer what portion of the chest x-ray global procedure each office performed to avoid overpayment. The imaging center reports code 70101 with HCPCS Level II modifier TC, *Technical component.* The physician's office reports the same code with modifier 26, *Professional component.* When the physician owns the equipment, purchases the supplies, and employs the technician, it is appropriate to report the global code without either modifier TC or 26. Finally, modifier 26 should not be appended to procedure codes that inherently represent only the professional component.

EXAMPLE 4.3

A polysomnography (sleep study) was performed on a 6-year-old patient at a certified sleep center. A physician who is not associated with the sleep center reviewed the diagnostic data and provided an interpretation of the findings and a written report. Because both the sleep center and the physician are reporting the same procedure code, for the same patient, to the same insurance payer, modifiers are needed to explain who provided the professional service and who provided the technical component:

- The sleep center bills the insurance payer for the services it provided with codes 95810 - TC, *Polysomnography; age 6 years or older, sleep staging with 4 or more additional parameters of sleep, attended by a technologist - Technical Component*.
- The reviewing physician reports 95810 - 26, *Polysomnography; age 6 years or older, sleep staging with 4 or more additional parameters of sleep, attended by a technologist - Professional Component*.

Think Like a Coder

Desmond is a registered health information technician (RHIT) who works as a coder in an orthopedic office. While having lunch in the break room, he hears the radiologist discussing with a coworker that the x-ray machine has been down for 2 days. He learns that patients who needed x-rays on Monday and Tuesday had to go to the imaging center on the first floor to get the x-rays done and bring the film back to the doctors to review. How does this affect how Desmond codes his records? What, if anything, should Desmond do?

Desmond spoke with his supervisor, who verified that what Desmond heard was true. Desmond will need to append modifier 26, *Professional component*, to x-ray codes for services on Monday and Tuesday because the physicians only interpreted the x-ray images. Knowingly billing the entire radiographic procedure when only the professional services were provided is fraud. Desmond took the time to verify the information and exhibited excellent coding ethics.

Modifier 27, *Multiple Outpatient Hospital E/M Encounters on the Same Date*

Modifier 27 is used when a patient receives multiple E/M services performed by the same or different physicians in the same or multiple outpatient hospital settings. Append modifier 27 to the second (and any subsequent) E/M code when more than 1 E/M service is provided. This will indicate that the second E/M service is a "separate and distinct E/M encounter" from the service previously provided that same day in the same or different hospital outpatient setting. Do not use modifier 27 to report multiple E/M services performed by the same physician on the same day in physician offices.

Modifier 32, *Mandated Services*

Modifier 32 is used for services related to mandated consultation and/or related services specifically requested by a third party, such as a disability determination examination. Examples of mandated services are examinations requested by government agencies or employers. Do not use modifier 32 when a patient seeks a second opinion for personal reasons, not specified by a third party.

Modifier 33, *Preventive Services*

Modifier 33 identifies preventive services without **cost sharing** (the patient pays no copay, deductible, or coinsurance). Do not report modifier 33 when reporting services specifically identified as preventive, such as E/M codes 99381 through 99397 that report preventive office visits. If multiple preventive services are performed on the same day, modifier 33 is appended to each preventive service or procedure code. Modifier 33 is also appended to preventive diagnostic procedures that are reported as surgical procedures because the physician collects a biopsy specimen or removes a polyp during the procedure. The modifier indicates that the procedure started as a preventive procedure. The example below shows how modifier 33 may be used.

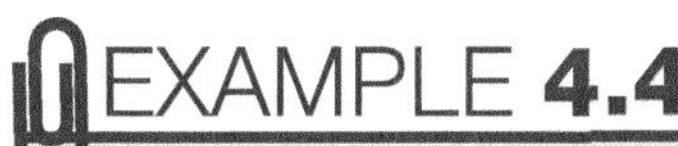

EXAMPLE **4.4**

A female patient had a screening colonoscopy (a visual exam of the colon) that resulted in a polypectomy (removal of polyps). Modifier 33 is appended to the polypectomy code, and the coder reports 45384 - 33, *Colonoscopy, flexible; with removal of tumor(s), polyp(s), or other lesion(s) by hot biopsy forceps - Preventive services*.

Coding for CMS

Medicare does not accept modifier 33. For a Medicare patient, if a diagnostic examination such as a colonoscopy leads to a surgical procedure such as a polypectomy, report the appropriate CPT® surgical code and append HCPCS modifier PT, *Colorectal cancer screening test; converted to diagnostic test or other procedure*.

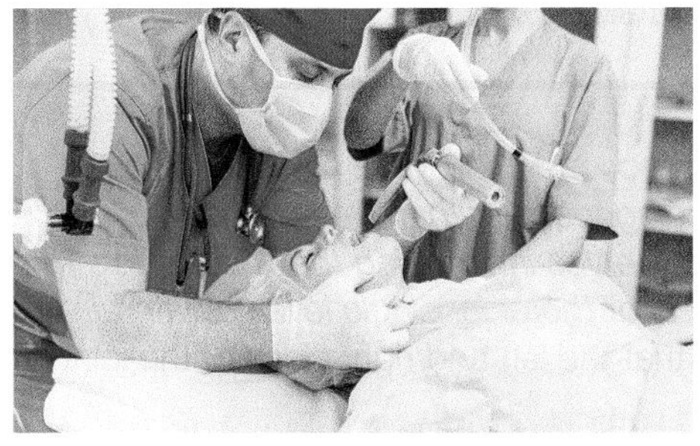

If a surgeon or assistant surgeon who is performing the procedure also administers general or regional anesthesia or moderate (conscious) sedation, modifier 47 may be used.

Modifier 47, *Anesthesia by Surgeon*

Anesthesia codes typically include a package of services rendered by an anesthesiologist (discussed in Chapter 7). Modifier 47 is used when the surgeon or assistant surgeon who is performing the procedure also administers general or regional anesthesia or moderate (conscious) sedation. Do not report for local anesthesia. Do not use modifier 47 if the surgeon is monitoring general anesthesia performed by an anesthesiologist, resident, or intern.

EXAMPLE 4.7

A physician performed a diagnostic flexible transoral esophagogastro-duodenoscopy (EGD). The procedure code includes the visual examination of the esophagus, stomach, and duodenum. During the procedure, the physician decided not to examine the duodenum due to the patient's excessive discomfort. Because the duodenum was not examined and a repeat procedure is not planned, the physician reports code 43235 - 52, *Esophagogastroduodenoscopy, flexible, transoral; diagnostic, including collection of specimen(s) by brushing and washing, when performed (separate procedure) - Reduced services*.

Modifier 53, *Discontinued Procedure*

When a physician determines that a surgical or diagnostic procedure should not be continued because it threatens the well-being of the patient, modifier 53 is appended to the discontinued procedure. Modifier 53 is used only when a procedure has been canceled or discontinued *after anesthesia* is administered for the specific reason of extenuating circumstances. For example, a patient may become hypotensive (develop low blood pressure) or experience arrhythmia (an irregular heartbeat) during the surgery. To preserve the life of the patient, the procedure is discontinued and the surgeon's attention turns to stabilizing the patient. If multiple procedures are scheduled, report only the procedure that was started and none of the other scheduled procedures that were not attempted.

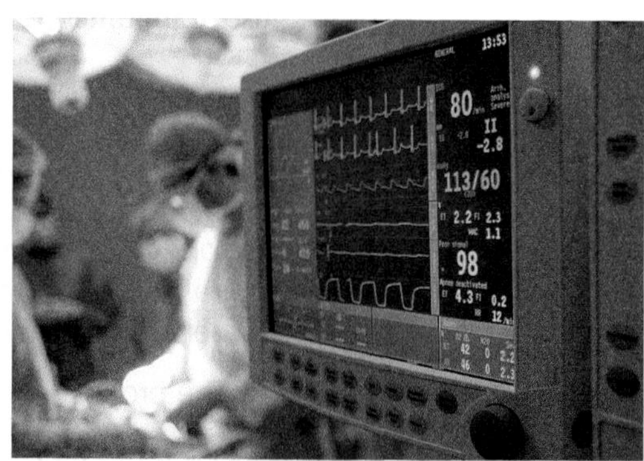

If a patient becomes hypotensive or experiences an arrhythmia during surgery, the procedure may be discontinued and would require modifier 53.

Modifier 54, *Surgical Care Only*

When a physician performs a surgical procedure and a different physician from a different physician practice provides preoperative and/or postoperative management, the surgeon appends modifier 54 to the surgical code to indicate that a reduction in reimbursement is warranted.

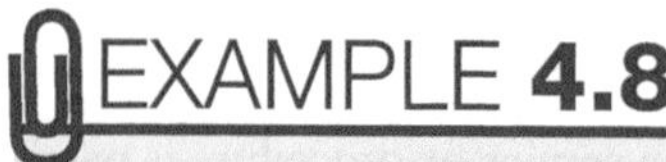

EXAMPLE 4.8

Dr. Jones performed an emergency appendectomy (a removal of the appendix) on a male patient who went to the hospital for severe abdominal pain. Dr. Jones referred the patient to Dr. Smith for postoperative care. Dr. Jones reported the "surgical package" code with modifier 54: 44950 - 54, *Appendectomy - Surgical care only*, which indicates that the surgeon performed only the surgery and did not provide the postoperative care.

Modifier 55, *Postoperative Management Only*

When a physician performs the postoperative management after another physician performs the surgical procedure, the physician who provides the postoperative care reports modifier 55 with the surgical procedure code. When modifier 55 is attached, dates of service must reflect the dates care was started and stopped. Modifier 55 applies only to procedures with 10- or 90-day global periods.

Modifier 56, *Preoperative Management Only*

Modifier 56 is used when a physician performs the preoperative care and evaluation and another physician performs the surgical procedure. When splitting care, the physician who provides the preoperative care appends modifier 56 to the surgical procedure code. Modifier 56 applies only to procedures with 10- or 90-day global periods.

LET'S TRY ONE **4.3**

Fill in the blank with the appropriate modifier.

1. A physician excised a 0.6-cm benign lesion on a patient's face and a 0.7-cm lesion on the nose. Which modifier would be appended to the secondary procedure? _____
2. A patient received postoperative care from a physician who did not perform the surgery. _____
3. A patient develops tachycardia after the administration of anesthesia. The surgeon cancels the procedure and the patient is sent to recovery. _____

Modifier 57, *Decision for Surgery*

Modifier 57 is used when an E/M service results in the initial decision to perform surgery. This modifier is used only with E/M codes when the service represents the initial decision to perform a major surgical procedure with a global period of 90 days. Preoperative services, including E/M services, provided on the day before or day of a major surgery are part of the surgical package and may not be billed separately. However, when the initial decision to perform a major surgery is made on the day of or day before the surgery, the associated E/M service may be reported by appending modifier 57 to the appropriate E/M code. When E/M services are provided on the same day as the initial decision for a minor surgery with a 0- to 10-day global period, use modifier 25, *Significant, separately identifiable evaluation and management service by the same physician or other qualified health care professional on the same day of the procedure or other service.*

Think Like a Coder

Deondre is a certified coding specialist (CCS) who works for an ophthalmologist. Dr. Johnson performs cataract surgeries. Deondre is coding a record in which Dr. Johnson documents that the patient is scheduled for cataract surgery the next day. The procedure has a 90-day global period. The electronic health record (EHR) system allows Deondre to review the previous date of service from 2 weeks ago. He reviews the patient's medical record and discovers that the decision for the surgery was made during the previous visit. Is modifier 57 needed for the date of service before the surgery? Was it appropriate for Deondre to look at the previous visit?

Modifier 58, *Staged or Related Procedure or Service by the Same Physician or Other Qualified Health Care Professional During the Postoperative Period*

Some conditions require more than 1 procedure, performed at different surgical sessions, to fully treat the patient. For example, some gastric bypass procedures are performed in 2 stages (see Chapter 13). Modifier 58 is used to identify the second planned surgery when performed by the same surgeon, during the same global period as the original procedure. NCCI Edits will provide guidance when assigning this modifier.

The procedure must meet the following requirements:

- A staged procedure is planned at the time of the original procedure.
- A staged procedure is more extensive than the original procedure.
- Therapy following a diagnostic surgical procedure is included.
- A second or related procedure is performed during the postoperative period.

EXAMPLE **4.9**

A patient had a large sacral ulcer. Debridement of the ulcer was performed on June 8. At the time of this debridement, the surgeon planned to treat the ulcer with a skin graft at a later date. On June 20, a split thickness graft was performed to treat the ulcer site.

The debridement was reported on June 8 with CPT® code 11043. The split thickness graft was reported on June 20 with code 15100 and modifier 58.

Modifier 59, *Distinct Procedural Service*

Under certain circumstances, the physician may need to indicate that a procedure or service was distinct or independent from other services performed on the same day. Modifier 59 is used to identify procedures/services that are not normally reported together but are appropriate under the circumstances.

The following criteria may represent appropriate uses of modifier 59:

- a different operative session;
- a different procedure or surgery;
- a different site or organ system;
- a separate incision or excision;
- a separate lesion;
- a separate injury not ordinarily encountered or treated the same day by the same individual.

Do not append modifier 59 to E/M codes. Do not use modifier 59 when a more descriptive modifier is available to clarify the services provided. NCCI Edits will provide guidance when assigning this modifier.

Coding for CMS

CMS states modifier 59 may be used to identify:

- different encounters;
- different anatomic sites;
- distinct services.

CMS has established 4 HCPCS modifiers (referred to collectively as X{EPSU} modifiers) to define specific subsets of modifier 59:

- XE, Separate encounter—a service that is distinct because it occurred during a separate encounter;
- XP, Separate practitioner—a service that is distinct because it was performed by a different practitioner;
- XS, Separate structure—a service that is distinct because it was performed on a separate organ/structure;
- XU, Unusual nonoverlapping service—the use of a service that is distinct because it does not overlap usual components of the main service.

CMS continues to recognize modifier 59 in many instances; however, it prefers that more specific modifiers, such as X{EPSU} modifiers, are used instead of modifier 59 whenever possible. Modifier 59 is the modifier of last resort.

For more specific instructions on modifier 59 and the X{EPSU} modifiers, read the CMS Manual System Transmittal 1422 at http://Coding.ParadigmEducation.com/Transmittal.

Modifier 62, *Two Surgeons*

When 2 surgeons work together as primary surgeons performing distinct part(s) of a single reportable procedure, each surgeon should report his or her distinct operative work by adding modifier 62 to the single procedure code. Each surgeon reports the procedure using the same procedure code. Additional and/or add-on procedures performed during the same surgical session may be reported with separate code(s) without modifier 62. Each surgeon dictates his or her own operative report. If a cosurgeon acts as an assistant in the performance of an additional procedure(s) during the same surgical session, do not use modifier 62.

Modifier 63, *Procedure Performed on Infants Less Than 4 kg*

Modifier 63 is used to report procedures performed on neonates and infants up to a present body weight of 4 kg. Modifier 63 may be reported with surgery codes 20000 through 69990. This modifier may not be reported with E/M, anesthesia, radiology, pathology/laboratory services, or medicine codes.

CONCEPTS CHECKPOINT **4.5**

Indicate if the statement is true or false.

1. _____ Modifier 58 is used only during the global period of the original procedure.
2. _____ If a cosurgeon acts as an assistant in the performance of additional procedure(s) during the same surgical session, use modifier 62.

List 3 appropriate uses of modifier 59.

3. ____________
4. ____________
5. ____________

Modifier 66, *Surgical Team*

Modifier 66 is used when a complicated single procedure requires more than 2 surgeons of different specialties. For example, a kidney transplant could involve the services of a general surgeon, a urologist, and/or a vascular surgeon to remove the diseased kidney, to implant the donated kidney, and to transplant the ureters. The procedure is reported by each surgeon, and each participating physician appends modifier 66 to the CPT® code. Most insurance payers require prior authorization for team surgery.

Modifier 73, *Discontinued Outpatient Hospital/Ambulatory Surgery Center (ASC) Procedure Prior to the Administration of Anesthesia*

Due to extenuating circumstances or those that threaten the well-being of the patient, the physician may cancel a surgical or diagnostic procedure subsequent to the patient's surgical preparation, which may include any sedation that has been given and transport to the operative facility but prior to the administration of anesthesia. Under these circumstances, the intended service that is prepared for, but canceled, can be reported by its CPT® code and modifier 73. The elective cancellation of a service prior to the administration of anesthesia and/or surgical preparation of the patient should not be reported. This modifier is appropriate only to report in outpatient settings or ambulatory surgery centers.

Modifier 74, *Discontinued Outpatient Hospital/Ambulatory Surgery Center (ASC) Procedure After Administration of Anesthesia*

Due to extenuating circumstances or those that threaten the well-being of the patient, the physician may terminate a surgical or diagnostic procedure after the administration of anesthesia or after the procedure was started. Under these circumstances, the procedure started but terminated can be reported by its usual CPT® code and the addition of modifier 74. The elective cancellation of a service prior to the administration of anesthesia and/or surgical preparation of the patient should not be reported.

Modifier 76, *Repeat Procedure by Same Physician or Other Qualified Health Care Professional*

Modifier 76 is used when the service or procedure is repeated the same day or during the postoperative period by the same physician. Medicare considers 2 physicians in the same group with the same specialty performing services on the same day as the same physician. Do not report modifier 51 for clinical laboratory tests on the same day.

Modifier 77, *Repeat Procedure by Another Physician or Other Qualified Health Care Professional*

Modifier 77 is used when the service or procedure is repeated the same day or during the postoperative period by a different physician. Modifier 77 may also be appended to x-ray and electrocardiogram (ECG) codes when the professional component is repeated by another physician, or the patient has 2 or more tests and more than 1 physician provides the interpretation and report. The following example is used by Medicare.

EXAMPLE **4.10**

A patient was admitted to the hospital and received 4 chest x-rays on a single day. The health record documentation shows the services were medically necessary, and 4 different radiologists provided an interpretation and report for each of the tests. The providers would append modifier 77 to the procedure code.

Modifier 78, *Unplanned Return to the Operating Room for a Related Procedure During the Postoperative Period*

In some circumstances, a physician may need to indicate that another procedure that is related to but not a repeat of the initial procedure was performed during the post-operative period of the initial procedure. Modifier 78 is used only when the related procedure is performed due to complications with the primary procedure. To report modifier 78, the procedure must be performed in an operating room. NCCI Edits will provide guidance when assigning this modifier.

EXAMPLE **4.11**

A partial colectomy (surgical removal of the large intestine) was performed on a Medicare patient in the hospital on March 1. The postoperative period for this procedure is 90 days. On March 15, the patient returned to the operating room for secondary suturing of the abdominal wall. The secondary suturing was related to the original surgery. The codes reported would be 44140, *Colectomy, partial; with anastomosis*; and 49900, *Suture, secondary, of abdominal wall for evisceration or dehiscence*. Modifier 78 would be appended to code 49900; the surgeon would report 44140 and 49900 - 78.

Modifier 79, *Unrelated Procedure or Service by the Same Physician or Other Qualified Health Care Professional During the Postoperative Period*

A physician may need to indicate that the performance of a procedure or service during the postoperative period was unrelated to the original procedure. If 2 or more unrelated procedures are performed during the global period, modifier 79 is appended to *all* unrelated procedures. When modifier 79 is reported, a new global period begins. NCCI Edits will provide guidance when assigning this modifier.

EXAMPLE **4.12**

A 75-year-old Medicare patient underwent cataract surgery on the right eye on May 14. The procedure code selected was 66984 - RT, *Extracapsular cataract removal with insertion of intraocular lens prosthesis, manual or mechanical technique - Right side*. On day 15 of the postoperative period, the patient complained of pain in the right eye. After examination, the surgeon discovered that the retina had detached, and the patient returned to the operating room for the repair. Code 67107 - *Repair of retinal detachment; scleral buckling (such as lamellar scleral dissection, imbrication or encircling procedure), including, when performed, implant, cryotherapy, photocoagulation, and drainage of subretinal fluid* would be reported with modifier 79; the coder would report 67107 - RT - 79.

Modifier 80, *Assistant Surgeon*

An "assistant at surgery" is a physician who actively assists the surgeon in charge of a case in performing a surgical procedure. Both surgeons report the procedure code, and modifier 80 is reported by the assistant surgeon who assists during the entire procedure. The assistant surgeon must be a licensed physician to report modifier 80. If the assistant at surgery is a physician assistant or a nurse practitioner, use HCPCS modifier AS, *Physician assistant, nurse practitioner, or clinical nurse specialist services for assistant at surgery*. Not all procedures qualify for the use of an assistant at surgery; refer to the MPFS for guidance on assigning modifier 80.

Modifier 81, *Minimum Assistant Surgeon*

Modifier 81 is used when the primary surgeon did not expect to need assistance from another surgeon, but circumstances during surgery arose that required another surgeon. Report only when an assistant surgeon was used for a short amount of time. The procedure code is reported by both physicians. The assistant surgeon appends modifier 81 to the procedure code.

Modifier 82, *Assistant Surgeon (When Qualified Resident Surgeon Not Available)*

When an assistant to surgery is required in a teaching hospital, a qualified resident surgeon must be utilized. If a qualified resident surgeon is not available, a licensed surgeon may assist with the surgery. This assistant surgeon reports the procedure code with modifier 82 appended. Documentation must support that a resident surgeon was unavailable for the procedure. Modifier 82 is applicable only for procedures in teaching facilities. If a teaching facility does not have an approved training program related to the medical specialty required for a surgical procedure, modifier 82 is reported by the assistant surgeon. Assistant surgeons are not allowed for some procedures, and coders should reference the MPFS prior to appending modifier 82.

Modifier 90, *Reference (Outside) Laboratory*

Physicians use modifier 90 when laboratory procedures are performed by a party other than the treating or reporting physician. Append modifier 90 to laboratory work when the physician bills the patient directly for laboratory tests that were performed in an outside laboratory. Not all payers recognize this billing method. Coders should consult their payer contract or payer manuals prior to billing.

Modifier 91, *Repeat Clinical Diagnostic Laboratory Test*

In the course of treatment of the patient, it may be necessary to repeat the same laboratory test on the same day to obtain subsequent (multiple) test results. Under these circumstances, the laboratory test performed can be identified by its usual procedure code and the addition of modifier 91. NCCI edits will provide guidance when assigning this modifier.

Modifier 91 is not intended to report test reruns for the following purposes:

- to confirm initial results;
- due to testing problems with specimens or equipment;
- for any other reason when a normal, one-time, reportable result is all that is required.

Modifier 91 may not be used when there is a HCPCS or a CPT® code that describes a series of results.

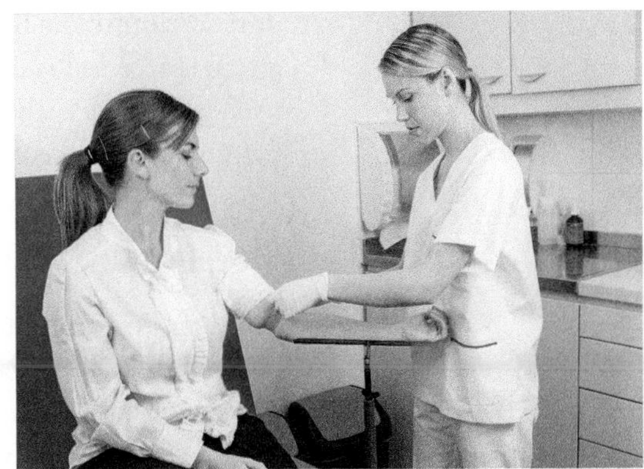

When laboratory tests are repeated, such as when monitoring a patient on a blood thinner medication, modifier 91 may need to be appended to the procedure code.

EXAMPLE **4.13**

A patient was on Coumadin, a blood thinner medication. The physician ordered a weekly prothrombin time blood test to monitor effects of the medication on the patient. The first test indicated the results were out of range. The physician instructed the patient to increase his dosage and return to the office at the end of the day for a repeat test. The patient returned just before closing and had a second test. The results were within range.

In addition to reporting the code for the office visit, the physician also reports code 85610, *Prothrombin time*. Modifier 91 is appended to the second listed 85610.

Modifier 92, *Alternative Laboratory Platform Testing*

Modifier 92 is used when laboratory testing is performed using a kit or transportable instrument that wholly or partially consists of a single-use, disposable analytical chamber. CMS recognizes modifier 92 only when used to report the use of portable HIV tests that provide instant results. Coders should check with commercial payer policy prior to reporting modifier 92. Testing location is not significant when reporting this modifier.

CMS recognizes modifier 92 when reported with the following HIV test codes:

- 86701, *Antibody; HIV-1*;
- 86702, *Antibody; HIV-2*;
- 86703, *Antibody HIV-1 and HIV-2*, single result.

Modifier 95, *Synchronous Telemedicine Service Rendered Via a Real-time Interactive Audio and Video Telecommunications System*

Modifier 95 is reported with appropriate CPT® codes to certify that the beneficiary was physically located at an eligible originating site during the telehealth service. Eligible originating sites include Rural Health Clinics and a county outside of a Metropolitan Statistical Area.

Patients with end stage renal disease (ESRD) may receive dialysis, a mechanical procedure to cleanse the blood, several times a week. The location where the patient's vein or artery is accessed is called a *vascular access*. When reporting Modifier 95 with an ESRD telehealth service, the provider certifies that they conducted a minimum of 1 physical examination of the vascular access site per month.

Modifier 96, *Habilitative Services*

Modifier 96 is reported when a service or procedure that may be either habilitative or rehabilitative in nature is provided for habilitative purposes. **Habilitative services** are offered to help patients develop, maintain, and/or improve skills that assist with functions for daily living and then keep and/or improve those learned skills.

Modifier 97, *Rehabilitative Services*

Modifier 97 is reported with the appropriate service or procedure that may be either habilitative or rehabilitative in nature is provided for rehabilitative purposes. **Rehabilitative services** help patients maintain, regain, or improve skills and functions for daily living that were affected due to an injury, illness, or disability.

Modifier 99, *Multiple Modifiers*

Modifier 99 is reported when more than 1 modifier is required to fully describe altered services or procedures. Modifier 99 is listed first, followed by the other modifiers in numerical order. Always list modifiers that affect reimbursement as the first modifier following modifier 99. For example, if a procedure required the reporting of modifiers

51, 59, and 80, the coder would report modifier 99, followed by the other modifiers in the following order:

- 99, *Multiple modifiers*;
- 51, *Multiple procedures*;
- 59, *Distinct procedural service*;
- 80, *Assistant surgeon*.

Prior to reporting modifier 99, review the payer's claim submission policy. Some payer systems allow for multiple modifiers without reporting modifier 99.

LET'S TRY ONE **4.4**

Fill in the blank with the appropriate modifier.

1. Each surgeon reports modifier _____ when performing team surgery.
2. Dr. Adams performed a procedure in the morning and the procedure needed to be repeated in the afternoon. Dr. Adams was not available so Dr. Brown performed the same procedure on the same day as the original surgery. Dr. Adams reports the procedure with modifier _____.

HCPCS Modifiers

HCPCS Level II modifiers are 2-character alphabetic or alphanumeric codes used to report everything from anatomical locations of procedures to maintenance of medical equipment. HCPCS modifiers may be reported with CPT® and HCPCS Level II codes.

The HCPCS Level II codebook does not categorize the modifiers and instead lists them alphabetically. Within the alphabetic list, modifiers related to specific services are grouped together; for example, A1 through A9 all relate to wound dressings. Coders must become familiar with modifiers that are common to their coding specialties.

There are more than 300 HCPCS modifiers. A full description of HCPCS modifiers is located in the HCPCS Level II codebook. HCPCS modifiers approved for hospital outpatient services and procedures are also listed in the front cover of the CPT® codebook.

Guidelines for Reporting Multiple HCPCS Modifiers

Coding Clicks

To learn more about pricing and informational modifiers, visit the Wisconsin Physicians Service Insurance Corporation (WPS) Medicare website at http://Coding.ParadigmEducation.com/WPS.

When reporting multiple HCPCS modifiers, it is important to distinguish between pricing modifiers and informational modifiers. **Pricing modifiers** affect payment of services and determine the allowance of services billed and should always be placed in the first modifier field. Table 4.4 lists pricing modifiers. **Informational modifiers** provide additional information; may state whether a service is reasonable and necessary; and should be used in the second, third, or fourth modifier field. List pricing modifiers that affect reimbursement first in alphanumeric order, then list informational modifiers in alphanumeric order. CPT® and HCPCS Level II modifiers may be reported together, in which case always report modifiers that affect reimbursement first, followed by the informational modifiers.

Table 4.4 HCPCS and CPT® Pricing Modifiers

Modifier	Description
AA	*Anesthesia service performed personally by anesthesiologist*
AD	*Medical supervision by a physician: more than four concurrent anesthesia procedures*
AS*	*Physician assistant, nurse practitioner, or clinical nurse specialist services for assistant at surgery*
KD**	*Drug or biological infused through DME*
QK	*Medical direction of two, three, or four concurrent anesthesia procedures involving qualified individuals*
QW	*CLIA waived tests*
QX	*CRNA service: with medical direction by a physician*
QY	*Medical direction of one CRNA by an anesthesiologist*
QZ	*CRNA service: without medical direction by a physician*
TC	*Technical component*
26	*Professional component*
50*	*Bilateral procedure* performed at the same session on an anatomical site
53	*Discontinued procedure* (only when appended to procedure codes 45378, G0105, and G0121)
54*	*Surgical care only* (The surgeon is billing the surgical care only.)
55*	*Postoperative management only* (indicates a physician other than the surgeon is billing for part of the outpatient postoperative care) Or: Used by the surgeon when providing only a portion of the post-discharge postoperative care
62*	*Two surgeons* (each in a different specialty are required to perform a specific procedure)
66*	*Surgical team* surgeons
73*	*Discontinued outpatient hospital/ambulatory surgery center (ASC) procedure prior to the administration of anesthesia*
78*	*Unplanned return to an operating room for a related procedure during the postoperative period*
80*	*Assistant surgeon* (assistant at surgery service is provided by a medical doctor [MD])
81*	*Minimum assistant surgeon* (to identify minimum surgical assistant services; submitted only with surgery codes)
82*	*Assistant surgeon (when qualified resident surgeon not available)* (assistant at surgery service provided by a MD when there is no qualified resident available)

Abbreviations: CLIA, Clinical Laboratory Improvement Amendments; CRNA, certified registered nurse anesthetist; DME, durable medical equipment.

*These payment modifiers are not limited to the first position. (If there is another pricing modifier submitted that is required to be in the first modifier field, these modifiers should be in the second, third, or fourth modifier position.)

**If multiple pricing or payment modifiers are submitted, the KD modifier should be placed in the first modifier position field.

Source: Adapted from Wisconsin Physicians Service Insurance Corporation, "Pricing or Payment Modifier Fact Sheet," WPSMedicare.com, accessed January 10, 2015, at http://www.wpsmedicare.com/j8macpartb/resources/modifiers/pricingmodifiers.shtml. Reprinted with permission.

Ambulance Services Modifiers

Ambulance modifiers are different from other modifiers. Single alpha characters represent locations that are paired to report the origin and destination of the ambulance service as a single 2-character modifier. The first letter represents the location where the ambulance picked up or serviced the patient. The second character represents the final destination of the ambulance. Table 4.5 contains the list of single-character ambulance codes.

There are a few HCPCS modifiers that may be reported in conjunction with the ambulance modifiers. These modifiers are listed in Table 4.6.

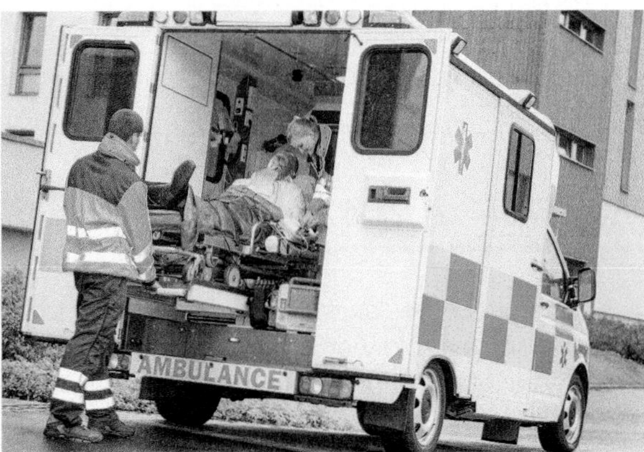

Ambulance modifiers are different from other modifiers and require knowing the origin and destination of the ambulance.

Table 4.5 HCPCS Single-Character Ambulance Codes

Code	Origin or Destination
D	Diagnostic or therapeutic site other than codes "P" or "H"
E	Residential, domiciliary, custodial facility, nursing home (other than 1819 facility)
G	Hospital-based dialysis facility (hospital or hospital related) that includes: • Hospital administered/hospital located • Nonhospital administered/nonhospital located
H	Hospital
I	Site of transfer (eg, airport, ferry, or helicopter pad) between modes of ambulance transport
J	Nonhospital-based dialysis facility • Nonhospital administered/nonhospital located • Hospital administered/hospital located
N	Skilled nursing facility (SNF) (1819 facility)
P	Physician's office (includes HMO nonhospital facility, clinic, etc.)
R	Residence
S	Scene of accident or acute event
X	Destination code only. Intermediate stop at physician's office en route to the hospital (includes HMO nonhospital facility, clinic, etc.)

Table 4.6 HCPCS Modifiers Reportable With Ambulance Modifiers

Modifier	Description
GY	Use when billing for a statutorily excluded service. Example: Patient transport is for a noncovered condition that does not meet the definition of any Medicare benefit. The provider is expecting a denial.
QL	Use when the patient is pronounced deceased after the ambulance is called but before transport. Ground providers can bill a basic life support service along with the QL modifier.
GM	Use when more than 1 patient is transported in an ambulance and document details of the transport; can be used by both ground and air transports.
GA	The provider or supplier has provided an Advance Beneficiary Notice of Noncoverage (ABN) to the patient.
GZ	The provider or supplier expects a medical necessity denial but did not provide an ABN to the patient.

EXAMPLE **4.14**

St. Francis Hospital Ambulance Service responded to an emergency call to the residence of a 65-year-old woman with severe chest pains. The ambulance service arrived at the patient's home, provided basic life support, and transported her to the hospital. The HCPCS code is A0429, *Ambulance service, basic life support, emergency transport (BLS-Emergency)*; append HCPCS ambulance modifier RH (origin is R, *Residence*, and destination is H, *Hospital*).

Advance Beneficiary Notice of Noncoverage (ABN) Modifiers

Coding Clicks

Coders rarely complete ABN forms, but they do correlate modifiers with the status of the forms when an ABN is associated with a claim. Therefore, it is useful to review the instructions on completing the form. Read the Medicare Learning Network booklet on how to complete the ABN form at http://Coding.ParadigmEducation.com/ABN.

An **Advance Beneficiary Notice of Noncoverage (ABN)** is a standard notice that a healthcare provider or vendor must give to a Medicare beneficiary before providing certain services or procedures that Medicare may deem not medically necessary or reasonable. By signing the completed form, the patient acknowledges that (a) they are aware that the healthcare provider recommended the service, procedure, or item; (b) they have been notified of the cost of the item; (c) they understand that Medicare may not reimburse the provider or vendor; and (d) they either agree or disagree to accept the services, procedure, or item. If they agree, the provider or vendor may bill the patient directly if the services are not reimbursed. If they refuse the service, procedure, or item, the form is kept for documentation that the physician recommended a specific service or procedure. Figure 4.3 illustrates the official CMS ABN, Form CMS-R-131.

The ABN form is valid only when the following criteria are met:

- The ABN is issued prior to the procedure, service, or item rendered to the beneficiary.
- The ABN is issued in a timely manner so that the content of the form may be discussed and all of the patient's questions and concerns can be addressed.
- All areas of the ABN that require completion by the provider or vendor are filled in prior to the patient reviewing and signing the form.

Figure 4.3 Advance Beneficiary Notice of Noncoverage (ABN)

A. Notifier: ______________

B. Patient Name: ______________ **C. Identification Number:** ______________

Advance Beneficiary Notice of Noncoverage (ABN)

NOTE: If Medicare doesn't pay for **D.** ______________ below, you may have to pay.
Medicare does not pay for everything, even some care that you or your health care provider have good reason to think you need. We expect Medicare may not pay for the **D.** ______________ below.

D.	**E. Reason Medicare May Not Pay:**	**F. Estimated Cost**

WHAT YOU NEED TO DO NOW:

- Read this notice, so you can make an informed decision about your care.
- Ask us any questions that you may have after you finish reading.
- Choose an option below about whether to receive the **D.** ______________ listed above.

Note: If you choose Option 1 or 2, we may help you to use any other insurance that you might have, but Medicare cannot require us to do this.

G. Options: **Check only one box. We cannot choose a box for you.**

☐ **OPTION 1.** I want the **D.** ______________ listed above. You may ask to be paid now, but I also want Medicare billed for an official decision on payment, which is sent to me on a Medicare Summary Notice (MSN). I understand that if Medicare doesn't pay, I am responsible for payment, but **I can appeal to Medicare** by following the directions on the MSN. If Medicare does pay, you will refund any payments I made to you, less co-pays or deductibles.

☐ **OPTION 2.** I want the **D.** ______________ listed above, but do not bill Medicare. You may ask to be paid now as I am responsible for payment. **I cannot appeal if Medicare is not billed.**

☐ **OPTION 3.** I don't want the **D.** ______________ listed above. I understand with this choice I am **not** responsible for payment, and **I cannot appeal to see if Medicare would pay.**

H. Additional Information:

This notice gives our opinion, not an official Medicare decision. **If you have other questions on this notice or Medicare billing, call** 1-800-MEDICARE **(1-800-633-4227/**TTY: **1-877-486-2048).**
Signing below means that you have received and understand this notice. You also receive a copy.

I. Signature:	**J. Date:**

According to the Paperwork Reduction Act of 1995, no persons are required to respond to a collection of information unless it displays a valid OMB control number. The valid OMB control number for this information collection is 0938-0566. The time required to complete this information collection is estimated to average 7 minutes per response, including the time to review instructions, search existing data resources, gather the data needed, and complete and review the information collection. If you have comments concerning the accuracy of the time estimate or suggestions for improving this form, please write to: CMS, 7500 Security Boulevard, Attn: PRA Reports Clearance Officer, Baltimore, Maryland 21244-1850.

Form CMS-R-131 (03/11) Form Approved OMB No. 0938-0566

Print Form

Modifiers GA, GX, GY, or GZ are reported with a procedure or service code to identify the status of an ABN form. The ABN modifiers do not appear on the ABN form; rather, they are reported on the insurance claim for Medicare patients, as shown in Table 4.7.

Table 4.7 Claim Modifiers Associated With ABN Use

ABN Status	Modifier to Report	Modifier Description
An item/service is expected to be denied as not reasonable and necessary and a mandatory ABN is on file	GA	*Waiver of liability statement issued as required by payer policy, individual case*
A voluntary ABN is issued for a service Medicare never covers as statutorily excluded or does not meet the definition of any Medicare benefit; you may use this modifier in combination with modifier GY	GX	*Notice of liability issued, voluntary under payer policy*
Medicare statutorily excludes the service, procedure, or item, or it is not a Medicare benefit; you may use this modifier in combination with modifier GX	GY	*Item or service statutorily excluded, does not meet the definition of any Medicare benefit or, for non-Medicare insurers, is not a contract benefit*
Medicare will deny payment of the item or service due to a lack of medical necessity and no ABN was issued	GZ	*Item or service expected to be denied as not reasonable and necessary*

Modifier Q6, *Service Furnished by a Locum Tenens Physician*

A **locum tenens physician** is a substitute physician when a regular physician is not able to care for a patient due to extenuating circumstances. A "regular physician" is the physician who is normally scheduled to see a patient. A locum tenens physician generally has no practice of his or her own and offers services to a regular physician as an independent contractor. The regular physician may bill and receive payment from a third-party payer for the substitute's services. Modifier Q6, *Service furnished by a locum tenens physician*, is appended to all reported codes representing the services or procedures provided by the substitute physician. All services and procedures are billed under the absent physician's National Provider Identification (NPI) number.

A substitute physician's services are reimbursable under the following circumstances:

- A physician agrees to see patients of another physician under a per-diem or similar fee-for-time arrangement.
- The regular physician is not available to provide patient services.
- The Medicare patient is scheduled to see the absent physician.
- Short-term (fewer than 60 days) coverage is provided by the substitute physician.
- Modifier Q6 must be used with the procedure code to identify the services as substitute physician services.

If the absent physician has patients in the hospital, the substitute may treat those patients in the hospital only if he or she is credentialed by that hospital where the patient is being treated. If a substitute physician does not have privileges at the hospital, the absent physician must make other arrangements for the care of the hospitalized patients.

EXAMPLE **4.15**

Patients were scheduled with their regular physician, Dr. Smith, who took a leave of absence due to extenuating circumstances. Dr. Jones, who is working as a locum tenens, treats all patients scheduled with Dr. Smith during Dr. Smith's absence. He bills using Dr. Smith's National Provider Identification and appends modifier Q6 to each CPT® or HCPCS Level II code for the procedures he performed.

RED FLAG

Do not submit the technical component separately when 1 physician performs both the professional and technical components on the same day. The single global CPT® code is reported without a modifier.

Modifier TC, *Technical Component*

Modifier TC, *Technical component*, identifies that only the technical component of a global procedure was provided. A global procedure is a procedure that clearly defines both the technical component and the professional component used to complete the procedures. When only the technical component was performed and the most accurate procedure code available is a global code, report the global code and append modifier TC. If a code exists that describes only the technical component of a procedure, do not append modifier TC. CPT® modifier 26 identifies the professional component of a global procedure.

Procedures that have technical components are found in the following CPT® sections:

- Surgery;
- Pathology and Laboratory;
- Radiology;
- Medicine.

EXAMPLE 4.16

A polysomnography (sleep study) was performed at a certified sleep center. A physician who is not associated with the sleep center interpreted the findings and created a written report. The certified sleep center reports 95811 - TC, *Polysomnography - Technical component*, and the physician reports 95811 - 26, *Polysomnography - Professional component*.

Modifier 59 Subset Modifiers

Modifier 59 subset modifiers are used instead of appending modifier 59 to a CPT surgical code. Appending modifier 59 allows the provider to request reimbursement for procedures that are not typically billed together. By appending the appropriate subset modifier, insurance payers can quickly identify why the 2 procedures are reported separately. Refer back to the CPT modifier section of this chapter to review modifier 59 guidelines.

The subset of modifiers that can be used instead of modifier 59 are:

- XE, *Separate encounter*, a service that is distinct because it occurred during a separate encounter;
- XP, *Separate practitioner*, a service that is distinct because it was performed by a different practitioner;
- XS, *Separate structure*, a service that is distinct because it was performed on a separate organ/structure;
- XU, *Unusual non-overlapping service*, the use of a service that is distinct because it does not overlap usual components of the main service.

HCPCS Laterality Modifiers

HCPCS Level II **laterality modifiers** are used to report anatomical location—that is, the side of the body on which a procedure was performed. For example, LT, *Left side*, is considered a laterality modifier. HCPCS Level II and CPT® codes do not specify laterality in the code descriptions. To identify laterality, a HCPCS modifier must be appended to the procedure code. Below is a list of laterality modifiers.

RT, *Right side* (used to identify procedures performed on the right side of the body);

LT, *Left side* (used to identify procedures performed on the left side of the body);

LC, *Left circumflex coronary artery*;

LD, *Left anterior descending coronary artery*;

LM, *Left main coronary artery*;

RC, *Right coronary artery*;

RI, *Ramus intermediate coronary artery*;

E1, *Upper left, eyelid*;

E2, *Lower left, eyelid;*

E3, *Upper right, eyelid;*

E4, *Lower right, eyelid;*

FA, *Left hand, thumb;*

F1, *Left hand, second digit;*

F2, *Left hand, third digit;*

F3, *Left hand, fourth digit;*

F4, *Left hand, fifth digit;*

F5, *Right hand, thumb;*

F6, *Right hand, second digit;*

F7, *Right hand, third digit;*

F8, *Right hand, fourth digit;*

F9, *Right hand, fifth digit;*

TA, *Left foot, great toe;*

T1, *Left foot, second digit;*

T2, *Left foot, third digit;*

T3, *Left foot, fourth digit;*

T4, *Left foot, fifth digit;*

T5, *Right foot, great toe;*

T6, *Right foot, second digit;*

T7, *Right foot, third digit;*

T8, *Right foot, fourth digit;*

T9, *Right foot, fifth digit.*

LET'S TRY ONE **4.5**

Match the HCPCS modifier with the correct scenario.

1. _____ E2
2. _____ TC
3. _____ Q6
4. _____ GZ

a. Radiology performs the x-ray and sends it to the physician to interpret and create a written report.

b. Dr. Jones is a locum tenens physician working in place of Dr. Smith.

c. The physician closes a wound on the lower left eyelid.

d. An ABN was not completed by the nurse or the patient for a service that was not covered by Medicare.

Chapter Summary

- Modifiers are the 2-character codes that are sometimes added to CPT® or HCPCS codes when the procedure, service, or item was altered from the code description. Modifiers supply payers with more information about services or procedures performed.
- NCCI Edits are a tool that helps to prevent unbundling of services and procedures. CMS publishes Medicare edits in the National Correct Coding Initiative Policy Manual for Medicare Services.
- Unbundling occurs when multiple CPT® codes are reported instead of the single code that represents the complete procedure.
- CPT® modifiers inform the insurance payer that the description of the reported code has been altered. CPT® modifiers consist of 2 numeric characters.
- The postoperative period is the time after the procedure. Global periods range from the day before a procedure to the end of the postoperative period, depending on the procedure.
- An Advance Beneficiary Notice of Noncoverage (ABN) is a standardized notice that a healthcare provider or vendor must give to a Medicare beneficiary before providing certain services or procedures that Medicare may deem not medical necessary or reasonable.
- A locum tenens physician is a substitute physician. Locum tenens are used when a regular physician is not able to care for a patient due to extenuating circumstances.
- A global procedure has a clearly defined technical component and professional component used to complete the procedure.

Navigator

Access interactive chapter review exercises, practice activities, flash cards, and study games.

Chapter 5

Using the Health Record to Report Codes

Fast Facts

- Physicians see an average of 50–99 patients per week and generate approximately 975 new pages of paperwork each week.
- A 2013 survey conducted by the Health Information and Management Systems Society (HIMSS) showed that 70% of physicians agreed that health information technology (HIT) applications, such as electronic health records (EHRs), improved their ability to care for patients.
- The survey also found that 80% of physicians agreed that with EHRs, they were more easily able to process data and improve access to information contained in patient records.

Source: http://hitconsultant.net

Crack the Code

Review the sample procedure note to find the correct code. You may need to return to this exercise after reading the chapter content.

PROCEDURE NOTE: Incision and drainage, infected cyst, left external ear

This 28-year-old male developed a lump anterior to his left ear over the last week. It is painful to him. Denies fever or chills. Inspection of the ear area reveals a 2-cm size lump just in the pre-auricular area of the external ear. It is tender to palpation; it is fluctuant. No cellulitis or erythema is present. Area is cleansed, local infiltration with 1% Xylocaine for anesthesia is performed. Area is incised with a #11 blade. A large amount of purulent material is expressed. Samples taken for culture and sensitivity. Loculations are broken up. Incision is irrigated and Iodoform is packed. Band-Aid applied. Patient advised to return to have packing removed in 1 day.

answer: 69000-LT

Learning Objectives

5.1 Define the health record and explain the types of content the health record contains.

5.2 Define and provide examples of the different types of clinical documentation.

5.3 Explain the standards and regulations related to clinical documentation.

5.4 Define the parts of the operative report.

5.5 Practice abstracting information from an operative report and explain how to report codes based on that information.

5.6 Explain the benefits of reporting codes from EHRs.

5.7 Explain how various forms of technology have improved the process of reporting medical codes.

Chapter Outline

Understanding the Health Record

A **health record**, also known as a **medical record**, is a legal document that contains descriptions of all the products and services provided to a patient. The format of a health record can be paper, electronic, or a combination of paper and electronic formats referred to as a **hybrid record**. An **electronic health record (EHR)** collects patient data in a computerized format designed to facilitate sharing across a continuum of healthcare entities. Figure 5.1 illustrates a typical EHR screen. The location of data in paper and electronic records may vary, but the type of information contained in each format is standardized.

Healthcare providers are responsible for maintaining accurate and complete health records for all of their patients. Health records contain a vast amount of clinical, administrative, financial, and legal data:

- **clinical data:** the documentation of the care provided to the patient (these data are used as a communication tool among providers to ensure continuity of patient care;

Figure 5.1 EHR Charts Screen

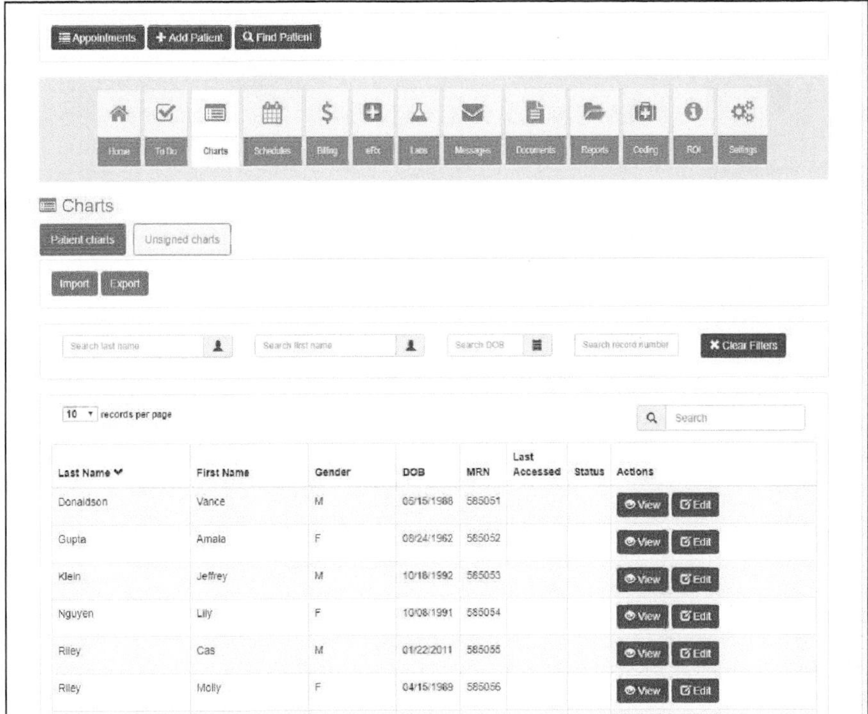

- **administrative data:** patient demographic information needed to provide patient care and for billing and reimbursement;
- **financial data:** the information about who is responsible for payment for the treatment provided;
- **legal data:** the patient's consent for treatment and the provider's notice of privacy practices.

Maintaining complete health records is important for ensuring continuity of care and also for complete and accurate billing. All treatment and/or supplies provided to a patient must be recorded in the health record; otherwise, the patient and his or her insurance company will not be charged and the healthcare facility will not be reimbursed. Medical codes may only be reported based on the documentation in the health record. This chapter will focus on administrative data and the content and structure of clinical data, as these forms of data are most relevant to coding.

Administrative Data

Administrative data includes identifying information such as the patient's full name, address, date of birth, gender, marital status, place of employment, insured status, payment arrangements, and other personal details that the facility or provider wishes to collect. Verification of administrative and financial data is the first step in the **revenue cycle,** the time frame that comprises the patient encounter through the final bill for services. This information should be verified at each patient visit, as bills sent to the wrong address or insurance company will delay reimbursement. Figure 5.2 is an example of a registration form used to collect administrative data in a healthcare facility.

Figure 5.2 Patient Registration Form

For Office Use Only:
MRUN: ________
Registrar: ______

EMC
Medical Center

EMC MEDICAL CENTER

Patient Registration Form

PATIENT INFORMATION

Patient's Last Name / First / Middle Initial		Type of Care: ❑ Inpatient ❑ Maternity ❑ Outpatient ❑ Same-Day Surgery ❑ Surgery	
Race / Marital Status / Religion / Primary Language		Date of Birth (mm/dd/yyyy)	Date of Scheduled Visit
Physician's Last Name / First Name		❑ Female ❑ Male	Social Security No.
Patient's Street Address / Apt. No.		City / State	ZIP
Home Phone ( ) / Work Phone ( ) / Cell Phone ( )		Visit Reason or Diagnosis	Admission Date
Temporary Address / Apt. No.		City / State	ZIP
Patient's Current Employer Name	Employer Address	City / State	ZIP
Employer Phone ( )	Patient's Occupation	Employment Status: ❑ Not Employed ❑ Full Time ❑ Part Time ❑ Student ❑ Retired and Date:	
Full Name of Emergency Contact	Relationship	Home Phone ( )	Work Phone ( )
Have you ever been a patient at EMC Medical Center? ❑ Yes ❑ No		If yes, when was your last visit?	Under what name?

Guarantor

Last Name / First / Middle Initial		Relationship	Date of Birth (mm/dd/yyyy)
Street Address / Apt. No.		❑ Female ❑ Male	Marital Status / Social Security No.
City / State / ZIP	Home Phone ( )	Work Phone ( )	Cell Phone ( )
Employer Name	Employer Address	City	State / ZIP
Employer Phone ( )	Occupation	Employment Status: ❑ Not Employed ❑ Full Time ❑ Part Time ❑ Student ❑ Retired and Date:	

Insurance Information

Primary Insurance Name		Name of Insured (exactly as it appears on card)	
Insurance Billing Address / City		State / ZIP	Phone No. ( )
Policy No. / Group No.	Plan Code	State / Effective Date	Expiration Date
Subscriber's Full Name	Subscriber's Soc. Sec. No.	Subscriber's Date of Birth (mm/dd/yyyy)	❑ Female ❑ Male
Subscriber's Employer Name (if self-employed, company name)	Relation to Insured	Subscriber's Employment Status: ❑ Not Employed ❑ Full Time ❑ Part Time ❑ Student ❑ Retired and Date:	
Subscriber's Employer Address / City		State / ZIP	Phone No. ( )

Effective Date (mm/dd/yyyy)
________ ❑ Part A (Hospital Benefit)
________ ❑ Part B (Medical Benefit)

Effective Date   State

Name of Insured (exactly as it appears on card)

State   ZIP   Phone No. ( )

State   Effective Date   Expiration Date

No.   Subscriber's Date of Birth (mm/dd/yyyy)   ❑ Female ❑ Male

Subscriber's Employment Status: ❑ Not Employed ❑ Full Time ❑ Part Time ❑ Student ❑ Retired and Date:

State   ZIP   Phone No. ( )

Date of Accident: (mm/dd/yyyy)   Claim No.

Phone No. ( )   Insurance Name

State   ZIP   Phone No. ( )

Advance Directive

Do you have an Advance Directive, such as a Living Will or Durable Power of Attorney for Healthcare? ❑ Yes ❑ No

Please specify the type: ________________________________

*** *If yes, please bring a copy at the time of your admission.* ***

Self-Pay

* If insured but your procedure is not covered or verified by your plan, a deposit is required at the time of admission.

* If you do not have insurance, please call our *EMC Financial Services at (XXX)-XXX-XXXX* before your scheduled arrival date to discuss financial terms.

Additional Information

Do you need special accommodations, such as Translation, Visual Aid, etc.? ❑ Yes ❑ No

*** *If yes, please specify so that prior arrangements can be made for the day of your visit.* ***

❑ Language Interpreter ____________ ❑ Sign Language Interpreter ❑ Visual Aid ❑ Other: ____________

Practice Professionalism

A long-time front desk clerk at Dr. Goodman's office does not ask patients who have recently been seen to verify their personal and insurance information when they check in for their next visit. She claims it wastes time because there are never any changes. Imagine you are Dr. Goodman's newly hired coding specialist. How will you explain the importance of the verification process to the front desk clerk?

Clinical Data

Every diagnosis and procedure related to caring for a patient must be documented in the health record. This collective body of documentation is known as **clinical data**. Clinical data may include a patient's medical history, physical information, progress notes, procedure and operative notes, anesthesia notes, pathology reports, and diagnostic reports. Providers are responsible for maintaining complete and accurate clinical data for every patient they treat, and they must meet certain standards regarding documentation of care to maintain licensure, certification, and/or accreditation by external healthcare organizations.

History and Physical

A basic component of any health record is the patient's medical history and results of a physical examination, known collectively as the **history and physical (H&P)**. A complete medical history includes a **chief complaint** (the reason the patient is seeking care, as identified by the patient), a history of the present illness, a history of past illnesses and surgeries, social and personal history, family medical history, and a review of systems. The **review of systems (ROS)** is a question-and-answer session between the provider and the patient—no physical examination is performed in this step—and it can include a complete review of every body system or be specific to the chief complaint. Figure 5.3 provides an example of an electronic review of systems form that may be used in obtaining a medical history. The **physical examination** is the provider's evaluation of the patient's physical condition. Like the review of systems, the physical examination can cover the entire body or be limited to the system related to the chief complaint. You will learn about each component of the history and physical and how to report related codes in Chapter 6.

Progress Notes

Progress notes are brief summaries written by physicians to document a patient's care and the patient's response to treatment. When writing progress notes (on paper or electronically), providers often employ the **SOAP note** format, an acronym representing the *subjective*, *objective*, *assessment*, and *plan* categories of information. These categories include several different types of documentation:

- The **subjective documentation** is a statement, in the patient's or family's own words, describing how the patient is feeling or why he or she is seeing the provider. It also includes pertinent or significant portions of past medical history, medications, and family/social history.

Figure 5.3 Review of Systems Form

Page 1 of 2

NPI#

Email Form

Print Form

EMC Medical Center

REVIEW OF SYSTEMS

PATIENT INFORMATION

Last Name Smith MI W First Name John Age 37

Address 1234 Main Street

Male

City Los Angeles State CA Zip Code 79567

Female

Email JSmith@smith.emcp.net Referred by Mr. Andrew Baker

Home # 915-555-0150 Cell # 915-555-0173 Work # Ext.

SSN# 000-45-6789 Date of Birth 12-15-1980 Driver's License # C123456789

MEDICAL INFORMATION

FOR THE FOLLOWING CONDITIONS PLEASE CHECK ○ **Past conditions** ☐ **Present conditions**

GENERAL

○ ☐ Recent weight gain	○ ☐ Recent weight loss	○ ☐ Fatigue	○ ☐ Rheumatic Fever
○ ☐ Loss of sleep	○ ☐ Loss of appetite	○ ☐ Polio	○ ☐ Cancer of any kind

INTEGUMENTARY (SKIN)

○ ☐ Skin problems	○ ☐ Skin rashes	○ ☐ Psoriasis	○ ☐ Skin cancer
○ ☐ Slow healing	○ ☐ Discolorations	○ ☐ Change in moles	○ ☐ Scars
○ ☐ Bruise easily	○ ☐ Itching	○ ☐ Change in skin color	○ ☐ Sores

NEUROLOGICAL

○ ☐ Light headed/dizzy	○ ☐ Fainting	○ ☐ Disorientation	○ ☐ Weakness
○ ☐ Memory loss	○ ☐ Concussion	○ ☐ Loss of coordination	○ ☐ Numbness
○ ☐ Difficulty speaking	○ ☐ Headaches	○ ☐ Difficulty walking	○ ☐ Tingling
○ ☐ Multiple Sclerosis	○ ☐ Migraines	○ ☐ Stroke	○ ☐ Tremors
○ ☐ Parkinson's disease	○ ☐ Epilepsy/seizures	○ ☐ Alzheimer disease	○ ☐ Disk problem

EYES, EARS, NOSE, AND THROAT

○ ☐ Vision problems	○ ☐ Glaucoma	○ ☐ Ear pain	○ ☐ Sore throat
○ ☐ Blurred vision	○ ☐ Hearing loss	○ ☐ Mouth sores	○ ☐ Nose bleeds
○ ☐ Double vision	○ ☐ Ear noises	○ ☐ Hoarseness	○ ☐ Dental problems

ENDOCRINE

○ ☐ Hypothyroidism	○ ☐ Hyperthyroidism	○ ☐ Diabetes	○ ☐ Goiter

RESPIRATORY

○ ☐ Coughing	○ ☐ Pneumonia	○ ☐ Superficial breathing	○ ☐ Bronchitis
○ ☐ Coughing up blood	○ ☐ Difficulty breathing	○ ☐ Chest pain	○ ☐ Emphysema
○ ☐ Chronic cough	○ ☐ Asthma	○ ☐ Tuberculosis	○ ☐ Lung cancer

Last Name Smith First Name John Date April 16, 2017 __________ Patient Signature

---

Email Form

Print Form

Center

STEMS

○ **Past conditions** ☐ **Present conditions**

☐ High blood pressure	○ ☐ Shortness of breath
☐ Low blood pressure	○ ☐ Perfuse sweating
☐ High triglycerides	○ ☐ Nausea
☐ High cholesterol levels	○ ☐ Vomiting

☐ Constipation	○ ☐ Blood in stool
☐ Diarrhea	○ ☐ Mucus in stool
☐ Hiatal hernia	○ ☐ Pancreatitis
☐ Colitis	○ ☐ Colon cancer

		☐ Kidney infection	○ ☐ Kidney stones
○ ☐ Blood in urine	○ ☐ Incontinence	○ ☐ Sexual difficulty	○ ☐ Loss of libido

HEMATOLOGIC (BLOOD)

○ ☐ Anemia	○ ☐ Bleeding disorder	○ ☐ Sickle Cell Anemia	○ ☐ Lymphoma

MUSCULOSKELETAL

○ ☐ Arthritis	○ ☐ Head injury	○ ☐ Cancer	○ ☐ Muscle pain
○ ☐ Osteoarthritis	○ ☐ Neck injury	○ ☐ Muscle weakness	○ ☐ Gout
○ ☐ Rheumatoid arthritis	○ ☐ Back injury	○ ☐ Osteoporosis	○ ☐ Scoliosis
○ ☐ Bone spurs	○ ☐ Spinal trauma	○ ☐ Muscular Dystrophy	○ ☐ Lupus
○ ☐ Broken bones	○ ☐ Birth trauma	○ ☐ Scheuermann's disease	○ ☐ Spina bifida
○ ☐ Compression fracture	○ ☐ Birth defects	○ ☐ Joint pain	○ ☐ Spondylolisthesis

ALLERGIC/IMMUNOLOGIC

○ ☐ Catch colds easily	○ ☐ Frequent sinus trouble	○ ☐ Frequent influenza	○ ☐ Fever
○ ☐ HIV	○ ☐ AIDS	○ ☐ Allergies	○ ☐ Hay fever

WOMEN ONLY

○ ☐ Irregular periods	○ ☐ Nipple discharge	○ ☐ Premenstrual depression
○ ☐ Hot flashes	○ ☐ Menstrual cramps	○ ☐ Lumps in breasts
○ ☐ Vaginal discharge	○ ☐ Abnormal pap smear	○ ☐ Hysterectomy

Men only

○ ☐ Burning on urination	○ ☐ Nightly urination	○ ☐ Prostrate trouble
○ ☐ Difficulty starting urine	○ ☐ Dripping after urination	○ ☐ Prostate cancer

Last Name Smith First Name John Date April 16, 2017 __________ Patient Signature

Healthcare Provider Notes: For Office Use Only

Type in additional notes here

Provider Name Austin Inge Title DC Date April 16, 2017 __________ Provider Signature

- The **objective documentation** includes data such as the patient's vital signs, physical exam findings, and diagnostic test results.
- The **assessment** documents the provider's evaluation of the patient and includes his or her diagnosis or assessment of the situation (eg, "patient is in satisfactory condition").
- The **plan for care** (or **care plan**) documents any medications, tests, and medical or surgical interventions required to treat the patient's condition. It also includes the plan for follow-up and patient education.

Figure 5.4 shows a SOAP note for a postoperative visit in electronic format.

Figure 5.4 Electronic SOAP Note for a Postoperative Visit

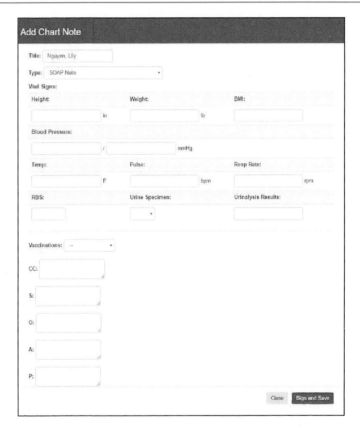

Procedure Notes and Operative Reports

Any procedure or service performed for a patient requires documentation not only for continued care of the patient but for coding and reimbursement purposes. Some simple procedures may be documented in a progress note; however, procedures requiring special facilities or equipment will be documented in a procedure note or operative report. In a **procedure note**, a provider briefly describes a simple procedure in narrative form, or he or she may use a specific procedure-note template if the facility's protocol calls for it.

More complex procedures that require the use of an operative facility are documented in an **operative report**, which records diagnoses, names of healthcare personnel involved in the procedure, findings, a procedure description, details of specimens, and blood loss.

Operative reports must provide the following information:

- name of patient;
- date of service;
- names of the surgeons and/or assistants who participated in the procedure;
- type of anesthesia used and who administered the anesthesia;
- preoperative diagnosis;
- postoperative diagnosis;
- name of the procedure performed;
- findings of the procedure;
- a description of the procedure itself and the events that occurred during the course of the procedure;
- descriptions of specimens removed;
- estimated blood loss;
- complications (frequently this section will read "none");
- date and time report was recorded (to confirm that the note was recorded prior to moving the patient to the next level of care).

Figure 5.5 is an example of an operative report. The appearance and content of the operative report will vary based on the procedure performed. For example, an operative report for an extensive abdominal surgery may be much longer than a report for a simple wart removal, because the greater complexity of the abdominal operation necessitates greater documentation. An operative report should be written or dictated immediately after a procedure is completed to ensure accuracy and provide the best continuity of care. Using the content of the operative note to report procedure codes will be discussed later in this chapter.

Anesthesia Notes

Anesthesia is the administration of gases or drugs to block pain and sensation, which allows a patient to tolerate an otherwise painful procedure or surgery. Although the operative report contains information about the anesthesia provided to the patient, the anesthesiologist or anesthetist administering the anesthesia for a procedure also completes a separate **anesthesia note**. The anesthesia note documents the anesthesia drugs provided to the patient, including their doses and method of administration, the vital signs of the patient while under anesthesia, and any other services provided such as a blood transfusion. Anesthesia notes may also include any complications relating to anesthesia administration. You will learn more about types of anesthesia services and how to report codes for them in Chapter 7.

Pathology Reports

A **pathologist** examines patient specimens to provide a diagnosis to the physician. After examining a specimen that has been sent for evaluation, the pathologist completes a **pathology report**. This report includes a description of the specimen

Figure 5.5 Sample Operative Report

DATE OF PROCEDURE	12/01/2019
PREOPERATIVE DIAGNOSIS	2 x 2-cm mass lesion of neck, right side, posterior triangle
POSTOPERATIVE DIAGNOSIS	2 x 2-cm mass lesion of neck, right side, posterior triangle
PROCEDURE PERFORMED	Excisional biopsy of 2 x 2-cm lesion of neck, right side
BLOOD LOSS	Minimal
SURGEON	Inez Gosling, MD
ANESTHESIA	General endotracheal

INDICATIONS AND FINDINGS AT OPERATION

A 6-year-old Hispanic male was followed by the pediatrician for a mass lesion on the right neck. During that time, the lesion intermittently increased and decreased in size. The patient was given a course of oral antibiotics twice. Therefore, because of the persistent mass lesion, the patient was seen in the office. The mother denied any systemic signs, and the patient was active. His appetite was good and he had not lost any weight. However, because of the possibility that the lesion might be a malignant melanoma, an excisional biopsy was recommended. At operation, findings were consistent with a hyperplastic lymph node. Although the node did not look malignant, a specimen was sent to pathology.

DESCRIPTION OF PROCEDURE

The patient was placed in a supine position and given general anesthesia. He was positioned so that the neck was slightly hyperextended. The operative field was prepped with Betadine solution and draped in the usual fashion observing sterile technique. A transverse incision along the skin crease was made. This incision was brought down to the subcutaneous tissue and platysma. The mass lesion was identified and subsequently excised. The soft tissue attachment of the lymph node was clamped and ligated with 3-0 chromic catgut to reduce the possibility of seroma. The specimen was submitted for histopathology. The subcutaneous tissue and platysma were approximated with interrupted 3-0 chromic catgut and the skin was closed by continuous 5-0 Vicryl. Steri-Strips were placed and sterile dressing applied. The patient tolerated the procedure well.

following both a **gross exam** (conducted with the naked eye) and a **microscopic exam** (conducted under a microscope), as well as a diagnosis based on the findings. While each specimen is evaluated individually, the evaluation of multiple specimens from 1 procedure may be documented in the same pathology report (unless the facility's protocol requires that a separate report be provided for each specimen). Figure 5.6 is an example of a pathology report describing a malignant lesion from the colon and lymph nodes. Certain procedure codes are assigned based on whether a lesion is **benign** (not harmful) or **malignant** (invasive, progressively worsening), so you should always read the pathology report before reporting a code. You will learn more about pathology and laboratory coding in Chapter 19.

Figure 5.6 Sample Pathology Report

SURGICAL PATHOLOGY REPORT

DIAGNOSIS

Right colon, segmental resection

1. Invasive poorly differentiated adenocarcinoma of the colon, 3.5 cm in greatest dimension, invading the muscularis propria and into the pericolic fat
2. Tumor present in lymphatic spaces
3. Surgical resection margins are free from tumor involvement
4. 2 of 15 lymph nodes with metastatic adenocarcinoma

GROSS EXAMINATION

Specimen labeled "Right Colon." Specimen is a short ileocolectomy specimen. The colon segment, which appears to be predominately cecum, measures 8 cm in length. At the ileocecal valve, there is a low fungating mass measuring 3.5 cm in diameter. This puckers the underlying serosa. There is an attached small ellipse of apparent small-bowel mucosa, which does not appear contiguous with the rest of the segment and appears adherent with a staple line measuring approximately 2.5 cm in length. This segment measures less than 6 mm in length. Segments of cecal tumor with this adherent eccentric small bowel is submitted in cassettes 1 and 2. Tumor at the ileocecal valve, which represents the deepest invasion, is submitted in cassettes 3 through 5. Tumor does appear to extend through the bowel wall. The proximal and distal margins are grossly negative for tumor (cassette 6). Cassette 7 shows tumor at the ileocecal valve where tumor is very close to and may involve the adjacent ileum by continuity. Pericolonic lymph nodes are cleared in chloroform. All lymph nodes found are submitted entirely.

MICROSCOPIC EXAMINATION

Sections of the right colon show an invasive, poorly differentiated colon adenocarcinoma with direct extension to involve the terminal ileum. Two lymph nodes are involved by metastatic adenocarcinoma, and the adenocarcinoma extends through the muscularis propria into the pericolonic adipose tissue. The surgical resection margins are negative for malignancy and dysplasia.

SPECIMEN

Right colon

CLINICAL DATA

Carcinoma colon

Diagnostic Reports

Diagnostic reports communicate the results from procedures such as laboratory tests and radiological exams and help a provider make decisions about a patient's condition and treatment. Two common types of diagnostic reports included in a patient's health record are laboratory reports and radiology reports.

Laboratory reports contain results from laboratory tests performed on blood, urine, and other specimens from the patient. Many common laboratory tests such as a complete blood count (CBC) and lipid panels are generated using automated laboratory equipment. These machines are able to interface with the EHR system to post results in the patient's health record immediately upon completion. Figure 5.7 is an example of an EHR interfacing with automated laboratory equipment. In a paper-based system, laboratory reports may be printed and placed in a patient's health record. When a lab test requires interpretation from a pathologist or other specially trained physician, these interpretations are documented by the physician and become part of the patient's health record as well.

Figure 5.7 EHR Lab Screen

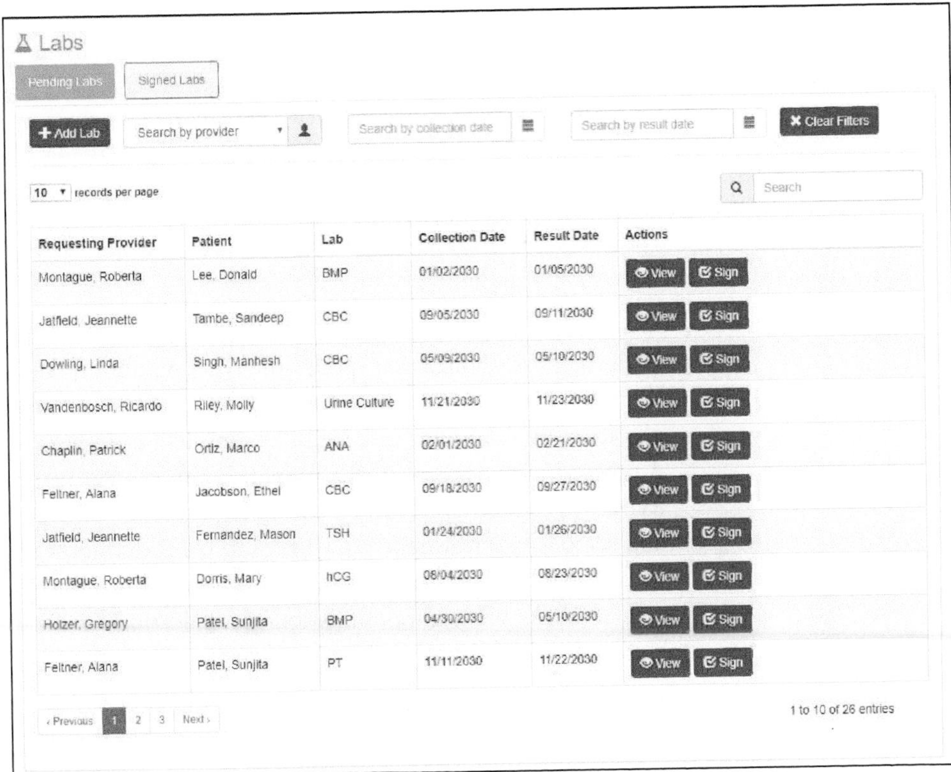

Labs

Pending Labs | Signed Labs

+ Add Lab | Search by provider | Search by collection date | Search by result date | ✖ Clear Filters

10 records per page | Search

Requesting Provider	Patient	Lab	Collection Date	Result Date	Actions
Montague, Roberta	Lee, Donald	BMP	01/02/2030	01/05/2030	View Sign
Jatfield, Jeannette	Tambe, Sandeep	CBC	09/05/2030	09/11/2030	View Sign
Dowling, Linda	Singh, Manhesh	CBC	05/09/2030	05/10/2030	View Sign
Vandenbosch, Ricardo	Riley, Molly	Urine Culture	11/21/2030	11/23/2030	View Sign
Chaplin, Patrick	Ortiz, Marco	ANA	02/01/2030	02/21/2030	View Sign
Feltner, Alana	Jacobson, Ethel	CBC	09/18/2030	09/27/2030	View Sign
Jatfield, Jeannette	Fernandez, Mason	TSH	01/24/2030	01/26/2030	View Sign
Montague, Roberta	Dorris, Mary	hCG	08/04/2030	08/23/2030	View Sign
Holzer, Gregory	Patel, Sunjita	BMP	04/30/2030	05/10/2030	View Sign
Feltner, Alana	Patel, Sunjita	PT	11/11/2030	11/22/2030	View Sign

‹ Previous 1 2 3 Next ›

1 to 10 of 26 entries

Many labs interface with the EHR system and post results to the patient's record immediately.

Radiology reports describe radiologists' findings and provide radiologic interpretations. Figure 5.8 shows a sample radiology report. A radiologist views and interprets x-rays and magnetic resonance images (MRIs) and issues a report of his or her findings. For example, if a radiologist sees an increased density in a patient's lower lung on a radiograph of the chest, the interpretation may state that the findings are consistent with pneumonia. Radiologists often perform "supervision and interpretation" of images to provide guidance for a surgeon during a procedure. The radiologist will generate a separate report for this service. Radiologists may also perform procedures in the radiology department such as needle biopsies or embolization vascular procedures. These procedures may be described in the radiology report.

Figure 5.8 Sample Radiology Report

X-RAY OF THE CHEST, TWO VIEWS

CLINICAL HISTORY
Cough, congestion.

FINDINGS
Posteroanterior and lateral views of chest reveal no evidence of active pleural or parenchymal abnormality. There are diffusely increased interstitial lung markings consistent with chronic bronchitis. Underlying pulmonary fibrosis is not excluded. The cardiac silhouette is normal. The mediastinum and pulmonary vessels appear normal. Aorta appears normal.

IMPRESSION
No evidence of acute pulmonary pathology. Diffusely increased interstitial lung markings consistent with chronic bronchitis. Underlying pulmonary fibrosis is not excluded.

Standards and Regulations Related to Clinical Data

Each state has statutes that specify the types of clinical data that healthcare facilities must document in order to maintain licensure. For example, Wisconsin requires that physicians in long-term care facilities complete a progress note for each patient visit. A progress note documents the provider's clinical observations of the patient. Collectively, progress notes form a chronological report of a patient's medical condition and response to treatment. Another example is that most states require nursing staff to document all information related to the administration of medication—a patient's refusal to take medication, omission of medication, errors in the administration of medication, and drug reactions.

In order to receive payment for treatment of Medicare and Medicaid patients, the **Centers for Medicare and Medicaid Services (CMS)** requires that facilities and providers meet the conditions of participation set forth in federal regulations. CMS requires that health records be complete, accurate, readily accessible, and organized. To ensure that a facility meets the CMS requirements, health records are audited by a survey conducted by a state agency on behalf of CMS or by another organization such as the **Joint Commission** or the **Center for Improvement in Healthcare Quality**. The Joint Commission is an accrediting organization that has been approved by CMS as having standards and a survey process that exceed federal requirements. If a healthcare organization meets the Joint Commission's accreditation standards, CMS accepts that the conditions of participation for CMS have also been met. CMS then awards the facility **deemed status** to authorize the organization to participate in and receive payment from the Medicare and Medicaid programs.

Coding Clicks

For more information about the Joint Commission's accreditation programs, visit http://jointcommission.org.

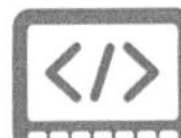

Coding for CMS

The Joint Commission, a CMS-approved accrediting organization, sets a variety of standards for facilities and providers. For example, the Joint Commission requires that the operative report contain sufficient information to

- identify the patient;
- identify the surgeon and any assistants;
- support the diagnosis;
- justify the treatment;
- document the postoperative course and results; and
- promote continuity of care.

Other organizations have also proposed guidelines for clinical documentation. The **National Committee on Vital and Health Statistics (NCVHS)** developed a list of 42 core data elements and definitions for use in a variety of healthcare settings. The **American Health Information Management Association (AHIMA)** developed a core data set for physician practices with elements for history and physicals, problem lists, and other data elements used by physicians.

CONCEPTS CHECKPOINT **5.1**

Choose the best answer for the following multiple-choice questions.

1. The review of systems can be found in the
   a. progress note.
   b. SOAP note.
   c. history and physical.
   d. operative report.
2. Administrative data contains
   a. a patient's personal information.
   b. data related to test results.
   c. physician notes.
   d. clinical information.
3. Notice of privacy practices is part of the
   a. administrative data.
   b. clinical data.
   c. financial data.
   d. legal data.
4. An operative report must contain
   a. preoperative and postoperative diagnoses.
   b. the name of the surgeon.
   c. a description of the procedure itself.
   d. All of the answers are correct.
5. Which organization accredits healthcare facilities?
   a. The American Health Information Management Association
   b. The Joint Commission
   c. The National Committee on Vital and Health Statistics
   d. All of the answers are correct.

Reporting Codes Based on the Health Record

You can think of reporting a medical code as summarizing an episode of patient care with numbers instead of words. As a CPT® coder, you will be required to sift through the data in a patient's health record to extract the pertinent information for reporting the appropriate code(s). In the health information management field, this process is referred to as **abstracting**.

The type of facility and/or practice specialty (such as anesthesia or plastic surgery) for which you are working will determine the part of the health record from which you will abstract information to report codes. If you are coding for anesthesiologists or other professionals providing only anesthesia services, you may need to review only the anesthesia record. If you are coding for an ambulatory (outpatient) surgery center, you may need to review many different types of clinical data related to the patient's episode of care, such as the history and physical, operative reports, anesthesia notes, pathology reports, radiology reports, and other diagnostic studies.

As mentioned earlier, you will learn how to read and interpret data from the history and physical examination and report related evaluation and management codes in Chapter 6 of this textbook. Because the Surgery section is by far the largest section in the CPT® codebook, this chapter will focus on interpreting and abstracting information from operative reports in order to report CPT® surgery codes.

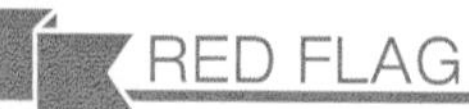

Always read the entire operative report before deciding what procedure(s) should be coded.

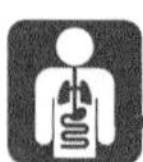

A&P Review

From your previous A&P studies, you will recall that the integumentary structures occur in layers. From the outermost layer, these structures are the epidermis and dermis (or skin), subcutaneous tissue, fascia, and muscle. The layers correlate with the CPT® codebook criteria for debridement based on depth.

Exploring the Parts of the Operative Report

Figure 5.9 shows an operative report for the debridement of necrotic tissue in the fascia and muscle. The most important parts of the introductory section of the report are labeled with headings as is typical with operative report formats. Underlining has been added to the operative technique section of the figure to indicate the key data that will be abstracted. Guidelines for abstracting data from this operative report in order to report codes are provided following the figure.

Abstracting Data From the Operative Report

A walk-through of Figure 5.9 will identify the data relevant to the coding process.

Procedures performed: The surgeon lists the procedures that were performed. Note that each procedure listed may not need a separate code. In this case, the surgeon lists 3 procedures: incision and drainage; debridement of necrotic tissue, fascia, and muscle; and irrigation and drainage. As you will learn in Chapter 9, incision and drainage and irrigation and drainage are components of debridement and therefore should not be reported with separate codes. You need to report only the appropriate code for debridement.

Preoperative and postoperative diagnoses: The preoperative and postoperative diagnoses follow the surgeon's list of procedures. The **preoperative diagnosis** is the indication for the procedure, and the **postoperative diagnosis** is the impression from the surgeon after the surgery has been performed. The postoperative diagnosis may be the

Figure 5.9 Abstracting Data From the Operative Report: Debridement of Necrotic Tissue

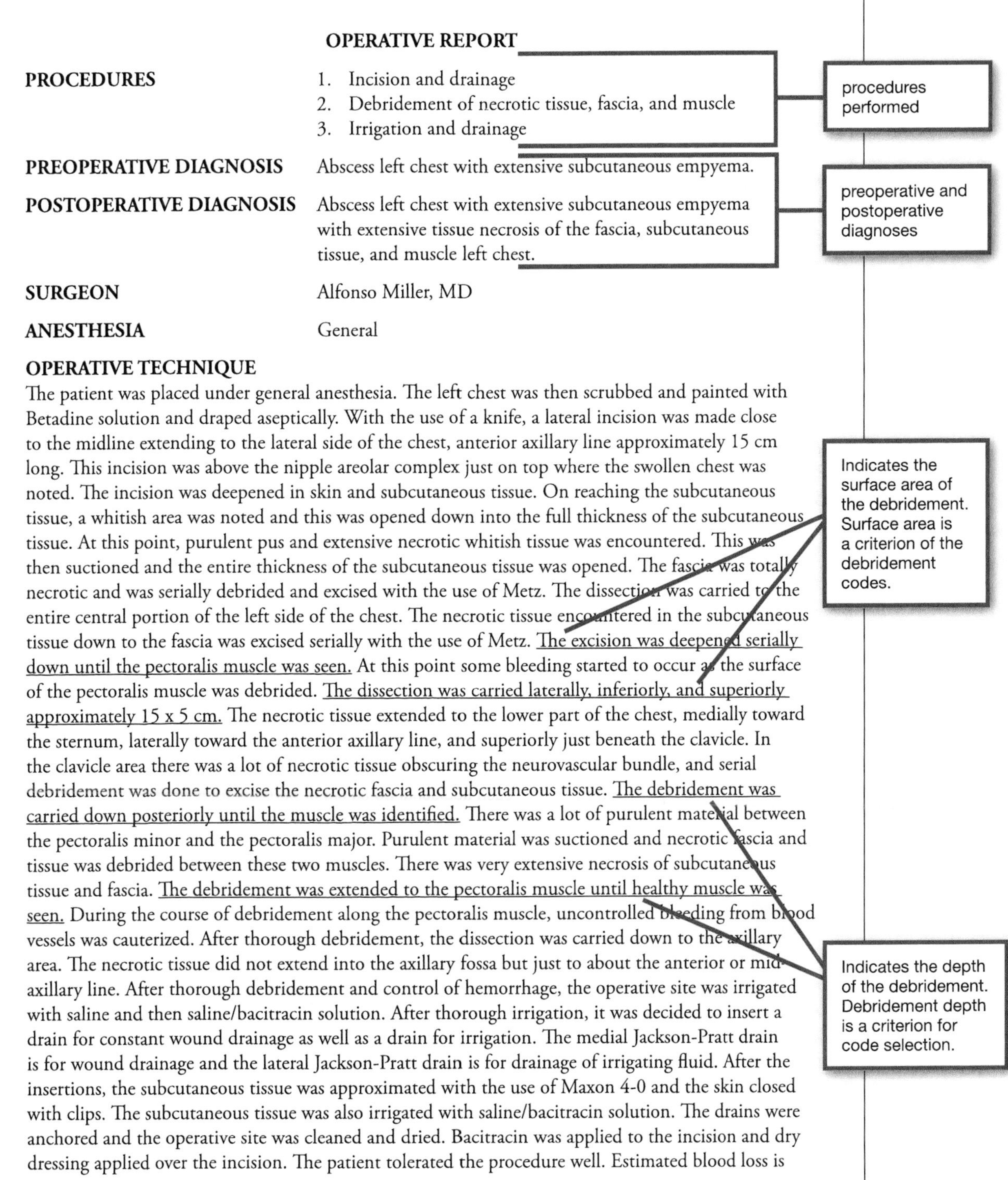

OPERATIVE REPORT

PROCEDURES
1. Incision and drainage
2. Debridement of necrotic tissue, fascia, and muscle
3. Irrigation and drainage

PREOPERATIVE DIAGNOSIS Abscess left chest with extensive subcutaneous empyema.

POSTOPERATIVE DIAGNOSIS Abscess left chest with extensive subcutaneous empyema with extensive tissue necrosis of the fascia, subcutaneous tissue, and muscle left chest.

SURGEON Alfonso Miller, MD

ANESTHESIA General

OPERATIVE TECHNIQUE

The patient was placed under general anesthesia. The left chest was then scrubbed and painted with Betadine solution and draped aseptically. With the use of a knife, a lateral incision was made close to the midline extending to the lateral side of the chest, anterior axillary line approximately 15 cm long. This incision was above the nipple areolar complex just on top where the swollen chest was noted. The incision was deepened in skin and subcutaneous tissue. On reaching the subcutaneous tissue, a whitish area was noted and this was opened down into the full thickness of the subcutaneous tissue. At this point, purulent pus and extensive necrotic whitish tissue was encountered. This was then suctioned and the entire thickness of the subcutaneous tissue was opened. The fascia was totally necrotic and was serially debrided and excised with the use of Metz. The dissection was carried to the entire central portion of the left side of the chest. The necrotic tissue encountered in the subcutaneous tissue down to the fascia was excised serially with the use of Metz. The excision was deepened serially down until the pectoralis muscle was seen. At this point some bleeding started to occur as the surface of the pectoralis muscle was debrided. The dissection was carried laterally, inferiorly, and superiorly approximately 15 x 5 cm. The necrotic tissue extended to the lower part of the chest, medially toward the sternum, laterally toward the anterior axillary line, and superiorly just beneath the clavicle. In the clavicle area there was a lot of necrotic tissue obscuring the neurovascular bundle, and serial debridement was done to excise the necrotic fascia and subcutaneous tissue. The debridement was carried down posteriorly until the muscle was identified. There was a lot of purulent material between the pectoralis minor and the pectoralis major. Purulent material was suctioned and necrotic fascia and tissue was debrided between these two muscles. There was very extensive necrosis of subcutaneous tissue and fascia. The debridement was extended to the pectoralis muscle until healthy muscle was seen. During the course of debridement along the pectoralis muscle, uncontrolled bleeding from blood vessels was cauterized. After thorough debridement, the dissection was carried down to the axillary area. The necrotic tissue did not extend into the axillary fossa but just to about the anterior or mid-axillary line. After thorough debridement and control of hemorrhage, the operative site was irrigated with saline and then saline/bacitracin solution. After thorough irrigation, it was decided to insert a drain for constant wound drainage as well as a drain for irrigation. The medial Jackson-Pratt drain is for wound drainage and the lateral Jackson-Pratt drain is for drainage of irrigating fluid. After the insertions, the subcutaneous tissue was approximated with the use of Maxon 4-0 and the skin closed with clips. The subcutaneous tissue was also irrigated with saline/bacitracin solution. The drains were anchored and the operative site was cleaned and dried. Bacitracin was applied to the incision and dry dressing applied over the incision. The patient tolerated the procedure well. Estimated blood loss is scanty.

procedures performed
preoperative and postoperative diagnoses
Indicates the surface area of the debridement. Surface area is a criterion of the debridement codes.
Indicates the depth of the debridement. Debridement depth is a criterion for code selection.

Figure 5.12 Thyroid Lobectomy Code Abstracted From Operative Report

60225	Total thyroid lobectomy, unilateral; with contralateral subtotal lobectomy, including isthmusectomy

At first glance, it may seem impossible to know which information from an operative report is relevant to reporting the appropriate code(s), but identifying the relevant data will get easier once you learn more about the codebook and practice reporting codes.

You will find that due to the differences in procedures, the information needed to report the appropriate codes varies widely. For example, code 20900, *Bone graft, any donor area; minor or small* from the Musculoskeletal System subsection of the Surgery section is not specific to an anatomical site and is used for obtaining a bone graft from any bone in the body; the only information needed to report this code would be that a bone graft was obtained. In contrast, code 21044, *Excision of malignant tumor of mandible,* also from the Musculoskeletal System subsection, is used to report a very specific procedure and may be used only if all the conditions set out in the code were performed. You will learn what information is required to assign each type of procedure code as you work through this textbook and complete the practice exercises.

CONCEPTS CHECKPOINT **5.2**

Answer true or false to each the following statements.

1. _____ The preoperative diagnosis is the reason or indication for the procedure.
2. _____ The preoperative and postoperative diagnoses will always be the same.
3. _____ Reading a narrative of the events that took place during surgery is necessary to assign an appropriate code.
4. _____ The anesthesiologist will not provide a separate report for anesthesia services.
5. _____ The pathologist will provide an evaluation for each specimen submitted.

LET'S TRY ONE **5.1**

Read the operative report and then answer the questions that follow.

OPERATIVE REPORT

PROCEDURE PERFORMED	Drainage of generalized peritonitis, appendectomy
PREOPERATIVE DIAGNOSIS	Acute appendicitis
POSTOPERATIVE DIAGNOSIS	Ruptured appendicitis with peritonitis
BLOOD LOSS	Minimal
SURGEON	Yusooff Adamson, MD
ANESTHESIA	General

INDICATIONS AND FINDINGS AT OPERATION

This 47-year-old white male was in good general health until around 6 o'clock the previous evening, when he started having right lower-quadrant abdominal pains. He was nauseated and felt like he had to have a bowel movement, but could not. The pain continued and was progressive, such that the patient was seen in the emergency department. A CT scan of the abdomen was positive for acute appendicitis and the white blood count was elevated. Therefore, around 5:30 in the morning, this surgical consultation was requested and the patient was scheduled for surgery.

At the operation, the findings were consistent with peritonitis. Cultures and sensitivities for aerobic and anaerobic organisms were requested. The peritonitis was drained and appendectomy was done. The appendix was perforated at the mid third. The right gutter and pelvis was copiously irrigated with saline and at least 1000 cc was used. The wound was approximated primarily. Sterile dressing was applied. The family was advised of the patient's condition and warned about the possibility of wound infection.

OPERATIVE TECHNIQUE

With the patient in the supine position, the patient was given general endotracheal anesthesia. The operative field was prepared with Betadine solution and draped in the usual fashion observing sterile technique. The patient was given 2 grams Ancef IVPB. A right lower abdominal incision was made. This incision was brought down to the subcutaneous tissue and fascia. The muscle layers were split along their fibers and the abdomen was entered. Suddenly, there was yellowish fluid that was encountered, and cultures and sensitivities for aerobic and anaerobic organisms were requested.

By sharp and blunt dissection and by digital exploration, the acutely inflamed and ruptured appendix was identified. An appendectomy was done. The patient was doubly ligated with 2-0 chromic catgut and the mesoappendix was ligated with 2-0 chromic catgut to complete the appendectomy. I could see a periphery at the middle third of the specimen, which was submitted for histopathology. The appendiceal stump was electrocauterized. Subsequently the operative site was copiously irrigated with saline until the return flow was clear; at least 1000 cc of normal saline was used. As soon as hemostasis was satisfactory, the peritoneum was approximated by continuous 0 PDS. The muscle layers were approximated with 0 PDS continuous and interrupted and the subcutaneous tissue closed by 3-0 chromic catgut. The skin was approximated with skin staples. Sterile dressing was applied. The patient tolerated the procedure well.

1. What procedure(s) was performed? ________________
2. What are the preoperative and postoperative diagnoses? ________________
3. Does the documentation in the body of the report describe the procedures that the surgeon listed in the introductory section of the report? ________________

Technological Advances in Coding

RED FLAG

Regardless of the format of the health record, you must always read and code from the documentation itself, taking care not to make assumptions if documentation is not present.

In this chapter, you have learned that the health record is where all the information regarding services provided to a patient is stored. As you learned in Chapter 1, while all healthcare providers used to maintain **paper records**, which consist of hard-copy forms stored in physical file folders, most providers now store their patients' health information in computer systems, known as EHRs. The creation and adoption of EHRs has brought positive changes, as well as challenges, to the field of medical coding.

Think Like a Coder

When some patient information is stored on paper and some is stored electronically, the health record is referred to as a *hybrid record*. What do you think might be some of the benefits to coding from a hybrid record? What challenges might it create?

Benefits of Coding From Electronic Health Records

The coding process itself is the same whether you are coding from paper, electronic, or hybrid health records. However, there are some benefits of coding from an EHR.

While a paper record must be physically located and therefore can be used by only 1 person at a time, EHRs are instantly available and can be accessed by more than 1 user from any location with an Internet connection. For example, coders who work for billing and coding companies that report codes for multiple facilities often do so remotely. These coding professionals log into a **documentation review program** to review health records; this allows them to view various health records without having to access multiple EHR systems.

Another advantage to EHRs is that all notes in an EHR are typed, so none of the issues related to handwritten notes exist—coders do not have to attempt to interpret poor penmanship or risk assigning the wrong code if a note is illegible. Figure 5.13 illustrates the difference between a handwritten and an electronic note.

EHRs also lead physicians and other providers to create higher-quality documentation because electronic records use templates, checklists, and prompts to ensure the information is complete. If an EHR does contain unclear or incomplete information, physician queries (requests for clarification or more documentation) can be generated through the EHR system, which will then notify the physician so that he or she can review and respond in a timely manner. All of these benefits cause the coding portion of the revenue cycle to be much shorter when EHRs are used, ultimately leading to lower costs and faster reimbursement for medical facilities.

Figure 5.13 Handwritten Versus Electronic Note

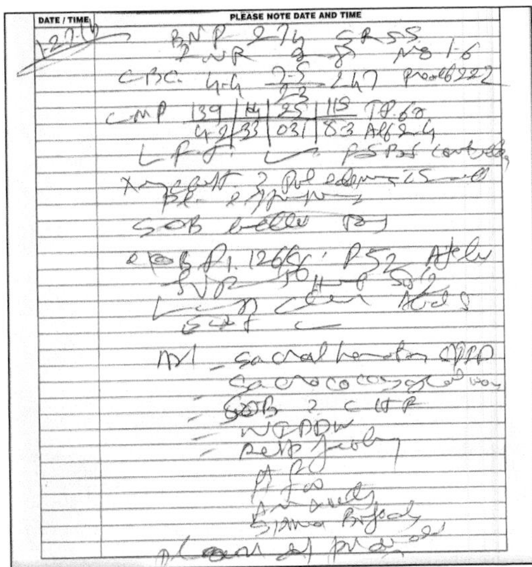

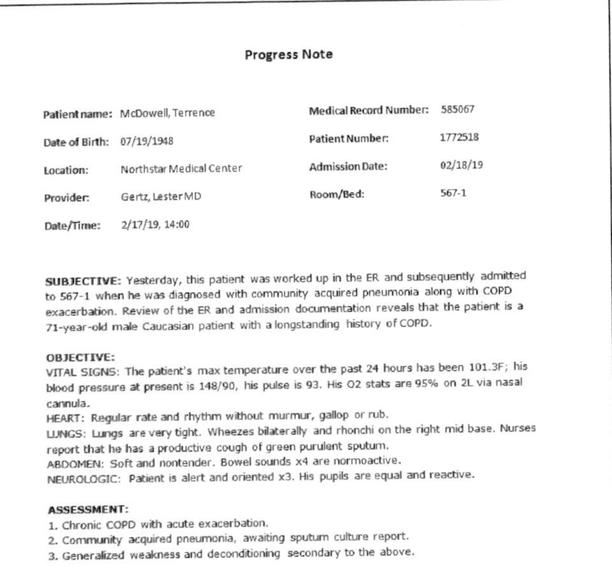

Progress Note

Patient name: McDowell, Terrence
Date of Birth: 07/19/1948
Location: Northstar Medical Center
Provider: Gertz, Lester MD
Date/Time: 2/17/19, 14:00

Medical Record Number: 585067
Patient Number: 1772518
Admission Date: 02/18/19
Room/Bed: 567-1

SUBJECTIVE: Yesterday, this patient was worked up in the ER and subsequently admitted to 567-1 when he was diagnosed with community acquired pneumonia along with COPD exacerbation. Review of the ER and admission documentation reveals that the patient is a 71-year-old male Caucasian patient with a longstanding history of COPD.

OBJECTIVE:
VITAL SIGNS: The patient's max temperature over the past 24 hours has been 101.3F; his blood pressure at present is 148/90, his pulse is 93. His O2 stats are 95% on 2L via nasal cannula.
HEART: Regular rate and rhythm without murmur, gallop or rub.
LUNGS: Lungs are very tight. Wheezes bilaterally and rhonchi on the right mid base. Nurses report that he has a productive cough of green purulent sputum.
ABDOMEN: Soft and nontender. Bowel sounds x4 are normoactive.
NEUROLOGIC: Patient is alert and oriented x3. His pupils are equal and reactive.

ASSESSMENT:
1. Chronic COPD with acute exacerbation.
2. Community acquired pneumonia, awaiting sputum culture report.
3. Generalized weakness and deconditioning secondary to the above.

Think Like a Coder

A new physician, Dr. Bignell, has joined the group practice where Terri is a coder. Terri has been unable to code several of Dr. Bignell's recent surgeries due to lack of detail in the operative notes. Dr. Bignell uses vague terminology such as "small lesion" instead of providing the lesion's measurements. How should Terri address this issue?

Coding Software

In addition to making health records more complete and easier to access, technology is also helping modern coders improve their accuracy. An **encoder** is a software tool that a coding specialist uses to locate appropriate codes. Encoders can be used with any type of EHR system. Some encoders are logic based, and others are knowledge based. To use a **logic-based encoder**, the coding specialist enters a main term and then answers a series of questions so that the encoder can provide the appropriate code. A **knowledge-based encoder** has a format similar to the codebook, meaning that the coder must have knowledge of the CPT® codebook's guidelines and Index to successfully use the encoder. Encoder software not only helps coders save time in locating codes, it also includes National Correct Coding Initiative (NCCI) edits to alert the coder of inappropriate code combinations or illogical codes. Encoders usually include or are linked to other software such as **groupers** (programs that sort codes into groups for prospective payment system calculations) and billing software for offices and facilities. Encoders will send the selected codes automatically to these programs. Encoders are useful tools to assist the coding process and make it more efficient and accurate, but are not a substitution for coding knowledge and skill.

Coding Clicks

Read an article detailing how CAC technology is changing health care and coding on the American Health Information Management Association (AHIMA) website at http://Coding.ParadigmEducation.com/CAC.

In an EHR environment, **computer-assisted coding (CAC)** may be used. CAC is a software program that analyzes text from EHR documentation and assigns codes accordingly. Note that the use of a CAC program does not mean that the coding process is entirely automated. A coding specialist must edit the codes assigned by the software before the claim is processed for billing purposes.

The health record contains a vast amount of information. As you have read, coding specialists must abstract pertinent information from the record to appropriately assign codes. A good understanding of health documentation is an essential skill for a coding specialist. You may want to refer back to this chapter to review these important concepts as you work through the rest of the book.

Chapter Summary

- The health record contains clinical, administrative, financial, and legal data.
- The format of a health record can be paper, electronic, or a combination of paper and electronic formats known as a *hybrid record.*
- Clinical data is the documentation of the care provided to the patient.
- Administrative data includes the patient's personal details necessary for the business end of providing health care such as address and place of employment. Verifying this information regularly is a vital part of an efficient revenue cycle.
- Financial data indicates who is responsible for paying for the treatment provided to the patient.
- Legal data consists of the consent for treatment and notice of privacy practices.
- In the *history and physical* component of the health record, the history documents the patient's current and past health history, and the physical examination is the provider's evaluation of the patient's physical condition.
- A *review of systems* documents the question-and-answer session between the provider and the patient.
- A *progress note* is used to document the patient's care and how well the patient is responding to treatment. Providers often use the SOAP format.
- A *procedure note* is used to document a simple procedure that does not warrant the completion of an operative report.
- An *operative report* must include: the patient's preoperative and postoperative diagnoses, names of surgeons and/or assistants, normal and abnormal findings, a description of the operative procedure and any events that occur during the course of the procedure, descriptions of specimens removed, type of anesthesia used, and estimated blood loss.
- An *anesthesia note* is a form of clinical documentation usually completed by an anesthesiologist or anesthetist that describes the type, dose, and method of anesthesia administered during a procedure.

- A *pathology report* includes a gross and microscopic description of a specimen.
- A *diagnostic report* communicates the results from procedures such as a laboratory test and a radiological exam.
- Providers and facilities must meet certain standards regarding documentation of care to maintain licensure, certification, and/or accreditation by external healthcare organizations.
- The Joint Commission is an accrediting organization that has been approved by the Centers for Medicare and Medicaid Services (CMS) as having standards that exceed federal requirements. If a healthcare organization meets the Joint Commission's standards, CMS awards the facility *deemed status.*
- *Abstracting* is the process of extracting specific data elements from a patient's health record to report the appropriate codes.
- Analyzing operative reports to abstract information into codes is a learned skill. The most important parts of an operative report are the procedure(s), the preoperative and postoperative diagnoses, and the operative technique. Each procedure listed by the surgeon in an operative report may not need a separate code.
- The electronic health record (EHR) is a technological advancement over paper records that facilitates document sharing, billing automation, and a shorter revenue cycle. A *documentation review program* allows coding professionals to review multiple heath records without having to log into multiple EHR systems.
- An *encoder* is a software tool that a coding specialist uses to locate appropriate codes. There are two types of encoders: logic based and knowledge based.
- *Computer-assisted coding (CAC)* is software that analyzes EHR documentation and assigns codes accordingly. Coding specialists must verify codes provided by the software before they can be submitted for billing purposes.

Navigator

Access interactive chapter review exercises, practice activities, flash cards, and study games.

Chapter 6

Evaluation and Management Services Coding

Fast Facts

- Patients who are treated with respect by their doctors report higher levels of satisfaction and are more likely to comply with doctors' orders.
- A Mayo Clinic study reveals that patients want doctors who are confident, empathetic, humane, personal, forthright, respectful, and thorough.

Source: http://emedexpert.com

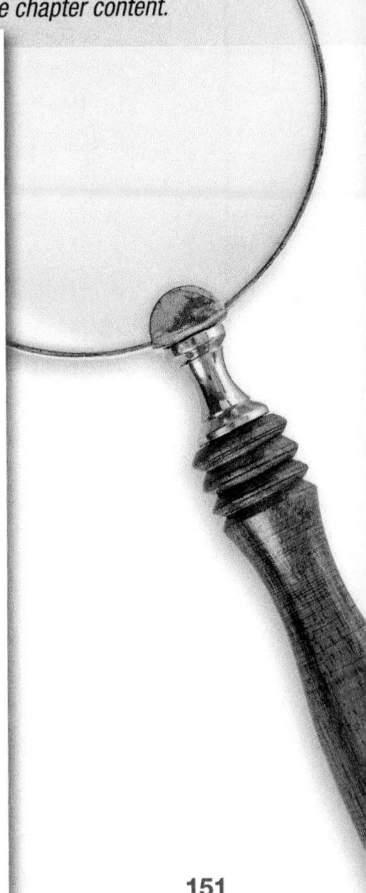

Crack the Code

Review the sample progress notes to find the correct E/M code. You may need to return to this exercise after reading the chapter content.

AUTHOR: Sandeep Dhaliwal, MD
SUBJECTIVE: Emma Ernst, a 10-year-old female established patient who presents for a camp physical exam. Patient/parent deny any current health-related concerns.
VITAL SIGNS:
BP 105/69
Pulse 77
Temp 98.8 (Oral)
Resp 18
Ht 4'7"
Wt 100 lb
SpO2 97%
Alert, cooperative, well-hydrated, appears well
GAIT: Normal, including heel, toe, tandem, squat
SKIN: Normal, no lesions or rashes
EYES: Pupils equal, round, reactive to light. EOMs intact.
EARS: TMs normal, auditory acuity grossly normal
MOUTH: No oropharyngeal congestion, exudates, filings present, no lesions
NECK: Supple, no adenopathy
LUNGS: Clear to auscultation
HEART: Regular rate and rhythm, no murmurs, clicks, gallops. Peripheral pulses normal S_1 S_2 in standing sitting supine.
ABDOMEN: Soft, nontender, no masses or organomegaly
NEURO: Cranial nerves intact, reflexes normal and symmetric
SPINE: Normal, symmetric
ASSESSMENT: Satisfactory camp physical
PLAN: Permission granted to participate in camp activities without restrictions. Form signed and returned to patient.

answer: 99393

Learning Objectives

6.1 Identify categories and subcategories in the Evaluation and Management (E/M) section of the CPT® codebook.

6.2 Identify the numerical range of E/M codes in the CPT® codebook.

6.3 Provide examples of the terms *patient status*, *type of service*, and *place of service* as used within the E/M section.

6.4 Define and differentiate a "new patient" and an "established patient."

6.5 Explain when time can be a key component in choosing the appropriate code.

6.6 Identify the 7 components of level of service that must be considered before assigning a code from the E/M section.

6.7 Understand the 3 key components of level of service used in assigning E/M codes.

6.8 Define and differentiate the terms *counseling*, *consultation*, and *concurrent care*.

6.9 Apply documentation guidelines in selecting the proper level of service in the history, examination, and medical decision-making aspects.

6.10 Apply the instructional notes and guidelines of the E/M section in selecting the proper setting and/or category of codes to use when coding for E/M services.

6.11 Identify the appropriate modifiers when assigning codes from the E/M section.

6.12 Assign appropriate E/M codes to case examples.

Chapter Outline

- **I.** Introduction to Evaluation and Management Coding
  - **A.** History of Evaluation and Management Codes
- **II.** Evaluation and Management Services Guidelines
  - **A.** Classification of Evaluation and Management Services
  - **B.** Definitions of Commonly Used Terms
    - **i.** New and Established Patient
    - **ii.** Chief Complaint
    - **iii.** Concurrent Care and Transfer of Care
    - **iv.** Counseling
    - **v.** History
    - **vi.** Levels of Evaluation and Management Services
    - **vii.** Nature of Presenting Problem
    - **viii.** Time
  - **C.** Unlisted Service
  - **D.** Special Report
  - **E.** Clinical Examples
  - **F.** Instructions for Selecting a Level of Evaluation and Management Service
    - **i.** History Key Component
    - **ii.** Examination Key Component
    - **iii.** Medical Decision-Making Key Component
    - **iv.** Contributing Components
- **III.** Organization of the Evaluation and Management Codes
  - **A.** Office or Other Outpatient Services (Codes 99201-99215)
  - **B.** Hospital Observation Services (Codes 99217-99226)
  - **C.** Hospital Inpatient Services (Codes 99221-99239)
  - **D.** Consultations (Codes 99241-99255)
  - **E.** Emergency Department Services (Codes 99281-99288)
  - **F.** Critical Care Services (Codes 99291-99292)
  - **G.** Nursing Facility Services (Codes 99304-99318)
  - **H.** Domiciliary, Rest Home (eg, Boarding Home), or Custodial Care Services (Codes 99324-99337)
  - **I.** Domiciliary, Rest Home (eg Assisted Living Facility), or Home Care Plan Oversight Services (Codes 99339-99340)
  - **J.** Home Services (Codes 99341-99350)
  - **K.** Prolonged Services (Codes 99354-99360; 99415-99416)
  - **L.** Case Management Services (Codes 99366-99368)
  - **M.** Care Plan Oversight Services (Codes 99374-99380)
  - **N.** Preventive Medicine Services (Codes 99381-99429)
  - **O.** Non-Face-to-Face Services (Codes 99441-99449)
  - **P.** Special Evaluation and Management Services (Codes 99450-99456)
  - **Q.** Newborn Care Services (Codes 99460-99463)
  - **R.** Delivery/Birthing Room Attendance and Resuscitation Services (Codes 99464-99465)
  - **S.** Inpatient Neonatal Intensive Care Services and Pediatric and Neonatal Critical Care Services (Codes 99466-99486)
  - **T.** Cognitive Assessment and Care Plan Services (Code 99483)
  - **U.** Care Management Services (Codes 99487-99490)
  - **V.** Psychiatric Collaborative Care Management Services (Codes 99492-99494)

Introduction to Evaluation and Management Coding

Evaluation and management (E/M) codes describe services that a physician or other qualified healthcare professional provides to evaluate patients and manage their care. In addition to physicians, "qualified healthcare professionals" include the following types of providers:

- nurse practitioners;
- clinical nurse specialists;
- certified nurse midwives;
- physician assistants.

E/M codes (99201 through 99499) are listed first in the tabular portion of most CPT® codebooks because these codes are reported frequently. E/M codes describe the intensity or complexity of the service provided to the patient during an encounter. The level of history, comprehensiveness of the physical examination, and the medical decision-making process is predictive of the value of that service provided. In other words, the more comprehensive the service, the more reimbursement received. Time is another way to measure the level and value of service provided, as well as other considerations that will be discussed in detail in this chapter.

History of Evaluation and Management Codes

Coding Clicks

The CMS web page "Documentation Guidelines for Evaluation and Management (E/M) Services" provides online access to the 1995 guidelines at http://Coding.ParadigmEducation.com/1995 and the 1997 guidelines at http://Coding.ParadigmEducation.com/1997.

The American Medical Association (AMA) has continued to develop the CPT® code set since its inception in 1966, as described in Chapter 2. New and more detailed E/M codes were created in 1992 to assist in selecting the most appropriate E/M level. Providers and claims reviewers had many disagreements regarding the application of the E/M codes. The Health Care Financing Administration (HCFA), now known as the Centers for Medicare and Medicaid Services (CMS), and the AMA issued the *1995 Documentation Guidelines for Evaluation and Management Services* to clarify the use of E/M codes. These guidelines still required interpretation and did not meet both the payers' and providers' needs. HCFA/CMS and AMA created a revised edition of the documentation guidelines in 1997 that were intended to be implemented in 1998 but were not. In 2001, CMS announced an indefinite hold on further collaboration with the AMA to refine the guidelines. This text will discuss the guidelines further and will primarily refer to the 1995 edition, which will be cited as the *1995 Documentation Guidelines*.

Evaluation and Management (E/M) Services Guidelines

The CPT® codebook Evaluation and Management section begins with a subsection titled "Evaluation and Management (E/M) Services Guidelines." These guidelines provide vital information for using E/M codes organized by the following topics that will be explored in this chapter:

- Classification of Evaluation and Management Services;
- Definitions of Commonly Used Terms;
- Unlisted Service;
- Special Report;
- Clinical Examples;
- Instructions for Selecting a Level of Evaluation and Management Service.

Classification of Evaluation and Management Services

E/M codes are classified into categories that describe the type of service, place of service, and patient status. Categories (such as office or outpatient visits) are then further divided into headings to identify the patient status (new or established) and the type of service from problem-focused to comprehensive.

Definitions of Commonly Used Terms

The E/M Guidelines define commonly used terms in the codes to reduce subjective interpretation and increase consistency in reporting. These terms are defined below.

New and Established Patient

A **new patient** is someone who has not received any face-to-face service from the physician, or any other physician or other qualified health professional in the exact same specialty who belongs to the same group practice, within the past 3 years. Advanced practice nurses and physician assistants who work with physicians are considered to be in the same specialty as the physicians they work with.

An **established patient** is someone who is not considered a new patient. Established patients have received face-to-face services from the physician or other qualified health professional in the exact same specialty within the past 3 years. Figure 6.1 illustrates how one can determine the status of a patient as either new or established.

Chief Complaint

The **chief complaint** is the reason for the encounter. The chief complaint is usually documented in the patient's own words. It is a statement that describes the symptom or problem that caused the patient to seek care.

Figure 6.1 Decision Tree for Distinguishing New Versus Established Patients in a Group Practice

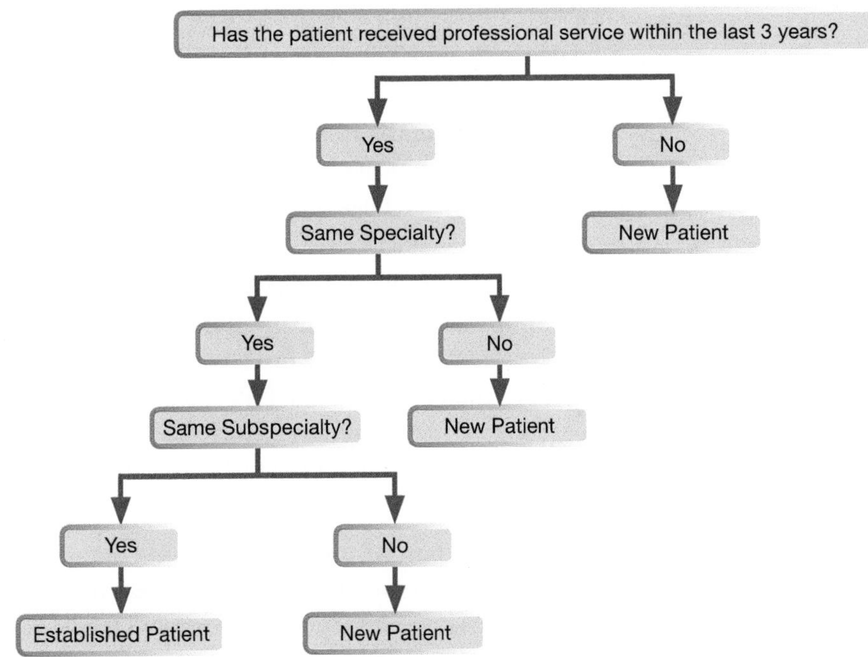

Concurrent Care and Transfer of Care

Concurrent care occurs when a patient is seen by more than 1 provider on the same date of service. Many third-party payers limit reimbursement of E/M codes to 1 physician per day unless the physicians have different specialties and the E/M services are medically necessary. For example, a hospital inpatient may have services on the same calendar day from a nephrologist for chronic kidney disease, as well as services from an oncologist for breast cancer. Since these are 2 different specialists who are providing services to the patient for different diagnoses, no special reporting is required.

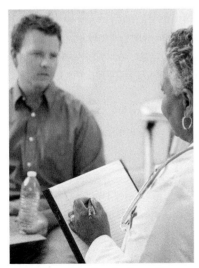
Doctors may review test results and discuss treatment options with the patient. This is considered counseling.

A **transfer of care** occurs when a physician gives the responsibility of providing services to a patient to another physician who explicitly agrees to accept this responsibility. A physician may transfer management of some or all of a patient's problems to another physician. A transfer of care is not considered a consultation, in which an opinion is provided but the responsibility of management remains with the original physician.

Counseling

Counseling is a discussion with the patient and/or family regarding the patient's care and treatment options. Counseling may include reviewing results of diagnostic tests, recommending tests to be performed, discussing the patient's prognosis, identifying the risks and benefits of treatment options, giving instructions for treatment and follow-up, explaining the importance of compliance with care management, discussing risk-factor reduction, and providing patient and/or family education. The time spent counseling the patient must be documented in the health record to be considered a factor in assigning E/M codes.

History

Documentation of a patient's history is represented by several component histories that a provider collects from a patient. The provider's fact-finding is documented as family history, history of present illness, past history, social history, and review of systems.

Family History **Family history** documents the diseases of biological family members that may place the patient's health at risk or may be hereditary. The health status or cause of death of parents, siblings, and children should be included in the family history.

History of Present Illness The **history of present illness (HPI)** is the chronological description of the development of the patient's current illness. The HPI includes the patient's description of the first sign or symptom of the illness until the present time. The documentation of the HPI should include the location, quality, severity, timing, context, and modifying factors affecting the presenting problem. The HPI is categorized as brief or extended based on the number of elements documented.

Past History A **past history** documents any of the patient's previous illnesses, injuries, treatments, hospitalizations, and surgeries. The patient's allergies, immunization status, dietary status, reproductive history, and medication use may also be documented in the past history.

Social History The **social history** documents the social factors that may affect the patient's health. This includes the patient's use of tobacco, alcohol, and drugs; level of education; occupational history and current employment; military history; sexual history; living arrangements; and any other factors that the provider identifies as relevant. Figure 6.2 illustrates a typical social history form in an electronic health record (EHR) system.

Review of Systems The **system review** or **review of systems (ROS)** is a series of questions asked by the provider to obtain information from the patient about his or her current condition. The CPT® codebook identifies 14 elements of a system review and the extent of elements documented is used to determine the level of history affecting the code assignment. The ROS will be discussed in more detail in the history section of this chapter.

Levels of Evaluation and Management Services

The **levels of E/M services** describe variations in the scope of services rendered and are the qualifying factors that distinguish codes within their respective categories and subcategories. A group of related codes may have from 3 to 5 levels. The levels are determined by 7 basic components that will be discussed in detail later in this chapter: history, examination, medical decision-making, counseling, coordination of care, nature of presenting problem, and time.

Figure 6.2 Social History in an Electronic Health Record

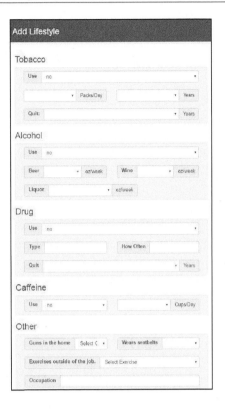

Nature of Presenting Problem

E/M codes describe 5 types of presenting problems: minimal, self-limited or minor, low severity, moderate severity, and high severity. A **minimal** problem is one that may not require the presence of a physician to treat. A **self-limited** or **minor** problem is transient, and it is not likely to alter the patient's health status permanently or has a good prognosis if the patient is compliant with medical treatment. A problem with **low severity** has a low risk of morbidity (disease) without treatment, little to no risk of mortality (death), and an expected full recovery without any functional impairment. A problem of **moderate severity** has a moderate risk of morbidity without treatment, a moderate risk of mortality without treatment, an uncertain prognosis, or a higher risk of prolonged functional impairment. A presenting problem of **high severity** has a high-to-extreme risk of morbidity and mortality without treatment. A presenting problem of high severity has a higher risk of severe, prolonged functional impairment.

Time

Time is a factor in the description of many E/M codes. AMA studies determined the time and work involved for typical E/M services, and the times presented in the code descriptors are averages to be used for comparison only. Time alone is not used as a determination of code selection with some exceptions that will be discussed later in this chapter. The time component includes intraservice time, which for office and outpatient visits is face-to-face time with the patient, and for hospital and other inpatient visits includes all unit or floor time spent in the care and management of the patient.

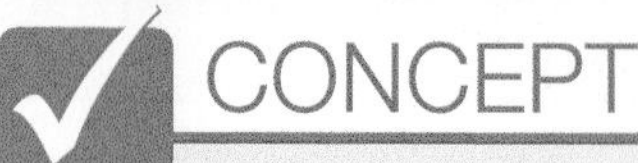

CONCEPTS CHECKPOINT 6.1

Fill in the blank to complete the following sentences.

1. The patient's use of alcohol and tobacco is documented in the ______________.
2. A presenting problem with little to no risk of mortality is considered ______________.
3. A statement in the patient's own words of the reason for the encounter is the ______________.
4. An established patient has been seen within the past ______________ years.
5. The cause of death of a patient's parent would be documented in the ______________.

Unlisted Service

An E/M service may be provided that has no available code to properly describe what was done. This section of the codebook has 2 codes that may be used, for an unlisted preventive medicine service or an unlisted E/M service. Additional reporting requirements apply as described below.

Special Report

CPT® guidelines include the use of special reports when an unusual service is provided. A service that is reported with an unlisted code may require a special report to show that the service was medically necessary and appropriate. When reporting an unlisted E/M code, the special report should contain the patient's final diagnosis, a description of the complexity of the symptoms, physical findings, results of diagnostic and therapeutic procedures, and any expected follow-up care.

Clinical Examples

Appendix C in the CPT® codebook provides clinical examples of the more common E/M codes. The examples in Appendix C describe typical patient scenarios intended to help providers understand the meaning of the code descriptions so the correct code is selected.

Instructions for Selecting a Level of Evaluation and Management Service

As described earlier, levels of E/M service distinguish codes within code families. In the AMA codebook, the red headings in the Instructions for Selecting a Level of Evaluation and Management Service subsection present a step-by-step method for selecting the level of service within a family of codes:

1. Review the reporting instructions for the selected category or subcategory.
2. Review the level of E/M service descriptors in the selected category or subcategory.
3. Determine the extent of history obtained from the health record.
4. Determine the extent of examination performed from the health record.

5. Determine the complexity of medical decision-making.
6. Select the appropriate level of E/M service.

Seven components must be considered before selecting the level of service. These components are reflected in the documentation in the health record, which must support the E/M code reported for the service. History, examination, and medical decision-making are considered the **key components**. These key components appear as bulleted items in the code descriptions. Counseling, coordination of care, the nature of the presenting problem, and time are considered **contributing components**. These components are summarized in the code descriptions, with the time component specified. Using the health record to determine these components is discussed in detail below.

History Key Component

The first key component in selecting the level of service is the history. The **history** component of the E/M code includes the chief complaint; the HPI; the ROS; and past medical, family, and social histories (PFSH). Reviewing the documentation in the health record for each of these elements will identify the extent of the history obtained. The history can then be categorized as 1 of 4 types, which differentiate the E/M codes:

- **problem-focused**—requires the chief complaint and a brief HPI or problem;
- **expanded problem-focused**—requires the chief complaint, a brief HPI, and a problem-pertinent ROS, which pertains only to the chief complaint;
- **detailed**—requires the chief complaint, an extended HPI, problem-pertinent ROS extended to include a review of a limited number of additional body systems, and a pertinent PFSH directly related to the patient's current problems;
- **comprehensive**—requires the chief complaint; an extended HPI; an ROS related to the problem identified in the HPI plus a review of all additional body systems; and complete PFSH.

Table 6.1 shows the progression of elements required for each type of history.

Table 6.1 Type of History Correlated With History Elements

Type of History	History Elements			
	Chief Complaint	History of Present Illness (HPI)	Review of Systems (ROS)	Past, Family, and/or Social History (PFSH)
Problem-focused	Required	Brief	N/A	N/A
Expanded problem-focused	Required	Brief	Problem pertinent	N/A
Detailed	Required	Extended	Extended	Pertinent
Comprehensive	Required	Extended	Complete	Complete

Adapted from: Centers for Medicare and Medicaid Services. *1995 Documentation Guidelines for Evaluation and Management Services.* Medicare Learning Network, 1995, p. 4. http://www.cms.gov/Outreach-and-Education/Medicare-Learning-Network-MLN/MLNEdWebGuide/Downloads/95Docguidelines.pdf, CMS.gov. Accessed February 1, 2015.

The chief complaint is required for all types of history. The HPI, ROS, and PFSH elements will be detailed in the following paragraphs.

History of Present Illness As shown in Table 6.1, the HPI is correlated with all 4 types of history. An HPI is a timeline of the development of the patient's illness that can be categorized as brief or extended based on the number of components it includes. Table 6.2 shows the 8 components of an HPI. A brief HPI contains up to 3 components, while an extended HPI will have 4 or more components documented.

Table 6.2 History of Present Illness Components

HPI Component	Definition
Location	The place on the body where the symptom or pain is occurring
Quality	Characteristics of the symptom or pain (fullness, bloating, sharp, stabbing, etc.)
Severity	The level of pain on a scale of 1 to 10, or a measure of how difficult the pain is to endure
Duration	The length of time the symptom has lasted (hours, days, weeks, etc.)
Timing	The time of day the symptom or pain occurs (only at night, first thing in the morning, etc.)
Context	The situation in which the symptom or pain occurs (after eating, while exercising, etc.)
Modifying factors	Activities that make the symptom or pain better or worse
Associated signs and symptoms	Other signs or symptoms that are present at the same time

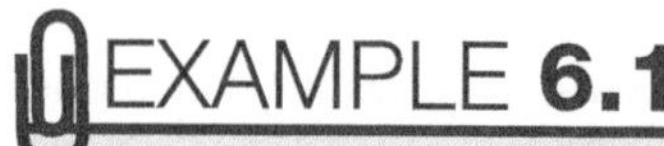

EXAMPLE **6.1**

A 46-year-old female presented to her physician's office with the chief complaint of dizziness. The physician documented the HPI:

> The dizziness is worse on bending over or with movement. She has no symptoms of tinnitus or cold, nor loss of consciousness; her only complaint is dizziness upon movement. She has been dizzy for 4 days.

This HPI is categorized as brief because it includes the following 3 documented components:

1. Modifying factors: dizziness is worse on bending over or with movement;
2. Timing: dizziness upon movement;
3. Duration: 4 days.

Review of Systems As Table 6.1 shows, the review of systems is relevant to 3 types of history that determine the E/M code:

- An expanded problem-focused type of history requires a **problem-pertinent ROS**, which involves the review of 1 body system related to the patient's current problem.
- A detailed type of history requires an **extended ROS**, which involves the review of 1 body system that is related to the patient's current problem as well as additional body systems. Therefore, an extended ROS requires from 2 to 9 systems.

- A comprehensive type of history requires a **complete ROS**, which involves 10 or more body systems. The physician may document positive responses as well as pertinent negative responses for each system.

The following body systems are recognized in the *1995 Documentation Guidelines*:

- constitutional (vital signs, general appearance);
- eyes;
- ears, nose, mouth, throat;
- cardiovascular;
- respiratory;
- gastrointestinal;
- genitourinary;
- musculoskeletal;
- integumentary;
- neurological;
- psychiatric;
- endocrine;
- hematologic/lymphatic;
- allergic/immunologic.

Past, Family, and Social History Documentation of the patient's PFSH is correlated with only 2 types of history. As you can see from Table 6.1, PFSH is not required for a problem-focused or expanded problem-focused history but only for a detailed or comprehensive history. A **pertinent PFSH** correlated with a detailed type of history is a review of the history area (past, family, and social) that is directly related to the presenting problem. A **complete PFSH** correlated with a comprehensive type of history requires a review of at least 2 of the 3 areas; some E/M categories would require a review of all 3 areas.

Determining the Level of History To determine the level of history documented, the coder must consider all 3 of the elements—HPI, ROS, and PFSH. Most coding specialists and auditors use an audit tool to help break down the required elements. The portion of the audit tool containing the history component is shown in Figure 6.3. The tool is a table consisting of 1 column that tracks all the history elements and 4 columns that correlate the elements to the level of history. This table facilitates a step-by-step analysis of the history documented in the health record:

1. Review the health record and use the check boxes in the first column to note the HPI, ROS, and PFSH information in the documentation.
2. Quantify the information for each history element—HPI, ROS, and PFSH—by checking 1 of the boxes in the next 4 history level columns to determine if the element qualifies as problem-focused, expanded problem-focused, detailed, or comprehensive.
3. Combine the HPI, ROS, and PFSH levels to assess the total history key component: If the level of each element is not the same, the history component is assigned to the lowest category documented. For example, if documentation equates to an extended HPI, an extended ROS, and a pertinent PFSH, these levels are not the same. Because the extended HPI falls under the comprehensive history level, but the extended ROS and pertinent PFSH fall under the detailed history level, the history is considered detailed.

Figure 6.3 Evaluation and Management History Audit Tool

SUPPLIES: Pre-Audit Post-Audit		PROBLEM-FOCUSED	EXP PROBLEM-FOCUSED	DETAILED	COMPREHENSIVE
History Final Result for History (3 of 3 required)	HPI: 3 CHRONIC CONDITIONS ❑ Location ❑ Context ❑ Quality ❑ Severity ❑ Modifying factors ❑ Duration ❑ Timing ❑ Associated signs and sx ________ ________ ________		❑ Brief (1-3)		❑ Extended (4 or more)
	ROS: ❑ Constitutional (weight loss, etc.) ❑ Integumentary (skin, breast) ❑ GU ❑ Allergy/immunology ❑ Eyes ❑ Respiratory ❑ Musculo ❑ "All others negative" ❑ ENM&T ❑ Card/Vasc ❑ Neurological ❑ Hem/Lymph ❑ GI ❑ Psychiatric ❑ Endo	❑ None	❑ Pertinent to problem (1 system)	❑ Extended (2-9 systems)	❑ Complete (10 or more systems or some systems with statement "all others negative")
	PFSH areas: ❑ Past history (the patient's past experiences with illness, operations, injuries, and treatments) ❑ Family history (a review of medical events in the patient's family, including diseases that may be hereditary or place the patient at risk) ❑ Social history (an age-appropriate review of past and current activities)		❑ None	❑ Pertinent (1 history area)	❑ Complete *(2 or 3 history areas)

* Complete PFSH 2 Hx areas (a) establish pts. office (outpatient) care, domiciliary care, home care; (b) emergency dept.; (c) subsequent nursing facility care. Circle Hx and exam type with appropriate grid and under level of service complete 3 Hx areas: (a) new pts. office (outpatient) care; domiciliary care; home care; (b) consultations; (c) initial hospital care; (d) hospital observation; and (e) comprehensive nursing facility assessment.

CONCEPTS CHECKPOINT **6.2**

Fill in the blank to complete each of the following statements.

1. A ____________ history does not require an ROS.
2. A ____________ history requires a complete PFSH.
3. An extended ROS must include at least ____________ systems.
4. Documentation in the HPI that includes a description of the location, severity, and timing of the patient's pain is considered to be ____________.
5. A description of what makes a symptom better or worse is called a(n) ____________ factor.

Examination Key Component

The examination is the second key component in selecting the level of service. The **physical examination** is a medical evaluation of a patient's body to determine the patient's health status for wellness or disease. Documentation of the examination uses the portions specified in the *1995 Documentation Guidelines* shown in Table 6.3.

According to the *1995 Documentation Guidelines*, the level of the physical examination component of the E/M service depends on the number of body areas or organ systems examined and the nature of the presenting problem. The levels are categorized into 4 types of examination:

- **problem-focused**—a limited exam of only the affected body area or organ system;
- **expanded problem-focused**—a limited exam of the affected body area or organ system and other symptomatic or related organ systems;
- **detailed**—an extended exam of the affected body area(s) as well as 2 to 7 other symptomatic or related organ systems;
- **comprehensive**—a complete examination of a single system or a general multisystem exam of 8 or more body systems.

Table 6.3 Physical Examination Body Areas and Organ Systems Specified in the *1995 Documentation Guidelines for Evaluation and Management Services*

Body Areas	Organ Systems
Head, including the face	Constitutional (vital signs, general appearance)
Neck	Eyes
Chest, including breasts and axillae	Ears, nose, mouth, and throat
Abdomen	Cardiovascular
Genitalia, groin, buttocks	Respiratory
Back, including spine	Gastrointestinal
Each extremity	Genitourinary
	Musculoskeletal
	Skin
	Neurologic
	Psychiatric
	Hematologic/lymphatic/immunologic

Source: Centers for Medicare and Medicaid Services. *1995 Documentation Guidelines for Evaluation and Management Services.* Medicare Learning Network, 1995, pp. 9-10. http://www.cms.gov/Outreach-and-Education/Medicare-Learning-Network-MLN/MLNEdWebGuide/Downloads/95Docguidelines.pdf, CMS.gov. Accessed February 1, 2015.

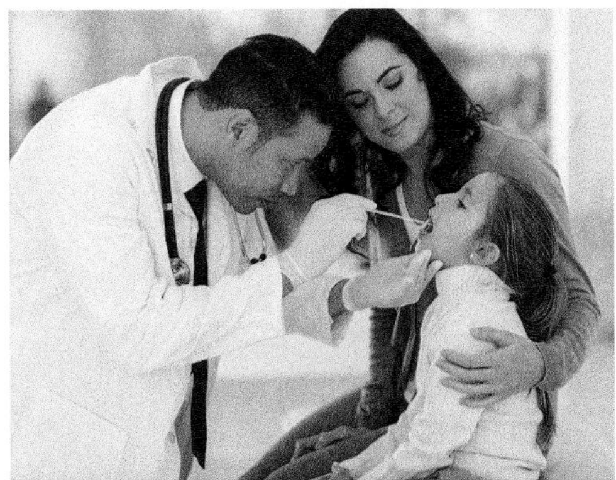

A physician will examine the patient to check for wellness or disease. The physician may focus only on the chief complaint or may do a comprehensive exam.

The 1997 content and documentation requirements for the level of examination are more specific and detailed than the 1995 guidelines. The 1997 documentation guidelines include criteria for general multisystem examinations as well as single-organ system specialty examinations (such as cardiovascular or eye). The content or individual elements of the examination pertaining to that body area or organ system are identified in the 1997 guidelines by bullets (•). As mentioned previously, providers may use either set of guidelines. In general, while most providers use the 1995 guidelines, the 1997 guidelines may be more appropriate for particular specialties or patients. The general multisystem examination content and documentation requirements are shown in Figure 6.4.

As with the history component, most coding specialists and auditors use an audit tool to help break down the required examination components. The portion of the audit tool containing the examination component is shown in Figure 6.5. The tool is a table consisting of 1 column that tracks all the exam elements and 4 columns that correlate the elements to the level of history. This table facilitates a step-by-step analysis of the examination documented in the health record:

1. Review the health record and use the check boxes in the first column to note the body area(s) and/or organ system(s) examined.
2. Quantify the information for each exam element—body area and organ system—by checking 1 of the boxes in the exam level component to determine if the element qualifies as problem-focused, expanded problem-focused, detailed, or comprehensive. The first row of boxes corresponds to the 1997 documentation guidelines and the second row to the 1995 guidelines.

Figure 6.4 General Multisystem Examination Content and Documentation Requirements in the *1997 Documentation Guidelines for Evaluation and Management Services*

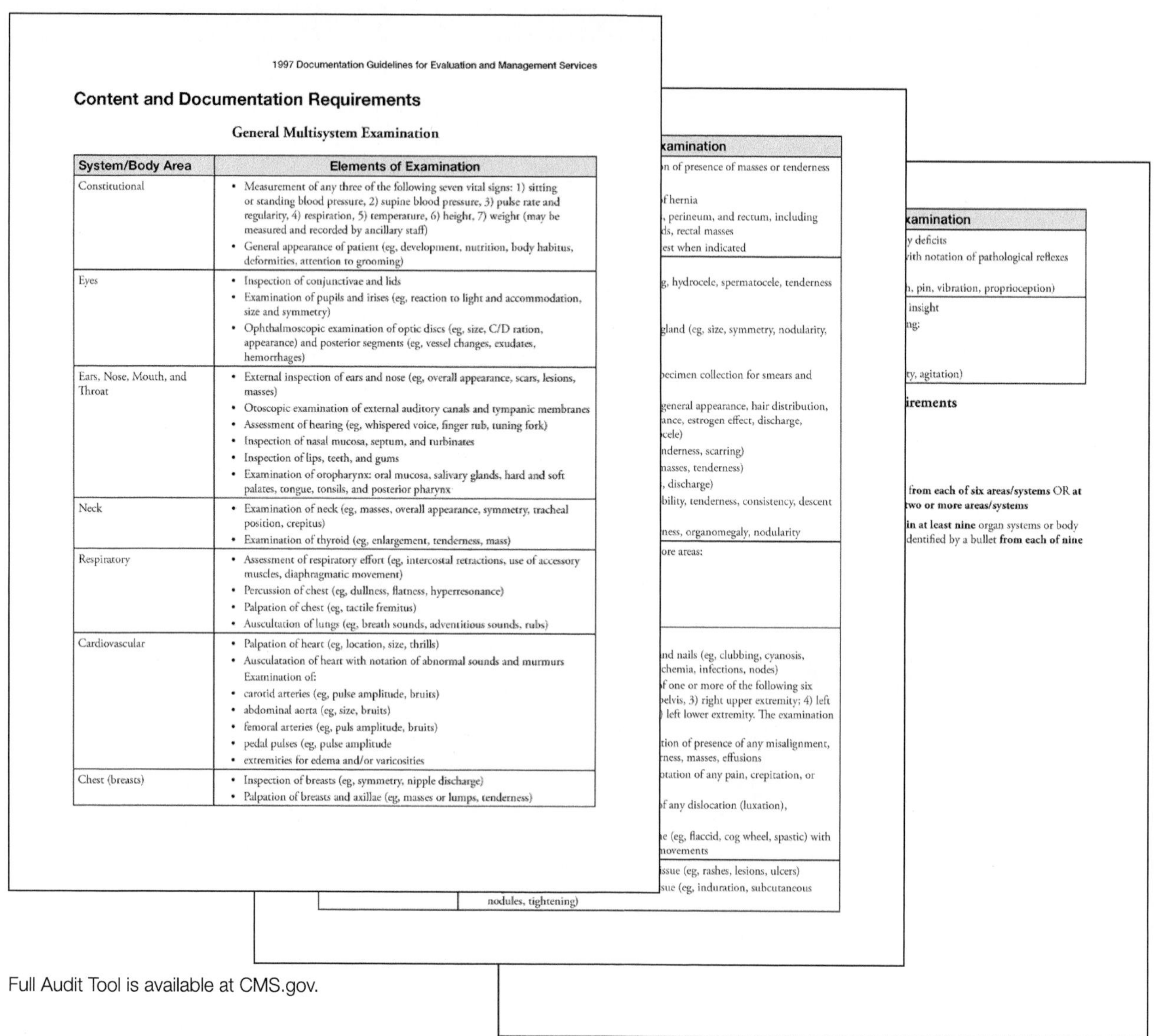

1997 Documentation Guidelines for Evaluation and Management Services

Content and Documentation Requirements

General Multisystem Examination

System/Body Area	Elements of Examination
Constitutional	• Measurement of any three of the following seven vital signs: 1) sitting or standing blood pressure, 2) supine blood pressure, 3) pulse rate and regularity, 4) respiration, 5) temperature, 6) height, 7) weight (may be measured and recorded by ancillary staff) • General appearance of patient (eg, development, nutrition, body habitus, deformities, attention to grooming)
Eyes	• Inspection of conjunctivae and lids • Examination of pupils and irises (eg, reaction to light and accommodation, size and symmetry) • Ophthalmoscopic examination of optic discs (eg, size, C/D ration, appearance) and posterior segments (eg, vessel changes, exudates, hemorrhages)
Ears, Nose, Mouth, and Throat	• External inspection of ears and nose (eg, overall appearance, scars, lesions, masses) • Otoscopic examination of external auditory canals and tympanic membranes • Assessment of hearing (eg, whispered voice, finger rub, tuning fork) • Inspection of nasal mucosa, septum, and turbinates • Inspection of lips, teeth, and gums • Examination of oropharynx: oral mucosa, salivary glands, hard and soft palates, tongue, tonsils, and posterior pharynx
Neck	• Examination of neck (eg, masses, overall appearance, symmetry, tracheal position, crepitus) • Examination of thyroid (eg, enlargement, tenderness, mass)
Respiratory	• Assessment of respiratory effort (eg, intercostal retractions, use of accessory muscles, diaphragmatic movement) • Percussion of chest (eg, dullness, flatness, hyperresonance) • Palpation of chest (eg, tactile fremitus) • Auscultation of lungs (eg, breath sounds, adventitious sounds, rubs)
Cardiovascular	• Palpation of heart (eg, location, size, thrills) • Ausculatation of heart with notation of abnormal sounds and murmurs Examination of: • carotid arteries (eg, pulse amplitude, bruits) • abdominal aorta (eg, size, bruits) • femoral arteries (eg, puls amplitude, bruits) • pedal pulses (eg, pulse amplitude • extremities for edema and/or varicosities
Chest (breasts)	• Inspection of breasts (eg, symmetry, nipple discharge) • Palpation of breasts and axillae (eg, masses or lumps, tenderness)

Full Audit Tool is available at CMS.gov.

Figure 6.5 Evaluation and Management Examination Audit Tool

				PROBLEM-FOCUSED	EXP PROBLEM-FOCUSED	DETAILED	COMPREHENSIVE
Exam	Body areas: ❑ Head, including face ❑ Abdomen ❑ Neck ❑ Each extremity	❑ Chest, including breast and axillae ❑ Back, including spine ❑ Genitalia, groin, buttocks	1997	❑ 1-5 bullets	❑ 6-11 bullets	❑ 12+ bullets	❑ Complete bullet system
	Organ systems: ❑ Constitutional (eg, vital, gen. app.) ❑ Resp ❑ Psych ❑ Skin ❑ Eyes ❑ GU	❑ Ears, nose, mouth, throat ❑ Musculoskeletal ❑ GI ❑ Hem/Lymph/Imm ❑ CV ❑ Neurological	1995	❑ 1 area or system	❑ 2-7 systems	❑ 2-7 systems or 1 in detail	❑ Complete (2 or 3 history areas)

EXAMPLE 6.2

A 65-year-old female presented to her physician's office complaining of abdominal pain. The physician completed a physical exam and documented findings as shown below.

General: This patient is alert and oriented, not in distress. Height 5'3", weight 140 pounds. T 98.5, P 77, R 18, BP 150/88.

HEENT: Head atraumatic, normocephalic. Nose and throat clear. Pupils equal, round, reactive to light.

Neck: Soft, no thyromegaly.

Chest and lungs: Symmetrical on expansion. Clear breath sounds bilaterally. No rales or wheezing.

Heart: Regular rate and rhythm.

Abdomen: Soft. Normoactive bowel sounds. Positive tenderness below the umbilicus. No palpable mass.

Extremities: No gross deformities.

Skin: Looks well hydrated, no rashes or open wounds.

This exam is considered comprehensive because 8 or more systems were examined: constitutional; eye; ear, nose, mouth, and throat; respiratory; cardiovascular; gastrointestinal; musculoskeletal; and skin.

CONCEPTS CHECKPOINT 6.3

Match the type of examination in the first column to the required elements in the second column.

1. _____ problem-focused exam
2. _____ expanded problem-focused exam
3. _____ detailed exam
4. _____ comprehensive exam

a. Extended, 2 to 7 systems
b. Limited, 2 to 7 systems
c. General, 8 or more systems, or complete exam of single system
d. Limited, 1 area or system

Medical Decision-Making Key Component

Medical decision-making is the third key component in selecting the level of service. **Medical decision-making (MDM)** refers to the complexity of establishing a diagnosis and/or selecting a management strategy. The documentation guidelines point out some general factors that indicate decision-making complexity. Decision-making for a problem that has already been diagnosed is easier than that for an undiagnosed problem. Another factor is the patient's progress. Problems that are resolving are less complex than those that are worsening.

Documenting the thought process makes MDM one of the more difficult key components. Providers must document the diagnosis and treatments they considered as well as all the data they reviewed to make the plan of care. The MDM component is measured in 3 elements, which will be discussed in depth:

- number of diagnoses or management options;
- amount and/or complexity of data to be reviewed;
- risk of significant complications, morbidity, and/or mortality.

Number of Diagnoses or Management Options The first element in assessing MDM complexity is the number and types of problems and their associated possible treatment options that are evaluated and reviewed during the patient encounter. The documentation of the presenting problem will differ based on whether a diagnosis has already been established or is yet unknown. With an established diagnosis, the documentation should state whether the problem is improving (well controlled, resolving, or resolved) or worsening (inadequately controlled, failing to change as expected). Without an established diagnosis, the documentation will reflect an assessment stated as a "possible," "probable," or "rule out" diagnosis, or as a differential diagnosis. A **differential diagnosis** is distinguishing a disease from others with similar signs or symptoms. Management decisions are documented as treatment options that may include patient instructions, nursing instructions, therapies, and medications. The provider characterizes the number of diagnoses or management options on a scale—minimal, limited, multiple, or extensive—at his or her discretion, as the documentation guidelines do not quantify the numbers of diagnoses or options in each category.

Amount and/or Complexity of Data to Be Reviewed The second element in assessing MDM complexity is the amount and/or complexity of the data to be reviewed. Data review can become complicated by evaluating a number of diagnostic tests and imaging studies, ordering and reviewing old medical records, or consulting sources other than the patient. For example, reviewing an image or tracing and not just reviewing the report is considered a factor that increases the amount of data to be reviewed. The 1995 and 1997 documentation guidelines describe how the review of diagnostic tests may be documented. Written prior to the widespread use of computer-based records, some of the guidelines are specific to paper-based records, such as the idea that a provider can document the review of a test by initialing and dating the report that contains the test results.

The data review is rated on a subjective scale: minimal or none, limited, moderate, or extensive. These categories are not defined in the documentation guidelines, and the provider has discretion. Figure 6.6 shows the MDM component of an audit tool. The left grid provides a worksheet to assign values to the 3 elements. Box A tracks diagnoses and management options, where points are assigned to problems. This numeric value is referenced to Box C, where a *minimal or none* level would be 1 item or less, a *limited* amount of data would be 2 items, a *moderate* amount would be 3 items, and an *extensive* amount would be 4 or more items.

EXAMPLE 6.3

A 21-year-old male came to the office as a new patient with complaints of recurrent stomach pain. The physician reviewed the lab results of a general health panel consisting of a comprehensive metabolic panel and a complete blood count that was brought in by the patient. The physician initialed and dated the paper copy of the lab report. The physician also ordered an abdominal ultrasound for the patient and requested old records from the patient's previous physician. Using Box B in Figure 6.6, the amount of data to be reviewed would encompass 3 categories: clinical lab tests, radiology, and decision to obtain old records. Awarding 1 point for each of those categories, the total score of 3 would reflect on line B in Box C a value of *moderate* for the amount and complexity of data to be reviewed.

Figure 6.6 Evaluation and Management Examination Audit Tool, Medical Decision-Making Detail

Medical Decision-Making

Box A:
Number of Diagnosis or Management Options (N x P + R)

Problems to Exam Physician	Number	Points	Result
Self-limited or minor (stable, improved, or worsening)	Max = 2	1	
Est. problem—stable, improved		1	
Est. problem—unstable		2	
New problem—no additional work-up planned	Max = 1	3	
New problem—additional work-up planned		4	
Bring total to line A in Final Result for MDM Total			

Box B:
Amount and/or complexity of data to be reviewed

			Points
Review and/or order of clinical lab tests			1
Review and/or order of tests in radiology section of CPT®			1
Review and/or order of tests in the medicine section of CPT®			1
Discussion of test results with performing physician			1
Discussion to obtain old records and/or obtain history from someone other than patient and/or discussion of case with another healthcare provider			2
Independent visualization of image, tracing, or specimen itself (not simply review of report)			2
Bring total to line B in Final Result for MDM Total			

Box C: Final result for complexity of medical decision-making: 2 of 3 required

A	Number of diagnoses or management options	<1 Minimal	2 Limited	3 Multiple	>4 Extensive
B	Amount and complexity of data to be reviewed	<1 Minimal	2 Limited	3 Multiple	>4 Extensive
C	Risk of complications and/or morbidity or mortality	Minimal	Low	Moderate	High
	TYPE OF DECISION-MAKING	STRAIGHT FORWARD	LOW COMPLEX	MODERATE COMPLEX	HIGH COMPLEX

Risk Level	Presenting Problem(s)	Diagnostic Procedure(s) Ordered	Management Options Selected
Minimal	• One self-limited or minor problem; eg, cold, insect bite, tinea corporis	• Laboratory tests requiring venipuncture • Chest x-rays • ECG/EEG • Urinalysis • Ultrasound; eg, echo • KOH prep	• Rest • Gargles • Elastic bandages • Superficial dressings
Low	• Two or more self-limited or minor problems • One stable chronic illness; eg, well-controlled hypertension or on-insulin dependent diabetes, cataract, BPH • Acute uncomplicated illness or injury; eg, cystitis, allergic rhinitis, simple sprain	• Physiological test not under stress; eg, pulmonary function tests • Noncardiovascular imaging studies with contrast; eg, barium enema • Superficial needle biopsies • Clinical laboratory tests requiring arterial puncture • Skin biopsies	• Over-the-counter drugs • Minor surgery with no identified risk factors • Physical therapy • Occupational therapy • IV fluids without additives
Moderate	• 1 or more chronic illnesses with mild exacerbation, progression, or side effects of treatment • 2 or more stable chronic illnesses • Undiagnosed new problem with uncertain prognosis; eg, lump in breast • Acute illness with systemic symptoms; eg, pyelonephritis, pheumonitis, colitis • Acute complicated injury; eg, head injury with brief loss of consciousness	• Physiologic test under stress; eg, cardiac stress test • Diagnostic endoscopies with no identified risk factors • Deep needle or incisional biopsy • Cardiovascular imaging studies with contrast and no identified risk factors; eg, arteriogram, cardiac catheterization • Obtain fluid from body cavity; eg, lumbar puncture, thoracentesis, culdocentesis	• Minor surgery with identified risk factors • Elective major surgery (open, percutaneous, or endoscopic) with no identified risk factors • Prescription drug management • Therapeutic nuclear medicine • IV fluids with additives • Closed treatment of fracture or dislocation without manipulation
High	• 1 or more chronic illnesses with severe exacerbation, progression, or side effects of treatment • Acute or chronic illnesses or injuries that pose a threat to life or bodily function; eg, multiple trauma, acute MI, pulmonary embolus, severe respiratory distress, progressive severe rheumatoid arthritis, psychiatric illness with potential threat to self or others, peritonitis, ARF • An abrupt change in neurologic status; eg, seizure, TIA, weakness, or sensory loss	• Cardiovascular imaging studies with contrast with identified risk factors • Cardiac electro-physiological tests • Diagnostic endoscopies with identified risk factors • Discography	• Elective major surgery (open, percutaneous, or endoscopic) with identified risk factors • Emergency major surgery (open, percutaneous, endoscopic) • Parental controlled substances • Drug therapy requiring intensive monitoring for toxicity • Decision not to resuscitate or to deescalate care because of poor prognosis
Bring results to line C in Final Result for Medical Decision-Making			

Risk of Complications and/or Morbidity or Mortality The third element in assessing MDM complexity is the level of risk of significant complications and/or morbidity or mortality. This risk is categorized as minimal, low, moderate, or high. The *1995 Documentation Guidelines* include a table that assesses levels of risk for 3 categories: the presenting problem(s), the diagnostic procedure(s), and the possible management options. This table has been reproduced as the right grid in the audit tool shown in Figure 6.6. The highest level assigned to any category determines the level of risk of complications and/or morbidity or mortality. For example, if the nature of the presenting problem is minor and considered to be in the *minimal* risk category, but the management option was an order for physical therapy in the *low* risk category, the higher level (in this case, *low* instead of *minimal*) would be used in determining the MDM.

Selecting the Medical Decision-Making Level To help put together the 3 elements that determine MDM complexity, the *1995 Documentation Guidelines* contains a chart that shows the progression of elements required for each level of MDM, as shown in Table 6.4. Two of the 3 elements must be met or exceeded to qualify for the level.

Table 6.4 *1995 Documentation Guidelines* Elements Correlated With Level of Medical Decision-Making

Level of Medical Decision-Making	Elements of Medical Decision-Making (2 of 3 elements must be met or exceeded)		
	Number of Diagnoses or Management Options	**Amount or Complexity of Data to Be Reviewed**	**Risk of Complications and/or Morbidity or Mortality**
Straightforward	Minimal	Minimal or none	Minimal
Low Complexity	Limited	Limited	Low
Moderate Complexity	Multiple	Moderate	Moderate
High Complexity	Extensive	Extensive	High

CONCEPTS CHECKPOINT 6.4

Answer the following questions.

1. List the 3 elements in MDM. ______________
2. How many of the 3 elements in MDM must be met or exceeded to qualify for a particular level? ______________
3. How is the level of risk of complications and/or morbidity or mortality determined if the elements are of differing values? ______________

</> Coding for CMS

When choosing an E/M code based on time spent counseling and/or coordinating care, CMS requires documentation of both the length of time for the entire visit and face-to-face time spent with the patient. The length of time spent on procedures that have a separate CPT® code are not factored into the time for the selected visit code.

Contributing Components

To define the level of E/M service, in addition to the 3 key components of the history, the examination, and the MDM, there are contributing components, which include counseling, coordination of care, the nature of the presenting problem, and time. These factors may not all be relevant to each patient encounter.

Counseling is a discussion with the patient and/or family regarding the patient's care and treatment options. **Coordination of care** is the deliberate organization of the patient's care between the physician and another caregiver, whether it be another physician, health professional, or facility, to ensure that the patient's needs are met. Time is an average unit of work involved in a service. When counseling and/or coordination of care comprises more than 50% of the patient encounter, time is considered the controlling factor in selecting the appropriate E/M level. The time spent counseling the patient or family and/or coordinating care must be documented in the health record. However, the nature of the presenting problem may dictate a higher-level E/M code when it affects the ability of the provider to complete the H&P exam. For example, a patient may arrive unconscious with an unknown diagnosis and be unable to provide a history to the physician.

Organization of the Evaluation and Management Codes

E/M codes are used to report the providers' assessment and supervision of medical conditions and are the most frequently reported CPT® codes. Therefore, they are typically the first set of codes listed in a CPT® codebook. E/M codes are divided into subsections by the place or type of service provided, as shown in Table 6.5.

The place of service (such as office or nursing facility) or type of service (such as office visit or case management services) represents the primary division of E/M codes. Instructional notes accompany many of these subsections and should be read carefully before selecting codes. Many E/M codes are further categorized by whether the service is for a new or established patient (as in office visits) or whether the service is for an initial visit or a subsequent visit (as inpatient hospital services). The final organizational principle is the level of service. In general, before the E/M code can be selected, the coding specialist must determine the place and type of service, if the patient was new or established, and the level of E/M service as discussed previously. This process will be discussed as it relates to each codebook subsection.

Office or Other Outpatient Services (Codes 99201-99215)

E/M services provided in an office or other outpatient setting are reported with codes 99201 through 99215. Outpatient settings include physician offices, clinics, and other ambulatory facilities. These codes are divided into new or established patients using the definitions given earlier in this chapter. New patients have 5 levels of visit codes ranging from 99201 at the simplest level to 99205 at the most comprehensive level. New patients must meet or exceed all the requirements of the 3 key components of history, examination, and MDM.

Table 6.5 Evaluation and Management Subsections and Corresponding Codes

Subsection	Code(s)
Office or Other Outpatient Services	99201-99215
Hospital Observation Services	99217-99220; 99224-99226
Hospital Inpatient Services	99221-99223; 99231-99239
Consultations	99241-99255
Emergency Department Services	99281-99288
Critical Care Services	99291-99292
Nursing Facility Services	99304-99318
Domiciliary, Rest Home (eg, Boarding Home), or Custodial Care Services	99324-99337
Domiciliary, Rest Home (eg, Assisted Living Facility), or Home Care Plan Oversight Services	99339-99340
Home Services	99341-99350
Prolonged Services	99354-99360; 99415-99416
Case Management Services	99366-99368
Care Plan Oversight Services	99374-99380
Preventive Medicine Services	99381-99429
Non-Face-to-Face Services	99441-99449
Special Evaluation and Management Services	99450-99456
Newborn Care Services	99460-99463
Delivery/Birthing Room Attendance and Resuscitation Services	99464-99465
Inpatient Neonatal Intensive Care Services and Pediatric and Neonatal Critical Care Services	99466-99486
Cognitive Assessment and Care Plan Services	99483
Care Management Services	99487-99490
Psychiatric Collaborative Care Management Services	99492-99494
Transitional Care Management Services	99495-99496
Advance Care Planning	99497-99498
General Behavioral Health Integration Care Management	99484
Other Evaluation and Management Services	99499

EXAMPLE **6.4**

A 68-year-old male visited the physician office for the first time with complaints of itchy, red bumps on his forearms. The physician documented the following office progress note:

CC: Itchy, red bumps on both forearms

HPI: This 68-year-old male noticed these bumps shortly after weeding his garden 2 days ago. He noticed the bumps appeared over several hours. The bumps are itchy and red and cover most of the forearm area. Their appearance has not changed.

Exam: Normal, healthy-appearing adult male. Raised, red bumps on both forearms. Skin otherwise intact, no cuts or bruising.

Assessment and plan: Contact dermatitis. Apply cool, wet compresses. Apply OTC anti-itch cream. Avoid working in the garden unless wearing long sleeves. No need for follow-up unless condition worsens.

The coding specialist for this physician's office noted that this is a new patient. Therefore, the range of codes from which to select is 99201 through 99205. To choose the correct code requires analyzing the 3 key components in the progress note to determine the E/M level of service. The table below shows the analysis.

Selecting the E/M Level of Service With 3 Key Components

Key Component	Progress Note Documented Elements	Analysis of E/M Level
History	• Chief complaint: Itchy, red bumps on forearms • History of present illness: Brief, 1-3 elements documented: – Timing: appeared over several hours – Context: started after gardening – Duration: lasted 2 days • Review of systems: Pertinent to problem (1 system) Integumentary • Past, family, and social history: None	This supports an expanded problem-focused level of history.
Examination	• Constitutional system: Normal, healthy appearing • Skin: Raised, red bumps on both forearms	This supports an **expanded problem-focused level of exam** (2-7 systems).
Medical Decision-Making	• Number of diagnoses or treatment options: This is a new problem with no additional workup planned: **moderate complexity** • Amount or complexity of data to be reviewed: None: **straightforward complexity** • Complication risk factors: One self-limited or minor problem, no additional tests ordered, over-the-counter remedy: considered **low complexity**.	The level of MDM requires the highest 2 out of 3 if all categories are not the same. Since this documentation is placed into straightforward, low, and moderate categories, the MDM element would be assigned to the low complexity level.

This is an office visit involving a new patient, and the E/M level of services would support code 99202, excerpted here to show the 3 key components of level of service:

> *Office or other outpatient visit for the evaluation and management of a new patient, which requires these 3 key components:*
>
> - *An expanded problem-focused history;*
> - *An expanded problem-focused examination;*
> - *Straightforward medical decision making.*

Since this is a new patient, 3 of 3 elements must be met or exceeded. The code's history and examination levels are both *expanded problem-focused* as documented in the progress note, and the MDM level of *straightforward* has been exceeded by the *low complexity* decision-making documented in the progress note. (While code 99203 has a *low complexity* level of MDM, the history and exam documented in the progress note are not detailed so do not meet the requirements of that code.)

EXAMPLE 6.5

An office visit was provided for a 45-year-old male patient, who is visiting from out of state and suffers from lichen planus. His medication was lost with his luggage, and he requires a refill of a topical steroid prescription. The physician documented the following progress note:

CC: Prescription refill

HPI: This 45-year-old male with a known diagnosis of lichen planus is visiting from out of state. Apparently, the airline lost his luggage, so he requests a refill of his prescription of Clobex lotion. The patient claims that Clobex helps with symptoms of redness and irritation.

Exam: His skin appears generally intact without bumps or lesions.

Assessment and plan: History of lichen planus. Prescription given for Clobex lotion 0.05%, apply twice daily.

The physician performed a problem-focused history and exam with straightforward MDM. This is reported with code 99201, excerpted here to show the 3 key components of level of service:

Office or other outpatient visit for the evaluation and management of a new patient, which requires these 3 key components:

- *A problem-focused history;*
- *A problem-focused examination;*
- *Straightforward medical decision making.*

Established patients also have 5 levels of visit codes ranging from 99211 at the lowest level to 99215 at the highest, most comprehensive level. Established patients have different requirements than new patients and must meet or exceed only 2 of the 3 key components. The first level for established patients (99211) does not require the presence of a physician or other qualified health professional and does not require a history, exam, or documentation of MDM. Code 99211 is reported for services such as dressing changes, suture removal, or a blood pressure check when performed by the nurse.

EXAMPLE 6.6

An office visit was provided for monitoring an established patient, a 50-year-old female with Type 1 insulin-dependent diabetes mellitus and stable coronary artery disease. The physician documented the following progress note:

CC: Feeling tired, occasional headaches

HPI: This 50-year-old female with a history of Type 1 IDDM and CAD presents with a complaint of feeling tired. Her blood sugars have been within acceptable range when she tests at home. She has been consistent with dosing.

ROS: Healthy-appearing female with no history of recent weight loss.

Exam: Vital signs WNL. Pulse 80 BPM; respirations 18; BP 120/79. Heart sounds WNL. Lungs sound normal.

Assessment and plan: Type 1 insulin-dependent diabetes mellitus: Continue with current insulin dosage on sliding scale.

Coronary artery disease: Stable. Continue to monitor diet and cholesterol.

Tiredness: Discussed sleep patterns, diet, and caffeine avoidance with patient.

Headaches: Suggested over-the-counter remedies.

Follow up if symptoms persist.

The physician performed an expanded problem-focused history and exam with low MDM. This is reported with code 99213, excerpted here to show the 3 key components of level of service:

Office or other outpatient visit for the evaluation and management of a new patient, which requires at least 2 of these 3 key components:

- *An expanded problem-focused history;*
- *An expanded problem-focused examination;*
- *Medical decision making of low complexity.*

LET'S TRY ONE **6.1**

An initial office visit was provided for a new patient, a 60-year-old male with a chief complaint of a recent change in bowel habits, weight loss, and abdominal pain. The physician performed a comprehensive history, a comprehensive exam, and MDM of moderate complexity. Which office or other outpatient service code would be appropriate for this visit? _____

Hospital Observation Services (Codes 99217-99226)

The codes in the hospital observation services category are used to report services for patients who are admitted to "observation status" in a hospital setting. Patients are typically placed in **observation status** when inpatient criteria for admission is not met, further testing is required, or it is unsafe to discharge the patient. Observation status is considered outpatient, and CMS and other payers have special rules for the number of hours and/or days that a patient may remain in observation status. In some facilities, the patient may be placed in a special observation area, but this is not a requirement to use observation services codes. If a patient is admitted to the hospital as an inpatient on the same day as observation services were provided, only the hospital inpatient services would be reported. Patients who are admitted and discharged on the same calendar date of service are reported with

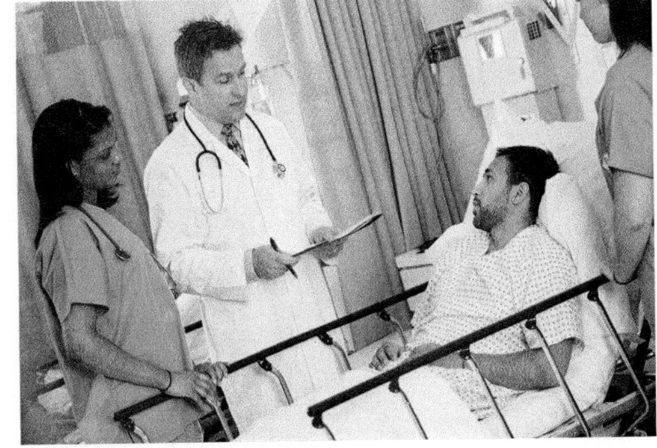

A patient is placed in observation status when criteria for admission is not met, further testing is required, or it is unsafe to discharge the patient.

a code from 99234 through 99236. Patients who are admitted and discharged on different calendar dates are reported with codes 99217 through 99226. Observation care codes may not be reported for patients placed in observation for postoperative recovery as this is considered part of the surgical package (services included in surgery codes). The surgical package will be discussed in greater detail in Chapter 8.

Codes 99218 through 99220 describe initial observation care, which is the first day of services. These codes are reported only once and require all 3 key components be met or exceeded, as shown in Figure 6.7.

Figure 6.7 Example of an Initial Observation Care Code

99218 Initial observation care, per day for the evaluation and management of a patient which requires these 3 key components:

- A detailed or comprehensive history;
- A detailed or comprehensive examination; and
- Medical decision making that is straightforward or of low complexity.

Counseling and/or coordination of care with other physicians, other qualified healthcare professionals, or agencies are provided consistent with the nature of the problem(s) and the patient's and/or family's needs.

Usually, the problem(s) requiring admission to outpatient hospital "observation status" are of low severity. Typically, 30 minutes are spent at the bedside and on the patient's hospital floor or unit.

Codes 99224 through 99226 are reported for subsequent observation care, which is the second or third day of services. Note that these codes are out of numerical sequence in the tabular list. Subsequent care codes, like established patient codes, require only 2 of the 3 key components to be met or exceeded for reporting. Code 99217 is reported for the day of discharge from observation services if the discharge is on a different date from the initial date of care. Code 99217 is used to report all the services provided on the day of discharge, including making the final examination, providing discharge instructions, and completing the discharge documentation.

EXAMPLE **6.7**

A 44-year-old male was admitted to observation complaining of chest pain. Cardiac enzymes and ECG were normal. A CT scan of the abdomen was completed, and it was determined that the patient had a hiatal hernia. The physician suggested that the pain was referred from the epigastric area and was not related to the heart. The physician completed a detailed history and detailed exam, and MDM was of moderate complexity. The patient was discharged the same calendar date as the admission. This would be reported with code 99234, as shown in Figure 6.8.

Figure 6.8 Example of an Observation or Inpatient Care Services Code

99234	Observation or inpatient hospital care, for the evaluation and management of a patient including admission and discharge on the same date, which requires these 3 key components: • A detailed or comprehensive history; • A detailed or comprehensive examination; and • Medical decision making that is straightforward or of low complexity. Counseling and/or coordination of care with other physicians, other qualified healthcare professionals, or agencies are provided consistent with the nature of the problem(s) and the patient's and/or family's needs. Usually the presenting problem(s) requiring admission are of low severity. Typically, 40 minutes are spent at the beside and on the patient's hospital floor or unit.

CONCEPTS CHECKPOINT **6.5**

Answer true or false to each of the following statements:

1. _____ Patients placed in observation status are considered inpatients.
2. _____ Two observation services codes are reported for patients admitted and discharged on the same date.
3. _____ Subsequent observation care codes require 2 of the 3 key components.
4. _____ If a patient is admitted as an inpatient on the same day that observation services were provided, only the inpatient services should be reported.
5. _____ Code 99217 is reported only if the discharge date is different from the admission date.

Hospital Inpatient Services (Codes 99221-99239)

Hospital **inpatients** are those patients who are formally admitted for treatment, usually requiring at least 1 overnight stay. Initial hospital care is reported with codes 99221 through 99223, which are reported for the first visit by the admitting physician. Any other E/M service provided on the day of admission is considered part of the initial hospital care service and may not be reported separately. The level of service that is reported by the admitting physician should take into consideration any other E/M services provided that day (such as an office visit prior to hospital admission) since these may not be reported separately.

Only 1 E/M code is reported per day. In the instance of an office visit and hospital visit in the same day, the higher level E/M code of the hospital visit should be reported. Initial hospital care codes require all 3 key components be met or exceeded. Subsequent hospital care codes 99231 through 99233 are reported for each subsequent day that the physician visits the patient. Subsequent care codes require 2 of the 3 key components. The instructional notes following each of the subsequent care codes are helpful in determining the level of service. The note following code 99231 states that the patient is usually stable, recovering, or improving. For code 99232, the patient is responding inadequately to therapy or has developed a minor complication. Code 99233 is reported when the patient is unstable or has developed a significant new problem.

RED FLAG

When reporting discharge day management, if the time spent is not documented, the code for 30 minutes or less (99238) must be reported.

Hospital discharge services are reported with codes 99238 or 99239 depending on the time spent by the physician for the service. Discharge management includes the final exam of the patient, instructions for continuing care, and preparation of discharge records. Code 99238 is reported for hospital discharge day management of 30 minutes or less, and code 99239 is reported for more than 30 minutes of service. Codes 99238 and 99239 are not reported for services when the patient is admitted and discharged on the same date.

EXAMPLE **6.8**

A 91-year-old female was complaining of hematuria, dysuria, and pyuria. She was in good health other than the current problem. Due to her extreme age, she was admitted for cystoscopy and IV antibiotics. The admitting physician performed a detailed history and exam, and the MDM was low. This service was reported with code 99221, excerpted here to show the 3 key components of level of service:

Initial hospital care, for the evaluation and management of a patient, which requires these 3 key components:

- *A detailed or comprehensive history;*
- *A detailed or comprehensive examination;*
- *Medical decision making that is straightforward or of low complexity.*

The next day, the patient spiked a fever, and the urine cultures were growing *Escherichia coli*. The patient was responding inadequately to IV therapy. The physician documented the change in her condition with an expanded problem-focused interval history, an expanded problem-focused exam, and moderate-complexity MDM. This service was reported with code 99232, excerpted here to show the 3 key components of level of service:

Subsequent hospital care for the evaluation and management of a patient, which requires at least 2 of these 3 key components:

- *An expanded problem-focused interval history;*
- *An expanded problem-focused examination;*
- *Medical decision making of moderate complexity.*

LET'S TRY ONE **6.2**

A 49-year-old male patient was seen on the second day of hospitalization. He was receiving IV antibiotics for pneumonia and was stable. The physician documented a problem-focused interval history, a problem-focused exam, and straightforward MDM. What is the appropriate code for this E/M service? _____

Consultations (Codes 99241-99255)

A **consultation** is a type of E/M service provided when a physician requests the advice and opinion of another physician. The consulting physician examines the patient and renders an opinion. Documentation in the health record must show the request from the initiating physician, and the findings of the consultation must be communicated back to the requesting physician. Consultations initiated by a patient or family member and not requested by a physician should not be reported with consultation codes. Consultation codes are reported only once unless another request is made for a new problem. Follow-up visits are reported using the appropriate codes for established patients' office visits or the appropriate subsequent care codes for facility visits. Consultations are reported with codes 99241 through 99245 for outpatients and 99251 through 99255 for inpatients. All consultation codes require all 3 key components. There is no distinction between new and established patients for consultation codes.

EXAMPLE **6.9**

A 60-year-old man was seen in consultation in the cardiologist's office for complaints of dyspnea, fatigue, and lightheadedness. He had a prior history of pacemaker insertion 6 years ago. He also had a history of mitral regurgitation. A comprehensive H&P examination was performed with the recommendation that the patient be admitted to the hospital for pacemaker interrogation and an echocardiogram to rule out pacemaker malfunction or valvular origin for his complaints. MDM was high. This service would be reported with code 99245, excerpted here to show the 3 key components of level of service:

Office consultation for a new or established patient, which requires these 3 key components:

- *A comprehensive history;*
- *A comprehensive examination;*
- *Medical decision making of high complexity.*

</> Coding for CMS

Medicare has eliminated reimbursement for consultation codes. CMS instructs physicians to report consultation services using the new or established outpatient office visit codes or the appropriate hospital care codes.

Emergency Department Services (Codes 99281-99288)

The emergency department (ED) services codes should be reported only by hospital-based EDs that are open 24 hours a day for patients who need immediate medical attention. Urgent care centers should not report ED services codes. There are 5 levels of ED visit codes, which all require 3 of the 3 key components. The lowest level, code 99281, is typically used when the presenting problem is self-limited or minor and requires a problem-focused history and exam and straightforward MDM. The highest level of ED visit codes, 99285, is reported when the presenting problem is of high severity and poses an immediate significant threat to life or physiologic function. A patient's condition may make it impossible for the physician to perform the

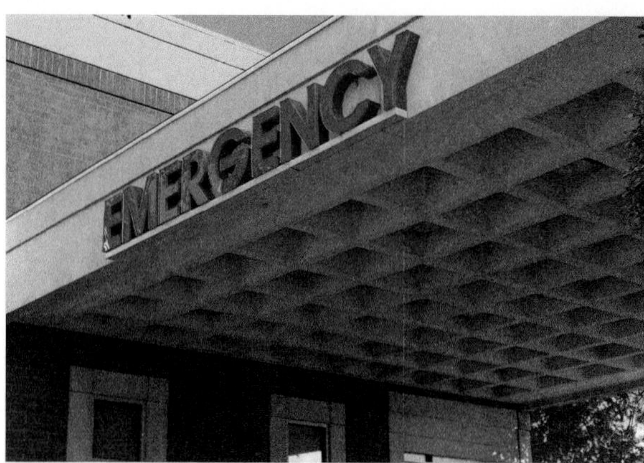

Emergency department services codes should be reported only by hospital-based emergency departments for patients who need immediate medical attention.

required comprehensive history and physical exam, but code 99285 may still be reported due to the high severity of the presenting problem, as noted in the code description in Figure 6.9.

Figure 6.9 Example of an Emergency Department Visit Code

99285 Emergency department visit for the evaluation and management of a patient, which requires these 3 key components within the constraints imposed by the urgency of the patient's clinical condition and/or mental status:

- A comprehensive history;
- A comprehensive examination;
- Medical decision making of high complexity.

Counseling and/or coordination of care with other physicians, other qualified healthcare professionals, or agencies are provided consistent with the nature of the problem(s) and the patient's and/or family's needs.

Usually, the presenting problem(s) are of high severity and pose an immediate significant threat to life or physiologic function.

EXAMPLE **6.10**

A 23-year-old female arrived at the ED after being found by her roommate in an unconscious state. A drug overdose, possible suicide attempt, was suspected. Because of the patient's clinical condition and mental status, a history could not be obtained. A comprehensive exam was completed, and MDM was of high complexity. This ED visit is reported with code 99285.

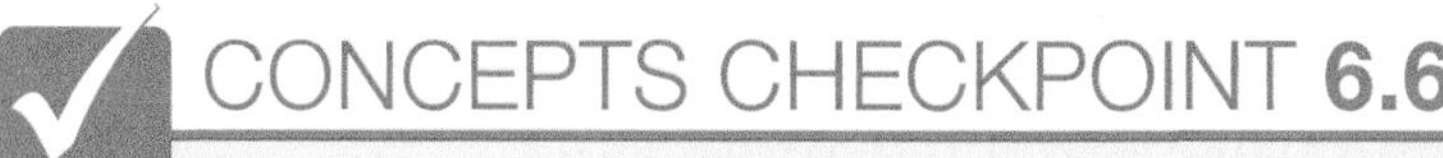

CONCEPTS CHECKPOINT **6.6**

Using the tabular portion of your codebook, answer the following questions:

1. Which of the 5 codes in the ED category has a low-to-moderate severity of presenting problem? _____
2. Which of the 5 codes in the ED category has a high severity of presenting problem, requiring urgent evaluation but not posing an immediate significant threat to life or physiologic function? _____
3. Should services provided in urgent care centers be reported with ED service codes? If not, why not? _______________

Critical Care Services (Codes 99291-99292)

Critical care service codes 99291 and 99292 are time based and used to report services provided for a patient who is critically ill or critically injured. CPT® guidelines define a critical illness or critical injury as one that impairs 1 or more vital organ systems such that there is a high probability of imminent or life-threatening deterioration in the patient's condition. Codes 99291 and 99292 are used to report the total time spent with the patient providing critical care services for each calendar day, even if the time is not continuous. For time spent with the patient in critical condition to be considered, the physician must not provide services to any other patient during that same period of time. The place of service is not required to be a critical care unit; critical care services may be provided in any area as long as the requirements are met. Many services are bundled into the critical care E/M codes for reporting by professionals, as shown in the list below. Facilities may report these services separately:

- interpretation of cardiac output measurement;
- chest x-rays;
- pulse oximetry;
- blood gases;
- gastric intubation;
- temporary transcutaneous pacing;
- ventilator management;
- vascular access procedures.

The first 30 to 74 minutes of critical care are reported with code 99291. Each additional 30 minutes is reported with code 99292. Critical care services of less than 30 minutes on any given date are reported with the appropriate E/M code. The tabular contains a table that illustrates the correct reporting of critical care services, reprinted as Table 6.6. The term *total duration* refers to the aggregate of time spent with the patient providing critical care services per calendar day.

Table 6.7 Selection Criteria for Transitional Care Management Services Codes

Type of Medical Decision-Making	Face-to-Face Visit Within 7 Days	Face-to-Face Visit Within 14 Days
Moderate complexity	99495	99495
High complexity	99496	99495

These codes may be reported only once every 30 days, and only 1 individual may report these services. Transitional care management services provided during the postoperative period may not be reported by the same individual reporting the surgery code but may be reported by another individual who provides the services.

Advance Care Planning (Codes 99497-99498)

Advance care planning codes are used to report the discussion and counseling provided regarding advance directives. An **advance directive** is a legal document that contains the patient's wishes regarding medical treatment and life-supporting measures. An advance directive may also be a durable power of attorney for health care, which gives another person the right to make medical decisions for the patient when the patient is unable to express his or her wishes or lacks the decision-making capacity. Another example of a written advance directive is a living will. Codes for advance care planning are time based and are reported in 30-minute increments, code 99497 for the first 30 minutes and add-on code 99498 for each additional 30 minutes spent in discussion and explanation of advance directives. Other E/M codes may be reported with 99497 and 99498.

EXAMPLE **6.16**

An established patient, a 72-year-old female, visited her physician's office for medication management. The physician completed a detailed history and exam. After the office visit, the patient returned with her daughter to discuss completion of an advance directive with her physician. The discussion lasted approximately 30 minutes. These services would be reported with code 99214 for the established patient office visit reflecting the detailed history and exam level and code 99497 for the discussion of advance directives.

LET'S TRY ONE **6.6**

A 65-year-old male patient who was recently diagnosed with colon cancer visited his physician for advance care planning. The patient, his wife, and the physician spent 1 hour discussing advance directives. How is this service reported? ____

Index Insider

E/M codes can be found in a variety of ways in the Index. The quickest way is to search under the main term *Evaluation and Management* and then the subterm for the service you wish to report. Another way to locate E/M codes is to start with the main term that describes the place of service, such as *Nursing Facility Services*. A third way is to start in the Index with the type of patient, such as *Established Patient*. Starting with the main term for the type of service, such as *Discharge Services*, is another way to locate E/M codes.

General Behavioral Health Integration Care Management (Code 99484)

General behavioral health integration care management code 99484 appears out of numerical sequence and is reported by the supervising physician or other qualified healthcare professional for services that are provided by clinical staff. Code 99484 is reported for at least 20 minutes of clinical staff time on case management services for behavioral health conditions. The services must be directed by the physician and include an assessment and treatment plan. Other E/M services provided by the physician may be reported separately. Code 99484 is reported once per calendar month and may be used in any outpatient setting.

Other Evaluation and Management Services (Code 99499)

The last E/M code is 99499, *Unlisted evaluation and management service.* In the unlikely event that a physician provides an E/M service for which no other E/M code is appropriate, code 99499 may be reported. Reporting of an unlisted code requires additional documentation or a special report sent along with the claim to third-party payers.

Evaluation and Management Modifiers

An E/M service may have been altered by a specific circumstance and require the addition of a CPT® or HCPCS modifier for reporting. A complete description of CPT® modifiers can be found in Appendix A in the CPT® codebook. Chapter 4 explains the use of modifiers in detail.

CPT® Modifiers

The following is a list of the more common CPT® modifiers used with E/M codes.

- 24, *Unrelated Evaluation and Management Service by the Same Physician or Other Qualified Health Professional During a Postoperative Period*;
- 25, *Significant, Separately Identifiable Evaluation and Management Service by the Same Physician or Other Qualified Health Care Professional on the Same Day of the Procedure or Other Service*;
- 32, *Mandated Services*;
- 55, *Postoperative Management Only*;
- 56, *Preoperative Management Only*;
- 57, *Decision for Surgery*.

HCPCS Modifiers

The following is a list of the more common HCPCS modifiers used with E/M codes.

- AI, *Principal physician of record* (admitting physician);
- FP, *Service provided as part of a family planning program*;
- GC, *This service has been performed in part by a resident under the direction of a teaching physician*;
- Q5, *Service furnished by a substitute physician under a reciprocal billing arrangement*;
- Q6, *Service furnished by a locum tenens physician.*

Instructions for Reporting Evaluation and Management Codes

This chapter gives a general overview of E/M codes and the guidelines for reporting them. Figure 6.12 provides a diagram to guide you through the process of reporting E/M codes.

Figure 6.12 Process for Locating and Reporting E/M Codes

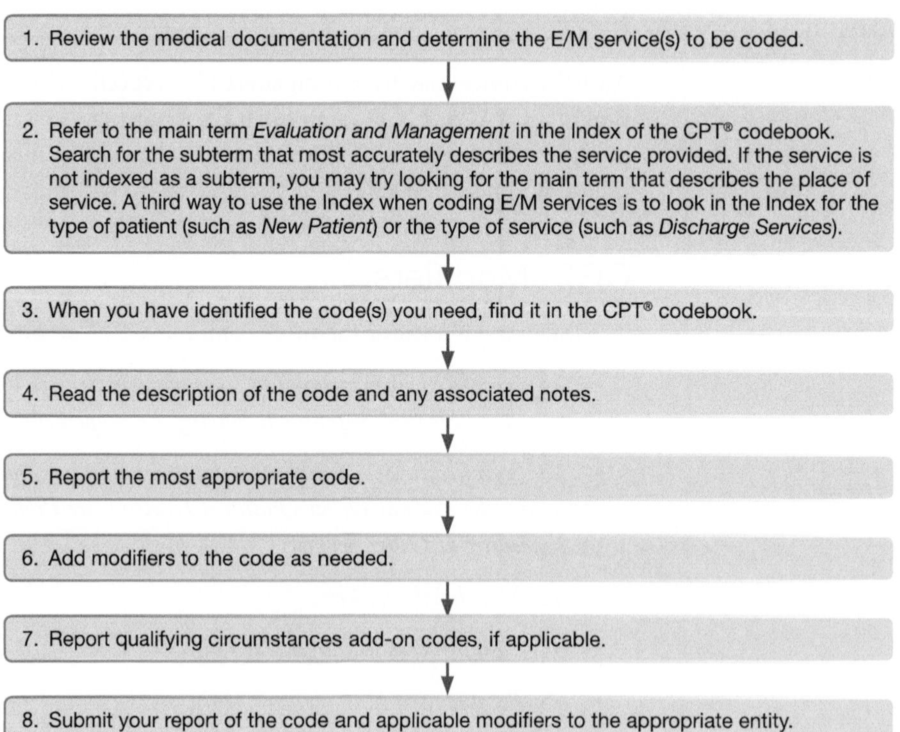

1. Review the medical documentation and determine the E/M service(s) to be coded.
2. Refer to the main term *Evaluation and Management* in the Index of the CPT® codebook. Search for the subterm that most accurately describes the service provided. If the service is not indexed as a subterm, you may try looking for the main term that describes the place of service. A third way to use the Index when coding E/M services is to look in the Index for the type of patient (such as *New Patient*) or the type of service (such as *Discharge Services*).
3. When you have identified the code(s) you need, find it in the CPT® codebook.
4. Read the description of the code and any associated notes.
5. Report the most appropriate code.
6. Add modifiers to the code as needed.
7. Report qualifying circumstances add-on codes, if applicable.
8. Submit your report of the code and applicable modifiers to the appropriate entity.

Chapter Summary

- Evaluation and Management (E/M) codes (99201-99499) describe the intensity or complexity of the service provided to the patient during an encounter.
- The level of history, examination, and medical decision making (MDM) are considered the key components in selecting an E/M code.
- The level of the history component reflects the chief complaint, history of present illness (HPI), review of systems (ROS), and past, family, and social histories (PFSH).
- The level of the physical examination component depends on the number of body areas or organ systems examined and the nature of the presenting problem.
- The level of the MDM component is measured in 3 elements: (1) the number of diagnoses or management options, (2) the amount and/or complexity of data to be reviewed, and (3) the risk of significant complications, morbidity, and/or mortality.
- In addition to the 3 key components of history, exam, and MDM that define the levels of E/M service, contributing components include counseling, coordination of care, the nature of the presenting problem, and time.
- E/M codes are divided into place of service (such as office or nursing facility) or type of service (such as office visit or case management services). Many E/M codes are further categorized by whether the service is for a new or established patient (as in office visits) or whether the service is for an initial visit or a subsequent visit (as with inpatient hospital services).
- A new patient is someone who has not received any face-to-face service from the physician, or any other physician or other qualified health professional in the exact same specialty who belongs to the same group practice, within the past 3 years.
- An established patient is someone who is not considered a new patient.
- In general, before the E/M code can be selected, the coding specialist must determine the place and category of service; the status of the patient as new or established; and the levels of history, exam, and MDM.

Navigator

Access interactive chapter review exercises, practice activities, flash cards, and study games.

Chapter 7

Anesthesia Coding

Fast Facts

- *Anesthesia* comes from the Greek word *anaisthesia*, or "loss of feeling."
- According to a 2002 study done at the University of Louisville in Kentucky, redheads require on average 20% more anesthesia than individuals with other hair colors.
- Alternative ways to create anesthesia include icing the affected body part, hypnosis, and acupuncture.

Sources: http://science.howstuffworks.com, http://funtrivia.com

Crack the Code

Review the sample operative report to find the correct anesthesia code. You may need to return to this exercise after reading the chapter content.

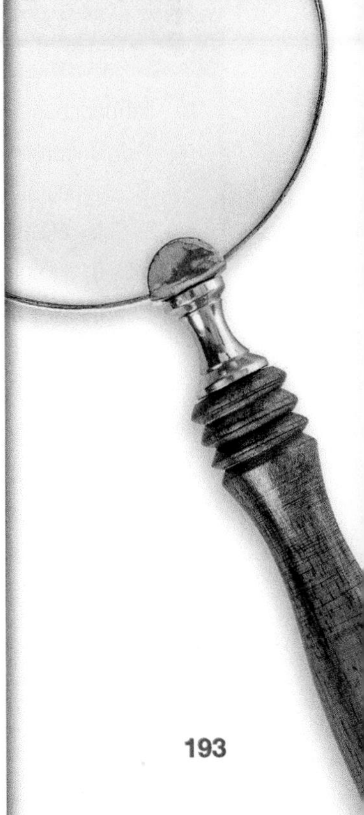

SURGEON: Gregory Smythe, MD

PREOPERATIVE DIAGNOSIS: Chronic right lower quadrant pain with complex right ovarian cyst

POSTOPERATIVE DIAGNOSIS: Chronic right lower quadrant pain with complex right ovarian cyst, pathology pending

OPERATION: Laparoscopic right salpingo-oophorectomy

ANESTHESIA: General endotracheal anesthesia

ESTIMATED BLOOD LOSS: Minimal

IV FLUIDS: 850-mL crystalloid

SPECIMENS: Right tube and ovary with cyst intact

OPERATIVE FINDINGS: The uterus was previously surgically removed. The left tube and ovary were normal in size and in character with some filmy adhesions from ovary to sidewall left intact. Also, some adhesions from colon in the posterior cul-de-sac deemed to be causing discomfort and left intact. The right ovary had an area of erythema overlying a small cyst. It did not have any external papulations or excrescences. The cyst was removed intact without rupture or exposure to abdomen.

answer: 00840

Learning Objectives

7.1 Define *anesthesia* and *anesthesiology*.

7.2 List the types of medical professionals who may administer and/or assist with anesthesia services.

7.3 Identify and provide examples of different types of anesthesia and anesthesia services.

7.4 Define key terms related to reporting codes for anesthesia services.

7.5 Identify the location and organization of anesthesia codes in the CPT® codebook.

7.6 Define *anesthesia time*, explain how it relates to HIPAA and third-party payers, and explore how it may be used to calculate fees.

7.7 List the services included in the anesthesia package and explain the difference between usual and unusual services.

7.8 Explain when supplies and materials should be coded separately.

7.9 Describe anesthesia services that may be reported using additional codes.

7.10 Explain when a special report is required.

7.11 Identify physical status modifiers and explain how they are used with anesthesia codes.

7.12 Identify some of the most common CPT® and HCPCS Level II modifiers used with anesthesia codes and explain when and why they are included.

7.13 Define anesthesia rules when multiple procedures are performed during 1 operative episode.

7.14 Define *qualifying circumstances* and explain when these add-on codes are used in reporting anesthesia services.

7.15 Locate the Other Procedures subsection and explain when codes from this subsection may be reported.

7.16 Demonstrate the ability to assign appropriate anesthesia codes.

Chapter Outline

- **I.** Introduction to Anesthesia
  - **A.** Understanding Anesthesiology
  - **B.** Types of Anesthesia and Anesthesia Services
    - **i.** General Anesthesia
    - **ii.** Regional Anesthesia
    - **iii.** Local Anesthesia
    - **iv.** Moderate (Conscious) Sedation
    - **v.** Monitored Anesthesia Care
- **II.** Anesthesia Terminology
- **III.** Organization of the Anesthesia Section
- **IV.** Guidelines for Reporting Anesthesia Codes
  - **A.** Time Reporting
  - **B.** Anesthesia Services
  - **C.** Supplied Materials
  - **D.** Separate or Multiple Procedures
  - **E.** Special Report
  - **F.** Anesthesia Modifiers
    - **i.** Physical Status Modifiers
    - **ii.** CPT® Modifiers
    - **iii.** HCPCS Level II Modifiers
  - **G.** Qualifying Circumstances
  - **H.** Using Other Procedures Codes (01990-01999)
- **V.** Instructions for Reporting Anesthesia Codes
- **VI.** Anesthesia Coding Resources
- **VII.** Chapter Summary

Introduction to Anesthesia

What is anesthesia? Think about the meanings of its word parts that you learned in medical terminology: *an-* means without, *-esthes* means sensation or feeling, and *-ia* means condition or state of being. Together they form the term *anesthesia*, a condition of being without sensation or feeling. **Anesthesia** is the administration of gases or drugs that inhibit pain and sensation during procedures and surgical operations.

Understanding Anesthesiology

Anesthesiology is the practice of medicine dedicated to the relief of pain and the care of the surgical patient before, during, and after surgery. Anesthesiology is practiced by *medical professionals known as anesthesiologists, certified registered nurse anesthetists (CRNAs), and anesthesiologist assistants (AAs).* **Anesthesiologists** are licensed physicians who administer anesthesia and manage its effects on vital functions during surgery. In the operating room, the anesthesiologist continuously assesses the patient to monitor heart rate, breathing, blood pressure, body temperature, and body fluid balance. The anesthesiologist also ensures that the patient's level of consciousness is appropriate for surgery. The Centers for Medicare and Medicaid Services (CMS) identifies both CRNAs and AAs as **nonphysician anesthetists**. CRNAs and AAs work under the medical direction of the anesthesiologist. In some cases, a surgeon may be the sole anesthesia provider. Coders should understand the different types of anesthesia and the different professionals who may report services involving the administration of anesthesia.

When a patient undergoes a procedure requiring anesthesia, typically the surgeon reports a code for the surgical procedure, and the anesthesiologist or nonphysician anesthetist reports an anesthesia code for the anesthesia service that was provided during surgery. However, any physician or healthcare provider performing anesthesia services can report anesthesia codes as long as they follow the reporting guidelines. You will learn more about the guidelines for reporting anesthesia codes later in this chapter.

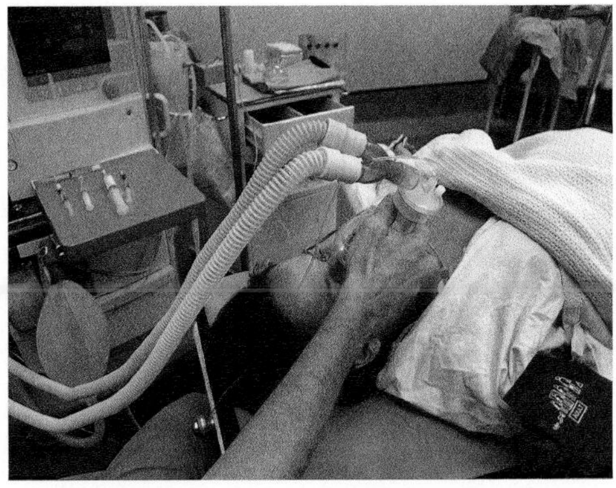

Anesthesiologists ensure that a patient's level of consciousness is appropriate for surgery.

Types of Anesthesia and Anesthesia Services

Anesthesia makes it possible to perform otherwise painful procedures such as surgery. Anesthetic drugs work on the peripheral nervous system, which is responsible for detecting sensations such as pain. Anesthetic drugs (for general anesthesia) also work on the central nervous system to induce loss of consciousness. Anesthesia is divided into three main types: general anesthetic drugs, which produce a loss of conscious sensation of pain throughout the entire body; regional anesthetic drugs, which block pain in a large area of the body; and local anesthetic drugs, which temporarily block pain in a small area of the body. Figure 7.1 shows the types of anesthesia and the parts of the body that are affected.

Figure 7.1 Three Types of Anesthesia

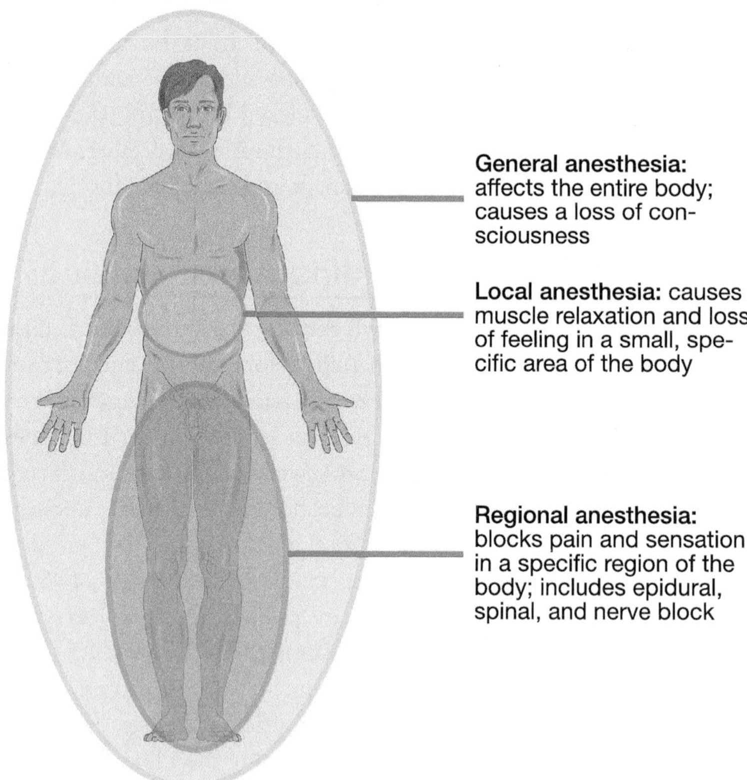
General anesthesia: affects the entire body; causes a loss of consciousness
Local anesthesia: causes muscle relaxation and loss of feeling in a small, specific area of the body
Regional anesthesia: blocks pain and sensation in a specific region of the body; includes epidural, spinal, and nerve block

> **RED FLAG**
>
> Remember that anesthesia codes are reported based on the anatomical site of the procedure or the nature of the procedure performed, and that not all types of anesthesia can be reported.

> **Coding Clicks**
>
> Visit http://Coding.ParadigmEducation.com/AnesthesiaCartoon to view a fun video cartoon of a discussion between an anesthesiologist and an orthopedic surgeon.

The anesthesiologist or other health professional providing anesthesia services will select the appropriate anesthesia for the patient based on the patient's condition and the surgical procedure. The ideal type of anesthesia is the 1 that poses the fewest risks to the patient while allowing him or her to tolerate the sensations and remain still for the procedure, but there may be other considerations as well. For example, a patient with a neck tumor may not be an appropriate candidate for general anesthesia, which requires **intubation** (the placement of a tube in the trachea).

When you work with anesthesia codes, 1 of the most important things to understand is that you will report codes based on the anatomical site of the procedure or the nature of the procedure performed, not the type of anesthesia given. Within the CPT® code set, anesthesia codes are assigned for the administration of general and regional (epidural, spinal, and nerve block) anesthesia. Local anesthesia, which is not coded, will be discussed later.

General Anesthesia

General anesthesia affects the entire body and causes a loss of consciousness. Bodywide, the skeletal muscles relax. Breathing slows, respiratory mucus production increases, and urination stops. Cardiac function also slows, causing a decrease in blood pressure (a condition that intravenous fluids are usually given to counteract). The patient has no memory of the event upon recovery. General anesthesia can be given by injection, inhalation, or instillation. General anesthesia requires close monitoring by the anesthesiologist or anesthetist and is used for both minor and major invasive surgical procedures. Children are often given general anesthesia when they are unable to cooperate during a procedure due to pain or anxiety.

Regional Anesthesia

Regional anesthesia blocks pain and sensation in a specific region of the body. Common types of regional anesthesia include epidural anesthesia, spinal anesthesia, and nerve block anesthesia.

Epidural anesthesia is most commonly used for obstetric patients during labor and delivery. An anesthetic drug such as bupivacaine, chloroprocaine, or lidocaine is injected into the epidural space of the spinal cord. The drug blocks the nerve impulses to the lower half of the body, thereby numbing any sensation in that region. Figure 7.2 illustrates the placement of the needle in the epidural space for the injection of the anesthetic.

Figure 7.2 Epidural Anesthesia Injection

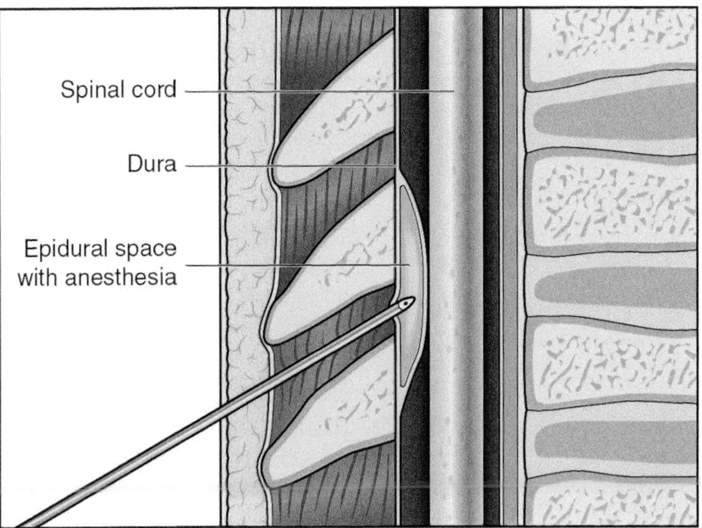

Spinal anesthesia is similar to epidural anesthesia in its effect on a large area of the body. Spinal anesthetics such as bupivacaine, chloroprocaine, or lidocaine are injected into the cerebral spinal fluid and are used for procedures on the genitals, urinary tract, and other areas of the lower body.

Nerve block anesthesia is an injection that works to block pain reception in the nerve bundles related to the surgical area without affecting the patient's brain or breathing. The patient remains conscious and is often given a sedative for relaxation. The tissue into which the anesthetic, such as lidocaine or bupivacaine, is injected may be located some distance from the surgical site. For example, a patient undergoing knee or hip surgery may be given a peripheral injection of anesthetic into the major nerves in the thigh. This numbs only the leg into which the anesthetic is injected and does not affect the other leg. The patient usually recovers faster and with fewer complications from this type of anesthesia than from general anesthesia.

Local Anesthesia

Local anesthesia affects only a small, specific area of the body, causing loss of pain, loss of feeling, and loss of temperature sensation, as well as muscle relaxation. A patient receiving local anesthesia may lose the ability to recognize his or her body's position in the area of the injection; however, the patient does not lose consciousness and can remember everything that happens during the procedure.

Local anesthesia is usually administered as a direct injection into tissue near the surgical site. The anesthesia drug blocks a specific group of nerves in a small area so the patient will not feel pain during the procedure. Novocain, a brand-name drug commonly administered during dental procedures, is a commonly used local anesthetic.

As mentioned earlier in this chapter, there are no CPT® codes assigned for local anesthesia, and it is not a separately reportable service. Administration of local anesthesia is bundled into the CPT® code for the procedure. Therefore, you should not report a code from the Anesthesia section of the CPT® codebook when only local anesthesia is used during a medical or surgical procedure.

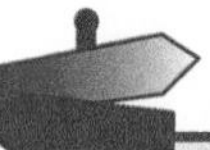

Learn Your Way

Sensing learners like to learn facts and are especially excited when they can tie the material they are learning to the real world. If you are a sensing learner, you may appreciate knowing some historical facts related to the topic of anesthesia. For example, many of the drug names for local anesthetics—lidocaine, bupivacaine, procaine, tetracaine—end with "caine" because they are chemically similar to the original local anesthetic: cocaine.

In 1884, an ophthalmologist named Carl Koller was the first physician to use cocaine as an anesthetic. His colleague Sigmund Freud suggested using cocaine for pain relief, and Koller discovered that the drug also produced tissue numbness. Cocaine was ideal for use in eye surgery during which the eye must remain still for a successful surgical outcome. It was later used in dentistry as well as other medical specialties.

EXAMPLE **7.1**

A 39-year-old male presented for an elective vasectomy. Before the surgeon made the first incision, a local anesthetic was injected into the scrotum. The surgeon then numbed the surgical area by bathing the vas deferens and nearby areas with an anesthetic agent. The vasectomy was completed, and the skin was closed. The code reported for this procedure is 55250, *Vasectomy, unilateral or bilateral*, from the Surgery section of the CPT® codebook. Administration of a local anesthetic was integral to the procedure and is not separately reportable; thus, an anesthesia code is not necessary.

LET'S TRY ONE 7.1

Should an anesthesia code be reported? Answer yes or no to each of the following scenarios.

1. A 16-year-old male presented to urgent care after cutting his hand on a broken glass while washing dishes. The 1.5-cm wound required a simple repair, for which the patient was given a local anesthetic to numb the area. The wound was then sutured closed. The code reported for this procedure was 12001, *Simple repair of superficial wounds of scalp, neck, axillae, trunk and/or extremities (including hands and feet); 2.5 cm or less.* _____
2. A 51-year-old female with varicose veins presented for vein stripping. The surgeon injected local anesthesia and performed a ligation and stripping of the short saphenous vein. The surgeon reported code 37718, *Ligation, division, and stripping, short saphenous vein.* _____
3. A 65-year-old male with a history of impotence presented for surgery to insert a penile prosthesis. After the patient received spinal anesthesia, the surgeon inserted a semirigid penile prosthesis without complication. The surgeon reported code 54400, *Insertion of penile prosthesis; non-inflatable.* _____

Moderate (Conscious) Sedation

Moderate sedation, also known as **conscious sedation**, is a state in which a patient is drowsy, relaxed, and able to respond to verbal commands. A combination of sedatives and analgesics is administered to achieve this state so that a patient can tolerate an uncomfortable procedure. Moderate sedation wears off after a short time and is therefore used for quick, minor procedures.

When it comes to reporting moderate (conscious) sedation, the anesthesia guidelines differentiate between a facility setting (such as a hospital, an ambulatory surgery center, or a skilled nursing facility) and a nonfacility setting (such as a physician office or freestanding imaging center). Moderate (conscious) sedation may be reported by the same physician who is also performing the diagnostic or therapeutic service with codes 99151 through 99153. In a facility setting, if a second physician other than the 1 performing the diagnostic or therapeutic service provides the moderate sedation, this service may be reported with a code from the 99155 through 99157 range of the Medicine section of the CPT® codebook. These codes are assigned based on the patient's age and the length of time he or she is under sedation. Reportable time begins with the administration of the sedating agent and ends when the continuous face-to-face presence of the physician ends. The time for preservice work, such as assessment of the patient, is not included in the total time for reporting moderate sedation.

In a nonfacility setting, such as a physician's office, codes 99155 through 99157 for moderate sedation may not be reported separately even if a second physician provides this service. This information is also provided in the Anesthesia guidelines at the beginning of the Anesthesia section in the CPT® codebook.

Monitored Anesthesia Care

Monitored anesthesia care (MAC) is a professional service that involves both the administration of sedatives and analgesics as well as the intraoperative monitoring of a patient's vital functions during a diagnostic or therapeutic procedure in anticipation of the need for general anesthesia. Like moderate (conscious) sedation, MAC involves the administration of drugs, but in contrast to moderate sedation, the anesthesia provider must be prepared to convert to general anesthesia if the patient develops any adverse effects during the surgical procedure. While moderate sedation generally does not induce the deep sedation that may compromise the patient's airway, the healthcare provider administering MAC must have the skill necessary to intubate if a transition to general anesthesia is needed. The professional performing MAC is also required to complete the preoperative assessment, prescribe and administer the anesthesia, and provide postanesthesia care. MAC is not a separately reportable service.

Coding for CMS

CMS defines the term *anesthesia* as "administration of a medication to produce loss of pain perception, voluntary and involuntary movement, autonomic function, and memory and/or consciousness." Medicare provides benefits for moderate (conscious) sedation and MAC that are reasonable and necessary in the circumstances. However, despite their anesthesia labels, CMS does not consider moderate (conscious) sedation, MAC, and local and topical anesthesia to be "anesthesia" due to their lack of systemic effects.

CONCEPTS CHECKPOINT **7.1**

Match the type of anesthesia in the first column to the description in the second column.

1. _____ epidural
2. _____ general
3. _____ local
4. _____ nerve block
5. _____ spinal

a. Affects the entire body, and the patient loses consciousness
b. Affects the lower half of the body and is used in obstetric procedures
c. A type of regional anesthesia injected into the cerebrospinal fluid
d. Direct injection that blocks nerve bundles related to the surgery site
e. Affects a small, specific part of the body

Anesthesia Terminology

To be able to accurately report anesthesia codes, you must be able to recognize and understand the terminology used in anesthesia documentation and in the Anesthesia section of the codebook. Table 7.1 defines some of the common terms used in anesthesia documentation, codes, and guidelines. Be sure to thoroughly review this information before beginning to report codes from the Anesthesia section.

Table 7.1 Common Anesthesia Terms

Term or Phrase	Meaning
conscious	Awake; aware of physical sensations and surroundings
systemic disease	Condition that affects multiple organs and tissues or the whole body
moribund	Describes a patient who is terminal (dying)
declared brain dead	Physician-diagnosed condition characterized by permanent, complete, irreversible cessation of brain function
total body hypothermia	Therapeutic treatment involving intentional reduction of body temperature to reduce tissue metabolism
controlled hypotension	Therapeutic treatment involving the intentional reduction of blood pressure to reduce blood loss
risk factor	Characteristic or condition of a patient that increases the possibility of developing disease, complications, or injury

Organization of the Anesthesia Section

Anesthesia codes are located in the second section of the CPT® codebook (following Evaluation and Management and preceding Surgery), and the code numbers range from 00100 through 01999. Because anesthesia codes are assigned by the American Medical Association (AMA) based on the anatomical site of the procedure or the type of procedure performed, the Anesthesia section is arranged by body sites in a head-to-toe sequence: the codes for procedures in and on the head are listed first, followed by neck procedures, and so on through the lower limbs and then the arms. The anatomical-site subsections are followed by subsections for radiological procedures, procedures related to burns, obstetric procedures, and other procedures not covered in any of the previous subsections. The subsections of the Anesthesia section and the codes they include are provided in Table 7.2.

Within each subsection, you will notice that most of the code descriptions begin with the word *Anesthesia*, which covers both general and regional anesthesia for the type of procedure indicated in the rest of the code description. Some anesthesia codes are broad, and some are more specific. For example, code 00500, *Anesthesia for all procedures on esophagus*, has a general description and might be reported for many different procedures. Conversely, code 00622, *Anesthesia for procedures on thoracic spine and cord; thoracolumbar sympathectomy*, is quite specific and can be used only for the procedures it describes.

Many chapters within this textbook, particularly the Surgery subsection chapters, will take you step-by-step through the various headings and categories in the codebook, pointing out common codes, important guidelines, and special considerations. Because anesthesia works differently than surgery, in that it is essentially the exact same service provided for procedures performed at different anatomical sites, this chapter does not require that level of detail. As long as you understand that general and regional are the only types of anesthesia that can be reported, that anesthesia codes are reported based on anatomical site (or by procedure, in the case of radiology, burn, obstetric, and certain other procedures), and that the codebook is organized to reflect this, you should be able to locate any anesthesia code you need.

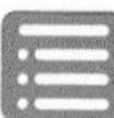

Index Insider

Under the main Index term *Anesthesia*, codes can be listed by anatomical site, procedure, or clinical condition. If you can't find a first-order modifying entry under *Anesthesia* for the name of the procedure you wish to code, you may find the procedure listed as a subterm under the relevant anatomical site or clinical condition.

Table 7.2 Subsections Within the Anesthesia Section of the CPT® Codebook

Anesthesia Subsection Name	Code Range
Head	00100-00222
Neck	00300-00352
Thorax (Chest Wall and Shoulder Girdle)	00400-00474
Intrathoracic	00500-00580
Spine and Spinal Cord	00600-00670
Upper Abdomen	00700-00797
Lower Abdomen	00800-00882
Perineum	00902-00952
Pelvis (Except Hip)	01112-01173
Upper Leg (Except Knee)	01200-01274
Knee and Popliteal Area	01320-01444
Lower Leg (Below Knee; Includes Ankle and Foot)	01462-01522
Shoulder and Axilla	01610-01680
Upper Arm and Elbow	01710-01782
Forearm, Wrist, and Hand	01810-01860
Radiological Procedures	01916-01936
Burn Excisions or Debridement	01951-01953
Obstetric	01958-01969
Other Procedures	01990-01999

CONCEPTS CHECKPOINT 7.2

Answer true or false to each of the following statements.

1. _____ CPT® anesthesia codes range from 00100 through 01999.
2. _____ The subsections of the Anesthesia section are organized by type of anesthesia.
3. _____ Anesthesia codes for burn procedures are not reported based on anatomical site.
4. _____ A conscious patient is aware of physical sensations.
5. _____ Total body hypothermia is the intentional elevation of body temperature for surgery.

Guidelines for Reporting Anesthesia Codes

Like all sections within the CPT® codebook, the Anesthesia section begins with a set of guidelines for selecting the codes. Reporting anesthesia services is different from reporting other services in the CPT® codebook, and the guidelines provide helpful information regarding the use of these codes. The most important differences involved in anesthesia coding will be covered in the following sections.

Time Reporting

RED FLAG

Medicare, Medicaid, and third-party payers often have different requirements when it comes to reporting anesthesia codes. Make sure to check these requirements before you begin reporting anesthesia codes from medical documentation.

The first subsection of the Guidelines covers time reporting as it relates to anesthesia. To understand this concept, a bit of background knowledge is helpful. As part of the Health Insurance Portability and Accountability Act of 1996 (HIPAA), the US Department of Health and Human Services (HHS) adopted specific code sets for diagnoses and procedures, and CPT® is 1 of the adopted code sets. Therefore, any entity that must comply with HIPAA rules and regulations (such as Medicare and Medicaid) must accept all valid CPT® codes. However, some payers, such as those involved with workers' compensation, are exempt from HIPAA. Because workers' compensation payers are exempt, they may ask that anesthesia services be reported using codes from the Surgery section, or they may create their own set of codes for billing anesthesia services. They may also require anesthesia time to be reported instead of codes so that fees can be calculated based on that time. Although a coding professional may not be required to calculate fees for billing purposes, it is helpful to understand how fees based on anesthesia time are determined.

Anesthesia fees are based on the complexity of the surgical procedure and the period of time during which anesthesia services are provided. **Anesthesia time** starts when the anesthesiologist begins to prepare the patient to receive services and ends when the anesthesiologist is no longer in personal attendance, at which point the patient may be placed in postoperative care. When multiple surgical procedures are performed during a single anesthesia session, the anesthesia code reported should represent the most complex procedure, and the time for all procedures should be combined. The **American Society of Anesthesiologists (ASA)** annually publishes a relative-value guide that contains the base values for anesthesia codes, physical status modifiers, and qualifying circumstances codes. A higher base value indicates a more complex procedure. Anesthesia time is calculated in units, with each payer determining the number of minutes in each time unit. Base units, time units, and modifying factors are added together and multiplied by a dollar amount (conversion factor; set by the anesthesia provider) to calculate the anesthesia fees.

EXAMPLE **7.2**

A 76-year-old female underwent a vaginal hysterectomy under general anesthesia. The anesthesia code for this procedure is 00944, *Anesthesia for vaginal procedures (including biopsy of labia, vagina, cervix or endometrium); vaginal hysterectomy*, with a base unit of 6 (according to the ASA's relative-value guide). The anesthesia time for the hysterectomy was 60 minutes, and the patient is a Medicare beneficiary, so 4 time units are reported (Medicare and Medicaid use 15-minute units). Because the patient is 76 years old, qualifying circumstances code 99100, *Anesthesia for a patient of extreme age, younger than 1 year and older than 70*, is also reported, which is a modifying factor for calculating fees. The anesthesia provider has set the conversion factor at $100. Therefore, the anesthesia fee is calculated using the following formula: 6 base units + 4 time units + 1 modifying factor x $100 = $1100.

LET'S TRY ONE **7.2**

A 38-year-old male underwent a surgical knee arthroscopy with medial meniscus repair under general anesthesia. The anesthesia time for this procedure was 45 minutes, and the patient is a Medicaid beneficiary. The anesthesia code reported for this procedure is 01400 *Anesthesia for open or surgical arthroscopic procedures on knee joint; not otherwise specified*, with a base unit of 4. The conversion factor is $100. What is the correct anesthesia fee for this service? _____

Coding for CMS

Medicare and Medicaid calculate anesthesia time in units of 15 minutes. For example, a procedure that required 60 anesthesia minutes would be reported as 4 units (60 ÷ 15 = 4). The *Medicare Claims Processing Manual* contains detailed information regarding billing for anesthesia.

Anesthesia Services

Although the next subsection of the Anesthesia Guidelines, Anesthesia Services, is short, there is 1 major point to understand about this topic, as it is 1 of the main ways anesthesia coding differs from other types of coding: when you report an anesthesia code, you are reporting a package of "usual" services. The introductory paragraphs of the Anesthesia Guidelines make a distinction between usual and unusual services, explaining that usual anesthesia care includes the following:

- a preoperative visit to assess the patient;
- anesthesia care during the procedure;
- administration of intravenous fluids or blood;
- the usual monitoring (eg, blood pressure, temperature, oximetry, capnography, electrocardiography, and mass spectrometry); and
- a postoperative visit to assess the patient's recovery from anesthesia.

You can think of a usual service as 1 that every anesthesia patient would receive and an unusual service as 1 not routinely associated with the administration of anesthesia. Unusual services may be coded separately. For example, when an anesthesiologist inserts a Swan-Ganz catheter during the operative episode, it is not considered to be a usual service associated with anesthesia, so it may be coded and reported for additional reimbursement.

As you learned in Chapter 5, the anesthesiologist or anesthetist administering the anesthesia for a procedure will complete a form of documentation called an *anesthesia note*. The anesthesia note documents the anesthesia drugs provided to the patient, including their doses and methods of administration, the patient's vital signs while under anesthesia, and any other services provided, such as blood transfusion. The anesthesia note provides the necessary details for determining whether the anesthesia services provided were usual or unusual so that you can report the appropriate code.

Supplied Materials

RED FLAG

Although you should be aware of separately reportable supplies and materials codes, these codes usually appear in a facility's chargemaster, so you would not be required to manually report them.

Supplies and materials commonly used in the administration of anesthesia are usually included in the anesthesia code and may not be reported separately. However, the Medicine section of the CPT® codebook contains a supplies and materials code that may be used in addition to an anesthesia code. Code 99070, *Supplies and materials (except spectacles) provided by the physician or other qualified health professional over and above those usually included with the office visit or other services rendered (list drugs, trays, supplies, or materials provided)*, is reported only when the supplies and materials used to provide the anesthesia care to the patient went above and beyond the usual. This code might be used to report items such as special dressings, sterile trays, sterile water, and wound irrigation equipment. Reimbursement for code 99070 varies—some payers accept this charge, but others do not cover it.

Separate or Multiple Procedures

Another distinctive feature of anesthesia coding is that unlike coding for surgical procedures, only 1 anesthesia code may be reported per **operative episode**, the continuous period that the patient is under anesthesia. If the patient undergoes multiple procedures during 1 episode, the Anesthesia Guidelines mandate that the anesthesia code reported should reflect the most complicated or resource-intensive procedure performed during that episode.

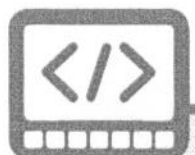

Coding for CMS

Coding Clicks

A list of the anesthesia base units can be found at http://Coding.ParadigmEducation.com/AnesthesiaBaseUnits.

According to the Medicare Claims Processing Manual, the coder should choose the procedure with the highest anesthesia base unit. An **anesthesia base unit** is a number assigned to each CPT® anesthesia code that reflects the difficulty and skill required to administer that form of anesthesia. Anesthesia base units range from 3 to 30: the higher the base unit, the more difficult the procedure. For example, code 00796, *Anesthesia for a liver transplant (recipient)*, has a base unit of 30, while code 00400, *Anesthesia for procedures on the integumentary system on the extremities, anterior trunk, and perineum; not otherwise specified*, has a base unit of 3. The higher base unit for the liver transplant is due to the fact that the procedure has a much greater risk of mortality or morbidity and thus requires greater skill from the anesthesiologist than a less invasive procedure on the skin, which has a lower risk to the patient. A listing of the base units associated with each CPT® anesthesia code is not included in the CPT® codebook published by the AMA but can be found on the CMS website.

Special Report

An anesthesia service that is reported with an unlisted anesthesia code (01999) or is rare or new may require a special report to show that the service was medically necessary and appropriate. The report should include information describing the procedure, the reason it was performed, the time and effort spent, and any special equipment that was used. CPT® guidelines mandate the use of special reports when *any* unusual service is provided—this guideline is not exclusive to anesthesia.

CONCEPTS CHECKPOINT 7.3

Answer true or false to each of the following statements.

1. _____ Supplies and materials commonly used in the administration of anesthesia are included in the anesthesia code and may not be reported separately.
2. _____ The anesthesia package includes a postoperative visit to assess the patient's recovery from anesthesia.
3. _____ The anesthesia package includes insertion of a Swan-Ganz catheter if the anesthesiologist performs this procedure while the patient is under anesthesia.
4. _____ If multiple procedures are performed while the patient is under anesthesia, it means that multiple operative episodes have occurred.
5. _____ A special report should be completed if a service is reported with an unlisted code.

Anesthesia Modifiers

As noted in the Anesthesia Guidelines, two-digit modifiers are attached to anesthesia codes to add more detail. Three types of modifiers are used when coding anesthesia procedures: physical status modifiers, CPT® modifiers, and HCPCS Level II modifiers.

Physical Status Modifiers

Physical status modifiers may be assigned by the anesthesia provider to indicate the patient's state of health and to help identify the level of complexity of the anesthesia service provided. These modifiers are represented by the letter *P* followed by a single digit from 1 through 6. The anesthesia physical status modifiers are defined in the Anesthesia Guidelines in the CPT® codebook:

- P1: a normal healthy patient;
- P2: a patient with mild systemic disease;
- P3: a patient with severe systemic disease;
- P4: a patient with severe systemic disease that is a constant threat to life;
- P5: a moribund patient who is not expected to survive without the operation; and
- P6: a declared brain-dead patient whose organs are being removed for donor purposes.

These 6 levels of physical status modifiers are consistent with the Physical Status Classification System created by the ASA. The anesthesiologist determines which classification best describes the patient.

EXAMPLE 7.3

A 55-year-old male patient with well-controlled diabetes mellitus underwent a transurethral resection of the prostate. The anesthesia code for this procedure is 00914, *Anesthesia for transurethral procedures; transurethral resection of prostate*, and the physical status modifier is P2, for a patient with mild systemic disease. The final format of the CPT® code should be 00914-P2.

</> Coding for CMS

The use of physical status modifiers is not always necessary. Some anesthesia providers will assign physical status modifiers to track patient outcomes, but Medicare and Medicaid do not accept physical status modifiers. Physical status modifiers may or may not affect reimbursement from third-party payers.

CPT® Modifiers

CPT® modifiers can also be used with anesthesia codes. A complete list of all modifiers applicable to CPT® codes is found in Appendix A of the codebook. Modifiers commonly used with anesthesia codes include: modifier 22, *Increased procedural service*; modifier 23, *Unusual anesthesia*; modifier 53, *Discontinued procedure*; modifier 59, *Distinct procedural service*; and modifier 74, *Discontinued out-patient hospital/ambulatory surgery center (ASC) procedure after administration of anesthesia*. Another related modifier to be aware of is modifier 47, *Anesthesia by surgeon*. However, this modifier cannot be used with the anesthesia procedure codes and is reported only with the surgery code.

Modifier 22: Increased Procedural Service When the work required to provide a service is substantially greater than typically required, modifier 22 is added to the anesthesia code. If the severity of the patient's condition increased the technical difficulty, intensity, or time involved in administering anesthesia, it is appropriate to assign modifier 22.

EXAMPLE 7.4

A trauma patient was brought to surgery for an exploration of a penetrating chest wound. The administration of general anesthesia was complicated by the location of the traumatic injury and the excessive blood loss. The anesthesiologist reported the service with code 00540-22, *Anesthesia for thoracotomy procedures involving lungs, pleura, diaphragm, and mediastinum (including surgical thoracoscopy); not otherwise specified - increased procedural service*.

Modifier 23: Unusual Anesthesia Modifier 23 is reported when a procedure that usually does not require anesthesia or requires only local anesthesia is done under general anesthesia. If there are unusual circumstances that require the patient to receive general anesthesia, it is appropriate to add modifier 23 to the anesthesia code.

EXAMPLE 7.5

An oncology patient who was in severe pain needed to receive radiation therapy. Radiation therapy usually does not require anesthesia, but because this patient could not remain still for the procedure due to pain, a general anesthetic was given to immobilize the patient. The anesthesiologist reported this service with code 01922-23, *Anesthesia for non-invasive imaging or radiation therapy - unusual anesthesia*.

Modifier 53: Discontinued Procedure Under certain circumstances, to ensure the patient's well-being, a physician may elect to terminate a surgical or diagnostic procedure that has already been started. Modifier 53 is used to indicate that a procedure was started but then discontinued. This modifier is not used if the procedure is canceled prior to the administration of anesthesia.

EXAMPLE 7.6

Two years after undergoing a total knee replacement, a 59-year-old patient returned to the operating room for a revision. The patient was placed under general endotracheal anesthesia, but after the incision was made and the orthopedic surgeon started the procedure, the patient's heart rate became irregular, causing the surgeon to discontinue the procedure. The anesthesiologist reported this episode with code 01402-53, *Anesthesia for open or surgical arthroscopic procedures on knee joint; total knee arthroplasty - discontinued procedure*.

Inside the OR

A Swan-Ganz catheter is a flow-directed venous catheter used to measure the heart's blood flow and function by monitoring pressure as well as taking blood samples and electrical recordings. When inserting and placing a Swan-Ganz catheter, the physician uses a central intravenous line to thread the catheter to the right heart, often through the femoral vein. It may also be inserted via the subclavian vein or internal jugular vein.

Modifier 59: Distinct Procedural Service Modifier 59 is used to indicate that a procedure or service is distinct or independent from another service provided on the same day. An anesthesiologist will use this modifier when he or she provides a separate service that is not included in the anesthesia package. In this case, reporting the second procedure code with modifier 59 attached indicates that the procedure was separate from the anesthesia.

Modifier 74: Discontinued Out-Patient Hospital/Ambulatory Surgery Center (ASC) Procedure After Administration of Anesthesia Modifier 74 is similar to modifier 53 in that it is used to indicate when the physician elects to terminate a surgical or diagnostic procedure after the administration of anesthesia. However, modifier 74 is used only in an outpatient hospital or ambulatory surgery center.

EXAMPLE 7.7

A 68-year-old male patient underwent a bypass graft procedure for which the surgeon requested the placement of a Swan-Ganz catheter to monitor the patient. The anesthesiologist inserted the Swan-Ganz catheter while the patient was under anesthesia during the operative episode. Placement of a Swan-Ganz catheter is not routinely associated with an anesthesia service, so this service must be coded and reported for additional reimbursement. The anesthesia code should be reported first, followed by the code for the Swan-Ganz catheter insertion with the modifier included: 93503-59, *Insertion and placement of flow directed catheter (eg, Swan-Ganz) for monitoring purposes - distinct procedural service.*

RED FLAG

When the surgeon administers general or regional anesthesia during a procedure, modifier 47 should be added to the end of the procedure code.

Coding Clicks

A list of the HCPCS Level II modifiers is available on the CMS website at http://Coding.ParadigmEducation.com/HCPCSModifiers.

Modifier 47: Anesthesia by Surgeon Modifier 47 is related to anesthesia, but is not 1 of the anesthesia code modifiers. Modifier 47 may be reported when regional or general anesthesia is provided by the surgeon instead of an anesthesiologist, CRNA, or AA. Modifier 47 cannot be reported with anesthesia procedure codes and is reported only with the surgery code.

HCPCS Level II Modifiers

HCPCS Level II modifiers may be required when reporting anesthesia services to Medicare and other third-party payers. A listing of Level II modifiers is available in Appendix A of the CPT® codebook. This list does not include descriptions of the modifiers. Descriptions are available from the CMS website. Examples of HCPCS Level II modifiers used for anesthesia procedures include the following:

- AA: anesthesia services performed personally by an anesthesiologist;
- AD: medical supervision by a physician, more than 4 concurrent anesthesia procedures;
- QK: medical direction by a physician of 2, 3, or 4 concurrent anesthesia procedures;
- QS: MAC;
- QX: CRNA's or AA's service with medical direction by a physician;
- QY: medical direction of 1 CRNA or AA by an anesthesiologist; and
- QZ: CRNA service without medical direction by a physician.

</> Coding for CMS

To receive proper reimbursement, a Medicare claim must include 1 (or more) of the modifiers AA, AD, QK, QX, QY, or QZ in the first field. Modifier QS must appear in the second field.

Qualifying Circumstances

Four add-on codes from the Medicine section of the CPT® codebook are included in the Anesthesia Guidelines, along with instructions for their reporting. These codes represent complications or circumstances that affect the nature of the anesthesia services reported; **qualifying circumstances** presented in these codes include the extraordinary condition of the patient, notable operative conditions, and/or unusual risk factors. As with all other add-on codes, a qualifying circumstances code may not be reported alone but should be reported as an additional procedure after the anesthesia code. More than 1 qualifying circumstances code may be assigned. Qualifying circumstances codes also carry a unit value for reimbursement by some third-party payers. The qualifying circumstances add-on codes are as follows:

- +99100, *Anesthesia for patient of extreme age, younger than 1 year and older than 70;*
- +99116, *Anesthesia complicated by utilization of total body hypothermia;*
- +99135, *Anesthesia complicated by utilization of controlled hypotension;* and
- +99140, *Anesthesia complicated by emergency conditions.*

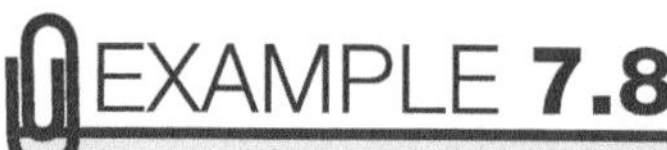

EXAMPLE **7.8**

An emergency department patient who had experienced a traumatic partial amputation of the arm was rushed to surgery. A complete medical history could not be obtained due to the patient's condition, and a delay in providing treatment to the patient would have been a threat to life and/or limb and would have affected patient outcome. In this situation, the administration of anesthesia can be considered complicated due to the fact that the surgery is an emergency and that there is no medical history available. Therefore, it is appropriate to report add-on code 99140, *Anesthesia complicated by emergency conditions*, in addition to the anesthesia code for the surgery.

CONCEPTS CHECKPOINT **7.4**

Answer true or false to each of the following statements.

1. _____ Qualifying circumstances codes replace anesthesia codes.
2. _____ A physical status modifier indicates the patient's state of health.
3. _____ Modifier 53 should be reported if a patient decided not to undergo a procedure.
4. _____ Modifier 22 should be reported when the amount or degree of difficulty of the work required by the physician was substantially greater than usual.
5. _____ Modifier 23 can be reported appropriately when a patient received spinal anesthesia.
6. _____ Modifier 47 can be used with anesthesia codes.

Using Other Procedures Codes (01990-01999)

> **RED FLAG**
>
> Be sure to choose the correct anatomical site! Code 62324 is reported for the placement of an epidural catheter to the cervical or thoracic region for continuous infusion of anesthetic, opioids, or other solution. Code 62326 is reported for the placement of an epidural catheter to the lumbar or sacral (caudal) region.

Although the Other Procedures subsection of codes is not specifically called out in the Anesthesia Guidelines, you should be aware of this subsection, which is located at the end of the Anesthesia section of the codebook. Codes from the Other Procedures subsection are used to report certain procedures that cannot be classified within any of the other subsections of the Anesthesia section. These procedures include services such as placing and monitoring epidural or subarachnoid catheters for continuous drug administration (code 01991). For example, code 01991 is reported when a patient undergoing extensive abdominal surgery receives epidural anesthesia via an epidural catheter during the surgical episode, and the catheter is left in place for continuous administration of medication to relieve pain after the surgery. If, in addition to the anesthesia given during surgery, the anesthesiologist afterward places an epidural catheter for pain relief only, as shown in Figure 7.3, placing the epidural catheter may be reported as a separate service (see codes 62324 and 62326, *Injection, including indwelling catheter placement, continuous infusion or intermittent bolus, epidural, subarachnoid, cervical, thoracic, lumbar, or sacral*). In both cases, code 01996, *Daily hospital management of epidural or subarachnoid continuous drug administration*, should be reported for each calendar day until the catheter is removed.

Figure 7.3 Placement of an Epidural Catheter

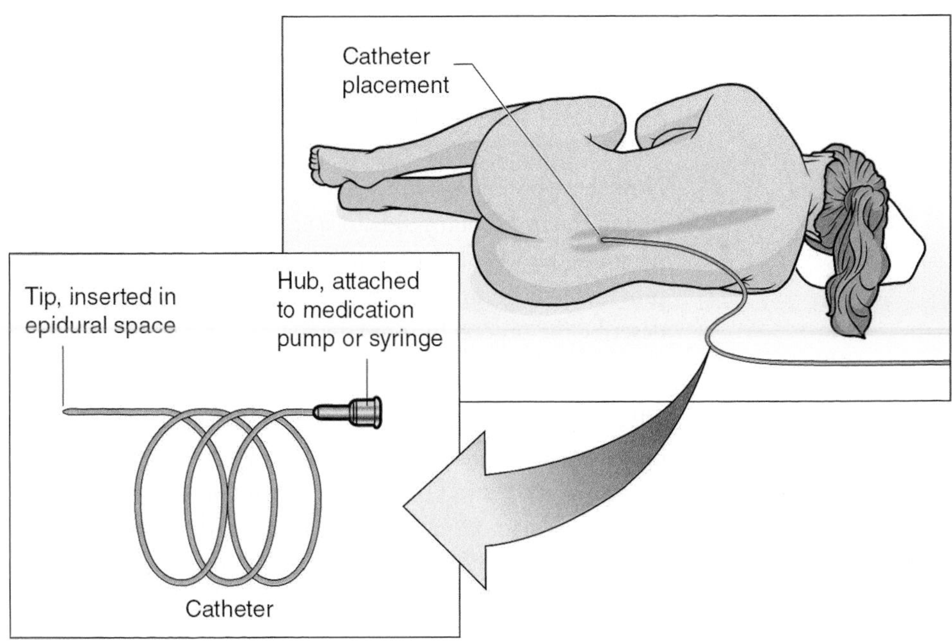

LET'S TRY ONE 7.3

After reading each scenario, answer yes or no to the question that follows.

1. A 62-year-old male underwent a radical retropubic prostatectomy under epidural anesthesia. Because of anticipated postoperative pain and the patient's history of low pain tolerance, the epidural catheter was left in place after the procedure was completed. Should the placement of the epidural catheter be reported as a separate procedure in addition to the code for the anesthesia? _____
2. A 45-year-old patient underwent a pelvic evisceration for an extensive malignancy under general anesthesia. The anesthesiologist inserted an epidural catheter for postoperative pain medication infusion. Should the placement of the epidural catheter be reported as a separate procedure in addition to the code for the anesthesia? _____
3. An anesthesiologist visited a patient the day after surgery under general anesthesia and managed the drugs administered through an epidural catheter that had been inserted for postoperative pain medication infusion. Should the anesthesiologist report a code for this visit? _____
4. A surgeon ordered a blood transfusion for a patient during surgery. The anesthesiologist gave the patient the transfusion. Should the anesthesiologist report a separate code for this service? _____
5. An anesthesiologist performed a postoperative assessment the day after surgery for a hospital inpatient. Should a code for this assessment be reported in addition to the code for the anesthesia service? _____

Instructions for Reporting Anesthesia Codes

Now that you understand what anesthesia is, how to find the codes necessary to report it, and the important guidelines and considerations associated with reporting anesthesia codes, how should you apply this information to reporting the codes? Figure 7.4 provides a diagram to guide you through this process, and the following paragraphs describe the process in more detail.

As stated earlier in the chapter, codes for anesthesia services are indexed in the CPT®codebook under the main term *Anesthesia* and then by a subterm based on the operative anatomical site, body system, type of procedure, name of procedure, surgical technique, or clinical condition. Begin your search for the appropriate code by referring to the main term *Anesthesia* in the Index and then searching for the subterm that most accurately describes the procedure performed. Some examples of various types of Index subterms and the codes indexed with them are as follows:

- operative anatomical site: Nose, 00160 through 00164;
- body system: Integumentary, with anatomical sites as subterms, comprising codes 00300 through 00400;
- type of procedure: Vascular Shunt, 01844;
- name of procedure: Nephrectomy, 00862;
- surgical technique: Arthroscopic Procedures, with anatomical sites as subterms, codes ranging from 01202 through 01830; and
- clinical condition: Arrhythmias, 00410.

Figure 7.4 Locating and Reporting Anesthesia Codes

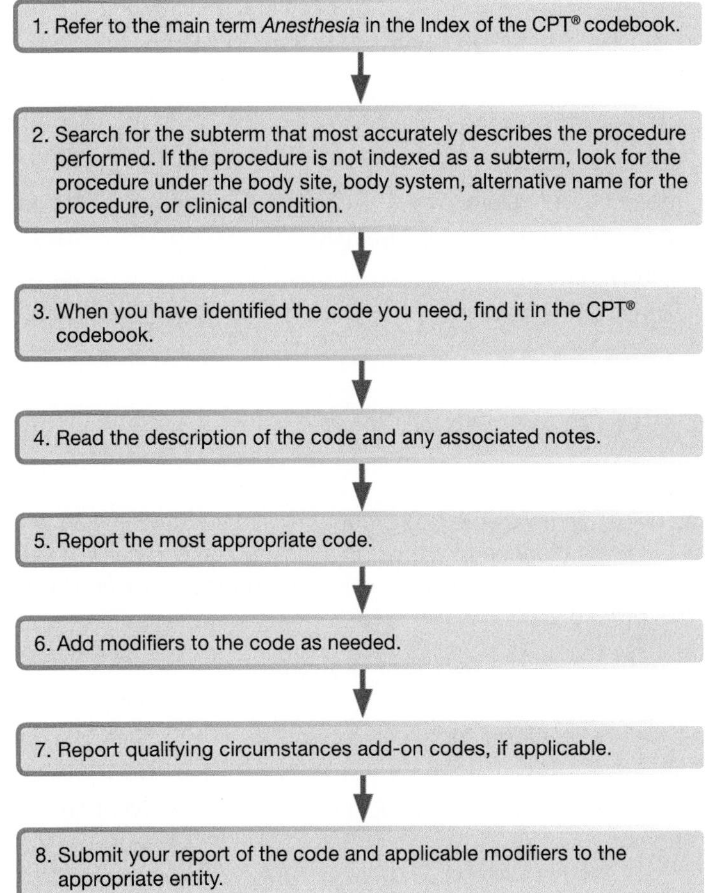

1. Refer to the main term *Anesthesia* in the Index of the CPT® codebook.
2. Search for the subterm that most accurately describes the procedure performed. If the procedure is not indexed as a subterm, look for the procedure under the body site, body system, alternative name for the procedure, or clinical condition.
3. When you have identified the code you need, find it in the CPT® codebook.
4. Read the description of the code and any associated notes.
5. Report the most appropriate code.
6. Add modifiers to the code as needed.
7. Report qualifying circumstances add-on codes, if applicable.
8. Submit your report of the code and applicable modifiers to the appropriate entity.

Once you have found the appropriate code or range of codes, refer to the corresponding section of the CPT® codebook to review your code selection. Carefully read the code description and any associated instructional notes before choosing a code. If multiple procedures were performed, be sure to choose the anesthesia code that reflects the most complex procedure (the procedure with the highest base unit). Assign modifiers as needed, as well as add-on codes for qualifying circumstances, if applicable.

EXAMPLE **7.9**

You are in search of the code for the anesthesia portion of an operation for a vaginal hysterectomy. Begin by referring to the main term *Anesthesia* in the Index. Find the subterm *Hysterectomy* and then, below that subterm, the subterm *Vaginal* with its code, 00944. Locate code 00944 in the Anesthesia section of the codebook. The description of code 00944 shares the base portion from code 00940, *Anesthesia for vaginal procedures (including biopsy of labia, vagina, cervix or endometrium)*, but the end portion of code 00944 is specific to a vaginal hysterectomy. Because this patient suffers from mild emphysema, you will also need to assign a physical status modifier of P2. The full code should be reported as 00944-P2.

CONCEPTS CHECKPOINT 7.5

Practice anesthesia coding by identifying the appropriate anesthesia code for each of the following procedures.

1. _____ needle biopsy of the thyroid
2. _____ cesarean section
3. _____ repair of cleft palate
4. _____ repair of ruptured Achilles tendon, without graft
5. _____ biopsy of the clavicle
6. _____ corneal transplant
7. _____ total cystectomy
8. _____ Whipple procedure
9. _____ vasectomy
10. _____ donor nephrectomy

LET'S TRY ONE 7.4

The parents of an 11-month-old boy brought him to the pediatrician when they noticed a bulging in the child's groin. He was diagnosed with an inguinal hernia, and a surgical intervention was scheduled. An inguinal hernia repair was successfully completed under general anesthesia. Answer the following questions related to this procedure.

1. What type of anesthesia was used for this procedure? _______________
2. Is this type of anesthesia separately reportable? _______________
3. How would you locate this procedure in the CPT® Index? _______________
4. Are there any qualifying circumstances in this scenario? _______________
5. Should a qualifying circumstance code be reported? _______________
6. What code(s) would the anesthesiologist report? _______________

LET'S TRY ONE 7.5

A 33-year-old female patient with type II diabetes underwent a tubal ligation under general anesthesia. Answer the following questions about this procedure.

1. What type of anesthesia was given? _______________
2. Is this a type of anesthesia that is separately reportable? _______________
3. How would you locate the code for this procedure in the Index? _______________
4. This patient has type II diabetes. Which physical status modifier should be applied? _______________
5. Are there any qualifying circumstances in this scenario? _______________
6. What code should be reported? _____

Anesthesia Coding Resources

Coding Clicks

Find answers to many coding-related questions at the American Society of Anesthesiologists's website at http://Coding.ParadigmEducation.com/ASA.

Many resources are available to assist you with anesthesia coding. One of these is called a **crosswalk** or **cross coder** (which may be a book or computer software), which links codes commonly used by anesthesiologists to corresponding CPT® surgical codes. Automated **encoders** also assist the coding professional, as discussed in Chapter 5. Another resource is the American Society of Anesthesiologists's website, http://asahq.org. This site contains a practice management section with answers to many coding questions. Finally, anesthesiologists and anesthetists are usually very familiar with the CPT® anesthesia codes, so don't be afraid to ask these medical professionals for their coding advice.

Chapter Summary

- CPT® codes are used to report anesthesia services when anesthesia (other than local) is provided.
- A package of services is included when an anesthesia code is reported. This package includes the usual care that accompanies the anesthesia service: preoperative and postoperative visits, administration of anesthesia during the surgical procedure, administration of IV fluids or blood, and monitoring the patient's vital signs.
- Anesthesia codes are assigned and reported based on the anatomical site or the type of procedure, not the type of anesthesia.
- The Anesthesia section of the CPT® codebook is arranged by body site, in a head-to-toe format. Codes for radiological procedures, burns, and obstetrical procedures are located near the end of the section.
- Only 1 anesthesia code should be reported per operative session.
- The 3 types of modifiers used with anesthesia codes are physical status modifiers, CPT® modifiers, and HCPCS Level II modifiers. These are reported along with the CPT® code to add more detail and/or describe unusual circumstances.
- There are 4 qualifying circumstances add-on codes that may be reported with anesthesia codes when anesthesia involves a patient of extreme age, total body hypothermia, controlled hypotension, or emergency conditions.
- Anesthesia codes may be found in the CPT® Index under the main term *Anesthesia* and the subterm that describes the procedure performed, the body site of the surgery, or the clinical condition.

Navigator

Access interactive chapter review exercises, practice activities, flash cards, and study games.

Chapter 8

Introduction to Surgery Coding

Fast Facts

- The word *surgery* comes from the Greek word *cheirourgen*, which means to work with one's hands.
- The earliest evidence of a surgical procedure was a trephination of the skull in 5000 BC. The primitive surgeon bored a hole in the patient's skull using flint or stone instruments.
- In 1897 Ludwig Rehn performed the first successful heart surgery.
- The first robot-assisted surgery was performed in 1985 with a robot called the Puma560. Today, robot-assisted surgeries are commonplace.

Sources: http://ncbi.nlm.nih.gov, http://encyclopedia.com

Crack the Code

Review the sample operative report to find the correct code. You may need to return to this exercise after reading the chapter content.

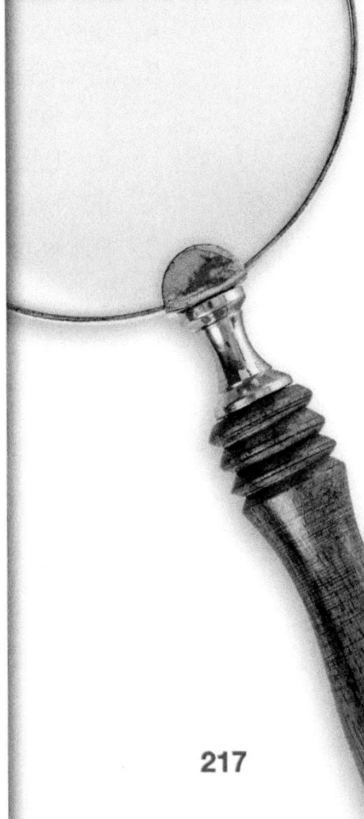

DATE OF PROCEDURE: 02/13/2019

PROCEDURE PERFORMED: Abdominal myomectomy

ANESTHESIA: General endotracheal anesthesia

SURGEON: Linda Dowling, MD

ASSISTANT: Pat Dorris, RN

IV FLUIDS: 1.2 L crystalloid

ESTIMATED BLOOD LOSS: 350 mL

URINE OUTPUT: 300 mL, clear throughout the case

FINDINGS: Included uniformly enlarged uterus secondary to uterine fibroids with uterine fibroid impinging upon the uterine cavity and normal-appearing adnexa bilaterally with normal-appearing fallopian tubes bilaterally

SPECIMEN: Included uterine fibroids

COMPLICATIONS: None

answer: 58140

Learning Objectives

8.1 Use suffixes to identify common surgical terminology.

8.2 Describe the organization of the Surgery subsections of the CPT® codebook.

8.3 Explain the use of guidelines, notes, and special instructions in the CPT® codebook.

8.4 Define the concept and parts of the surgical package.

8.5 Differentiate between the characteristics and code requirements of surgical techniques, including the different methods of surgical destruction.

8.6 Differentiate between follow-up care for diagnostic and therapeutic procedures.

8.7 Identify the location of codes for surgical supplies and materials.

8.8 Describe the reporting of more than 1 procedure or service in an operative episode by the use of add-on codes and modifiers listed in the Surgery section.

8.9 Identify CPT® and HCPCS modifiers commonly used with surgery codes.

8.10 Explain the separate procedure notation used in the CPT® codebook.

8.11 Identify when and how to use unlisted procedure codes.

8.12 Explain circumstances that require a special report.

Chapter Outline

I. Introduction to Surgery Coding
II. Surgical Terminology
III. Organization of the Surgery Section
- **A.** Surgery Headings and Categories
- **B.** Subsection Guidelines and Notes

IV. Surgery Guidelines
- **A.** Services
- **B.** CPT® Surgical Package Definition
  - **i.** Services Bundled in a Surgery Code
  - **ii.** Unbundling Surgical Codes
  - **iii.** Endoscopic and Laparoscopic Procedures
- **C.** Follow-up Care for Diagnostic Procedures
- **D.** Follow-up Care for Therapeutic Surgical Procedures
- **E.** Supplied Materials
- **F.** Reporting More Than 1 Procedure/Service
  - **i.** Add-on Codes
  - **ii.** Modifiers Used in Surgery Coding
- **G.** Separate Procedure
- **H.** Unlisted Service or Procedure
- **I.** Special Report
- **J.** Surgical Destruction

V. Instructions for Reporting Surgery Codes
VI. Chapter Summary

Introduction to Surgery Coding

The Surgery section is by far the largest section in the CPT®codebook. The Surgery codes represent surgical procedures and other services provided to a surgical patient, most of which are invasive procedures for diagnostic or therapeutic purposes that require the skill of a well-trained medical professional. The surgery codes range from 10021 through 69990. This chapter presents coding practices common to most surgery procedures. You will learn more about surgery codes for each body system in subsequent chapters in this book.

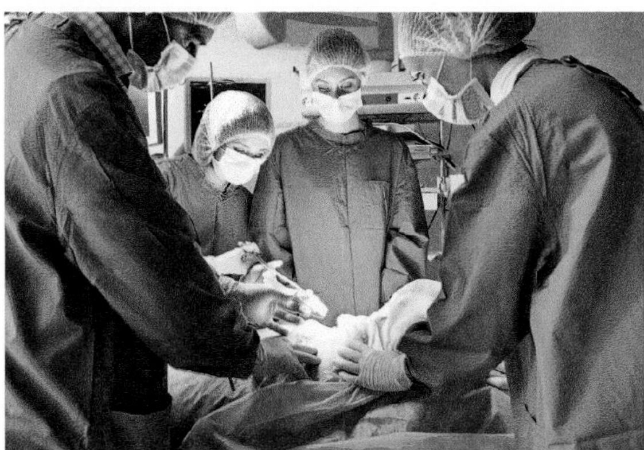

Surgical procedures require the skill of a well-trained medical professional. Surgery codes make up the bulk of the CPT® codebook.

Surgical Terminology

As you learned in Chapter 5, operative reports contain the surgeon's description of the procedure performed and any events that took place during the surgery. To be able to accurately report surgery codes, you must be able to recognize and understand the terminology used in surgery documentation. This means you must become familiar with common surgical suffixes and understand how to distinguish between similar terms. Often, the spelling of 2 surgical suffixes may vary by only 1 letter but indicate a completely different procedure. For example, at first glance, *colotomy* and *colostomy* might appear to be the same term, but if you look closely, you will notice that *colostomy* contains an *s* where *colotomy* does not. That 1 letter differentiates between 2 distinct procedures and indicates the type of procedure or technique performed. The suffix *-tomy* means to cut into or to make an incision, so a colotomy is an incision into the colon, whereas the suffix *-stomy* means to create an artificial opening, so a colostomy is the creation of an artificial opening in the colon. Table 8.1 defines and provides examples of some of the most common suffixes used in the names of surgical procedures. Be sure to thoroughly review this information before beginning to report codes from the Surgery section.

Table 8.1 Common Surgical Suffixes

Suffix	Meaning	Example
-ectomy	removal or excision	Appendectomy: removal of the appendix
-tomy	cutting operation	Laparotomy: an incision into the abdomen
-stomy	creation of an artificial opening	Colostomy: creation of an artificial opening in the colon
-plasty	surgical repair	Rhinoplasty: surgical repair of the nose
-pexy	surgical fixation or putting into place	Nephropexy: surgical fixation of a mobile kidney
-centesis	puncture to aspirate (draw out) fluid	Thoracocentesis: puncture of the thoracic cavity to draw out fluid
-scopy	visual examination using scope	Colonoscopy: visual examination of the colon using a colonoscope
-opsy	viewing	Biopsy: a procedure to view living tissue
-rrhaphy	a repair by suturing (stitching)	Colporrhaphy: repair of the vagina by suturing
-desis	surgical fusion	Arthrodesis: surgical fusion of a joint
-lysis	a separation	Adhesiolysis: separation of adhesions
-tripsy	surgical crushing	Lithotripsy: the crushing of stones located in the kidney, bladder, or ureter

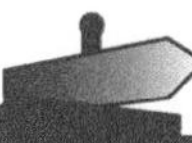

Learn Your Way

Learning new medical terms takes some memorization, and students respond to different strategies. Verbal learners may find it helpful to create flashcards for each of the common surgical suffixes, with the suffix on 1 side and the definition on the other.

Be sure to study the cards both ways—looking at the definition and naming the suffix, and looking at the suffix and stating the definition. Once you understand the meanings of the suffixes, you will be able to identify many surgical procedures.

CONCEPTS CHECKPOINT **8.1**

After memorizing the surgical suffixes, complete this checkpoint without looking at Table 8.1. Match the surgical suffixes in the first column to their definitions in the second column.

1. _____ *-ectomy*
2. _____ *-tomy*
3. _____ *-stomy*
4. _____ *-plasty*
5. _____ *-pexy*
6. _____ *-rrhaphy*
7. _____ *-centesis*
8. _____ *-tripsy*
9. _____ *-desis*
10. _____ *-scopy*

a. surgical repair
b. puncture to aspirate fluid
c. excision; to remove
d. surgical fixation
e. incision; to cut into
f. repair by suturing
g. creation of artificial opening
h. surgical fusion
i. to crush
j. visual examination using a scope

Organization of the Surgery Section

The Surgery section includes the Guidelines common to all surgical procedures, 18 subsections by body system, and a subsection containing 1 add-on code for microsurgical techniques that require the use of an operating microscope. Table 8.2 provides a list of the subsections of the Surgery section and their corresponding code ranges.

The first subsection after the Guidelines, General, has 2 codes (10021 and 10022) for fine needle aspiration. These codes are applicable to many different anatomical sites. For each body system subsection that follows, headings and categories group the subsection by body site and type of surgical procedure.

Table 8.2 Surgery Subsections and Corresponding Codes

Surgery Subsection	Code(s)
General	10021-10022
Integumentary System	10030-19499
Musculoskeletal System	20005-29999
Respiratory System	30000-32999
Cardiovascular System	33010-37799
Hemic and Lymphatic Systems	38100-38999
Mediastinum and Diaphragm	39000-39599
Digestive System	40490-49999
Urinary System	50010-53899
Male Genital System	54000-55899
Reproductive System Procedures	55920
Intersex Surgery	55970-55980
Female Genital System	56405-58999
Maternity Care and Delivery	59000-59899
Endocrine System	60000-60699
Nervous System	61000-64999
Eye and Ocular Adnexa	65091-68899
Auditory System	69000-69979
Operating Microscope	69990

Surgery Headings and Categories

Index Insider

Many of the surgical procedure categories (such as Exploration) are main entries in the CPT® Index, with anatomical site subterms providing the relevant codes.

The Surgery subsections by body system share an organizational scheme of headings and categories. The first heading generally indicates anatomical sites. The second category under the first heading indicates the types of surgical procedures. In general, within each body system subsection, the incision and excision codes are listed first, followed by introduction and removal, repair, destruction, and finally, other procedures.

Subsection Guidelines and Notes

At the beginning of many subsections within the Surgery section, you will see specific coding guidelines for that subsection. Make sure to read these guidelines thoroughly, as following them is mandatory to remain compliant with Health Insurance Portability and Accountability Act of 1996 (HIPAA) healthcare fraud and abuse policies. In addition, you should always read any notes that appear within a subsection before selecting a code from that subsection. These notes often include details not provided in the code descriptions.

Coding Clicks

For more information about HIPAA and the most up-to-date fraud and abuse legislation related to coding, visit the American Health Information Management Association's HIM Body of Knowledge website at http://Coding.ParadigmEducation.com/BoK. You must be an AHIMA member to access the Body of Knowledge.

For example, see the parenthetic note that appears below code 19364, *Breast reconstruction with free flap*, as shown in Figure 8.1. This note explains that code 19364 includes several procedures: harvesting of the flap, microvascular transfer, closure of the donor site, and inset shaping the flap into a breast. The note provides crucial information, as reporting those procedures separately would be fraudulent and a violation of HIPAA regulations. However, remember that submission of a code that is compliant with all guidelines, notes, and special instructions does not guarantee payment. Third-party payers determine the requirements for payment to providers.

Figure 8.1 Example of a Codebook Note in the Surgery Section

19364	Breast reconstruction with free flap
	(Do not report code 69990 in addition to code 19364)
	(19364 includes harvesting of the flap, microvascular transfer, closure of the donor site, and inset shaping the flap into a breast)

Surgery Guidelines

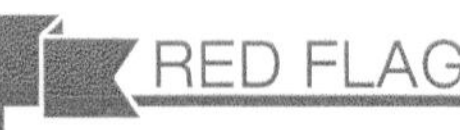

RED FLAG

Always read any notes that appear within a subsection before selecting a code from that subsection.

The Surgery Guidelines at the beginning of the Surgery section contain instructions and definitions that apply to all of the surgical CPT® codes. The Surgery Guidelines are organized into the following headings, which will be discussed in turn:

- Services
- CPT® Surgical Package Definition
- Follow-up Care for Diagnostic Procedures
- Follow-up Care for Therapeutic Surgical Procedures
- Supplied Materials
- Reporting More Than One Procedure/Service
- Separate Procedure
- Unlisted Service or Procedure
- Special Report
- Surgical Destruction

Services

Physician services that are not included in the surgical package described below are reported with codes from the Evaluation and Management section (99201 through 99499). Codes from the Medicine section's Special Services, Procedures, and Reports subsection (99000 through 99091) should be reported for other services or supplies and materials not included in the surgical package. These codes should be reported in addition to the code for the surgical procedure.

CPT® Surgical Package Definition

A surgical procedure consists of a sequence of services provided to a patient, from the preoperative consultation to the postoperative follow-up care. In CPT® coding, the **surgical package** is made up of the services and time involved in performing a normal, uncomplicated surgical service. These services that the surgeon provides (in addition to the surgical procedure itself) are bundled or "packaged" into the 1 surgery code. The Surgery Guidelines in the CPT® codebook list the services that are packaged in each CPT® surgery code, as shown in Figure 8.2.

Figure 8.2 CPT® Surgical Package Definition from the Surgery Guidelines

In defining the specific services "included" in a given CPT® surgical code, the following services related to the surgery when furnished by the physician and other qualified health care professional who performs the surgery are included in addition to the operation per se:

- Evaluation and Management (E/M) service(s) subsequent to the decision for surgery on the day before and/or the day of surgery (including history and physical)
- Local infiltration, metacarpal/metatarsal/digital block or topical anesthesia
- Immediate postoperative care, including dictating operative notes, talking with the family and other physicians or other qualified health care professionals
- Writing orders
- Evaluating the patient in the postanesthesia recovery area
- Typical postoperative follow-up care

Services Bundled in a Surgery Code

The surgical package concept assumes that all patients receiving the same type of surgery receive the same services and the same length of follow-up care. These services are not to be reported separately.

Evaluation and Management Service The diagnosis of a condition and the determination of the need for surgery precede the surgical package and are therefore not packaged into the surgery code. For example, the physician who evaluates the clinical problem may refer the patient to a surgeon. The surgeon who will render the services necessary to correct the problem initiates the surgical package. The preoperative assessment that is part of the surgical package is a typical E/M encounter on the date immediately prior to or on the date of the procedure and includes a history and physical. This E/M service is included in the surgical package.

EXAMPLE **8.1**

An obese 36-year-old woman presented to her family physician with a history of light-colored stools that followed an episode of abdominal pain after a heavy meal the night before. She experienced some nausea and vomiting but had begun to feel better. Her physician ordered an abdominal ultrasound that showed evidence of gallstones. She was diagnosed with cholecystitis and cholelithiasis and referred to as a *general surgeon*. The surgeon recommended the patient undergo a laparoscopic cholecystectomy, and the patient scheduled the procedure for the next day with the surgeon. On the day of the surgery, the usual preoperative assessment was performed prior to the patient being taken to the operating room. The patient's first visit with the surgeon was the decision for surgery and would be coded with the appropriate E/M code, with modifier 57 appended. The preoperative assessment on the day of surgery would be included in the surgical package.

Anesthesia and Moderate (Conscious) Sedation The anesthesia included in the surgical package is local and topical anesthesia, administered in the specific region of a minor surgical procedure. As discussed in Chapter 7, major surgical procedures can require general, regional, or nerve block anesthesia. By nature of the skilled services required for monitored anesthesia care, the administration of these types of anesthesia has codes that are reported separately by the anesthesia provider (located in the Anesthesia section of the codebook, 00100 through 01999).

Moderate (conscious) sedation is created by providing the patient with a combination of sedatives and analgesics to help him or her to tolerate an uncomfortable procedure. A consciously sedated patient is drowsy, relaxed, and able to respond to verbal commands. Moderate (conscious) sedation wears off after a short time and therefore is used only for minor procedures.

Immediate Postoperative Care After the surgical procedure has been completed and the patient has left the surgical suite, immediate postoperative care involves evaluating the patient in the postanesthesia recovery area, writing postoperative orders, and dictating operative notes. Immediate postoperative care also includes speaking to family members regarding the surgical findings and the plan of care for the patient.

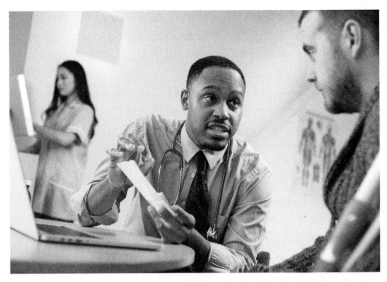

The surgical package helps ensure that patients return for follow-up care.

Follow-up Care One of the reasons for bundling services into a surgical package is to ensure that the patient returns for follow-up care. Often, patients who expect to be charged for additional appointments with a physician will not return to the office. However, knowing that follow-up visits are included in the overall surgery charge encourages patients to continue to receive care.

Including follow-up care in the surgical package also makes billing easier for the provider because it allows billers to report 1 CPT® code for an entire episode of care, no matter how many postoperative visits the patient receives during the global period. The **global period**, also known as **global days**, refers to the length of time over which a typical patient receives follow-up care for a surgical procedure, and this period is included in the surgical package. There is a defined number of days within a global period. You will learn more about this concept later in the chapter. When it is packaged into the surgery code, reimbursement for follow-up care is based on the code for the surgical procedure.

Unbundling Surgical Codes

RED FLAG

Reporting separate codes when 1 code could be used is considered fraudulent. The Office of the Inspector General has identified unbundling as a risk area that will be monitored specifically for Centers for Medicare and Medicaid Services patients.

Because surgical codes are intended to cover many components of a surgical procedure, it is inappropriate to code these components separately. **Unbundling** is the practice of using multiple codes when 1 code could sufficiently cover all the components of a service. This practice is not only unethical but also illegal.

Surgical operations may have many integral steps. Examples of minor components of a surgical procedure include the following services:

- local infiltration of medication;
- minor debridement (removal of dead tissue or foreign objects from a wound);
- obtaining a wound culture;
- exploration of the operative area;
- lysis of moderate adhesions;
- fulguration of bleeding points;
- closure of the surgical wound;
- application of dressings; and
- application of splints (musculoskeletal procedures).

Coding Clicks

The National Correct Coding Initiative (NCCI) was implemented to prevent duplicate payment for services that should have been reported with a single code (bundled). To view the NCCI policy manual that addresses issues related to the edits and standard surgical practice, visit http://Coding.ParadigmEducation.com/NCCI. The manual is updated annually.

These minor components are integral to the surgical procedure itself and should not be coded as separate procedures. Notes within the Surgery section also list components specific to certain procedure codes, as shown in Figure 8.3.

Figure 8.3 Components Specific to Procedure Codes

63090 Vertebral corpectomy (vertebral body resection), partial or complete, transperitoneal or retroperitoneal approach with decompression of spinal cord, cauda equina or nerve root(s), lower thoracic, lumbar, or sacral; single segment

63091 each additional segment (List separately in addition to code for primary procedure)

(Use 63901 in conjunction with 63090)

(Procedures 63081-63091 include discectomy above and/ or below vertebral segment)

(If followed by arthrodesis, see 22548-22812)

(For reconstruction of spine, use appropriate vertebral corpectomy codes 63081-63091, bone graft codes 20930-20938, arthrodesis codes 22548-22812, and spinal instrumentation codes 22840-22855)

EXAMPLE **8.2**

A 14-year-old male patient had an appendectomy. Removal of the appendix required an abdominal incision. After the appendix was removed, the incision was closed. The opening and closing of the abdominal incision was an integral minor component of the appendectomy procedure. The only code reported for this procedure is 44950, *Appendectomy*. Even though codes exist for incision and closure of abdominal incisions, these may not be reported in addition to the code for an abdominal surgery.

CONCEPTS CHECKPOINT **8.2**

Are the following services included in the CPT® surgical package? Answer yes or no to each service.

1. _____ local anesthesia
2. _____ general anesthesia
3. _____ an office visit 1 week prior to surgery
4. _____ immediate postoperative care
5. _____ assessing the patient in the recovery room
6. _____ obtaining a wound culture
7. _____ normal, uncomplicated care during the period of global days assigned to the procedure
8. _____ any and all E/M visits within the global days

Endoscopic and Laparoscopic Procedures

Endoscopic and **laparoscopic** surgeries provide an alternative to the traditional open technique, which requires a large incision and exposure of internal organs. Endoscopic surgeries use an **endoscope**, a tubular instrument with a light source designed for examining and performing surgeries on hollow body organs such as the stomach. The endoscope is inserted into the body through an opening such as the mouth or rectum. In a laparoscopic surgery, small incisions are made for passage of a **laparoscope**, an endoscope that is used for visual examination of the abdominal cavity, so that the surgery can be accomplished without opening the patient's abdomen. Compared to an open procedure, an endoscopic or laparoscopic procedure allows for a shorter recovery period, less postoperative pain, and reduced risk of infection for the patient; however, the procedures are technically demanding and may require a longer time to complete than an open approach to the same procedure.

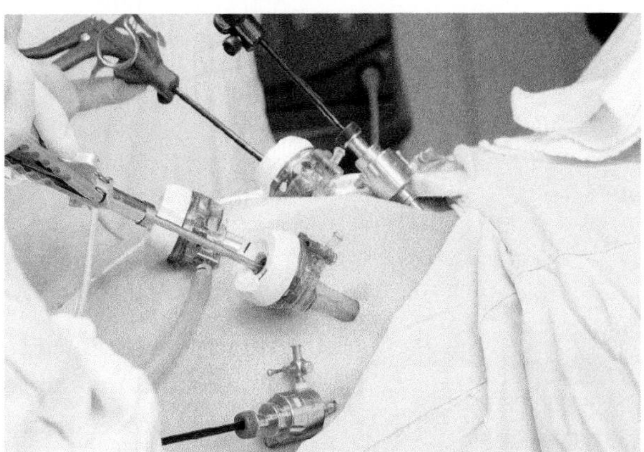

In a laparoscopic surgery, small incisions allow a laparoscope to pass through so that the surgery can be accomplished without opening the patient's abdomen.

Codes for endoscopic or laparoscopic surgery are found under the anatomical headings in the subsections of the Surgery section. Procedures performed using an endoscopic or laparoscopic approach must be reported with a code from the appropriate endoscopic or laparoscopic category under the anatomical site headings. Do not report the procedure using a code for the open technique. When the documentation indicates that a procedure was performed using a "scope," find the code located under the category provided for these procedures within the specific body systems in the tabular list. You can find these subheadings in the tables of contents that precede each surgery body system as blue entries under the red anatomical-site entries. Another way to find an endoscopic or laparoscopic procedure is by using the Index:

1. Look in the Index for the "scope" procedure listed as a main term, recognizable from the *-scopy* suffix (for example, *Anoscopy*, *Arthroscopy*, *Endoscopy*, *Laparoscopy*, *Thoracoscopy*).
2. Look for the relevant anatomical site indexed as a subterm.
3. Look under the anatomical site subterm for the surgical procedure you want to report and identify the code that describes the service.
4. Find the code in the tabular list by doing a numerical search.
5. Review the code, making sure that its description contains the use of a "scope."

EXAMPLE 8.3

A 45-year-old woman presented with chronic pain in her right lower abdomen that suggested an ovarian cyst. The patient had a history of hysterectomy (her uterus had been removed). A laparoscopy was scheduled. Under general endotracheal anesthesia, the previous laparoscopic incisions were opened, and laparoscopic trocars and ports were inserted to provide access to the surgical area. Using Metzenbaum scissors, the adhesions were taken down. No endometriosis was noted after dissecting away adhesions from the omentum and sigmoid colon to the right adnexa. The ovary was mobilized. A 4- to 5-cm ovarian cyst that appeared benign was excised and sent to pathology. A normal liver edge and normal gallbladder surfaces were noted. The pelvis was irrigated and hemostasis assured at all adhesiolysis sites and the ovarian cyst site. The procedure was well tolerated.

In this procedure, the lysis of adhesions was incidental to reaching the ovary to remove the cyst and would not be separately coded. The procedure documentation does not indicate that the adhesiolysis was extensive or difficult. The code reported for this procedure would be 58662, *Laparoscopy, surgical; with fulguration or excision of lesions of the ovary, pelvic viscera, or peritoneal surface by any method*.

RED FLAG

When surgery documentation indicates a service was performed laparoscopically but there is no code for the laparoscopic technique, do not report the code for the open technique—report the appropriate unlisted laparoscopic procedure code instead.

If a surgery is attempted as a laparoscopic procedure but must be converted to an open procedure, only the open procedure should be coded. Medicare refers to this as a **sequential procedure** and advises that the most invasive service be billed (in this case, the open procedure). The unsuccessful initial procedure should not be separately reported.

If no laparoscopic or endoscopic code exists for the procedure, an unlisted procedure code should be reported. The Surgery Guidelines contain a compilation of all of the surgery unlisted service or procedure codes including specific codes for unlisted procedures done with a "scope" (recognized by the suffix *-scopy*). For example, you can report code 58578, *Unlisted laparoscopy procedure, uterus*, for an unlisted laparoscopic procedure of the uterus. Unlisted procedure codes can be found in the Surgery Guidelines in anatomical order or in the Index in alphabetical order under the main term *Unlisted Services and Procedures*.

Coding for CMS

Publication 100-4, *Medicare Claims Processing Manual*, provides instructions for coding and billing for Medicare patients. The specific rule mentioned above for sequential procedures can be found in Publication 100-4, Chapter 12, section 30 under the heading "Correct Coding Policy." The entire manual can be found online by accessing the Internet-Only Manuals (IOMs) website at http://Coding.ParadigmEducation.com/IOMs.

LET'S TRY ONE 8.1

A 61-year-old female was found to have a small mass on her right kidney. She was taken to surgery where a laparoscopic partial nephrectomy was performed. What is the correct code for this procedure? _____

Follow-up Care for Diagnostic Procedures

The Surgery Guidelines indicate that follow-up care for diagnostic procedures (eg, diagnostic bronchoscopy performed to look for a cause of symptoms) includes only care related to recovery from the diagnostic procedure itself. Any other services provided after a diagnostic procedure (eg, services related to treating any conditions discovered by the diagnostic procedure) must be reported separately.

Follow-up Care for Therapeutic Surgical Procedures

As explained earlier in the chapter, the global period or global days refers to the length of time over which a typical patient receives follow-up care for a surgical procedure, and this period is included in the surgical package. The number of global days associated with a specific CPT® code is determined by each third-party payer, but many payers use the number of global days determined by the Centers for Medicare and Medicaid Services (CMS) for that procedure. Global days range from 0 to 90, depending on the complexity of the procedure. Typical global periods are 0, 10, 15, 45, or 90 days in length. Most major surgeries have a 90-day global period. Follow-up care for therapeutic procedures lasting longer than the allowed global period may be coded separately.

RED FLAG

The Medicine section of the CPT® codebook contains a code that describes a postoperative follow-up visit, 99024, and this code may be reported, but no charge is allowed for this visit. Coders should check with their respective facilities to see if it is necessary to report code 99024 for a postoperative follow-up visit. Some facilities may use this code for administrative purposes to track the number of patient visits related to surgery aftercare.

Inside the OR

In a laparoscopic cholecystectomy, a surgeon removes the gallbladder with the aid of a laparoscope. To begin the procedure, small incisions are made in the patient's abdomen, and the abdomen is inflated with carbon dioxide. A fiberoptic laparoscope with a camera and light source is inserted and used to examine the abdomen, while instruments are inserted through the other incisions. Clips are applied to the cystic duct and artery, and the gallbladder is removed. The small incisions are closed, and the procedure is completed.

Follow-up care for therapeutic surgical procedures (that is, repair or removal procedures as opposed to diagnostic procedures) includes only the normal, usual, uncomplicated service. Examples of additional services that may be reported separately include the following scenarios:

- A patient develops a complication such as a wound infection at the surgical site and requires additional care; any services and/or visits related to treatment of the infection may be reported separately.
- The surgeon provides care not related to the original surgery such as for a patient who during the postoperative period for a knee surgery complains of wrist pain and is seen by the same orthopedic surgeon who performed the knee surgery. Care for the wrist can be reported separately, as it is not included in the surgery package.

Modifier 24, *Unrelated evaluation and management service by the same physician during a postoperative period*, would be attached to the additional E/M service codes for both of the circumstances described above and may be reported during the postoperative period.

EXAMPLE 8.4

The surgeon's coding staff reported code 47562 for a laparoscopic cholecystectomy. According to the third-party payer for this patient, there are 90 global days associated with code 47562. Therefore, when the patient returned to the surgeon's office 1 week after the surgery for follow-up, there was no charge for the follow-up visit.

The patient returned the following week for suture removal. Again, code 99024 may be reported based on the policies of the facility, but there was no charge for this visit, as removal of sutures is included in typical postoperative follow-up care.

The codes reported by the surgeon for this patient's episode of care are the following:

- Date of surgery: 47562, *Laparoscopy, surgical; cholecystectomy*
- 1 week after surgery: 99024, *Postoperative follow-up visit (no charge)*
- 2 weeks after surgery: 99024, *Postoperative follow-up visit (no charge)*

Supplied Materials

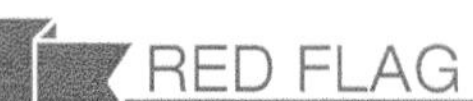

RED FLAG

Although you should be aware of separately reportable supplies and materials codes, these codes usually appear in a facility's chargemaster, so you would not be required to manually report them.

Supplies and materials commonly used in a surgical procedure are usually considered to be included in the surgery code and may not be reported separately. However, the Medicine section of the CPT® codebook contains a supplies and materials code that may be used in addition to a surgery code. Code 99070, *Supplies and materials (except spectacles) provided by the physician or other qualified health professional over and above those usually included with the office visit or other services rendered (list drugs, trays, supplies, or materials provided)*, is reported only when the supplies and materials used to perform the surgery went above and beyond the usual. This code might be used to report items such as special dressings, sterile trays, sterile water, and wound irrigation equipment. Reimbursement for code 99070 varies—some payers accept this charge, but others do not cover it.

Reporting More Than One Procedure/Service

The codebook has guidelines for reporting more than 1 procedure or service on the same date, during the same session, or during a postoperative period associated with a surgical package. Add-on codes and modifiers are used for these purposes.

Add-on Codes

As you have learned, **add-on codes** describe additional procedures or services that are related to the primary procedure performed and are reported in addition to the code for the primary procedure. These additional procedures are identified in the tabular list by a "+" symbol that precedes the code number, and a complete listing is found in

Appendix D of the CPT® codebook. Add-on code descriptors include the phrase "each additional" or "(List separately in addition to code for primary procedure)." Parenthetical instructions follow the code in the tabular list to "use in conjunction with" a specific other code or codes. These instructions mandate which codes may be used together. Figure 8.4 is an example of how the instructions appear in the tabular list.

Figure 8.4 Example of Add-on Code Instructions

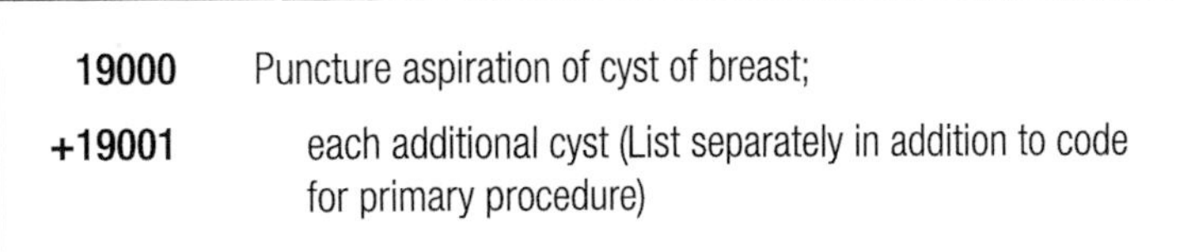

19000 Puncture aspiration of cyst of breast;

+19001 each additional cyst (List separately in addition to code for primary procedure)

Many add-on codes in the Surgery section identify additional areas or pieces of a body part, such as larger skin grafts in integumentary system procedures, additional veins or arteries in cardiovascular system procedures, and additional vertebral segments in the nervous system procedures. Table 8.3 shows examples of procedure codes associated with an add-on code. As with the format of the terminology in the codebook, the indented descriptions of the add-on codes pick up the common portion of the procedure above them, which is shown in the Table 8.3 column "Full Add-on Code Description."

Table 8.3 Examples of Surgical Add-on Codes

Procedure Code	Procedure Code Description	Add-on Code	Full Add-on Code Description
15200	*Full thickness graft, free, including direct closure of donor site, trunk; 20 sq cm or less*	15201	*Full thickness graft, free, including direct closure of donor site, trunk; each additional 20 sq cm, or part thereof (List separately in addition to code for primary procedure)*
36478	*Endovenous ablation therapy of incompetent vein, extremity, inclusive of all image guidance and monitoring, percutaneous, laser; first vein treated*	36479	*Endovenous ablation therapy of incompetent vein, extremity, inclusive of all image guidance and monitoring, percutaneous, laser; second and subsequent veins treated in a single extremity, each through separate access sites (List separately in addition to code for primary procedure)*
63081	*Vertebral corpectomy (vertebral body resection), partial or complete, anterior approach with decompression of spinal cord and/or nerve root(s); cervical, single segment*	63082	*Vertebral corpectomy (vertebral body resection), partial or complete, anterior approach with decompression of spinal cord and/or nerve root(s); cervical, each additional segment (List separately in addition to code for primary procedure)*

The rules for reporting procedural add-on codes are as follows:

- Add-on codes apply only to procedures performed by the same physician.
- Add-on codes are never reported first.
- Add-on codes are never reported alone.

- Because they are never reported alone, add-on codes are exempt from modifier 51, *Multiple procedures.*
- Before assigning an add-on code, be sure to read the tabular list for "use in conjunction with" notes.

LET'S TRY ONE **8.2**

A 55-year-old woman presented with 2 skin lesions on her arm. The physician performed a simple skin biopsy on each lesion and sent the specimens for pathological examination. What code(s) would be reported for this procedure? _____

CONCEPTS CHECKPOINT **8.3**

Answer true or false to each of the following statements.

1. _____ Procedures performed using a laparoscopic approach must be reported with a laparoscopic procedure code.
2. _____ If a procedure was unsuccessful using a laparoscopic approach and was successfully completed with an open approach in the same operative episode, only the code for the open approach should be reported.
3. _____ Separate procedure codes should never be reported.
4. _____ Supplies and materials commonly used in a surgical procedure are usually considered to be included in the surgery code and may not be reported separately.
5. _____ Add-on codes may be reported alone.

Modifiers Used in Surgery Coding

Many modifiers are available to use with codes from the Surgery section when services performed in the procedure are altered by circumstances. Both CPT® and HCPCS modifiers may be appropriately reported with CPT® surgery codes. Appendix A in the CPT® codebook lists all the CPT® modifiers with their descriptions and notes for their use. Anesthesia Physical Status modifiers are also listed in Appendix A as well as the Level I (CPT®) and Level II (HCPCS/National) modifiers approved for Ambulatory Surgery Center (ASC) Hospital Outpatient Use. To review the concept of modifiers, refer to Chapter 4 of this textbook.

Using CPT® Modifiers in Surgery Coding Table 8.4 presents some of the more common CPT® modifiers associated with the CPT® surgical package along with a brief description and explanations of circumstances in which the modifiers are used.

Within the various subsections of the Surgery section in the tabular list, you will notice notes and special instructions related to modifier usage for particular codes. These notes should be read and followed. As an example, Figure 8.5 shows the special modifier instruction for code 30465 in the Respiratory subsection of the Surgery section, a procedure involving the nasal passages of the nose. The code was developed to cover the procedure bilaterally. If the procedure is done unilaterally, modifier 52, *Reduced services,* must be reported since the procedure was done on only 1 side.

Table 8.4 CPT® Modifiers Commonly Used with Surgery Codes

CPT® Modifier	Brief Description	Use in Surgical Contexts
22	Increased procedural service	A surgery requires substantially more services than usually required.
24	Unrelated E/M service by the same physician during a postoperative period	The physician performed an unrelated E/M service during the postoperative period.
50	Bilateral procedure	A code assigned for a unilateral procedure is so modified to indicate the service was done on both sides.
51	Multiple procedures	Multiple procedures are performed on the same day, during the same surgical session.
52	Reduced services	A surgery requires substantially less services than usually required (as an example, append to a code assigned for a bilateral procedure to indicate the service was done on only 1 side).
53	Discontinued procedure	The physician elected to terminate a procedure for the patient's well-being.
54	Surgical care only	The surgeon bills for the surgery only, and postoperative care has been transferred to another physician.
55	Postoperative management only	A physician other than the surgeon assumes postdischarge care of a surgical patient.
56	Preoperative management only	A healthcare professional other than the surgeon performed the preoperative care.
58	Staged or related procedure by the same physician during the postoperative period	A procedure was planned prospectively at the time of the original procedure, a more extensive procedure was done than the original procedure, or therapy followed a diagnostic surgical procedure.
59	Distinct procedural service	Separate procedures were performed on the same day by the same physician.
62	Two surgeons	Two surgeons from different specialties are required to perform a specific procedure.
63	Procedure performed on infants less than 4 kg	Procedure performed on a neonate or infant weighing under 4 kg.
66	Surgical team	More than 2 surgeons from different specialties are required to perform a specific procedure.
73	Discontinued outpatient procedure prior to anesthesia administration	For hospital outpatient use when a procedure is cancelled due to extenuating circumstances after preparation of patient but before anesthesia administration.
74	Discontinued outpatient procedure after anesthesia administration	For hospital outpatient use when a procedure is canceled due to extenuating circumstances after anesthesia administration or after the procedure was started.
76	Repeat procedure by same physician	The surgeon who rendered the original service repeats the procedure.
77	Repeat procedure by another physician	A surgeon other than the original physician repeats the procedure.
78	Unplanned return to Operating/Procedure Room by the same physician for a related procedure during the postoperative period	A procedure related to the original procedure is performed in an operating room during the postoperative period.
79	Unrelated procedure by the same physician during the postoperative period	A procedure unrelated to the original procedure is performed during the postoperative period.
80	Assistant surgeon	An assistant surgeon works alongside the primary surgeon for a substantial portion of the operation, and the assistant surgeon reports the same surgical code as the primary surgeon with modifier 80 appended.
81	Minimum assistant surgeon	The services of an assistant surgeon who provides minimal services for a relatively short time.
82	Assistant surgeon when qualified resident not available	In certain facilities, a surgeon not designated as a qualified resident surgeon serves as assistant surgeon.

Figure 8.5 Example of a Special Modifier Code Instruction

30465	Repair of nasal vestibular stenosis (eg, spreader grafting, lateral nasal wall reconstruction) (30465 excludes obtaining graft. For graft procedure, see 20900-20926, 21210) (30465 is used to report a bilateral procedure. For unilateral procedure, use modifier 52)

Using HCPCS Modifiers in Surgery Coding Like CPT® modifiers, many of the most common HCPCS modifiers are listed in Appendix A of the CPT® codebook. Unlike CPT® modifiers that use only numbers, HCPCS modifiers use letters or a combination of numbers and letters. Table 8.5 presents some of the HCPCS modifiers most commonly used with CPT® procedure codes along with their descriptions, which are self-explanatory as they indicate anatomical sites. In addition to identifying the left and right sides of paired organs, there are also HCPCS modifiers to specify eyelids, fingers, and coronary arteries.

The modifiers RT (right side) and LT (left side) should be used when a procedure is performed on only 1 side of a paired organ (such as the eyes, ears, or breasts). However, the code that these modifiers are attached to must be specific to the body part. Reporting an RT or LT modifier with a CPT® code whose description includes multiple body parts would not be appropriate. If an identical procedure is completed on both parts of a paired organ, CPT® modifier 50, *Bilateral procedure*, should be assigned—do not use modifiers RT and LT together on the same code.

Coding Clicks

To view a complete list of HCPCS modifiers, visit http://Coding.ParadigmEducation.com/HCPCSModifiers.

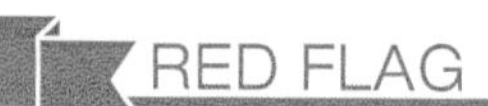

Do not use modifiers RT and LT together! If an identical procedure was performed on both sides, use modifier 50 to indicate a bilateral procedure.

Table 8.5 HCPCS Modifiers Commonly Used with Surgery Codes

HCPCS Modifier	Description
RT	*Right side*
LT	*Left side*
E1	*Upper left, eyelid*
E2	*Lower left, eyelid*
E3	*Upper right, eyelid*
E4	*Lower right, eyelid*
FA	*Left hand, thumb*
F1	*Left hand, second digit* (index finger)
F2	*Left hand, third digit* (middle finger)
F3	*Left hand, fourth digit* (ring finger)
F4	*Left hand, fifth digit* (little finger)
F5	*Right hand, thumb*
F6	*Right hand, second digit* (index finger)
F7	*Right hand, third digit* (middle finger)
F8	*Right hand, fourth digit* (ring finger)
F9	*Right hand, fifth digit* (little finger)

HCPCS Modifier	Description
LC	*Left circumflex coronary artery*
LD	*Left anterior descending coronary artery*
LM	*Left main coronary artery*
RC	*Right coronary artery*
RI	*Ramus intermedius coronary artery*
TA	*Left foot, great toe*
T1	*Left foot, second digit* (from great toe)
T2	*Left foot, third digit*
T3	*Left foot, fourth digit*
T4	*Left foot, fifth digit*
T5	*Right foot, great toe*
T6	*Right foot, second digit* (from great toe)
T7	*Right foot, third digit*
T8	*Right foot, fourth digit*
T9	*Right foot, fifth digit*

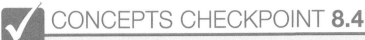

CONCEPTS CHECKPOINT 8.4

Answer true or false to each of the following statements.

1. _____ If an identical procedure is completed on both eyes, modifier 50 should be reported.
2. _____ If an identical procedure is completed on both eyes, modifiers RT and LT should be reported.
3. _____ An assistant surgeon should report services using modifier 62.
4. _____ Modifier TA may be assigned to a procedure completed on the left big toe.
5. _____ A procedure discontinued after the start of anesthesia should be reported with modifier 53.

Separate Procedure

In the CPT® codebook, you may see the phrase *separate procedure* noted in parentheses following the code description, as shown in Figure 8.6.

Figure 8.6 Example of a Separate Procedure Notation

44005	Enterolysis (freeing of intestinal adhesion) (separate procedure)

A code designated as a **separate procedure** indicates a procedure or service that is usually carried out as an integral component of a larger service but which may be reported separately under certain circumstances. You should view this notation as a warning that the code cannot be reported in addition to the code for the main procedure of which it is a component, and the procedure may be reported only if it is the only procedure performed, if it is carried out independently, or if it is considered to be unrelated and distinct from any other service being reported at that time.

Inside the OR

Enterolysis is the surgical separation of intestinal or abdominal adhesions, which are fibrous bands of tissue that form between organs and abdominal tissues, causing them to stick together. Patients who have had previous abdominal surgery often develop adhesions, which can become larger as time passes and may cause problems years after surgery. Enterolysis is an integral part of many abdominal procedures, because the surgeon must free the adhesions to get to the organs on which the therapeutic procedure is to be performed. For this reason, the code for enterolysis carries a separate procedure notation (as shown in Figure 8.6) and, in most cases, should not be reported on its own. Code 44005 may be reported alone if it is the only procedure that is performed, meaning that it was indeed a separate procedure.

Other cases in which separate procedure codes may be reported include the following scenarios:

- The service was provided in a different operative session.
- The service was provided as a different procedure or surgery.
- The service was performed on a different site or organ system.
- The service requires a separate incision.
- The service requires a separate excision.
- The service involves a separate lesion.
- The service involves an injury or area of injury separate from a group of extensive injuries.

If the service designated as a separate procedure is normally performed as part of a larger service but was done alone for a specific purpose, the separate procedure code may also be reported. Separate procedure codes may be reported alone or in addition to other procedure codes by attaching modifier 59, *Distinct procedural service*, to show that it was a distinct procedure. Always double-check the documentation to ensure that the separate procedure code meets the criteria listed above.

EXAMPLE **8.5**

A 19-year-old male sustained several lacerations after falling through a window. He was brought to the emergency room where a 2-cm laceration on his right arm was noted. A deeper wound in his back was bleeding profusely and required surgical exploration to determine the extent of penetration. He was taken to the OR, and an exploration of the back wound was performed. The arm laceration was also repaired with a layered closure. The exploration of the back wound was unrelated to the repair of the arm wound (a different body site) and therefore meets the criteria of a separate procedure. The codes reported for this episode of care are 20102, *Exploration of penetrating wound (separate procedure); abdomen/flank/back*, and 12031, *Repair, intermediate, wounds of scalp, axillae, trunk, and/or extremities (excluding hands and feet); 2.5 cm or less*.

Unlisted Service or Procedure

When a surgeon performs a procedure or service that is not specifically listed in the CPT® codebook, an **unlisted procedure code** may be reported. Unlisted procedure codes appear at the end of the anatomical subsections within the Surgery section and commonly end in *99*. You can reference the complete list of these codes in the Surgery Guidelines.

Use these codes only after thoroughly searching for a code for the specific procedure that was done. Although it may seem easier to just report an unlisted code, doing so comes with several drawbacks. Reporting unlisted procedure codes will result in delayed reimbursement, as a specific fee amount is not associated with an unlisted code. For an unlisted procedure to be considered for reimbursement, a special report must be provided with the claim, so you will have to send that documentation in addition to reporting the code.

EXAMPLE 8.6

A 42-year-old female with breast cancer undergoes a right partial mastectomy with an insertion of a cavitary evaluation device (for radiation therapy). This procedure would be reported with codes 19301, *Mastectomy, partial (eg, lumpectomy, tylectomy, quadrantectomy, segmentectomy*, and 19499, *Unlisted procedure, breast*. Code 19499 is 1 example of an unlisted procedure code. Since there is no specific code for the insertion of a cavitary evaluation device, an unlisted code is reported. Insertion of a cavitary evaluation device is not a typical part of a mastectomy, and so it may be reported as a separate procedure.

Special Report

CPT® guidelines include the use of special reports when an unusual service is provided. A service that is reported with an unlisted code or that is rare or new may require a special report to show that the service was medically necessary and appropriate. The report should include information describing the procedure, the need for the procedure, the time and effort, and any special equipment that was used in the service provided to the patient.

Surgical Destruction

When surgical destruction is used to remove lesions or tissue, the method of destruction is not usually listed. Most surgical codes for destruction include any method such as cryosurgery, destruction by laser or electricity, or chemical treatment. Separate code numbers are assigned in some circumstances such as 17340, *Cryotherapy (CO2 slush, liquid N2) for acne.*

Instructions for Reporting Surgery Codes

This chapter provided a general overview of surgery codes and the guidelines for reporting them. Chapters 9 through 17 will present more specifics when it comes to reporting codes for surgical procedures on each body system, but first it may be helpful to have an overall understanding of the steps involved in reporting surgery codes. If you have already read about how to report anesthesia codes in Chapter 7, the procedure for reporting surgery codes may seem familiar. Figure 8.7 provides a diagram to guide you through the process of reporting surgery codes, and the following paragraphs describe it in more detail.

As you have learned, CPT® codes may be indexed under the main term based on the operative anatomical site, type of procedure, name of procedure, surgical technique, or clinical condition. Begin your search for the appropriate code by referring to the main

Figure 8.7 Locating and Reporting Surgery Codes

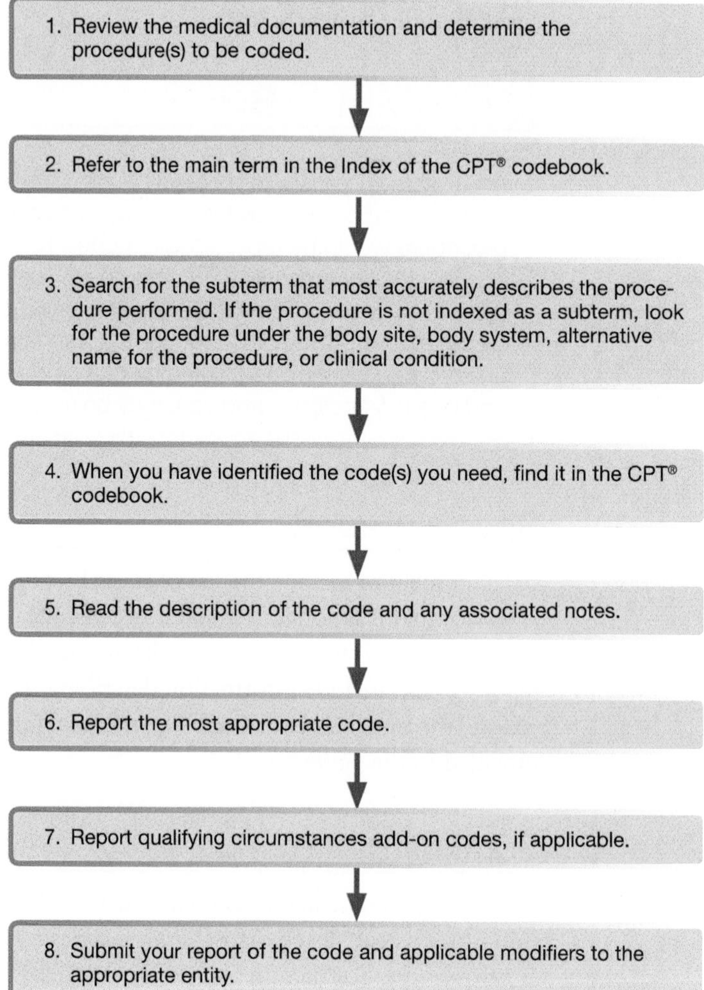
1. Review the medical documentation and determine the procedure(s) to be coded.
2. Refer to the main term in the Index of the CPT® codebook.
3. Search for the subterm that most accurately describes the procedure performed. If the procedure is not indexed as a subterm, look for the procedure under the body site, body system, alternative name for the procedure, or clinical condition.
4. When you have identified the code(s) you need, find it in the CPT® codebook.
5. Read the description of the code and any associated notes.
6. Report the most appropriate code.
7. Report qualifying circumstances add-on codes, if applicable.
8. Submit your report of the code and applicable modifiers to the appropriate entity.

term in the Index and then searching for the subterm that most accurately describes the procedure performed. Examples of various types of Index main terms and subterms for a mastectomy (excision of breast) are as follows:

- operative anatomical site: Breast, excision, mastectomy;
- type of procedure: Removal, breast;
- name of procedure: Mastectomy;
- surgical technique: Modified radical mastectomy; and
- clinical condition: Lesion, breast.

Once you have found the appropriate code or range of codes, refer to the corresponding section of the CPT® codebook to review your code selection. Carefully read the code description and any associated instructional notes before choosing a code.

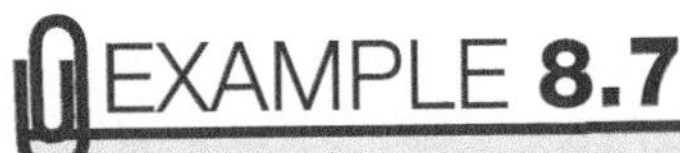

EXAMPLE **8.7**

You are in search of the code for a vaginal hysterectomy with a uterus weighing 300 g. Begin by referring to the main term *Hysterectomy*, and then, the subterm *Vaginal*. You will see code ranges 58260 through 58270, 58290 through 58294, 58550 through 58554 listed. Refer to the Surgery section, female genital system, locate code 58260, and begin reading the code descriptions. You may have to read through the descriptions for many of the codes listed in the Index until you locate the appropriate code for this procedure. The appropriate code for a vaginal hysterectomy with a uterus weighing 300 g is 58290, *Vaginal hysterectomy, for uterus greater than 250 g*.

LET'S TRY ONE **8.3**

Report codes for the following procedures:

1. Nonobstetrical colporrhaphy: _____
2. Reduction mammaplasty: _____
3. Thoracentesis with imaging guidance: _____

CONCEPTS CHECKPOINT **8.5**

Practice finding codes by listing at least 2 ways to find each of these procedures in the Index. Then choose the appropriate code for each of the following procedures.

1. ______________ needle biopsy of the thyroid
2. ______________ cesarean section, delivery only
3. ______________ repair of cleft lip, secondary
4. ______________ Whipple procedure
5. ______________ vasectomy

LET'S TRY ONE **8.4**

The parents of an 11-month-old boy brought him to the pediatrician when they noticed a bulging in the child's groin. He was diagnosed with an inguinal hernia, and a surgical intervention was scheduled. An inguinal hernia repair was successfully completed under general anesthesia. Answer the following questions related to this procedure.

1. What main term would lead to the code for this procedure in the CPT® Index?

   ____

2. What code(s) would the surgeon report?

   ____

Chapter Summary

- It is important to read medical documentation carefully before reporting codes. Attention to detail is vital as surgical codes are dependent on the site of surgery and the procedure performed, and many codes are differentiated by only a single word.
- The Surgery section of the CPT® codebook contains codes that represent surgical procedures and other services. Most of the codes are for invasive procedures.
- The procedure codes are arranged by body systems and the procedures within those systems.
- When reporting a surgery code, the services include normal, uncomplicated care given to the patient before, during, and after surgery. The CPT® guidelines define which specific services are included.
- Some surgery codes have a "separate procedure" notation indicating that the procedure is usually part of a larger procedure. These codes may be reported if the procedure was done alone or the procedure was unrelated and distinct from any other service being reported.
- Unlisted procedure codes may be reported if a surgeon performs a procedure not listed in the codebook. A special report should be provided if an unlisted code is used.
- Procedures accomplished using a laparoscopic or endoscopic approach must be coded as such. If no laparoscopic code exists, an unlisted laparoscopic procedure code is reported.
- Add-on codes are reported in addition to the code for the primary procedure performed. Add-on codes may not be reported alone.
- Moderate (conscious) sedation is included in many procedure codes and may not be reported separately if the code has the ⊙ symbol.
- There are many modifiers available to use with surgery codes. A complete listing is in Appendix A of the CPT® codebook.

Navigator

Access interactive chapter review exercises, practice activities, flash cards, and study games.

Chapter 9

Surgery Coding: Integumentary System

Fast Facts

- People shed approximately 40 pounds of skin over a lifetime and grow a new layer of skin every month.
- Hair can contain up to 14 different elements, including traces of gold.
- The arrector pili muscles contract in response to physical changes or emotions, causing goosebumps on your skin.
- Every year more than 2 million cases of skin cancer are diagnosed in the United States.

Sources: http://integumentarysystem.organsofthebody.com, http://info.visibilebody.com, http://cancer.org

Crack the Code

Review the sample operative report to find the correct integumentary system code. You may need to return to this exercise after reading the chapter content.

PROCEDURE PERFORMED: Application of Apligraf skin graft over ulcer site, right hallux

DESCRIPTION OF PROCEDURE: Attention was directed to the Apligraf skin graft, which was opened using aseptic technique and placed on the back OR table. At this time the skin graft was removed from the packaging and moistened with normal saline. The skin graft was then meshed manually using a #11 blade and making a small incision on the entire skin graft. At this time the shiny side of the skin graft was determined and noted to be the dermis side. The skin graft was then taken from the back table and applied over the ulceration site with the shiny side (the dermal side) against the ulcer site. Iris scissors were utilized to trim excess skin graft from the margins of the ulcer site. The skin graft was allowed to overlap the wound margin by 2 to 3 mm on all sides. Once the skin graft had been applied, a sterile cotton swab was used to try and remove all excess air from underneath the skin graft. 5-0 Nylon was used to stitch the skin graft to the good skin margins, leaving excess trail from the knot for application of bolster. Simple suturing technique was utilized. Adaptic was cut to the size of the wound and applied over the skin graft. The patient tolerated the procedure and anesthesia well.

answer: 15275

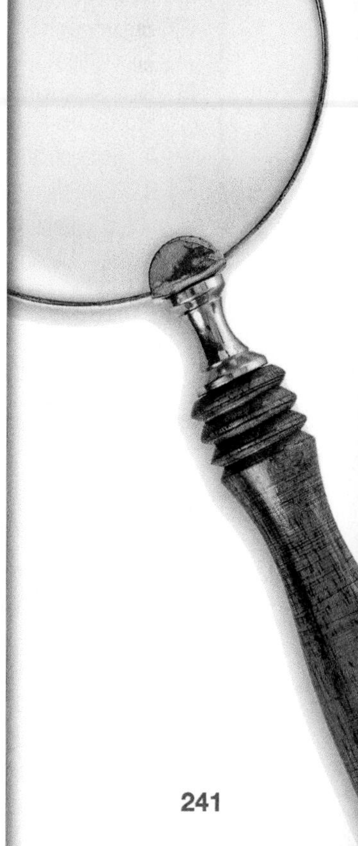

Learning Objectives

9.1 Describe the basic anatomy of the integumentary system.

9.2 Employ terminology for skin structures and surgical techniques.

9.3 Describe the arrangement of codes in the Integumentary System Surgery subsection and the surgical procedures specific to skin structures.

9.4 Differentiate between simple and complex incision and drainage procedures.

9.5 Determine when debridement procedures can be coded separately.

9.6 Identify the factors involved in coding the excision of lesions, and apply criteria based on benign or malignant characteristics, location, and size.

9.7 Differentiate between simple, intermediate, and complex skin repairs.

9.8 Differentiate between adjacent tissue transfers, free skin grafts, and flaps.

9.9 Apply methods for determining the surface area of burns.

9.10 Identify methods used in destruction of lesions.

9.11 Differentiate between various types of breast biopsies.

9.12 Differentiate between various types of mastectomy procedures.

9.13 Report codes for procedures on the skin, subcutaneous tissues, and accessory structures.

9.14 Report codes for procedures on the nails.

9.15 Report codes for breast procedures.

Chapter Outline

- **I.** Introduction to the Integumentary System
- **II.** Integumentary System Terminology
- **III.** Organization of the Integumentary System Surgery Subsection
- **IV.** Skin, Subcutaneous Tissues, and Accessory Structures Procedures (Codes 10030-11646)
  - **A.** Incision and Drainage
  - **B.** Debridement
    - **i.** Debridement for Eczematous or Infected Skin
    - **ii.** Debridement for Necrotizing Soft Tissue Infection
    - **iii.** Debridement of Wounds
  - **C.** Excision of Lesions
    - **i.** Benign and Malignant Characteristics of Lesions
    - **ii.** Site of Lesions
    - **iii.** Size of Lesions
    - **iv.** Wound Closure
- **V.** Nail Procedures (Codes 11719-11765)
- **VI.** Pilonidal Cyst Procedures (Codes 11770-11772)
- **VII.** Introduction Procedures (Codes 11900-11983)
- **VIII.** Repair (Closure) Procedures (Codes 12001-16036)
  - **A.** Repair Classifications: Simple, Intermediate, and Complex
  - **B.** Adjacent Tissue Transfer or Rearrangement
  - **C.** Skin Replacement Surgery
  - **D.** Surgical Preparation of Skin Graft Recipient Site
  - **E.** Reporting Codes for Skin Grafts
  - **F.** Reporting Codes for Flaps
    - **i.** Skin and/or Deep Tissue Flaps
    - **ii.** Other Flaps and Grafts
  - **G.** Other Procedures
  - **H.** Pressure Ulcers
  - **I.** Burns, Local Treatment
    - **i.** Lund-Browder Classification Method of Burn Estimating
    - **ii.** Escharotomy
- **IX.** Destruction Codes (17000-17999)
  - **A.** Destruction, Benign or Premalignant Lesions
  - **B.** Destruction, Malignant Lesions, Any Method
- **X.** Breast Procedures (Codes 19000-19499)
  - **A.** Incision
  - **B.** Excision
    - **i.** Types of Breast Biopsies
    - **ii.** Coding for Breast Biopsies
  - **C.** Introduction
  - **D.** Mastectomy Procedures
  - **E.** Repair and/or Reconstruction, Other Procedures
- **XI.** Chapter Summary

Introduction to the Integumentary System

The integumentary system is made up of the tissue that covers the body and includes skin, nails, and hair. This system protects the body by acting as a barrier to bacteria and other organisms, protecting against excessive water loss, and helping to regulate body temperature.

Developing a strong understanding of the layers of the skin is important, as many of the codes related to the integumentary system are reported depending on the depth of the procedure. As Figure 9.1 illustrates, the skin has 3 layers: the epidermis, dermis, and hypodermis (subcutaneous tissue).

- The **epidermis** is the outermost layer and consists of dead cells generated by the dermis.
- The **dermis** is the living, functioning layer of the skin, where blood vessels and nerves are active. The dermis contains sweat glands (that produce perspiration), sebaceous glands (that produce oil), and ceruminous glands (that produce earwax).
- The **hypodermis** or **subcutaneous tissue** is the innermost layer of the skin (*subcutaneous* means "under the skin"), and it connects the dermis to the underlying organs and tissues. This layer varies in thickness and is composed of **fascia** (fibrous connective tissue) and **adipose tissue** (fat).

Figure 9.1 Normal Skin Anatomy

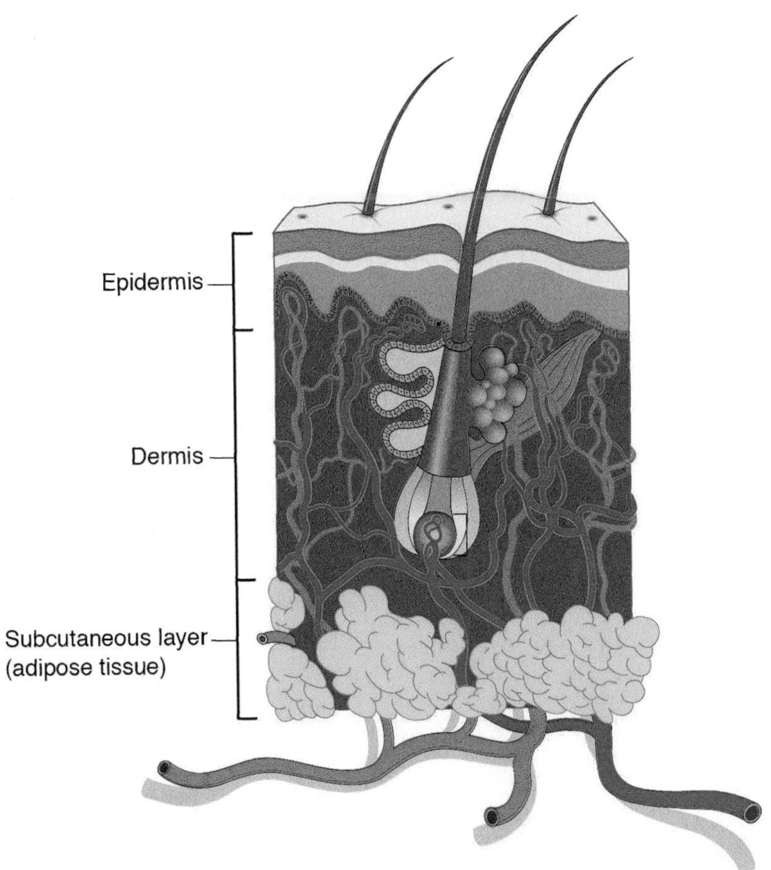

Integumentary System Terminology

In addition to the terms assigned to the different layers of the skin, there are a few other words and phrases commonly used to describe procedures of the integumentary system. Table 9.1 defines these terms.

Table 9.1 Integumentary System Structures and Surgical Terminology

Term	Definition
abscess	A localized collection of pus at the site of an infection; a cavity formed by liquefactive necrosis (the transformation of tissue into a liquid viscous mass) within solid tissue Procedures for abscesses generally also refer to other conditions such as carbuncles, furuncles, cysts, and suppurative hidradenitis.
ablation	Removal or destruction of function of a body part or area of tissue
autologous	Referring to a graft in which the donor and recipient areas are in the same person, ie, an autograft
avulsion	A tearing away or forcible separation
cryosurgery	Destroying a lesion through the use of extreme cold
cutane-	Word root that means "skin" Used with other word parts to indicate conditions relating to skin (eg, cutaneous, subcutaneous, fasciocutaneous, fibrocutaneous, percutaneous, myocutaneous)
cyst	A fluid-filled sac
debridement	Cleaning or removing tissue from a wound
dehiscence	Gaping or splitting of a sutured wound
destruction	Killing of tissue by electrocautery, laser surgery, chemicals, or other means
excision	Removing a lesion through the dermal layer; may include simple closure (stitching)
imaging modality	A type of imaging technology such as radiographic imaging, ultrasonography, or magnetic resonance imaging
incision and drainage	Cutting into and extracting fluid
localization device	A clip, metallic pellet, wire/needle, or other device inserted into tissue using image guidance to mark a biopsy site for greater accuracy
onycho-	Word root denoting a fingernail or toenail
paring	Removing thin layers of skin by peeling or scraping
repairing	Suturing (stitching up) a wound
shaving	Removing dermal or epidermal lesions horizontally or transversely, without full-thickness (epidermal and dermal) excision
skin graft	Transplanted tissue used to repair a defect
tissue transfer	A skin graft in which the piece of skin used for transplant is still partially attached to the donor site and is used to cover an adjacent defect

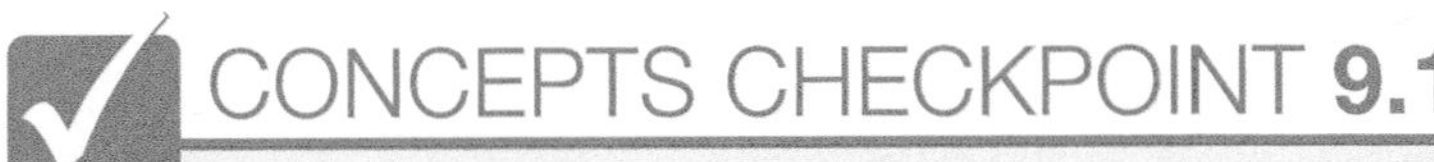

CONCEPTS CHECKPOINT 9.1

Match the terms in the first column with the definitions in the second column.

1. _____ debridement
2. _____ destruction
3. _____ excision
4. _____ paring
5. _____ shaving
6. _____ incision and drainage

a. To cut into and drain fluid
b. Killing of tissue by electrocautery, laser surgery, chemical treatment, or other means
c. Horizontal or transverse removal of a lesion without full excision
d. Cleaning or removing tissue from a wound
e. Removal of a lesion through the dermal layer that may include stitching
f. Removal of thin skin layers by peeling or scraping

Organization of the Integumentary System Surgery Subsection

The Integumentary System subsection of the Surgery section in the CPT® codebook includes codes for procedures on integumentary structures: the skin; subcutaneous tissue; accessory structures such as the hair, nails, and glands; and breast tissues. While not all of the integumentary procedures will be explained in detail in this chapter, some of the more common and more challenging codes you may be required to report are discussed in the upcoming sections. Table 9.2 provides all of the main headings within this subsection and the codes they include.

Table 9.2 Headings Within the Integumentary Subsection of the CPT® Codebook

Heading	Code Range
Skin, Subcutaneous, and Accessory Structures	10030-11646
Nails	11719-11765
Pilonidal Cyst	11770-11772
Introduction	11900-11983
Repair (Closure)	12001-16036
Destruction	17000-17999
Breast	19000-19499

Skin, Subcutaneous Tissues, and Accessory Structures Procedures (Codes 10030-11646)

Procedure codes that fall under the skin, subcutaneous tissues, and accessory structures (10030-11646) include introduction, removal, drainage, debridement, and excision of skin lesions. While not every code from this section will be covered, many of the more challenging codes will be described in the following sections.

Introduction and Removal

The first of the 3 codes under the introduction and removal heading (10030) describes image-guided fluid collection by catheter. Code 10030 is reported once for each individual collection of fluid drained with a separate catheter. Code 10030 is not to be reported with codes from the radiology section, such as 77002, *Fluoroscopic guidance for needle placement.*

Codes 10035 and 10036 are reported for soft tissue marker placement if a more specific code does not exist (such as 19287, which specifies marker placement in the breast). Code 10035 is reported once per target site even if more than 1 marker is placed there. Add-on code 10036 is reported in addition to 10035 if markers are placed at additional target sites. Code 10036 is reported for each additional lesion site where markers are placed.

Incision and Drainage

Incision and drainage (I/D) procedures involve cutting into the skin to remove fluid. The codes in this category are differentiated from one another based on whether the procedure is simple or complicated. Figure 9.2 shows an example of how the codes are structured for the level of difficulty and/or the number of sites. In the incision and drainage of an abscess, the surgeon makes a small incision through the skin and opens the abscess to drain the fluid. If the documentation indicates that the procedure was simple or performed on a single abscess, code 10060 should be reported. If the procedure was more complex (such as requiring closure at a later date) or was performed on multiple abscesses, code 10061 should be reported.

Figure 9.2 Example of Coding for Level of Complexity: Incision and Drainage of an Abscess

10060	Incision and drainage of abscess (eg, carbuncle, suppurative hidradenitis, cutaneous or subcutaneous abscess, cyst, furuncle, or paronychia); simple or single
10061	complicated or multiple

Figure 9.3 shows code 10180, *Incision and drainage, complex, postoperative wound infection.* In this procedure, the wound must be drained of the infected fluid and then irrigated; therefore, no simple code is available for the procedure. This procedure is always considered complex. The wound may or may not be closed at the time of the

procedure; if left open to allow for additional drainage, the closure is reported as indicated in the parenthetic note "for secondary closure of surgical wound," as shown in Figure 9.3.

Figure 9.3 Code for Incision and Drainage of a Postoperative Wound

10180	Incision and drainage, complex, postoperative wound infection (For secondary closure of surgical wound, see 12020, 12021, 13160)

Inside the OR

Infection is 1 reason that incision and drainage of a postoperative wound may be required. To treat an infected postoperative wound, the surgeon begins by removing the original surgical stitches or staples and, possibly, by making an additional incision into the site. Fluid is drained from the infected site, any necrotic (dead) tissue is removed, and the wound is irrigated. The wound may be packed with gauze and left open to be sutured closed at a later time, or it may be sutured immediately. A drain may be placed into the wound to allow any additional fluid to escape.

LET'S TRY ONE **9.1**

An obese 61-year-old female had an exploratory laparotomy with appendectomy. Postoperatively, the surgical wound dressing became soaked with foul-smelling fluid. The surgeon suspected a deep infection at the site of the surgical incision and performed an incision and drainage procedure. Infected fluid was drained from the wound, and the wound was sutured closed. What procedure code would be reported for this operative episode?_____

Debridement

Debridement refers to surgical excision procedures using forceps, scissors, scalpel, or dermatome to remove dead or infected tissue to promote healing and the growth of healthy tissue. Debridement may be required to treat many conditions, including infections, injuries, wounds, and ulcers.

Debridement for Eczematous or Infected Skin

The Debridement category in the tabular begins with codes for surgical procedures associated with skin disease management. Two codes for the debridement of eczematous or infected skin, codes 11000 and 11001, are differentiated by percentage of body surface treated, code 11000 for up to 10% and add-on code 11001 is reported for each additional 10%, or part thereof.

Debridement for Necrotizing Soft Tissue Infection

Necrotizing soft tissue infection is a rare but severe condition caused by bacteria such as streptococcus or methicillin-resistant Staphylococcus aureus (MRSA). This type of infection is often referred to as "flesh-eating" because the infection breaks down the flesh, causing tissue death, gangrene, and systemic disease. Necrotizing soft tissue infections can affect the skin, subcutaneous fat, fascia, and muscle tissue. A surgeon performing debridement to treat necrotizing soft tissue infection would open the infected area and remove the dead tissue to keep the infection from spreading. When performed in certain anatomical sites, this surgical treatment has specific codes:

- code 11004—the external genitalia and perineum;
- code 11005—the abdominal wall, with or without fascial closure;
- code 11006—the combined sites of external genitalia, perineum, and abdominal wall, with or without fascial closure. If an orchiectomy (removal of testicles) is also performed at this time, it is reported separately with code 54520, *Orchiectomy, simple (including subcapsular), with or without testicular prosthesis, scrotal or inguinal approach*;
- code 11008—removal of prosthetic materials in the abdomen. This code is an add-on code.

Debridement of other areas of the body due to necrotizing soft tissue infection is reported with codes 11042 through 11047.

Debridement of Wounds

For the care of open fractures, open dislocations, and other wounds, debridement codes are differentiated by depth of the anatomical site and size of the surgical surface.

Depth of Debridement Recalling what you know about anatomy, debridement codes are differentiated from 1 another based on the **debridement depth**, which is the tissue layer of the debridement site. The depths used in the CPT® codebook are listed below in order from superficial to deepest tissues:

1. skin surface: biofilm, epidermis, and dermis;
2. subcutaneous tissue;
3. muscle fascia;
4. muscle; and
5. bone.

Codes specific to each depth also include the tissue levels above the depth described in the code. See for example the wording in parentheses for code 11042, "*Debridement, subcutaneous tissue (includes epidermis and dermis, if performed)...*"

CPT® codebook parenthetic notes stipulate that some debridement codes for the first layer of depth—skin, which consists of the epidermis and dermis layers—are found in the Medicine section of the CPT® codebook:

(For debridement of skin, ie, epidermis and/or dermis only, see 97597, 97598)...

(Do not report 11042-11047 in conjunction with 97597-97602 for the same wound)

Coding Clicks

Biofilm is a slimy film of microorganisms adhering to the surface of a structure. For more information about the formation and purpose of biofilm, visit http://Coding.ParadigmEducation.com/Biofilm.

The codes to which these notes refer, 97597 through 97602, are Active Wound Care Management codes within the Medicine section of the tabular list. These codes would be reported for debridement of wound surface **biofilm** (a slimy film of microorganisms adhering to the surface of a structure) or the skin layers only (epidermis and dermis). For treatment of the same wound, codes 11042 through 11047 cannot be reported with codes 97597 through 97602.

Figure 9.4 shows an example of debridement codes that are reported only if the debridement is at the subcutaneous layer or deeper. The codes shown, 11010 through 11012, are for debridement at the site of an open fracture and/or an open dislocation at the subcutaneous tissue, muscle fascia, muscle, and bone levels.

Figure 9.4 Example of Codes for Debridement at the Subcutaneous Level or Deeper

11010	Debridement including removal of foreign material at the site of an open fracture and/or an open dislocation (eg, excisional debridement); skin and subcutaneous tissues
11011	skin, subcutaneous tissue, muscle fascia, and muscle
11012	skin, subcutaneous tissue, muscle fascia, muscle, and bone

EXAMPLE **9.1**

A 23-year-old male presented to the emergency department (ED) with an open fracture of the femur. He had been riding his motorcycle and lost control when he hit debris on the road. In addition to the fracture, the skin and soft tissue around the bone were damaged. An extensive wound excision and debridement down to the muscle level were necessary. All foreign bodies were removed from the wound, followed by prolonged cleansing of the wound. Excision of the contaminated skin and other tissue was completed to allow the orthopedic surgeon to provide the fracture care. The debridement procedure would be reported using code 11011, *Debridement including removal of foreign material at the site of an open fracture and/or an open dislocation (eg, excisional debridement); skin, subcutaneous tissue, muscle fascia, and muscle.*

Surface Area of Debridement The total wound area debrided at the deepest level should be used to assign the appropriate code. **Debridement surface area** describes, in square centimeters or percentage of body surface, the extent of the wound that was debrided. When a single wound is debrided, the code is assigned by the depth of the deepest tissue removed. When more than 1 wound is debrided, codes 11042 through 11046 provide the means to calculate and report the surface area of wounds that are at the same depth, as follows:

- Code 11042 is reported for the debridement of the first 20 sq cm or less of subcutaneous tissue (including the dermis and epidermis). Add-on code 11045 is reported 1 time for the debridement of each additional 20 sq cm or less.

RED FLAG

Watch for add-on codes that are out of numerical sequence in the Debridement category under the Skin, Subcutaneous, and Accessory Structures heading. For example, the add-on code 11045 appears before code 11043, and the add-on code 11046 appears before code 11044. Be on the lookout for the # symbol, which appears before these add-on codes to indicate that they have been resequenced.

- Code 11043 is reported for the debridement of the first 20 sq cm or less of muscle and/or fascia (including subcutaneous tissue, dermis, and epidermis). Add-on code 11046 is reported 1 time for the debridement of each additional 20 sq cm or less.
- Code 11044 is reported for the debridement of the first 20 sq cm or less of bone (including muscle and/or fascia, subcutaneous tissue, dermis, and epidermis). Add-on code 11047 is reported 1 time for the debridement of each additional 20 sq cm or less.

If there are multiple wounds that require different depths of debridement, a separate code should be reported for the debridement of each wound.

EXAMPLE 9.2

A physician performed a debridement of an infected wound of the subcutaneous tissue measuring approximately 1 × 2 cm on a patient's right foot. The physician then debrided a second infected wound of the subcutaneous tissue on the same foot measuring 2 × 2 cm. Because these 2 areas were debrided to the same depth (the subcutaneous layer), the surface areas can be added together to determine the total surface area that should be reported by using the following calculations:

Surface area of the first wound: 1 × 2 cm = 2 sq cm

Surface area of the second wound: 2 × 2 cm = 4 sq cm

Total surface area of both wounds: 2 + 4 sq cm = 6 sq cm

The correct code for these 2 debridement procedures is code 11042, *Debridement, subcutaneous tissue (includes dermis and epidermis, if performed); first 20 sq cm or less*. If the total surface area of the debridement had been greater than 20 sq cm, add-on code 11045 would have been used with the primary procedure code to report each additional 20 sq cm or less.

LET'S TRY ONE 9.2

Choose the correct code for each of the following scenarios.

1. Debridement of abdominal wall down to the muscle for a patient with necrotizing soft tissue infection
   a. 11004
   b. 11005
   c. 11043
   d. 11047
2. Debridement of 3 × 4-cm foot wound including epidermis, dermis, and subcutaneous tissue
   a. 11010
   b. 11011
   c. 11042
   d. 11043
3. Debridement of an open fracture at the base of the right thumb with removal of pieces of gravel at the muscle layer
   a. 11043
   b. 11044
   c. 11010
   d. 11011
4. What is the code for debridement of extensive eczematous skin approximately 15% of body surface? _____
5. What is the code for debridement of external genitalia for a flesh-eating bacterial infection? _____

Excision of Lesions

Excision is removal of a lesion through the dermal layer of the skin. Codes for excision of skin lesions include the administration of local anesthesia and **simple closure**, which is suturing (stitching) 1 layer of the skin. Each lesion excision is reported separately.

Codes for excision of skin lesions are covered in 2 categories under the Skin, Subcutaneous, and Accessory Structures heading in the Integumentary subsection: Excision—Benign Lesions and Excision—Malignant Lesions. In addition to whether the lesion is benign or malignant, codes for the excision of lesions are also determined by the location of the lesion (body site) and the size of the excised diameter (in centimeters).

Benign and Malignant Characteristics of Lesions

When assigning a code for removal of a skin lesion, the first step is to determine whether the lesion was benign or malignant, as shown in Figure 9.5. Read the pathology report to confirm the nature of the lesion. This will tell you which category to reference in the tabular list, Excision—Benign Lesions or Excision—Malignant Lesions. Table 9.3 lists the some of the most common types of benign and malignant skin lesions.

Figure 9.5 Benign or Malignant Lesion Decision Tree

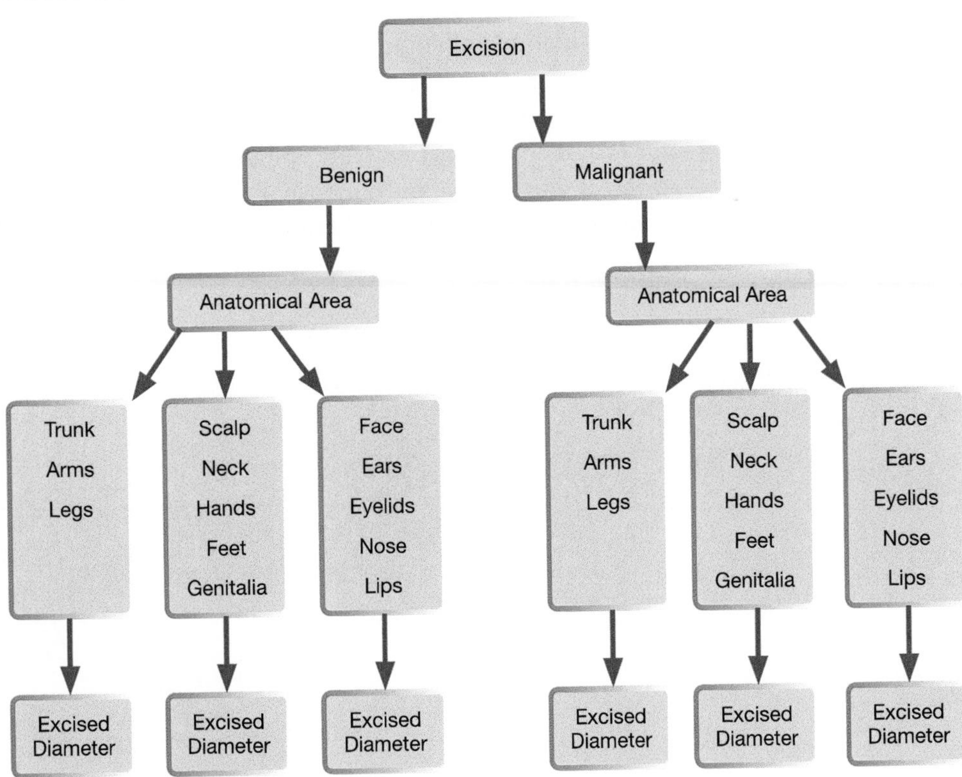

Table 9.3 Types of Benign and Malignant Skin Lesions

Benign Lesions	Malignant Lesions
seborrheic keratosis	basal cell carcinoma
senile lentigo	squamous cell carcinoma
cysts	melanoma
papular lesions	
granulomas	

Site of Lesions

The next step is to determine the family of codes that relate to the body site of the lesion excision. For both benign and malignant excisions, there are 3 groupings:

- trunk, arms, and legs;
- scalp, neck, hands, feet, and genitalia; and
- face ears, eyelids, nose, and lips (benign excisions add mucous membranes to this grouping).

Size of Lesions

> **RED FLAG**
> Remember to code each lesion excision separately. Calculate the excised diameter by adding the size of the margin to the size of the lesion.

Further narrow down the choice of codes based on the measurement of the lesion and the width of the margins prior to excision. The **margins** are the areas surrounding the lesion that are free from disease but are also excised to make sure all the diseased cells have been removed. The lesion itself should be measured at the greatest diameter, and the margins judged necessary for complete excision should be added to that measurement, as shown in Figure 9.6. The CPT® codebook contains some helpful graphics to guide you in the measuring of lesions.

Figure 9.6 Lesion Margin Measurement

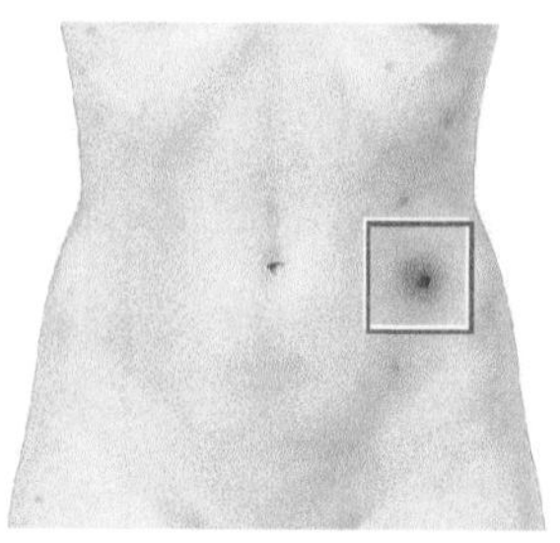

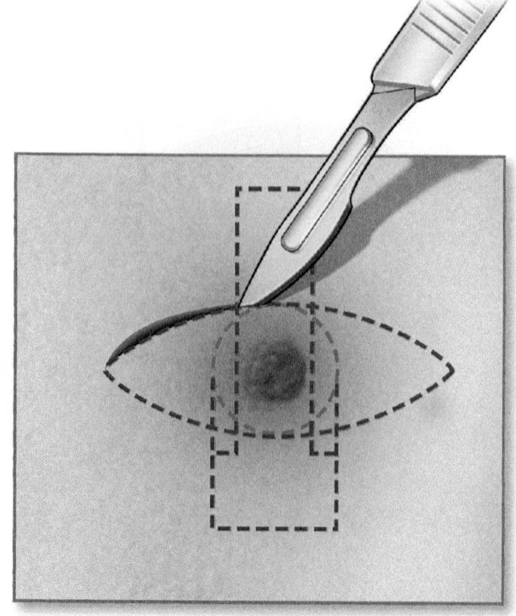

Wound Closure

Recall that excision of a skin lesion includes a simple closure, but more complicated skin closures should be coded separately. For example, a **layered closure** requires closure of both the skin and subcutaneous layers and is reported with the codes for intermediate wound repair (12031 through 12057). A **complex closure** may require **undermining** (surgically separating the skin from its underlying connective tissue), obtaining **hemostasis** (stopping bleeding), or placing sutures (stitching) to avoid distortion; a complex closure is reported with the codes for complex wound repair (13100 through 13153). Codes for lesion excisions cannot be reported with codes for adjacent tissue transfers (14000 through 14302). If an adjacent tissue transfer skin graft is performed at the time of the lesion excision, the lesion excision is included in the code for the tissue transfer and should not be reported separately. Tissue transfers and skin grafts will be discussed later in this chapter.

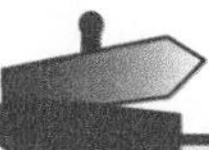

Learn Your Way

In the Index of Learning Styles, sequential learners prefer a logical approach and a good, clear explanation when attempting a new task. If you are a sequential learner, you may find that following a step-by-step plan when reporting codes makes the most sense. You can follow these steps to determine the appropriate code for an excision of a lesion.

1. Was the lesion benign or malignant?
2. Where was the lesion?
3. What was the size of the lesion plus the margins?
4. What type of closure was performed?

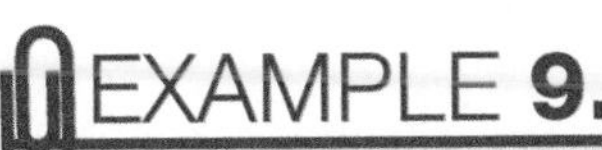

EXAMPLE 9.3

A 43-year-old woman presented to the outpatient surgery center for an excision of a lesion on her cheek that measured 2 cm in diameter and appeared to be benign. Seborrheic keratosis was suspected. After marking the area around the lesion (see Figure 9.7) and administering a local anesthetic, the surgeon made a full-thickness incision (through the dermis) and excised the lesion with a 0.2-cm margin on all sides. The wound was repaired using a single layer of sutures (see Figure 9.8). The pathology report confirmed the diagnosis of seborrheic keratosis.

To determine the code for this procedure, first note that the lesion was benign. Next note that the lesion was removed from the patient's cheek. Then calculate the excised diameter of the lesion by adding the lesion's measurement of 2 cm to the margins of 0.2 cm on either side of the lesion (2 cm + 0.2 cm + 0.2 cm = 2.4 cm). Finally, notice that the wound was closed with a simple closure. The combination of all of this documentation indicates code 11443, *Excision, other benign lesion including margins, except skin tag (unless listed elsewhere), face, ears, eyelids, nose, lips, mucous membranes; excised diameter 2.1 to 3.0 cm.*

Figure 9.7 Surgeon's Mark Around a Skin Lesion on the Face

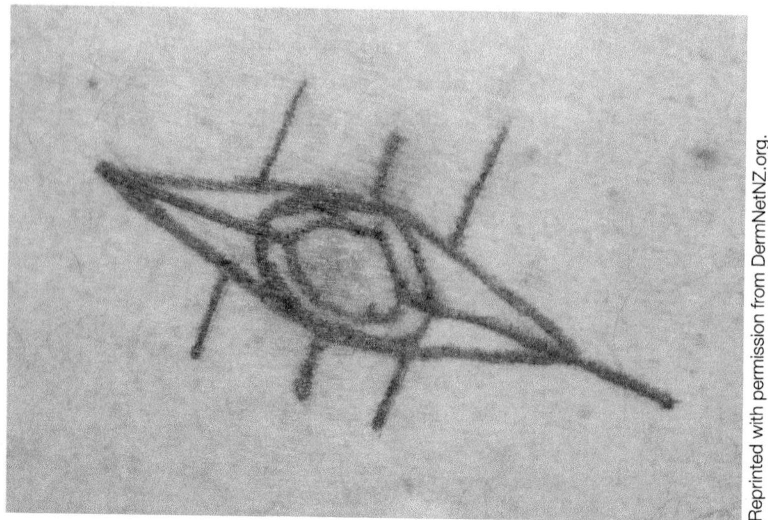

Reprinted with permission from DermNetNZ.org.

Figure 9.8 Sutured Incision After Removal of the Skin Lesion

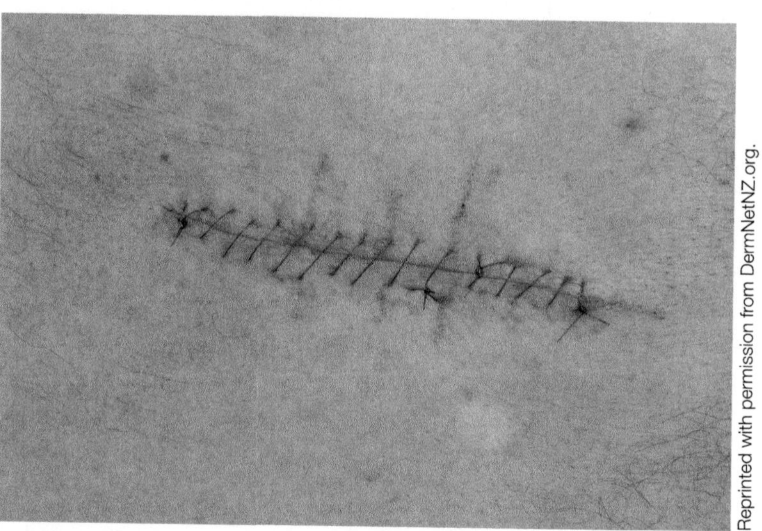

Reprinted with permission from DermNetNZ.org.

LET'S TRY ONE **9.3**

Write the correct code for each of the following procedures.

1. Excision of 4.0-cm benign lesion of leg, each margin was 0.5 cm; a simple closure was done: _____
2. Excision of 2.0-cm squamous cell carcinoma from the patient's forehead; each margin was 0.3 cm; a single-layer closure was performed: _____
3. Excision of a 2.5-cm lip lesion, malignant, and a 1.5-cm chest lesion, malignant; the surgeon used 0.3-cm margins on both lesions; simple closures were done on both sites: _____

Nail Procedures (Codes 11719-11765)

A review of the anatomy of the nail is shown in Figure 9.9. The procedures under the Nails heading of the Integumentary System Surgery subsection range from a simple trimming to a complex reconstruction of a nail bed with grafting. The codes vary widely in terms of the number of nails that can be involved in each procedure. For example, code 11720, *Debridement of nail(s) by any method(s); 1 to 5*, can be reported for 1 to 5 nails, but if 6 or more nails are debrided, then code 11721 should be reported. Code 11730, *Avulsion of nail plate, partial or complete, simple; single* can be reported only for a single nail; add-on code 11732 must be used for each additional nail plate.

Figure 9.9 Anatomy of the Nail

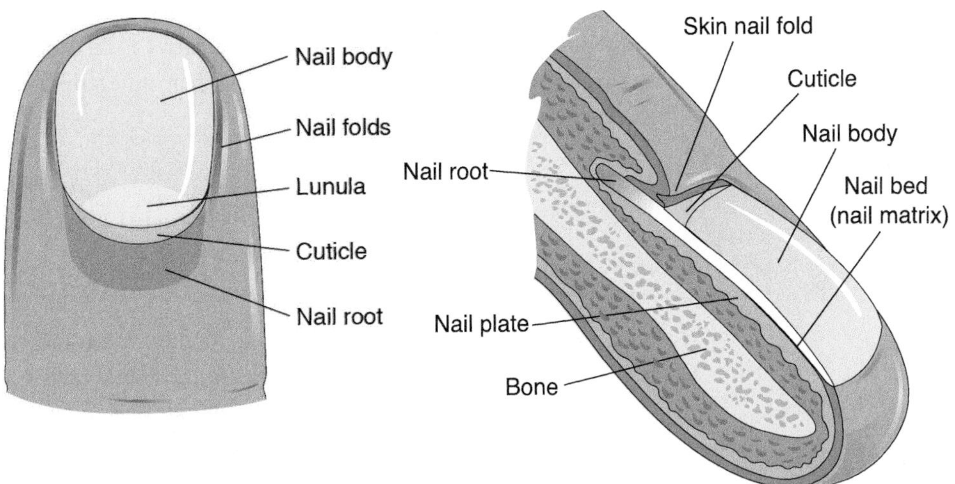

Patients with chronic onychomycosis (fungal infection in the nail) may require avulsion of the nail plate. In this procedure, the surgeon bluntly dissects the nail plate from the nail bed. Code 11730 is reported for a partial or complete nail avulsion for a single nail. Each additional nail plate avulsion is reported with add-on code 11732.

Patients with onychocryptosis (ingrown nail) and other chronic nail dystrophy may require an avulsion with matrixectomy. Excision of the nail plate and the nail matrix (nail bed) permanently removes a fingernail or toenail. In this procedure, the surgeon bluntly dissects and removes the nail plate. The matrix is then destroyed by chemical ablation, electrocautery, or laser. Partial or complete excision of the nail matrix is reported with code 11750.

Pilonidal Cyst Procedures (Codes 11770-11772)

A pilonidal cyst, also referred to as a *pilonidal sinus*, is a cyst that forms at the site of a hair follicle, typically in the coccyx area. There are 3 codes for simple, extensive, or complicated excisions. Excision of a small cyst or sinus requiring simple closure is reported with code 11770. A more extensive excision requiring layered closure is reported with code 11771. A sinus involving many subcutaneous extensions and requiring a more complicated excision is reported with code 11772. A complicated excision may be left open to heal or may require skin grafting, which is reported separately.

Introduction Procedures (Codes 11900-11983)

The codes under the Introduction heading represent a variety of procedures: intralesional injections; filling material injections such as collagen; therapeutic tattooing; and implantations into the skin layers. These are mostly self-explanatory, specialized procedures, but codes 11900 and 11901 carry some parenthetic instructions that are worth noting: these injection codes are not to be used for administration of local anesthetic or for intralesional chemotherapy. Preoperative local anesthetic injections are included in surgical procedures, and intralesional chemotherapy injections have codes located in the Medicine section of the codebook.

Repair (Closure) Procedures (Codes 12001-16036)

Under the heading Repair (Closure) are codes for wound repairs, adjacent tissue transfers, skin replacement surgery, skin grafts and flaps, excisions of ulcers, wound repair after excision of lesions, and burn treatments. The codebook provides helpful guidelines for these repair procedures that stipulate the closure materials used, define the classification of wound repair levels of complexity, and give instructions for reporting services. The guidelines under the Repair (Closure) heading are required reading for the categories of codes that follow.

Repair Classifications: Simple, Intermediate, and Complex

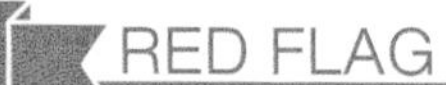

Wound repair that only uses adhesive strips is not reported separately but is considered to be an E/M service.

The first group of repair codes is for repair of wounds of the skin. There are 3 categories that contain codes used to report wound closure using sutures, staples, or tissue adhesives: Repair—Simple; Repair—Intermediate; and Repair—Complex. These codes can be reported alone or in combination with other wound repair codes. The guidelines that precede these categories state that wound repair using adhesive strips only is considered to be an evaluation and management (E/M) service.

A **simple repair** is a closure that involves only 1 layer of the skin. Simple repairs are commonly used on superficial wounds involving the epidermis and dermis, but they can also be used on wounds involving subcutaneous tissue, as long as there is no involvement of deeper structures. Choose the code appropriate for the anatomical site and length of the repair.

An **intermediate repair** is a layered closure of 1 or more of the deeper layers of subcutaneous tissue and superficial fascia in addition to the skin closure (dermal and epidermal layers). Intermediate repair codes may also be used when a single layer closure was done on wounds that were heavily contaminated and required extensive cleaning prior to closure. In an intermediate closure, the wound edges are undermined (separated from the dermal layer) to reduce tension and distortion. Buried, absorbable sutures are used to close the subcutaneous and dermal layers. Subcuticular (under the skin) sutures are used to close the epidermal skin edges. Choose the code appropriate for the anatomical site and length of the repair.

Inside the OR

There are many different types and brands of sutures. Absorbable sutures break down in the body, and nonabsorbable sutures are removed if on the skin or left in place if inside the body. There are braided (strands woven together) or nonbraided (single strand) sutures. Researching sutures on the Internet will yield many product descriptions and details for uses of particular suture types.

Complex repairs involve repairing wounds with more extensive methods than just a layered closure. Debridement of traumatic lacerations or avulsions (injuries in which a body structure is forcibly pulled off), extensive undermining, and use of stents or retention sutures in the closure of a wound would be reported as complex repairs. Complex repair may be required to avoid distortion in delicate areas such as the lip or eyelid. A layered repair of a laceration that required debridement of the wound edges before closure would also be coded as a complex repair.

All wound repair codes include the following services:

- local anesthesia;
- simple ligation of vessels in an open wound; and
- simple exploration of nerves, blood vessels, or tendons.

Extensive debridement or removal of contaminated tissue is not included and should be reported using the debridement codes. Repair of nerves, blood vessels, and tendons should also be reported under the appropriate codes for those systems.

Wound repair codes are assigned according to the type of repair, the length of the repair (in centimeters), and the anatomical site of the repair. When multiple wounds are repaired, the lengths of repairs of the same classification (simple, intermediate, or complex) that are located in the same anatomical grouping in the code description are added together. The total is used to determine the code.

EXAMPLE **9.4**

A patient presented to the ED with multiple lacerations of the extremities that required simple repair. A 3-cm wound was repaired on the lower leg, and a 4-cm wound was repaired on the thigh, both with a single layer of sutures.

To determine the code, note that these repairs are of the same classification (simple). Also note that both repairs were performed on the leg, which is an extremity. Therefore, you can add their lengths to determine the total length you will use to choose the code (3 cm + 4 cm = 7 cm). The combination of this documentation indicates code 12002, *Simple repair of superficial wounds of scalp, neck, axillae, external genitalia, trunk and/or extremities (including hands and feet); 2.6 cm to 7.5 cm*.

Make sure not to improperly combine wound repairs that have different classifications or anatomical locations. Remember:

- Wound repairs of different classifications may not be added together.
- Wound repairs of the same classification but different anatomical groupings in the code descriptions may not be added together.
- When more than 1 of the same classification of repairs is reported, it is appropriate to report multiple wound repair codes using the code for each anatomical group. Use modifier 51, *Multiple procedures*, on the second and subsequent codes.
- When more than 1 classification of wound repair is performed, the most complicated repair is reported first, and the less complicated repairs are reported as secondary procedures with modifier 59, *Distinct procedural service*.

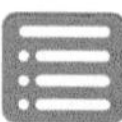

Index Insider

You can find codes for wound repairs in the Index in several ways: under the main term *Repair*, find the subterms *Skin* and *Wound*; under the main term *Skin*, find the subterm *Wound Repair*, and under the main term *Wound*, find the subterm *Repair*, under which many different anatomical sites are indexed.

EXAMPLE **9.5**

A 15-year-old male patient presented to the ED after tripping and falling while carrying a glass pitcher. He sustained multiple lacerations on both his hands and arms, 3 of which needed stitches. A simple repair was done on a 2.5-cm wound on the right hand, a 3.5-cm layered repair was done on the right arm, and a simple repair was done on a 2-cm left arm laceration.

Note that 2 of the repairs are classified as simple (as opposed to the layered repair) and appear in the same codebook anatomical grouping (the right hand and left arm are extremities). The lengths of these 2 repairs should be added together (2.5 cm + 2.0 cm = 4.5 cm) to determine the code: 12002, *Simple repair of superficial wounds of scalp, neck, axillae, external genitalia, trunk and/or extremities (including hands and feet); 2.6 to 7.5 cm*. The 3.5-cm layered repair of the arm is classified as an intermediate repair, so code 12032, *Repair, intermediate, wounds of scalp, axillae, trunk, and/or extremities (excluding hands and feet) 2.6 to 7.5 cm*, should be reported. An intermediate repair is more complicated than a simple repair, so code 12032 is reported before code 12002. Modifier 59, *Distinct procedural service*, should also be attached to the second repair code since it is of a different classification. This episode would be reported as 12032, 12002 - 59.

LET'S TRY ONE **9.4**

Select the correct code for each of the following procedures.

1. 1-cm simple wound repair of right index finger: _____
2. Layered closure of wound of foot, 4.2 cm: _____
3. Intermediate repair of laceration, left ear, 1.3 cm: _____

Adjacent Tissue Transfer or Rearrangement

Adjacent Tissue Transfer or Rearrangement is another category under the Repair (Closure) heading. These codes are used when a lesion or scar is excised and the resulting defect is repaired using a transfer of adjacent tissue. Some of the techniques are known as a *rotation flap, Z-plasty, W-plasty, V-Y plasty, advancement flap, or rotational flap procedures.*

Z-plasty, W-plasty, and V-Y plasty are named after the shape of the incision that is made as part of the procedure. As shown in Figure 9.10, in a **Z-plasty**, the letter Z is centered over the defect, and the 2 incisions at each end are equal in length to the center incision. This creates 2 flaps of skin, which are then rotated as indicated by the arrows in Figure 9.10. The result is that the original Z is rotated 90° and reversed.

Figure 9.10 Diagram of a Z-plasty

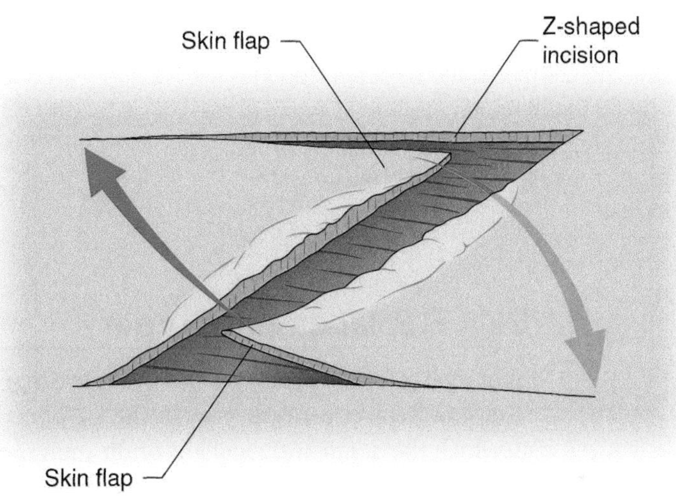

The adjacent tissue transfer codes are differentiated from 1 another by the anatomical site and the size of the defect being repaired. In this category, the CPT® codebook has guidelines that describe 2 "defects" that must be measured together to determine the code:

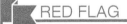

RED FLAG

The excision of a benign or malignant lesion cannot be reported separately if a tissue transfer type of repair was performed for closure of the defect created by the surgery. The tissue transfer codes include the lesion excision when performed.

- The **primary defect** is the site of the excision.
- The **secondary defect** is the site of the tissue being transferred to repair the primary defect.

The CPT® codebook contains helpful graphics that demonstrate how to measure these types of grafts to determine the appropriate code.

In a lesion excision, the size of the primary defect resulting from the excision and the size of the flap needed to perform the reconstruction are added together to determine the code. Codes for the adjacent tissue transfers or rearrangements (14000 through 14302) include the excision of the lesion and cannot be reported with codes for excision of benign lesions (11400 through 11446) or malignant lesions (11600 through 11646).

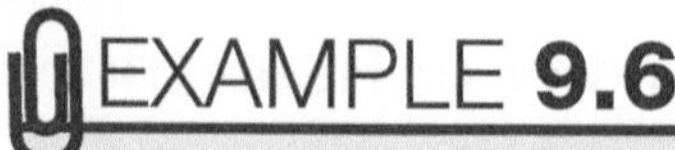

EXAMPLE 9.6

A 29-year-old female patient had a 2-sq-cm malignant neoplasm removed from her forehead. Z-plasty measuring 4 sq cm was used to repair this site.

Because the codes for adjacent tissue transfers (like Z-plasty) include the excision of benign or malignant lesions, the only procedure reported is the Z-plasty. The area was less than 10 sq cm on the patient's forehead, therefore code 14040, *Adjacent tissue transfer or rearrangement, forehead, cheeks, chin, mouth, neck, axillae, genitalia, hands and/or feet; defect 10 sq cm or less*, is reported.

CONCEPTS CHECKPOINT 9.2

Answer true or false to each of the following statements.

1. _____ Defects are measured and reported in square centimeters.
2. _____ Z-plasty, W-plasty, and V-Y plasty procedures are named after the shape of the incision.
3. _____ A code for the excision of a lesion should be reported in addition to the code for the adjacent tissue transfer.

Skin Replacement Surgery

Skin replacement surgery, also known as **skin grafting**, involves transplanting skin. The Skin Replacement category in the CPT® codebook contains codes for autografts, in which the donor and recipient of the grafted tissue are the same individual, and skin substitute grafts, in which the donor is different from the recipient.

An **autograft** is a skin graft taken from the patient's own skin. The surgeon takes healthy skin from 1 area of the body (the donor site) and moves it to an area needing repair (the recipient site). Once the procedure is complete, the autograft is permanent.

Skin grafts can be either split (partial) thickness or full thickness. A **split-thickness graft** contains the epidermis and a portion of the dermis of the donor site. A **full-thickness graft**, also known as a **free skin graft**, contains the entire epidermis and dermis layers. The difference in thickness between the 2 types of grafts is shown in Figure 9.11.

The donor site for a split-thickness skin graft heals spontaneously and does not require closure. The donor site from a full-thickness skin graft may be sutured together using a simple closure, which is included in the code and should not be reported separately. If the donor site requires a complex closure or a split-thickness skin graft, these procedures may be reported separately.

Figure 9.11 Split-Thickness Versus Full-Thickness Skin Grafts

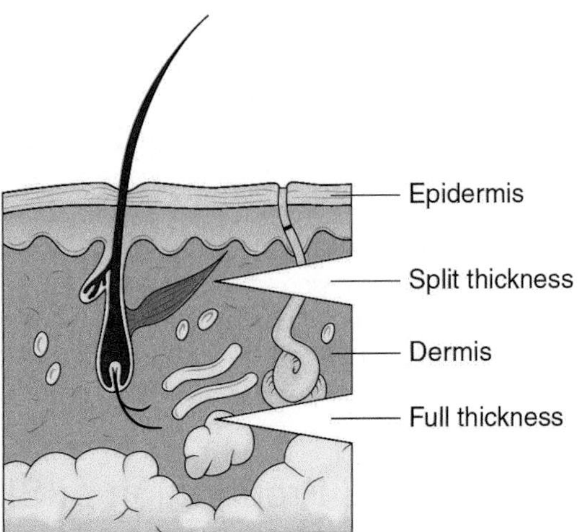

A **skin substitute graft** is a temporary wound closure used to promote healing until a permanent graft can be applied. Skin substitute grafts can be made of non-autologous human skin (skin from a different person's body), nonhuman skin, and/or biological products that form scaffolding for skin growth. Types of skin substitute grafts mentioned in the "Definitions" codebook guidelines for this category and the distinctions between the grafts are as follows:

- allograft—a graft originating from a donor who is genetically different from the recipient but of the same species, ie, human to human;
- homograft—a term used interchangeably with "allograft";
- tissue-cultured autograft—tissue grown from the recipient's own cells; and
- xenograft—a nonhuman skin graft or biologic wound dressing, eg, porcine tissue or pigskin.

Inside the OR

Epicel is a brand name for a cultured epidermal autograft that is grown in a lab from the patient's own keratinocytes (the predominant type of cells found in the epidermis) and mouse cells. Each sheet of Epicel consists of 2 to 8 cell layers of keratinocytes. Before they can be transplanted, these playing-card-sized sheets are attached to petrolatum gauze backing with stainless steel surgical clips. The Epicel skin substitute is trimmed to the size needed, placed over the prepared wound site, and sutured or stapled into place. Epicel is used for skin grafts in patients who have deep or full-thickness burns over 30% or more of their total body surface area (TBSA). It may be used alone or in conjunction with split-thickness autografts.

Epicel is considered a product for xenotransplantation (transplanting living cells between 2 different species) because it is grown by cocultivation with mouse cells.

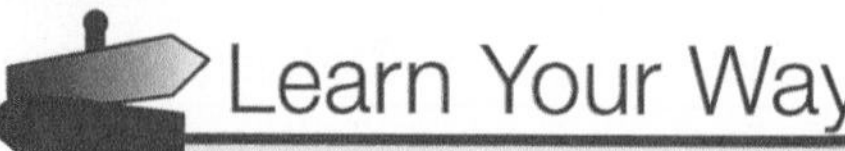

Learn Your Way

Reflective learners prefer concrete experience and reflective observation, and they choose to watch rather than do. If you are a reflective learner, observing a real-life skin graft procedure will appeal to you. The accompanying links show how skin grafts are performed. The first link is an animated video meant for patients who will receive skin grafts. The second link is a video of a real split-thickness skin graft surgery and is graphic in nature. Viewer discretion is advised.

http://Coding.ParadigmEducation.com/SkinGraft1

http://Coding.ParadigmEducation.com/SkinGraft2

Surgical Preparation of Skin Graft Recipient Site

Surgical preparation of the recipient site is a procedure in which nonviable tissue is removed by excision. The surgeon prepares the recipient's tissue to receive a graft by excising skin, subcutaneous tissue, scars, burn eschar (pieces of dead tissue), and lesions to provide a healthy tissue bed for the new skin. Codes 15002 through 15005 are used to report surgical preparation of a recipient site. Modifier 51, *Multiple procedures*, is not used with codes 15002 through 15005, as the guidelines state that they are to be coded in addition to the graft procedure. There are 2 criteria for code selection:

- the anatomical location with respect to the groupings given in the codes: 15002 and 15003 for trunk, arms, and legs; and 15004 and 15005 for face scalp, eyelids, mouth, neck, ears, orbits, genitalia, hands, feet, fingers, and toes;
- the size of the site, given in percentage of body area for infants and children younger than 10 years of age, and in square centimeters for adults.

If multiple recipient sites are prepared, the surface area of all wounds in the same anatomical grouping in the code description can be added together.

Reporting Codes for Skin Grafts

Codes for skin grafts are determined by the type of graft (autograft, split thickness, skin substitute, etc.), the anatomical site, and the surface area. Read the operative note carefully to obtain this information. The area of the graft is measured in square centimeters, and the codes have minimum baseline measurements ranging from 10 sq cm to 100 sq cm. Add-on codes are used to report additional surface area. Pay special attention to the code descriptions, which group anatomical areas similarly to those in the wound repair codes. Skin grafts are coded to the recipient site (where the graft is placed). The donor site (where the graft was taken from) does not affect code assignment.

EXAMPLE 9.7

A 25-year-old female requested that a 5 × 2-cm scar defect on her right cheek be removed and repaired for cosmetic purposes. The scar tissue was cut away and the site prepared for grafting. A full-thickness graft was harvested from her left thigh and placed on her cheek.

This procedure will require 2 codes, 1 for the preparation and 1 for the graft. See Figure 9.12.

Figure 9.12 Surgical Preparation and Skin Graft Codes

15004	Surgical preparation or creation of recipient site by excision of open wounds, burn eschar, or scar (including subcutaneous tissues), or incisional release of scar contracture, face, scalp, eyelids, mouth, neck, ears, orbits. genitalia, hands, feet and/or multiple digits; first 100 sq cm or 1% of body area of infants and children
15240	Full thickness graft, free, including direct closure of donor site, forehead, cheeks, chin, mouth neck, axillae, genitalia, hands, and/or feet; 20 sq cm or less

Reporting Codes for Flaps

Flap surgery is a procedure in which a piece of tissue still attached to the artery or vein at its base is set into the recipient site (injured area or defect). A graft or free flap is tissue that is moved from 1 body area to anther. The blood vessels can then be surgically reconnected at the recipient site.

Skin and/or Deep Tissue Flaps (Codes 15570-15738)

The surgical reconstruction procedures in the category Flaps (Skin and/or Deep Tissues) use pedicle flaps, either direct or tubed. For a tubed flap, the edges of a flap are sutured together to form a tube. A **pedicle flap** is full-thickness skin and subcutaneous tissue that has been harvested in the donor area to maintain an intact edge with its blood supply so that the tissue may be rotated or transferred to the adjacent recipient area. Figure 9.13 shows a pedicle flap graft on a woman's nose. The red area is the source (donor site) of the graft. If the donor area is repaired with skin grafts or flaps, a separate code may be reported.

Other Flaps and Grafts

In the category Other Flaps and Grafts, codes 15740 and 15750 are used for formation of an island pedicle flap. An **island pedicle flap** is a flap formed near but not immediately adjacent to the recipient site. The site is covered by a flap of skin and subcutaneous tissue that has been elevated to cover it. The tissue may also be transferred through a tunnel underneath the skin.

Figure 9.14 First-Degree, Second-Degree, and Third-Degree Burns

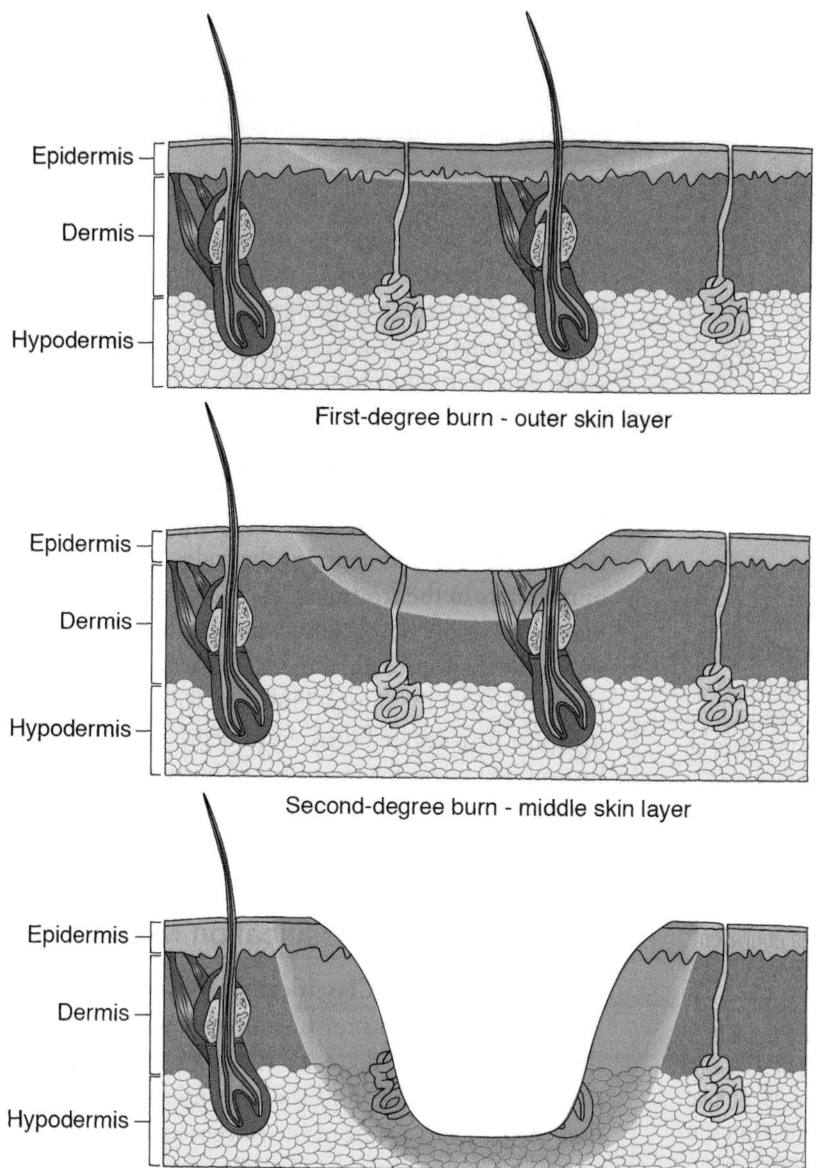

> **RED FLAG**
>
> Do not use debridement codes 11000 through 11047 to report debridement of burn wounds. Debridement of burns is reported with codes 16020 through 16030.

Escharotomy

Eschar is a leathery slough (ie, scab) resulting from a third-degree burn injury. Following a full-thickness burn, as the underlying tissues are rehydrated, they become constricted due to the eschar's lack of elasticity. In an **escharotomy**, the surgeon makes an incision through the eschar to expose the tissue below. This allows the underlying tissue to grow and expand and prevents burn-induced compartment syndrome (a serious condition of increased pressure in a muscle compartment) and further tissue injury.

Escharotomy is reported with code 16035 for the initial incision and 16036 for each additional incision. These codes are not specific to any particular body site. Escharotomy incisions are often performed bilaterally to release the constricting tissues and allow organs to maintain their normal function. Medial and lateral incisions may be made on an affected extremity. For a patient with burn eschar present on the chest or abdomen, transverse incisions are often made to allow the patient's chest to move for respiration.

Table 9.4 Lund-Browder Classification Method Table for Burn Estimates

Area	Percentage of Total Body Surface Area (TBSA) by Age						Burn Degree		Total
	Birth-1 Year	1-4 Years	5-9 Years	10-14 Years	15 Years	Adult	Second	Third	
Head	19%	17%	13%	11%	9%	7%			
Neck	2%	2%	2%	2%	2%	2%			
Anterior trunk	13%	13%	13%	13%	13%	13%			
Posterior trunk	13%	13%	13%	13%	13%	13%			
Right buttock	2.5%	2.5%	2.5%	2.5%	2.5%	2.5%			
Left buttock	2.5%	2.5%	2.5%	2.5%	2.5%	2.5%			
Genitalia	1%	1%	1%	1%	1%	1%			
Right upper arm	4%	4%	4%	4%	4%	4%			
Left upper arm	4%	4%	4%	4%	4%	4%			
Right lower arm	3%	3%	3%	3%	3%	3%			
Left lower arm	3%	3%	3%	3%	3%	3%			
Right hand	2.5%	2.5%	2.5%	2.5%	2.5%	2.5%			
Left hand	2.5%	2.5%	2.5%	2.5%	2.5%	2.5%			
Right thigh	2.5%	6.5%	8%	8.5%	9%	9.5%			
Left thigh	5.5%	6.5%	8%	8.5%	9%	9.5%			
Right leg	5%	5%	5.5%	6%	6.5%	7%			
Left leg	5%	5%	5.5%	6%	6.5%	7%			
Right foot	3.5%	3.5%	3.5%	3.5%	3.5%	3.5%			
Left foot	3.5%	3.5%	3.5%	3.5%	3.5%	3.5%			
Total									

CONCEPTS CHECKPOINT **9.3**

Answer true or false to each of the following statements.

1. _____ Using the Lund-Browder method, the right leg of an adult is considered to be 5% of his or her TBSA.
2. _____ To code multiple burns, each site is calculated and added together for the TBSA.
3. _____ Treatment of first-degree burns is reported with codes 16020 through 16030.
4. _____ Codes 16000 through 16036 refer to local treatment of burned surfaces.
5. _____ One code is assigned for each escharotomy incision performed.

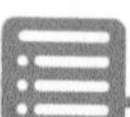

Destruction Codes (17000-17999)

Index Insider

Look for the subterm *Lesion* under the Index main entry *Destruction* to see a list of anatomical sites with lesion destruction codes.

Destruction is described as the ablation of lesions by any method, including electrosurgery, cryosurgery, laser treatments, and chemical treatments. Unlike lesion excision, the lesion is destroyed, and no specimen is sent to pathology for review. Lesions that may be destroyed include condylomata, papillomata, molluscum contagiosum, herpetic lesions, warts, milia, or other benign, premalignant, or malignant lesions. The destruction codes found in the Integumentary System codebook subsection are specific to skin, and lesion destruction codes specific to an organ or body structure are found in other subsections. Destruction codes include the administration of local anesthesia, but these types of procedures usually do not require closure of the skin.

Destruction, Benign or Premalignant Lesions

In coding for the destruction of benign and premalignant lesions, size and location are not factors. Codes are differentiated by the type and number of lesions destroyed. Code 17000, *Destruction (eg, laser surgery, electrosurgery, cryosurgery, chemosurgery, surgical curettement), premalignant lesions (eg, actinic keratoses); first lesion*, is reported for the first premalignant lesion destroyed. Add-on code 17003 is reported for each additional premalignant lesion destroyed, from 2 through 14 lesions. Since this is an add-on code, modifier 51, *Multiple procedures*, is not used. If 15 or more premalignant lesions are destroyed, code 17004 is reported instead of code 17000 and 17003. Code 17004 should not be reported with codes 17000 and 17003.

Destruction of cutaneous vascular proliferative lesions (such as a birth mark, port wine stain, salmon patch, or hemangioma) is reported with codes 17106 through 17108 based on the total square centimeters treated: 17106 for an area less than 10.0 sq cm, 17107 for 10.0 to 50.0 sq cm, and 17108 for over 50.0 sq cm. Like the other codes in this category, the size and location of cutaneous vascular proliferative lesions is not a factor in code assignment.

RED FLAG

Destruction of skin tags is reported with codes 11200 or 11201.

Destruction of benign lesions other than skin tags (small pieces of skin that protrude with a stalk) or cutaneous vascular proliferative lesions is reported with code 17110 or 17111. These codes are differentiated by the number of lesions destroyed—once again, lesion size and location are not factors in code assignment. Code 17110 is reported for destruction of up to 14 benign lesions, and code 17111 is reported when 15 or more benign lesions are destroyed.

</> Coding for CMS

When coding for destruction of malignant lesions, you may or may not have a pathology report to confirm that the lesion is malignant. The documentation by the provider stating that the lesion is consistent with that of a skin malignancy is sufficient for most insurances, including Medicare.

Destruction, Malignant Lesions, Any Method

Unlike benign and premalignant lesions, the codes for the destruction of malignant lesions are differentiated from 1 another by the size and location of the lesion, as shown in Figure 9.15. Each lesion destroyed is reported separately. Codes 17260 through 17266 are reported for lesions on the trunk, arms, or legs; codes 17270 through 17276 are reported for lesions on the scalp, neck, hands, feet, or genitalia; and codes 17280 through 17286 are reported for lesions on the face, ears, eyelids, nose, lips, or mucous membranes.

Figure 9.15 Malignant Lesion Size and Location Differentiation

Destruction

- Benign or Premalignant
  - Number of Lesions
- Malignant
  - Trunk, Arms, Legs
    - Diameter of Lesion
  - Scalp, Neck, Hands, Feet, Genitalia
    - Diameter of Lesion
  - Face, Ears, Eyelids, Nose, Lips, Mucous Membrane
    - Diameter of Lesion

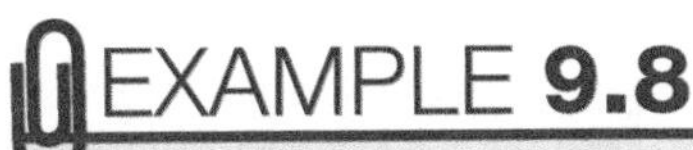

EXAMPLE **9.8**

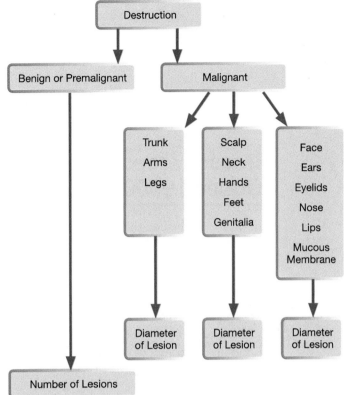

A 35-year-old balding male presented to the office for destruction of several squamous cell carcinomas on his forehead. Cryosurgery was used to destroy a 0.8-cm lesion on the right side of the forehead; a 0.4-cm lesion, approximately 1 cm inferior to the right forehead lesion; and a 1.2-cm lesion above the left eyebrow.

Destruction of these lesions requires 3 codes because 3 separate lesions were treated. All of the lesions were located on the face, the site described by the code family 17280 through 17286, *Destruction, malignant lesion (eg, laser surgery, electrosurgery, cryosurgery, chemosurgery, surgical curettement), face, ears, eyelids, nose, lips, mucous membrane*:

- The largest lesion destruction is reported first. The 1.2-cm malignant lesion destruction is reported with 17282, *lesion diameter 1.1 to 2.0 cm*.
- The 0.8-cm lesion destruction is reported next with 17281, *lesion diameter 0.6 to 1.0 cm*.
- The 0.4-cm lesion destruction is reported with 17280, *lesion diameter 0.5 cm or less*.

LET'S TRY ONE 9.6

Assign codes for each of the following scenarios.

1. Destruction of 3 premalignant facial lesions: _____
2. Destruction of squamous cell carcinoma on scalp, lesion diameter 0.7 cm: _____
3. Cryosurgical destruction of actinic keratoses, 16 lesions: _____

Breast Procedures (Codes 19000-19499)

The breasts, located on the front of the chest, are known as *mammary glands*. The structure of male and female breasts is essentially the same with the exception that female breasts contain milk-producing glandular structures and ducts that transport milk. The breast does not contain muscle; the breast tissue sits on top of the chest wall muscle and underneath the skin. Breasts do contain blood and lymphatic vessels. The areola is the darkened area of skin around the nipple. Breast is the last heading in the Integumentary System Surgery subsection of the CPT® codebook. It contains the codes for various procedures of the breasts, such as biopsies, removal of cysts, mastectomies, and breast reconstruction.

Incision

There are few codes in the Incision category. Codes 19000 and 19001 describe the puncture aspiration of cysts in the breast. Code 19020 is for a **mastotomy**, the incision into the breast, with exploration or drainage of abscess. Finally, code 19030 describes an injection procedure for **mammary ductogram** or **galactogram**, a special type of mammogram used for imaging the breast ducts.

Excision

Guidelines at the beginning of the Excision category describe coding the surgical breast procedures and detail the following: different types of breast biopsies associated with lesion removal, involving either image guidance or an open approach; the removal of benign or malignant cysts or lesions; the removal of chest wall tumors; and the gamut of mastectomies.

Types of Breast Biopsies

Various methods exist for obtaining breast biopsy specimens. The 2 basic types of biopsies are percutaneous (performed using a needle or punch) and open (performed by exposing the organs and tissues):

- Percutaneous methods include **puncture aspiration biopsies**, in which the surgeon uses a needle and a syringe to obtain a specimen, and **needle core biopsies**, in which the surgeon uses a small hollow instrument to puncture a lesion.

- Open biopsy procedures include **incisional biopsies**, which involve cutting into a lesion to obtain a specimen, and **excisional biopsies**, which involve the removal of the entire lesion.

Coding for Breast Biopsies

The breast biopsy and excision codes 19081 through 19086 are differentiated from 1 another by the technique—percutaneous needle versus open incisional—and the use of 1 of 3 types of image guidance—stereotactic mammography, ultrasound, or magnetic resonance imaging (MRI). For example, code 19081 describes a breast biopsy performed using mammography (x-ray) imaging to guide the surgeon to the site of the lesion. Stereotactic mammography uses x-rays taken from 2 different angles and a computer to pinpoint the exact location of the breast lesion. In this procedure, because the lesion is too small to feel, image guidance is used to mark the site of the lesion with a metallic clip or pellet so the surgeon can locate the lesion to biopsy it. If no image guidance is used during a biopsy, codes 19100 and 19101 are reported. When an open incisional biopsy is performed after placement of a marker or localization device (clip, metallic pellet, wire, needle, or radioactive seeds placed adjacent to the lesion to help the surgeon identify the site), the appropriate code for the image-guided placement of the localization device is reported.

Add-on codes are used when more than 1 biopsy or localization device placement is performed using the same imaging modality. If more than 1 biopsy is performed and the imaging modalities are different, each additional biopsy and modality should be reported separately. Separate codes exist for biopsies using stereotactic, ultrasound, and magnetic resonance guidance. Excision of a single breast lesion identified preoperatively by a radiological marker is coded as 19125. Each additional lesion separately identified by a marker is coded with 19126. Code 19126 must be used in conjunction with 19125 for additional lesion excisions.

Introduction

Codes 19281 through 19288 are used only for the placement of a localization device using image guidance—that is, without an image-guided biopsy. Codes 19296 through 19298 are similarly codes for the placement of catheters preparatory to administration of radiation therapy.

Mastectomy Procedures

A **mastectomy** is defined as removal of the breast. Patients with breast cancer commonly have this procedure. There are several types of mastectomies, and coding for these procedures depends on how much of the breast tissue was removed. Mastectomy codes are unilateral so the RT (Right side) or LT (Left side) modifiers should be used if the procedure is performed on 1 breast. If the procedure is done bilaterally, modifier 50, *Bilateral procedure*, should be applied. Figure 9.16 illustrates the amount of tissue removed in each procedure.

- When a lesion is excised and the defect created is repaired with a tissue transfer or rearrangement such as a Z-plasty, a separate code for the lesion excision is not reported. Only the code for the tissue transfer procedure is reported.
- Skin graft codes are differentiated by the type of graft, the recipient site, and the size.
- Preparation of the skin graft recipient site may require an additional code if nonviable tissue is removed by excision.
- Closure of the donor site may require an additional code if the donor area is repaired with skin grafts or flaps.
- Codes for treatment of burns (debridement and dressing) are assigned based on whether the burn is small, medium, or large—measurements determined by the percentage of the body surface affected.
- Codes for the destruction of benign and premalignant lesions are differentiated by the type and number of lesions destroyed.
- Breast biopsy codes are differentiated by technique and the type of imaging guidance used.
- Mastectomy codes are differentiated by the type of mastectomy performed.
- Breast reconstruction codes are based on 1 breast, and modifier 50 is appended for bilateral procedures.

Navigator

Access interactive chapter review exercises, practice activities, flash cards, and study games.

Chapter 10

Surgery Coding: The Musculoskeletal System

Fast Facts

- Babies have more bones than adults: a human infant has 300 bones and an adult human has 206. Some bones fuse together as we grow.
- The largest muscle in the human body is the gluteus maximus (found in the buttocks).
- People are taller in the morning and shorter in the evening because gravity causes compression on the discs between the vertebrae throughout the day. The discs return to normal during sleep.

Source: http://livescience.com

Crack the Code

Review the sample operative report to find the correct musculoskeletal system code. You may need to return to this exercise after reading the chapter content.

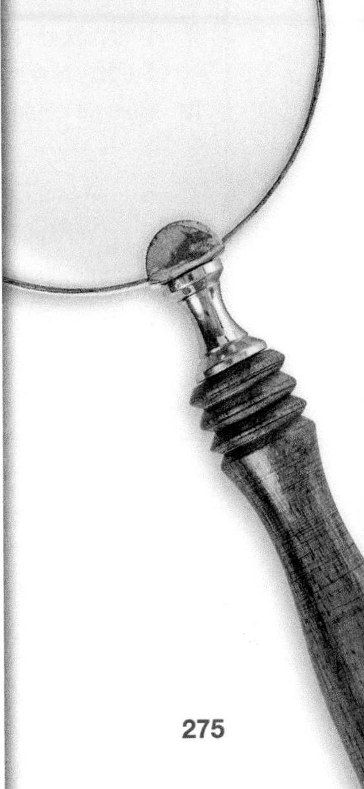

DATE OF OPERATION: 05/09/2019

PREOPERATIVE DIAGNOSIS: Right submandibular mass

POSTOPERATIVE DIAGNOSIS: Right submandibular mass

OPERATIVE PROCEDURE: Final needle aspiration biopsy, right submandibular mass (muscle)

SURGEON: Dr. Nelson

INDICATIONS: This is a 72-year-old female with a 2.5 cm mass in the right submandibular area. The mass has not been painful or tender and is not resolved with antibiotic therapy.

PROCEDURE: The patient was placed in the sitting position. The skin was cleansed with alcohol. Using a 10 cc syringe and a 22-gauge needle, a fine needle aspiration biopsy was performed and submitted for cytology. This procedure was repeated 2 more times. There were no complications, and the patient tolerated the procedure well.
A sterile Band-Aid was applied.

answer: 20206

Learning Objectives

10.1 Recognize the basic anatomical structures in the musculoskeletal system.

10.2 Identify specialized surgical terminology associated with the musculoskeletal system.

10.3 Describe the arrangement of codes in the Musculoskeletal System Surgery subsection.

10.4 Explain orthopedic repair and reconstruction techniques.

10.5 Describe the 3 types of fracture treatment (open, closed, and percutaneous).

10.6 Explain when cast applications and strapping codes are used.

10.7 Differentiate between partial and total arthroplasties.

10.8 Differentiate between a diagnostic and surgical arthroscopy.

10.9 Explain the importance of reviewing the full operative report when coding musculoskeletal system procedures.

10.10 Code the following types of musculoskeletal system procedures: wound exploration, injections, arthroplasty, fracture and/or dislocation treatment, repair and reconstruction operations, bunion repairs, casts and strapping procedures, and arthroscopies.

Chapter Outline

I. Introduction to the Musculoskeletal System
- **A.** Bones
- **B.** Ligaments, Joints, Bursa, Muscles, Tendons, and Fascia

II. Musculoskeletal System Terminology

III. Organization of the Musculoskeletal System Surgery Subsection

IV. General (Codes 20005-20999)
- **A.** Incision
- **B.** Wound Exploration—Trauma
- **C.** Excision
- **D.** Introduction or Removal
  - **i.** Tendon Sheath or Ligament Injections
  - **ii.** Trigger Point Injections
  - **iii.** Joint Aspirations and Injections
- **E.** Replantation
- **F.** Grafts (or Implants)
- **G.** Other Procedures

V. Anatomical Sites (Codes 21010-28899)
- **A.** Incision
- **B.** Excision
- **C.** Introduction or Removal
- **D.** Repair, Revision, and/or Reconstruction
  - **i.** Arthroplasty
  - **ii.** Eponyms for Surgical Procedures
  - **iii.** Foot Procedures
- **E.** Fracture Care
- **F.** Manipulation
- **G.** Arthrodesis
- **H.** Amputation
- **I.** Other Procedures

VI. Application of Casts and Strapping (Codes 29000-29799)

VII. Endoscopy/Arthroscopy (Codes 29800-29999)

VIII. Chapter Summary

Introduction to the Musculoskeletal System

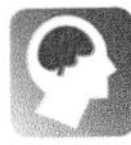

3-D
To explore the musculoskeletal system in the BioDigital Human, go to: http://Coding.ParadigmEducation.com/BioDigital_Skeleton and http://Coding.ParadigmEducation.com/BioDigital_Muscles.

The **musculoskeletal system** includes bones and joints as well as ligaments, tendons, muscle, bursa, fascia, and other soft tissues. Together, these elements provide the body with structure and support and allow it to move freely. Parts of the musculoskeletal system also provide protection for vital organs such as the heart and lungs.

Bones

Bones provide the body with structure and support, but they also serve many other functions. For example, without bones to attach to and pull on, the muscles would have a difficult time moving the parts of the body. Certain bones, such as the ribs and pelvis, do not directly provide movement but instead serve as a protection for vital organs such as the heart, lungs, and reproductive organs. Long bones, such as the femur, contain marrow, where new blood cells are formed. Bones play an essential role in the normal functions of many different body systems.

As a coder, it is important to know and remember the names and locations of all of the individual bones. This will not only make finding the correct code in the Musculoskeletal System subsection easier; it will also help you find codes in other sections, as many structures in the body are named after nearby bones. For example, the radial artery is so named because it is located near the radius, a lateral bone in the forearm; the ulnar nerve is so named because it is located near the ulna, a medial bone in the forearm. Figures 10.1 and 10.2 illustrate the bones in the human body from the anterior and posterior views.

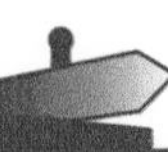

Learn Your Way

To learn the names and locations of individual bones, some students who are active or visual learners find it helpful to create a skeleton or handle a model of a human skeleton. Challenge yourself to recall the name of each bone. Disarticulate the skeleton and see if you can recognize the location of each individual bone to reassemble your skeleton model. Once you know the bones, you will more easily identify the anatomy and surgical procedures in the musculoskeletal system. Active or visual learners may also find it useful to interact with the BioDigital Human's musculoskeletal system, located at http://Coding.ParadigmEducation.com.BioDigital_Skeleton and http://Coding.ParadigmEducation.com/BioDigital_Muscles. The BioDigital Human allows you to view and manipulate three-dimensional human anatomy images to enhance your study of anatomy and physiology.

Figure 10.1 Human Bone Chart: Anterior View

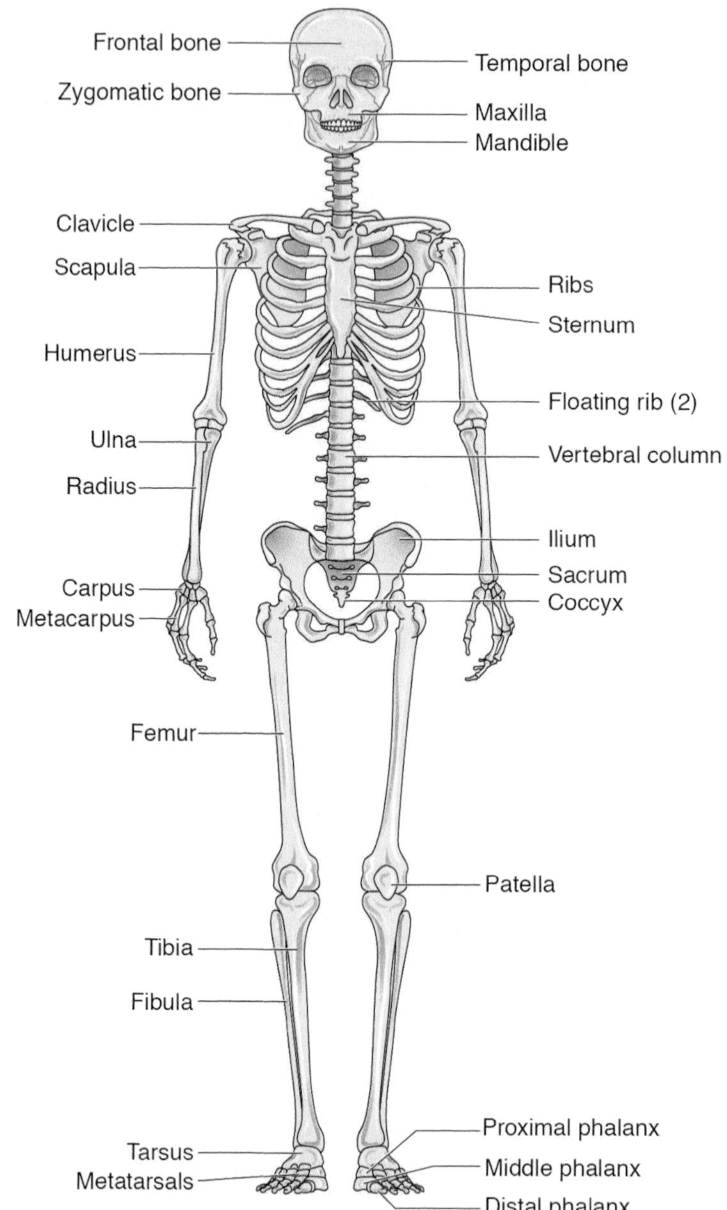

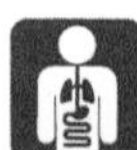

A&P Review

Soft spots or fontanelles on an infant's head allow the bones of the skull to move so the head can pass through the birth canal. The bones eventually get harder and form joints (called *cranial sutures*). The soft spots on an infant's head usually close by the age of 19 months.

Ligaments, Joints, Bursa, Muscles, Tendons, and Fascia

Ligaments are a tough fibrous tissue that connects bones, forming a joint. **Joints** occur where 2 bones meet. Some joints don't move much (such as the skull) and some freely move (such as the knee). Joints are sometimes called articulations and the ligaments referred to as *articular ligaments*. **Bursae** are fluid-filled sacs that allow for easy movement of the joints. **Muscles** pull on the joints, allowing movement. Muscles are connected to bones by **tendons**, which are cord-like tissues. **Fascia** is the connective tissue that surrounds muscles, blood vessels, and nerves.

Figure 10.2 Human Bone Chart: Posterior View

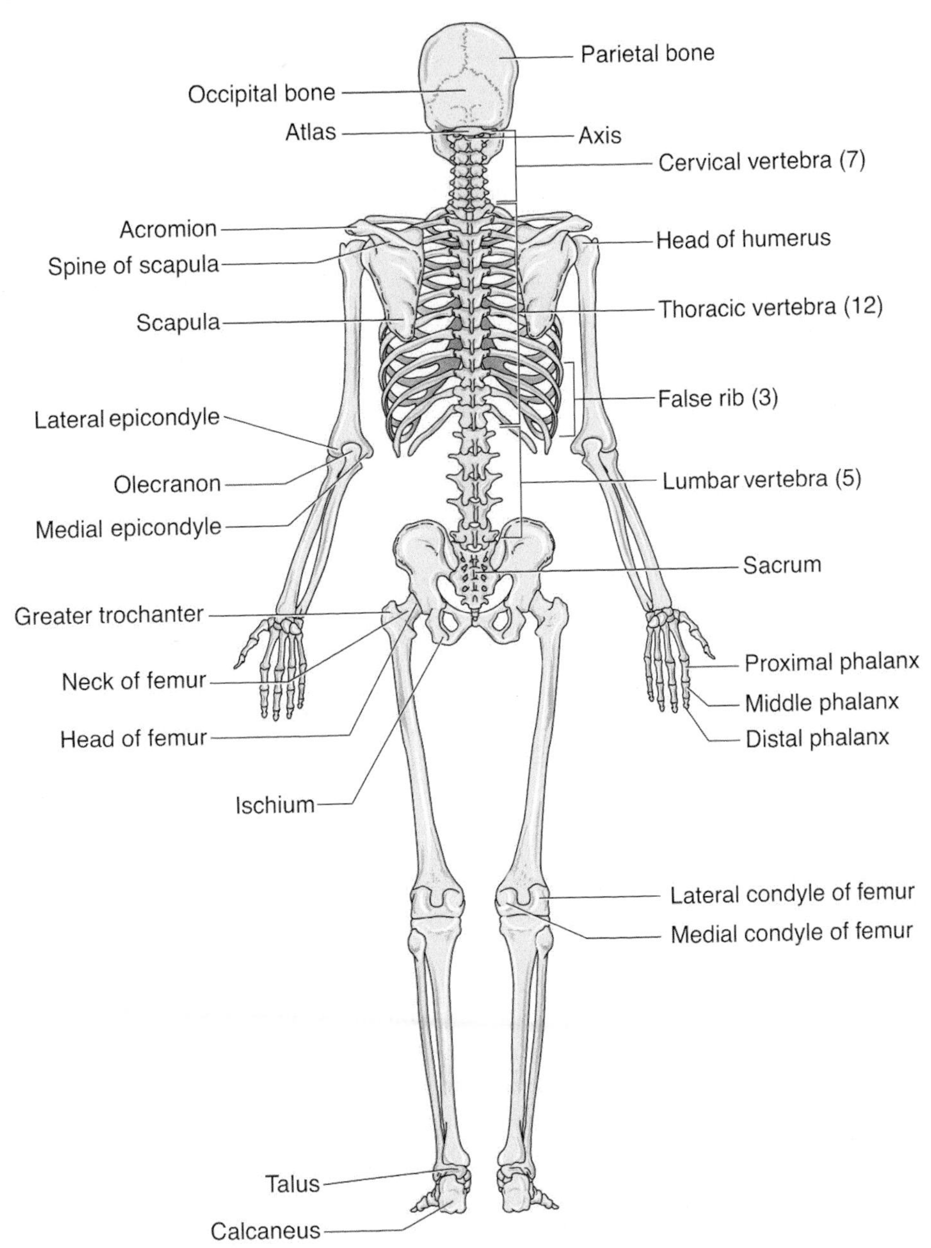

Musculoskeletal System Terminology

The Musculoskeletal System Surgery subsection in the CPT® codebook lists codes for many surgical procedures, ranging from limb replantation, joint replacement, and facial reconstruction to traumatic injury care, fracture repair, and lesion removal.

It is important to familiarize yourself with the specialized terminology before attempting to select codes. Some of the common terms related to procedures of the musculoskeletal system are listed in Table 10.1.

Table 10.1 Musculoskeletal System Terms and Definitions

Musculoskeletal System Term	Definition
arthrodesis	Surgical fixation or fusion of a joint
arthroplasty	Surgically repairing a joint by replacing, reshaping, reconstructing, or remodeling it
articular cartilage	A smooth layer of fibrous tissue that covers the contact surfaces of joints
bursa	A fluid-filled sac that allows for easy movement of joints
closed treatment	Fracture site that is not surgically opened and visualized
dislocation	An injury in which 1 or more bones separates from the joint
fascia	Connective tissue that surrounds muscles, blood vessels, and nerves
fixation	The placement of screws, rods, plates, or pins to hold a bone in place while healing
fracture	A break in a bone
ligament	Fibrous tissue that connects bone to bone
manipulation or reduction	Putting the fracture or dislocation back into the normal anatomical position
open treatment	Fracture site that is surgically opened and visualized
radical resection	Excision of tumor with wide margins of normal tissue
soft tissue	Supports or surrounds other structures in the body; includes ligaments, tendons, and fascia, among others
tendon	Band of fibrous tissue that connects muscle to bone
traction	Application of force to a limb for the purpose of straightening bones or relieving pressure

In addition, review Table 8.1, Common Surgical Suffixes, located on page 232, to understand how word parts that indicate procedures combine with those that indicate anatomical structures for specific surgical terminology found in the codebook Musculoskeletal System Surgery subsection.

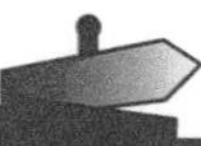

Learn Your Way

Learning new medical terms will take some amount of memorization. Students who are verbal learners find it helpful to create flash cards for each term. The cards should have the musculoskeletal system term on 1 side and the definition on the other. Be sure to study the cards both ways, looking at the definition and naming the term, and looking at the term and stating the definition. Electronic versions of these cards, and other key terms from this textbook, are located on the Course Navigator learning management system. Once you know the terms, you will more accurately identify the anatomy and surgical procedures in the musculoskeletal system.

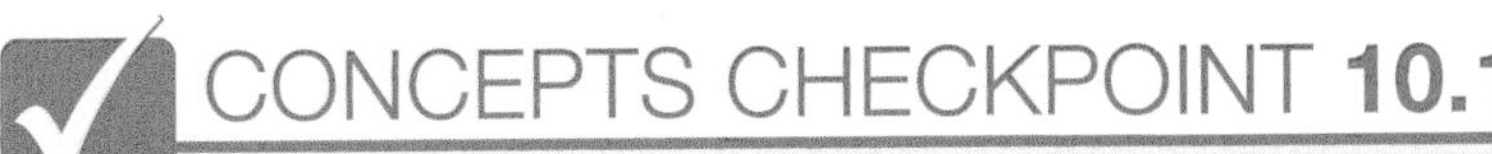

CONCEPTS CHECKPOINT 10.1

Match the term in the first column to the definition in the second column.

1. _____ closed treatment
2. _____ open treatment
3. _____ manipulation or reduction
4. _____ traction
5. _____ arthroplasty

a. The application of force to a limb
b. Words used interchangeably to mean the attempted restoration of a fracture or joint dislocation to its normal anatomical position
c. Fracture site that is not surgically opened and visualized
d. Reshaping or reconstructing a joint
e. Fracture site that is surgically opened and visualized

Organization of the Musculoskeletal System Surgery Subsection

The Musculoskeletal System begins with an introductory section containing definitions of code terminology developed by the AMA to reflect current orthopedic and surgical treatments. The definitions lay groundwork that will be helpful as a bridge from a legal medical record to its associated billing report and describe services that are included in procedures.

This introductory section provides definitions regarding orthopedic procedures. Orthopedic procedures that include application and removal of a cast and/or traction device are the following:

- closed treatment;
- open treatment;
- percutaneous skeletal fixation; and
- manipulation.

Following the definitions are observations on how procedural details are organized within the codes, as for example, this description of the elements of fracture codes:

> The codes for treatment of fractures and joint injuries (dislocations) are categorized by the type of manipulation (reduction) and stabilization (fixation or immobilization). These codes can apply to either open (compound) or closed fractures or joint injuries.

The introductory section closes with descriptions of 4 types of excision codes, with related information on code selection:

- excision of subcutaneous soft connective tissue;
- excision of fascial or subfascial soft tissue tumors;
- radical resection of soft connective tissue tumors; and
- radical resection of bone tumors.

With a few exceptions, the CPT® codebook organizes the codes in the Musculoskeletal System subsection of the Surgery section by anatomical sites in a top-down, center-out sequence: the head, the center of the body, the arms, the legs, the feet, and the toes. Within each anatomical grouping, the codebook arranges procedures by category in the following order:

- Incision
- Excision
- Introduction or removal
- Repair, revision, reconstruction
- Fracture, dislocation
- Manipulation
- Arthrodesis
- Amputation
- Other procedures

While not all of the musculoskeletal procedures will be explained in detail in this chapter, some of the more common and more challenging codes you may be required to report are discussed in the upcoming sections. Table 10.2 presents the main headings for this subsection and the codes organized under those headings.

Table 10.2 Headings Within the Musculoskeletal System Surgery Subsection of the CPT® Codebook

Heading	Code Range
General	20005-20999
Head	21010-21499
Neck (Soft Tissues) and Thorax	21501-21899
Back and Flank	21920-21936
Spine (Vertebral Column)	22010-22899
Abdomen	22900-22999
Shoulder	23000-23929
Humerus (Upper Arm) and Elbow	23930-24999
Forearm and Wrist	25000-25999
Hand and Fingers	26010-26989
Pelvis and Hip Joint	26990-27299
Femur (Thigh Region) and Knee Joint	27301-27599
Leg (Tibia and Fibula) and Ankle Joint	27600-27899
Foot and Toes	28001-28899
Application of Casts and Strapping	29000-29799
Endoscopy/Arthroscopy	29800-29999

General (Codes 20005-20999)

The first heading in the Musculoskeletal System subsection is titled "General," which indicates that the codes have application to multiple body sites. The categories of codes include wound explorations, excisional biopsies, injections and aspirations, replantation of limbs and digits, bone grafts, and miscellaneous ("Other") procedures. While not every code from this section will be covered, many of the more challenging codes will be described in the following sections.

Incision

Code 20005 is reported for an incision and drainage of soft tissue abscess involving the soft tissue below the deep fascia. In this procedure, the physician makes an incision directly over the abscessed area. The incision goes through the skin and fascia and allows the abscess to drain. The physician may leave a drain in place or insert packing into the area.

Wound Exploration—Trauma

Codes 20100 through 20103 describe surgical exploration of penetrating traumatic injuries—gunshot or stab wounds, for example—involving the neck, chest, abdomen, flank, back, or an extremity. Notes preceding the codes detail the anatomical structures included in the exploration: subcutaneous tissue, muscle fascia, muscle, and minor muscular or subcutaneous blood vessels. Exploration procedures include the following:

- surgical exploration of the wound (making an incision to inspect);
- enlargement of the wound (making an incision that extends the wound to inspect);
- debridement of the wound (cleaning out debris);
- removal of a foreign body from the wound (taking out something that does not belong like a piece of gravel or a bullet); and
- ligation or coagulation of minor vessels (tying off or otherwise stopping bleeding).

Do not use codes 20100 through 20103 under certain circumstances:

- If a wound repair does not require 1 of the procedures listed above, choose a simple, intermediate, or complex wound closure procedure from codes 12001 through 13160 in the Integumentary System subsection.
- If the wound involves major blood vessels or structures, report the specific codes that describe the repair of the vessel or structure instead.
- If a laparotomy (opening up the abdomen) or a thoracotomy (opening up the chest) is performed for wound exploration, only the laparotomy or thoracotomy would be reported because it is a larger, more difficult surgical procedure that would include exploration.

EXAMPLE 10.1

A 19-year-old male was stabbed in the neck during a fight. His physical examination was otherwise normal. Because of the depth and location of the wound, he was taken to the OR for exploration under general anesthesia. The stab wound was extended and the damage assessed. The carotid artery and internal jugular vein appeared normal and were not injured. No major blood vessels or structures needed repair. The wound was debrided, and the muscle, subcutaneous layers, and skin were sutured. This procedure should be reported with code 20100, *Exploration of penetrating wound (separate procedure); neck.*

Excision

One code for excision of epiphyseal bar (end of a long bone that becomes ossified to the main bone) and multiple biopsy codes are found under the excision heading. Code 20150, *Excision of epiphyseal bar, with or without autogenous tissue graft obtained through same fascial incision*, is a procedure performed on a long bone (femur, tibia, fibula) to treat partial epiphyseal arrest. Codes for biopsy of muscle and bone (20200 through 20245) are differentiated by the technique (needle, open) and the depth (superficial, deep). Open vertebral body biopsies are differentiated by the anatomical site, either thoracic (reported with 20250), or lumbar or cervical (reported with 20251).

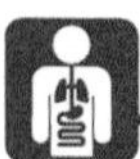

A&P Review

A tendon is a cord-like structure that attaches muscle to bone. The tendon origin is the proximal end of attachment (nearest the center of the body or the point of attachment of an extremity to the trunk). The insertion site of the tendon is the distal end (or away from the center of the body or point of attachment of the extremity).

Introduction or Removal

The Introduction or Removal category under the General heading includes codes 20500 through 20696 for therapeutic and diagnostic injection procedures, insertion of needles and catheters for subsequent therapy, removal of foreign bodies, joint aspiration, and application of external fixation devices.

Tendon Sheath or Ligament Injections

A common procedure in a physician's office is an injection of a therapeutic agent (usually a combination of an anesthetic and a corticosteroid) into tendons and ligaments to provide pain relief for the patient. Code 20550 is reported for single or multiple injections to a single tendon sheath, ligament, or aponeurosis (such as the plantar fascia, which supports the arch of the foot). Code 20551 is reported for single or multiple injections into a single tendon origin/insertion site. The tendon origin is the proximal end of attachment to the muscle, while the insertion site of the tendon is the distal end.

A&P Review

An aponeurosis is a flat sheet of dense fibrous connective tissue that connects a muscle to the body part that the muscle moves. Structurally similar to tendons and ligaments, *aponeurosis* is a term used to describe fascia. The aponeurosis that supports the arch on the bottom of the foot is commonly called the *plantar fascia*.

EXAMPLE 10.2

A 29-year-old male roofer presented to his physician complaining of neck and shoulder pain that he had been experiencing for several weeks. The physician suspected an inflammation of the acromioclavicular ligament, which attaches the acromion of the scapula to the clavicle. The patient did not respond to physical therapy, so a solution of an anesthetic and a corticosteroid was injected into the acromioclavicular ligament. This procedure should be reported with code 20550, *Injection(s); single tendon sheath, or ligament, aponeurosis (eg, plantar "fascia").*

LET'S TRY ONE **10.1**

Report the appropriate codes for each of the following scenarios.

1. A 54-year-old female office worker presented with complaints of persistent tennis elbow (lateral epicondylitis) due to frequent keyboard use. The physician injected a corticosteroid into the tendon. _____
2. A 62-year-old male gardener complained of persistent pain in his foot. The physician diagnosed plantar fasciitis and injected lidocaine and betamethasone into the plantar fascia. _____
3. A 43-year-old male presented with pain in his ankle. The physician performed a steroid injection into the tendon insertion site. _____
4. A patient complaining of right shoulder pain of several months' duration presented to his physician. The physician performed a single injection of a corticosteroid into the AC ligament in an attempt to ease the patient's pain. _____

Trigger Point Injections

Trigger points, also known as *muscle knots*, are spots of hypersensitive irritability within a band of muscle. They may form when acute or repetitive trauma overstresses the muscle fibers. The pain from 1 of these trigger points could be local (at the identified trigger point) or referred (in a different area than the trigger point). A physician identifies a trigger point by palpation or by using radiographic imaging and may choose to treat the trigger point with an injection of a therapeutic agent (anesthetic and corticosteroid). Figure 10.3 shows the codes for single or multiple trigger point injections, code 20552 for 1 or 2 muscles and code 20553 for 3 or more muscles. Codes 20552 and 20553 are reported only 1 time regardless of the number of injections.

Figure 10.3 Codes for Single or Multiple Trigger Point Injections

20552	Injection(s); single or multiple trigger point(s); 1 or 2 muscle(s)
20553	single or multiple trigger point(s), 3 or more muscle(s)

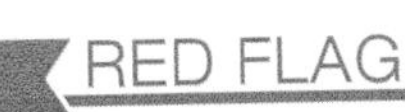

RED FLAG

You should report 1 tendon injection code for each injection site. Code trigger point injections based on the number of muscles injected, not the number of injections performed.

Coding for CMS

The Centers for Medicare and Medicaid Services (CMS) has issued a local coverage determination (LCD) for coverage criteria of "Injections—Tendon, Ligament, Ganglion Cyst, Tunnel Syndromes and Morton's Neuroma" (Medicare Coverage Database Number L24317). This document contains the diagnosis codes that meet medical necessity requirements. Injections into more than 2 sites in 1 session and frequent or repeated injections are likely to result in a request from CMS for health records.

Joint Aspirations and Injections

Another common procedure done in a physician's office is **arthrocentesis**, aspiration or draining of fluid from a joint. Joint aspiration and injection codes 20600 through 20611 are differentiated from one another by the size of the joint—small, intermediate, or major—and the use of ultrasound guidance. Figure 10.4 shows these codes. In the descriptor of the code, *and/or* indicates that the code includes either 1 or both of the procedures described (aspiration and injection). Therefore, if a physician aspirates fluid and then injects medication into the same joint, the code is reported only once. The drug injected is not included in the CPT® code, but it should be reported with a HCPCS Level II drug code.

Figure 10.4 Codes for Arthrocentesis

20600	Arthrocentesis, aspiration and/or injection, small joint or bursa (eg, fingers, toes); without ultrasound guidance
20604	with ultrasound guidance, with permanent recording and reporting
20605	Arthrocentesis, aspiration and/or injection, intermediate joint or bursa (eg, temporomandibular, acromioclavicular, wrist, elbow or ankle, olecranon bursa), without ultrasound guidance
20606	with ultrasound guidance, with permanent recording and reporting
20610	Arthrocentesis, aspiration and/or injection, major joint or bursa (eg, shoulder, hip, knee joint, subacromial bursa); without ultrasound guidance
20611	with ultrasound guidance, with permanent recording and reporting

LET'S TRY ONE **10.2**

Report the appropriate code(s) for each of the following procedures.

1. A 75-year-old male with bursitis of the knee presented to the office. The physician aspirated fluid and injected cortisone into the knee joint.

   _____

2. A 60-year-old female presented with a 3-month history of neck and back pain. The physician identified 3 trigger points by palpation. He performed 3 single lidocaine/corticosteroid injections on the 3 separate muscles. _____

3. A 40-year-old office worker suffering from pain and numbness due to carpal tunnel syndrome presented to the physician's office and received a cortisone injection into the carpal tunnel.

   _____

Replantation

Patients who have experienced traumatic amputation or severed digits or limbs may undergo a surgical reattachment of the body part. Codes 20802 through 20838 are used to report replantation when the body part was completely amputated. Replantation of incomplete amputations is reported with the specific codes for the repair of the bone, ligament, tendon, nerves, or blood vessels. Codes for replantation include reattachment of the severed nerves, blood vessels, tendons, muscles, and bones using sutures, wires, plates, or other fixation devices. Soft tissues and skin are joined with layered sutures. Replantation codes are differentiated by the body part with separate codes for the arm, forearm, hand, digits, thumb, and foot.

Grafts (or Implants)

Transplants of bone, cartilage, tendons, and fascia can help restore normal function after tissue is lost to injury or disease. Codes 20900 through 20939 describe the harvesting of autogenous (the patient's own) bone, cartilage, fascia lata (deep fascia of the thigh), tendons, and other tissues through separate incisions. These codes are reported separately in addition to the code for the transplant of the graft to the recipient site unless obtaining the graft is included in the code description for the primary procedure. Figure 10.5 contains an example of 1 such code under the Pelvis and Hip Joint codebook heading. Bone grafts obtained from a cadaver or bone bank are not reported using codes 20900 and 20902. Modifier 62, *Two Surgeons*, cannot be used with codes 20900 through 20938 as indicated in the tabular instructions.

Figure 10.5 Code for Bone Graft That Includes Obtaining the Bone Graft

27170	Bone graft, femoral head, neck, intertrochanteric or subtrochanteric area (includes obtaining bone graft)

Inside the OR

The harvesting of a small bone graft is reported with code 20900, *Bone graft, any donor area; minor or small (eg, dowel or button)*. In this procedure, the surgeon makes an incision over the donor site—that is, the area on the patient from which the autograft will be harvested. The incision is carried through the fascia and muscle, and the fascia and muscle are retracted. For a dowel graft or button graft, the surgeon uses special instrumentation to cut a circular piece of bone. The graft is then prepared for implantation. Finally, the incision is closed with sutures. If the graft is major (larger than a dowel or button), code 20902 should be reported instead.

Other Procedures

Procedures under the heading Other Procedures (codes 20950 through 20999) include bone grafts with microvascular anastomosis, ablation therapy for eradication for bone tumors, and an unlisted general musculoskeletal system procedure code (20999).

Anatomical Sites (Codes 21010-28899)

After presenting code categories that are broadly applicable to different body structures, the codebook presents categories for specific anatomical sites in the top down, center out scheme mentioned earlier. Categories of procedures specific to these sites will be presented next.

Incision

Procedure codes found under the Incision heading in any given anatomical site may include arthrotomy (creating an opening in a joint), incision and drainage of deep abscesses, and incision for contracture release. As a reminder, when an arthrotomy is performed as the operative approach, a separate code is not reported for that incision. Only the code for the surgical procedure that was accomplished is reported.

Excision

Procedure codes found under the Excision heading in any given anatomical site may include biopsies, excision of tumors or other musculoskeletal lesions, bones, and partial or radical resections.

Introduction or Removal

Procedure codes found under the Introduction or Removal heading in any given anatomical site may include codes for injection procedures for arthrography (images of a joint after being injected with contrast medium) and removal of foreign bodies, prosthesis, implants, and fixation devices. It should be noted that the neck and spine do not have a heading for introduction or removal, and these types of procedures are incorporated under other headings. Other codes such as manipulation, wrist under anesthesia (25259) are included under the introduction or removal heading.

Repair, Revision, and/or Reconstruction

The codes for repair, revision, and/or reconstruction appear under each anatomical heading with the exception of Back and Flank and Spine (Vertebral Column). The specialized spinal surgical techniques are categorized by different terminology. Codes located in the Repair, Revision, and/or Reconstruction category include many different surgical techniques. Some of the more common procedures are arthroplasties. Also discussed are the special challenges of coding procedures that are named for the person who originated the technique, as with bunion repairs.

Arthroplasty

Arthroplasty is the repair and/or replacement of a joint, a common orthopedic procedure performed on patients with osteoarthritis or degenerative joint disease when more conservative medical treatment is unsuccessful. Partial and total knee and hip replacements are very common types of arthroplasty in the United States—according to the Centers for Disease Control and Prevention (CDC), over a million knee and hip replacement operations were completed in 2010 alone. Figure 10.6 illustrates the steps for a total hip arthroplasty procedure.

Figure 10.6 Total Hip Arthroplasty

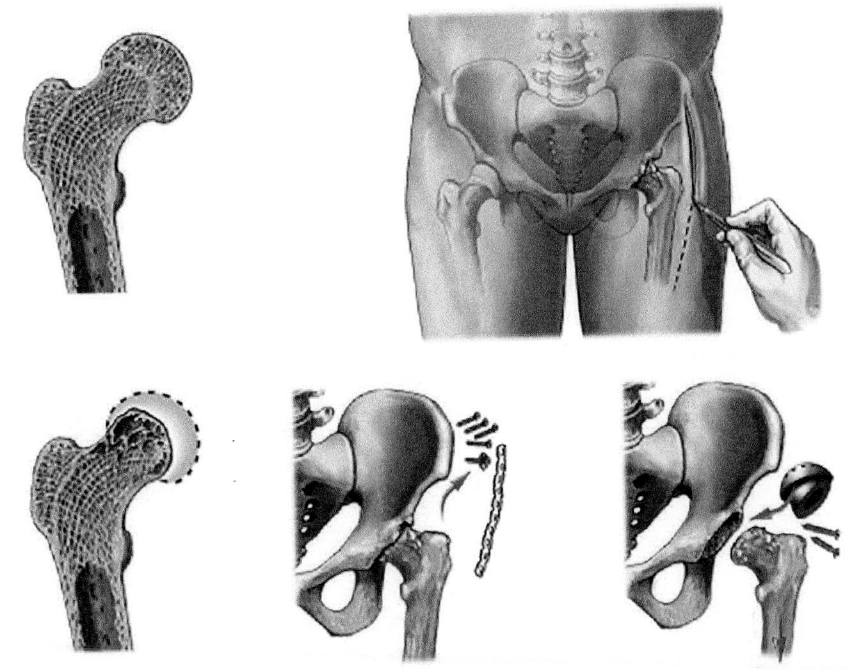

Inside the OR

To perform a total hip replacement, the surgeon makes an incision along the hip, exposing the joint capsule. The hip is dislocated and the femoral head is removed with a saw. Osteophytes are removed, the acetabulum is reamed out (the hole is widened), and the acetabular replacement is inserted. The femoral shaft is prepared and a stem is pounded into place. The hip is repositioned and the muscles reattached. The incision is repaired in layers and the procedure is completed. In a partial hip replacement, the femoral neck is removed and replaced, but the acetabulum is not.

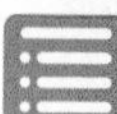

Index Insider

To find the code for a total hip replacement, complete the following steps:

1. Turn to the Index and find the main term *Arthroplasty*.
2. Look for the subterm *Hip* and then find the subterm *Total Replacement* under *Hip*. You will see code 27130 listed, as shown in Figure 10.7.
3. Turn to the tabular list and find code 27130. Read the description (shown in Figure 10.8) to determine if this is the correct code.
4. Report the code you have chosen along with any applicable modifier.

Arthroplasty codes for most anatomical headings throughout the Musculoskeletal System subsection are organized under the category Repair, Revision, and/or Reconstruction. Spinal arthroplasties that involve vertebral disc replacement are found in the Spinal Instrumentation category. Codes for arthroplasty may be indexed under the main term *Arthroplasty* or under the name of the specific joint. Figure 10.7 shows the arthroplasty entry in the Index. Figure 10.8 illustrates the code for total hip replacement.

Figure 10.7 Entry for Arthroplasty in the Alphabetic Index

Arthroplasty
Ankle 27700-27703
Elbow 24360-24363
    Revision 24370-24371
Hip 27132
    Partial Replacement 27125
    Revision 27134-27138
    Total Replacement 27130

Figure 10.8 Code for Total Hip Replacement Surgery

27130 Arthroplasty, acetabular and proximal femoral prosthetic replacement (total hip arthroplasty), with or without autograft or allograft

LET'S TRY ONE **10.3**

Read the following scenario and then answer the questions that follow.

A 55-year-old male underwent a right total knee replacement due to advanced osteoarthritis. A hinge prosthesis was used.

1. What code should be reported for this procedure? _____
2. What modifier should be used to indicate that this procedure was done on the right knee? _____

Eponyms for Surgical Procedures

Rather than describing a surgical procedure, some codes simply reference an **eponym**, a name of a person to whom a procedure is attributed. It becomes important to cross-reference the description of the service in the operative report with the codebook name for the operation. An example of a repair that has multiple eponymous procedure names is a hallux valgus correction, and the codebook provides illustrations to differentiate the surgical operations.

The medical term for *bunion* is **hallux valgus**, which refers to an enlargement of the base of the metatarsophalangeal joint of the big (great) toe. Bunions are sometimes caused by wearing shoes (such as high heels) that put pressure on the toes or squeeze them together. When this happens, the big toe may angle inward, causing the toes to overlap and creating pain and inflammation. A **bunionectomy** is a repair of a bunion by removing bone, which relieves pain and realigns the joint. Figure 10.9 shows before, during, and after images of a bunion repair procedure.

Figure 10.9 Bunion Repair Procedure

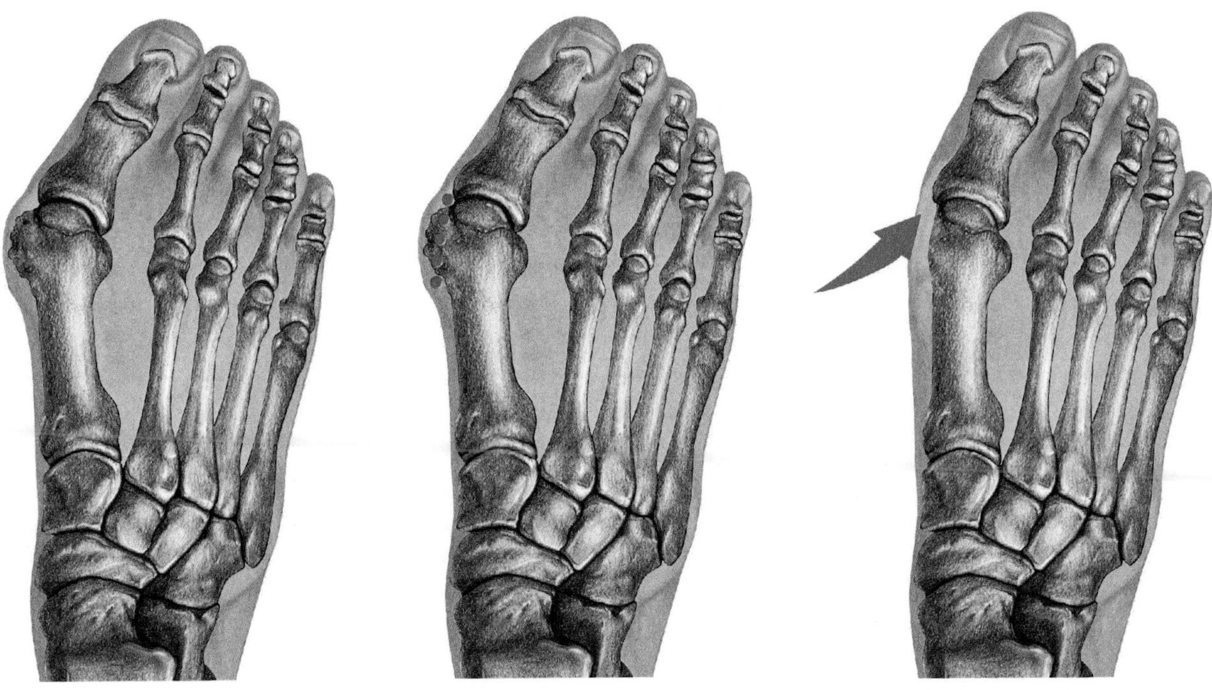

Bunion repair codes are differentiated from one another based on the complexity of the procedure and the use of implants. The CPT® codebook includes a wide range of bunion procedures (codes 28292 through 28299). Some may include revision of the metatarsal shaft, metatarsal head, or other surrounding structures. Use the illustrations in the CPT® codebook to guide your code assignment. A simple resection of the medial eminence is called a *Silver bunionectomy*, described in code 28292. A podiatric surgeon may also correct a bunion using a Chevron, Joplin, Keller, Lapidus, Mayo, McBride, or Mitchell type procedure. In these types of procedures, the surgeon first makes an incision along the medial aspect of the big toe. The incision is then deepened down to the metatarsophalangeal joint. At this point, each procedure has different elements that must be correlated with the operative report, as illustrated in the Keller, Mayo, and McBride techniques:

- In a Keller procedure, the base of the proximal phalanx and the medial eminence are resectioned. Kirschner wire (K-wire) may be used to hold the joint in place.
- In a Mayo procedure, the metatarsal head is removed, and excision of the medial exostosis is performed.
- In a McBride procedure, an incision is made between the first and second toe to release ligaments. The metatarsophalangeal joint is reduced, and the medial eminence is resected. A medial incision is made so the medial capsule of the joint can be imbricated (overlapped, like fish scales).

There are several ways to locate the codes for bunion repair. They may be found in the Index under the main term *Bunion Repair*, the name of the procedure (eg, *Keller*), or under the more general main terms *Repair* or *Toe*.

Foot Procedures

Another common foot procedure is a **cheilectomy**, which is a surgery performed to correct **hallux rigidus**, a stiffness caused by a bone spur that prevents movement in the big toe. Hallux rigidus is usually caused by arthritis. During a cheilectomy, a part of the lip of the first metatarsophalangeal joint is excised to remove the bone spurs and bone overgrowth that cause pain. Part of the metatarsal head is also removed. This procedure is reported with code 28289, *Hallux rigidus correction with cheilectomy, debridement and capsular release of the first metatarsophalangeal joint.*

LET'S TRY ONE **10.4**

Assign the correct code (and modifier, if applicable) for each of the following procedures.

1. Mayo bunionectomy, right foot: _____
2. Silver procedure with sesamoidectomy, right foot: _____
3. Hallux rigidus correction with joint implant, left foot: _____
4. Cheilectomy right foot and capsular release for hallux rigidus correction: _____

RED FLAG

Remember that fracture care is coded by treatment, not by the type of fracture.

Fracture Care

Fracture care codes are included in the Fracture and/or Dislocation category under each anatomical heading throughout the Musculoskeletal System subsection. Codes are differentiated by the site of the fracture and the use of manipulation and stabilization. In other words, codes are assigned according to the type of treatment given and not by the type of fracture. Important terms to know when reporting codes for fracture care include closed treatment, open treatment, and percutaneous skeletal fixation, defined in the guidelines at the beginning of the Musculoskeletal System subsection in the CPT® codebook and discussed below.

Caring for a fracture via **closed treatment** means that the surgeon does not expose the bone or directly view the fracture to provide care. The surgeon may treat the fracture by manipulating the fracture fragments into place without making an incision into the skin. Closed treatment is the preferred method of fracture care because it decreases the risk of infection and recovery time for the patient when compared to open treatment. The physician may choose local, regional, or general anesthesia, depending on the site of the fracture and the patient's condition. Closed reduction of the fracture may also take place prior to an open treatment. A **closed reduction** is the manipulation of the fractured bone to return it to the proper alignment by simply pushing the fracture back into place.

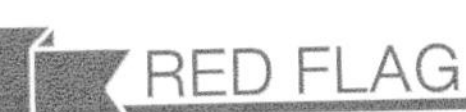

RED FLAG

The term *manipulation*, used throughout the Fracture and/or Dislocation category, has the same meaning as *reduction*.

Caring for a fracture via **open treatment** means that the fracture site is either surgically opened so that the surgeon can see the bone, or an incision is made away from the fracture site so that an internal fixation device can be inserted across the fracture site. In the latter instance, even if the fracture site itself is not opened and visualized, the treatment is still considered to be open. Surgeons may use **open reduction** when they are unable to reduce a fracture with closed treatment. An example is a **comminuted** fracture in which the bone is broken into more than 2 pieces.

Coding Clicks

Watch a video of the surgical repair of an ankle fracture at http://Coding.ParadigmEducation.com/AnkleFracture.

A third treatment option involves accessing areas of the body through the skin. **Percutaneous skeletal fixation** uses needle punctures in the placement of fixation devices. **Internal fixation** devices such as pins, screws, metal plates, wires, or rods are usually placed with the use of image guidance. Figure 10.10 shows a postoperative image of a patient with multiple fractures that have been repaired using several types of internal fixation: screws, rods, and nails. **External fixation** refers to using skeletal pins or screws attached to a device outside the skin to realign the bone. Figure 10.11 shows the use of external fixation for a fracture of the tibia and fibula.

Fracture care codes may be indexed under various main terms: *Fracture*, the name of the bone, or the procedure. For example, to find the code for an open reduction with internal fixation (ORIF) of the shaft of the tibia (27758), you may start in the Index with the main term *Fracture*, the main entry for the *Tibia* bone, or the main entry for *Fixation* procedures.

CONCEPTS CHECKPOINT **10.2**

Answer true or false to each of the following statements.

1. _____ The type of fracture (open, compound, or closed) does not have any coding correlation with the type of fracture care given.
2. _____ In an open treatment, the fracture site may be surgically opened to expose the bone.
3. _____ Manipulation has the same meaning as fixation, per the CPT® guidelines.

Figure 10.10 Postoperative Radiograph Showing the Use of Internal Fixation

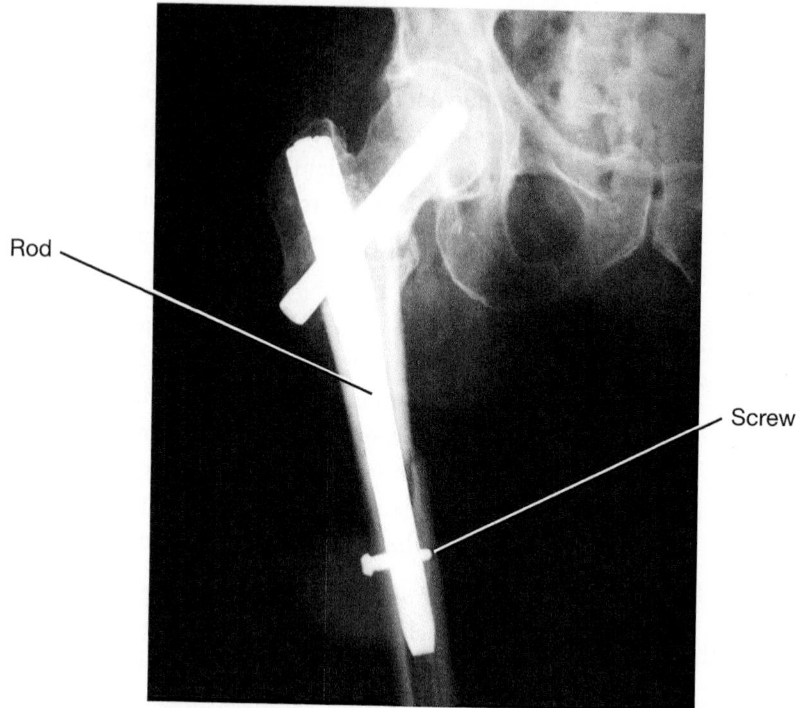

Figure 10.11 External Fixation for a Fracture of the Tibia and Fibula

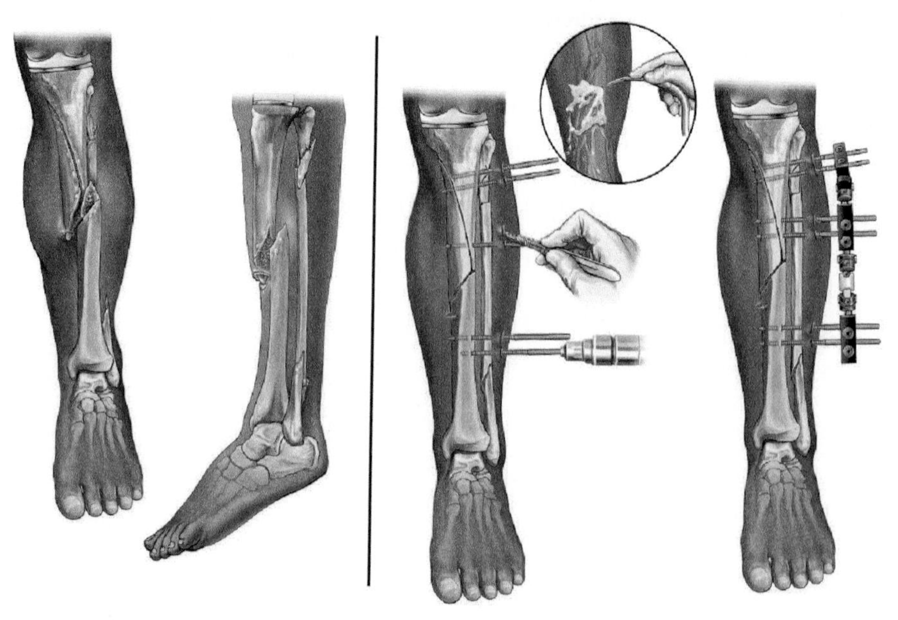

EXAMPLE 10.3

A 12-year-old girl presented to the emergency department (ED) complaining of pain in her right wrist and forearm after falling from her skateboard. A radiograph revealed slightly displaced fractures of the radial and ulnar shafts. The patient was referred to an orthopedic specialist for treatment. The orthopedic surgeon assessed the patient, performed a closed reduction, and applied a short-arm cast. Follow these steps to find the correct code for this procedure:

1. Turn to the Index and find the main term *Fracture*.
2. Look for the subterm *Radius* and then find the subterm *Closed Treatment* under *Radius*. You will see the range of codes 25560 through 25565.
3. Turn to the tabular list and locate the code range identified for closed treatment of a fracture of the radius. Read through the descriptions of codes 25560 and 25565 and determine which code best fits the scenario described above.

This patient had a closed reduction of a radial and ulnar shaft fracture, which means code 25565, *Closed treatment of radial and ulnar shaft fractures; with manipulation*, should be reported. The RT modifier is also assigned, as the documentation specifies that the right arm was fractured. The final code is formatted as 25565 - RT. The orthopedic surgeon would also charge the appropriate level of E/M code for this patient, as it was a new injury, with modifier 57 for decision for surgery.

LET'S TRY ONE 10.5

Read the scenario below and then answer the questions that follow.

A 44-year-old male fell off a tractor and fractured his right fibula and tibia shaft. He received open treatment, during which multiple screws were placed.

1. What code would be reported for this procedure? ______
2. What modifier is appropriate? ______

Manipulation

The procedure codes found under the Manipulation heading are reported when manipulation is performed under general anesthesia. Not all anatomical sites have a separate heading for manipulation procedures. Manipulation codes are not reported for fracture care. Manipulation may be performed when the patient has a stiff joint (also called a *frozen joint*). The physician pushes and pulls on the limb and may temporarily apply a traction device to help restore movement. For example, code 27860, *Manipulation of ankle under general anesthesia (includes application of traction or other fixation apparatus)*, is reported when the patient is placed under general anesthesia, and the physician maneuvers the foot, ankle, and leg to treat a stiff ankle.

Arthrodesis

Arthrodesis (joint fusion) that is performed as an open procedure (not arthroscopic) is reported with codes found under the Arthrodesis heading in the specific anatomical

exist. There are 19 separate codes for arthroscopic knee procedures, including synovectomy, meniscectomy, debridement, and repairs, and it is possible that a patient may undergo more than 1 procedure during an operative episode. Make sure to read the operative notes carefully to determine the specific procedures accomplished during the operative episode. It is not appropriate to report an arthroscopic procedure with a code for an open procedure. If an unlisted arthroscopic procedure is performed, code 29999, *Unlisted procedure, arthroscopy,* should be reported.

Inside the OR

A surgical arthroscopy with shaving of articular cartilage is shown in Figure 10.12. To perform this procedure, the surgeon makes a 1-cm incision on either side of the patellar tendon to insert the arthroscope. He or she then uses the arthroscope and a probe to identify lesions on the cartilage. The cartilage is debrided using a motorized suction cutter or shaver, the joint is flushed, and a temporary drain may be inserted. The incisions are closed with sutures and covered with sterile bandages.

Figure 10.12 Knee Arthroscopy With Shaving of Articular Cartilage

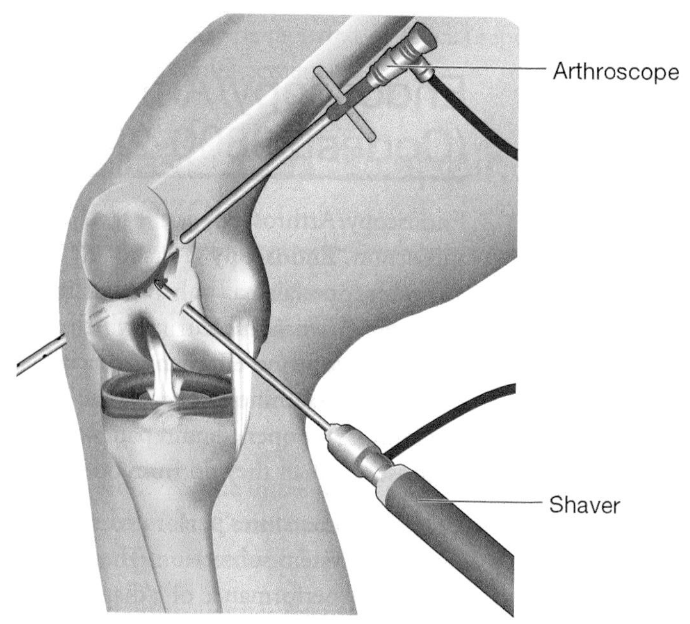

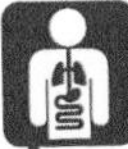

A&P Review

A retinaculum is a fibrous band of fascia that holds tendons in place to stabilize them. The knee contains 2 retinacula: the lateral retinaculum (located on the outer side of the kneecap) and the medial patellar retinaculum (located in the inner side of the kneecap, medial meaning the middle of the body).

Codes for arthroscopy are indexed under the main term *Arthroscopy*, the anatomical site, or the name of the specific procedure (eg, *Meniscectomy*). To find the code for the knee procedure described in *Inside the OR* on the previous page, you can look in the Index under several main terms, making sure you focus on the arthroscopic procedure:

- Under the main entry *Arthroscopy*, there are 2 subterms, *Diagnostic* and *Surgical*; you are looking for a surgical arthroscopic procedure, so find *Knee* under the subterm *Surgical*;
- Start with the main entry *Knee* and find the subterm *Arthroscopy* and its subterm *Surgical*.

In both locations, the Index lists codes from the Endoscopy/Arthroscopy heading. Do not search for the codes using a constituent of the surgical procedure—for example, under the main entry *Debridement*; this is not the main procedure performed, and the codes listed there will incorrectly lead you to open procedures. When a procedure was accomplished arthroscopically, always be sure you are choosing an arthroscopic code.

CONCEPTS CHECKPOINT **10.4**

Answer true or false to each of the following statements.

1. _____ Codes for surgical arthroscopy include the performance of diagnostic arthroscopy.
2. _____ It is never appropriate to report multiple arthroscopic procedure codes for the same operative episode.
3. _____ Codes for arthroscopy and arthrotomy cannot be reported together.

LET'S TRY ONE **10.6**

Read the scenario below and then answer the questions that follow.

A healthy 29-year-old football player presented to his physician with bilateral patellofemoral pain syndrome with patellar malalignment. He was taken to surgery, where bilateral arthroscopic retinacular releases were performed. After arthroscopic inspection, a Beaver blade was introduced through the anteromedial port. With this blade, the lateral retinaculum was released, providing satisfactory mobilization of the patella. The identical procedure was completed on the left and right knees.

1. What arthroscopic surgical procedure was completed in this scenario? _____
2. What is the correct code for this procedure? _____
3. Which CPT® modifier should be used to indicate that this was a bilateral procedure? _____

Chapter Summary

- Most of the codes in the Musculoskeletal System Surgery subsection are arranged by body site and then categorized by procedure.
- Wound exploration codes are used to report surgical exploration and enlargement of traumatic wounds involving subcutaneous tissue, muscle fascia, muscle, and minor blood vessels.
- Harvesting autogenous bone grafts through separate incisions may be reported in addition to the code for the graft unless otherwise specified in the code description.
- Multiple injections to tendons or trigger points may be reported with a single code.
- Joint aspiration and injection to the same location is reported with a single code, which depends on the size of the joint.
- Codes for arthroplasty are found under the Repair, Revision, and/or Reconstruction heading throughout the Musculoskeletal System Surgery subsection and are differentiated by anatomical site and use of implant material.
- Procedures may be described by an eponym, as in the case of bunion repair codes, which describe multiple techniques.
- Fracture care codes are assigned according to the anatomical site and the type of care given.
- Fracture care codes are differentiated by the type of manipulation and stabilization.
- Initial cast application is included in the fracture care codes. Replacement casts may be coded separately.
- Application of a cast or strapping to immobilize a fracture is coded separately when no fracture care is provided.
- A diagnostic arthroscopy is always included in a surgical arthroscopy and is not reported separately.

Navigator

Access interactive chapter review exercises, practice activities, flash cards, and study games.

Chapter 11

Surgery Coding: Respiratory System

Fast Facts

- While most people can hold their breath for only 30 to 60 seconds, some can do so for much longer. A man from Denmark holds the world record for holding his breath; he held his breath underwater for 22 minutes!
- Pranayama, an ancient form of yoga, comes from the Sanskrit word meaning "extension of the breath." The breathing exercises practiced in Pranayama may be beneficial in reducing stress.
- The average adult breathes between 12 and 20 times per minute.

Sources: Livescience, http://yogahealthcenter.net/pranayama

Crack the Code

Review the sample operative report to find the correct respiratory system code. You may need to return to this exercise after reading the chapter content.

PREOPERATIVE DIAGNOSIS:
Probable bronchiectasis, right lower lobe, rule out unusual infections

POSTOPERATIVE DIAGNOSIS:
Evidence of bronchitis, no other abnormality seen

OPERATION: Bronchoscopy with washings

PROCEDURE: The patient was taken to the endoscopy suite as an outpatient. The nose and hypopharynx were anesthetized with Pontocaine. Following satisfactory anesthesia, the bronchoscope was passed transnasally without difficulty. The hypopharynx, epiglottis, and cords were normal and moved normally. Trachea was normal without signs of deviation or compression. The carina was sharp and pulsatile. Both right and left tracheobronchial tree were inspected to the subsegmental level. There was some erythema and friability of the mucosa in the right middle and right lower lobe area and mild mucopurulent secretions. Other than the above findings, the tracheobronchial tree was normal without evidence of neoplasm or bleeding. Specimens were obtained for cytology and microbiologic studies. The patient tolerated the procedure well without complications.

answer: 31622

Learning Objectives

11.1 Recognize the anatomical structures in the respiratory system.

11.2 Explain specialized respiratory system surgical terminology.

11.3 Describe the arrangement of codes in the Respiratory System surgery subsection of the CPT® codebook.

11.4 Apply the use of symbols, guidelines, and instructional notes in coding respiratory procedures.

11.5 Apply appropriate modifiers when coding respiratory surgical procedures.

11.6 Differentiate between simple and extensive polyps.

11.7 Differentiate between an indirect and direct laryngoscopy.

11.8 Determine when codes that include the use of an operating microscope should be reported.

11.9 Differentiate between diagnostic and therapeutic procedures.

11.10 Explain the importance of reviewing the full operative report when coding respiratory surgical procedures.

11.11 Code respiratory system surgical procedures.

Chapter Outline

3-D
To explore the respiratory system in the BioDigital Human, go to: http://Coding.ParadigmEducation.com/BioDigital_Respiratory.

Introduction to the Respiratory System

The respiratory system is divided into the upper respiratory system and the lower respiratory system. The upper respiratory system is composed of the nose, nasal cavity, paranasal sinuses, and larynx. The lower respiratory system is composed of the trachea, bronchial tree, and lungs. Figure 11.1 shows the components of the respiratory system.

The **nose** is the protruding part of the human face where the nostrils are located and consists of cartilage, the nasal septum, and the nasal cavity. Around the nasal cavity is a network of sinuses, which the codebook refers to as the **accessory sinuses**.

The **larynx** lies between the pharynx and the trachea and contains the vocal cords. The **arytenoid cartilages** are a pair of pyramid-shaped structures that form part of the larynx where the vocal cords are attached. The **pharynx** is a large cavity formed by the facial bones, as shown in Figure 11.1. The pharynx is divided into the nasopharynx, the oropharynx, and the laryngopharynx. The **nasopharynx** lies posterior to the nasal cavity. The **oropharynx** is the area of the throat at the back of the mouth where the passageway for food and air and the tonsils are located. The tonsils are part of the lymphatic system and work with the adenoids of the nasopharynx to prevent organisms that cause infections from entering the lower respiratory system. The distal portion of the pharynx is the **laryngopharynx**. The **epiglottis** is a flap of cartilage attached to the muscles of the larynx. The epiglottis covers the trachea when a person swallows to prevent choking.

Figure 11.1 Components of the Respiratory System

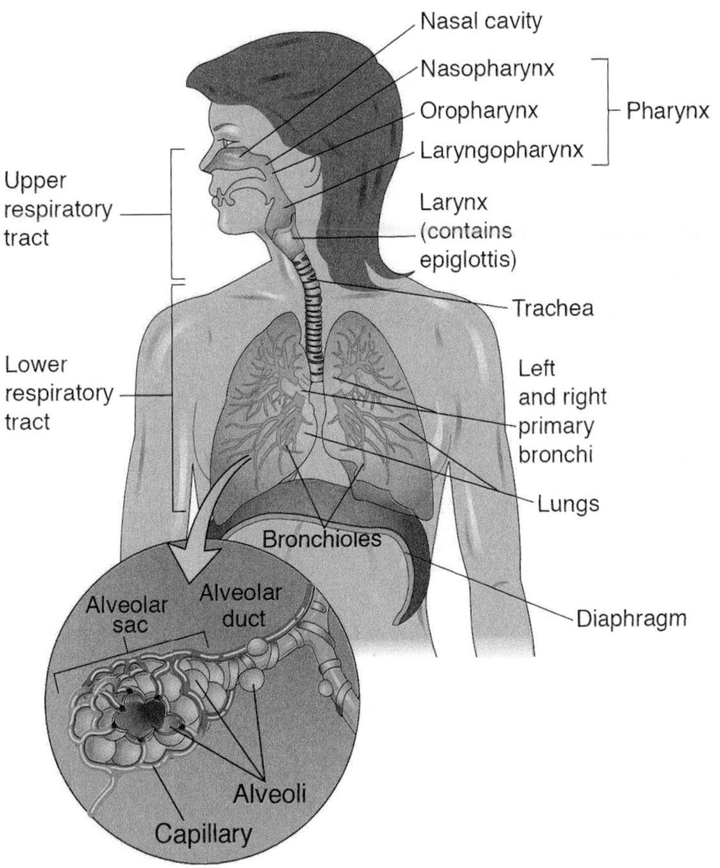

The **trachea** is the airway that connects the larynx to the **bronchi**. The bronchi conduct air into the lungs. The **lungs** are 2 organs that bring oxygen to the blood and remove carbon dioxide from the body. The right lung has 3 lobes and the left lung has 2 lobes. The **pleura** is the double-folded membrane that covers each lung and lines the thoracic cavity. The **diaphragm** is the muscular partition that separates the thoracic cavity from the abdominal cavity. Table 11.1 lists the structures in the respiratory system.

Table 11.1 Respiratory System Structures

Structure	Description
nose	Midface structure that includes the nostrils and nasal septum
sinuses	Air cavities within the cranial bone that open into the nasal cavity
larynx	Tube-shaped organ located between the pharynx and the trachea containing the vocal cords
pharynx	The throat, or cavity, behind the mouth
nasopharynx	The upper part of the throat behind the nose
oropharynx	The area of the throat at the back of the mouth
epiglottis	Flap of cartilage that covers the trachea while swallowing
trachea	The airway that connects the larynx to the primary bronchi
bronchi	The tubes that conduct air into the lungs
lungs	Two organs that bring oxygen to the blood and remove carbon dioxide
pleura	Membrane that covers each lung and lines the thoracic cavity
diaphragm	The muscular partition that separates the thoracic cavity from the abdominal cavity

Respiratory System Surgical Terminology

Table 11.2 presents anatomical terms, word roots, and terminology used frequently in documentation for procedures on the respiratory system.

Table 11.2 Respiratory System Surgical Terminology

Term	Definition
antrum	Cavity within a bone
antrotomy	Cutting through the antrum wall to make an opening in the sinus
bronchoscopy	Endoscopic inspection of the bronchial tree using a bronchoscope
embolectomy	Removal of blockage from vessels
endoscopy	Inspection of body organs or cavities using a lighted scope, placed through an existing opening or a small incision
lobectomy	Excision of a lobe of the lung
pneum/o	Word root meaning *lung* or *air*
polyp	Tumor-like growth on a stalk that bleeds easily and may become malignant
rhin/o	Word root meaning *nose*
thoracentesis	Surgical puncture of the thoracic cavity to remove fluid
thoracoscopy	Use of a lighted endoscope to view pleural spaces and thoracic cavity or perform surgical procedures
thoracostomy	Cutting into the chest cavity to place tube for drainage
thoracotomy	Surgical incision into the chest cavity

CONCEPTS CHECKPOINT 11.1

Match the term in the first column with the definition in the second column.

1. _____ antrotomy
2. _____ bronchoscopy
3. _____ endoscopy
4. _____ lobectomy
5. _____ thoracentesis

a. Excision of a lobe of the lung
b. Surgical puncture of the thoracic cavity to remove fluids
c. Inspection of body organs or cavities using a lighted scope, placed through an existing opening or through a small incision
d. Inspection of the bronchial tree using a bronchoscope
e. Cutting through the antrum wall to make an opening in the sinus

Organization of the Respiratory System Surgery Subsection

The codes in the Respiratory System subsection of the CPT® codebook are arranged by anatomical site from nose to lungs. Table 11.3 provides a list of the anatomical site headings and the associated code numbers.

Table 11.3 Headings Within the Respiratory System Surgery Subsection of the CPT® Codebook

Heading	Code Numbers
Nose	30000-30999
Accessory Sinuses	31000-31299
Larynx	31300-31599
Trachea and Bronchi	31600-31899
Lungs and Pleura	32035-32999

In general, under each anatomical site heading, codes are sequenced by procedural categories that can include Incision, Excision, Introduction, Repair, Removal of Foreign Body, Endoscopy, Destruction, and Other Procedures. This chapter will identify the types of surgical procedures within each category and discuss those procedures that are common or have multiple coding criteria.

Nose (Codes 30000-30999)

The shape of the nose is formed by the ethmoid bone and the nasal septum that separates the right and left nostrils.

Categories and Procedures for the Nose

Procedures and their codes found under the Nose heading are organized by the categories listed in Table 11.4.

Table 11.4 Nose Procedures and Codes

Codebook Category	Surgical Procedure(s)	Code(s)
Incision	Drainage of abscess or hematoma	30000-30020
Excision	Biopsy	30100
	Cyst, lesion, or polyp excision/destruction	30100-30118, 30124-30125
	Excision of structures	30120, 30130-30140
	Rhinectomy	30150-30160
Introduction	Injection, therapeutic	30200
	Displacement therapy	30210
	Insertion, nasal prosthesis	30220
Removal of Foreign Body	Removal of foreign body	30300-30320
Repair	Rhinoplasty	30400-30462
	Repair, nasal vestibular stenosis	30465
	Septoplasty	30520
	Repair, choanal atresia	30540-30545
	Lysis, intranasal synechia	30560
	Repair, fistula	30580-30600
	Dermatoplasty	30620
	Repair, nasal septum perforations	30630
Destruction	Ablation	30801-30802
Other Procedures	Control of hemorrhage	30901-30906
	Arterial ligation	30915-30920
	Therapeutic fracture	30930
	Unlisted procedure, nose	30999

Codes for treatment of traumatic nasal fractures are found in the Musculoskeletal System surgery subsection.

Coding Common Procedures of the Nose

Discussed here are 2 of the most common nasal surgery procedures, excision of polyps and rhinoplasty.

Excision of Polyps

Nasal polyps are soft, noncancerous growths that may block airway passages and prevent drainage, requiring removal. **Polypectomy** is excision of nasal polyps. A simple excision of easily removed polyps may be performed in an office setting and is reported with code 30110. Excision of nasal polyps that are extensive or more difficult to remove would normally require a facility setting (outpatient or ambulatory surgery center) and is reported with code 30115. Large polyps may be removed with the use of a wire snare: the snare stretches the polyp base, and then the snare or a scalpel is used to detach the polyp. Larger excisions may leave defects in the mucosa (mucous membrane lining); these defects are closed with sutures in a single layer. One code is reported regardless of the number of polyps removed. If the procedure is done bilaterally, modifier 50, *Bilateral procedure*, is reported.

EXAMPLE **11.1**

A 61-year-old male with a history of nasal polyps presented to his physician's office complaining of chronic allergies and loss of smell. A simple polypectomy was performed in the office removing 2 small polyps from inside the right side of the nose. This is reported with code 30110-RT, *Excision, nasal polyp(s); simple - right side*.

Rhinoplasty

Rhinoplasty is surgery to reshape the external and/or internal nose. Rhinoplasties may be performed using an open or closed technique. In an open procedure, the surgeon makes external skin incisions. In a closed procedure, the surgeon makes incisions within the nose. The approach to accomplish the rhinoplasty does not affect code assignment. Rhinoplasty codes located in the Repair category of the codebook are differentiated by the extent of the work done and whether it was a primary or secondary surgery.

A **primary rhinoplasty** is defined as the first time the patient has undergone rhinoplasty. The codes that pertain to these procedures are the following:

- Code 30400, *Rhinoplasty, primary; lateral and alar cartilages and/or elevation of nasal tip*, is reported when the surgeon reshapes cartilage. Fat may also be removed. The nasal tip may be elevated.
- Code 30410, *Rhinoplasty, primary; complete, external parts including bony pyramid, lateral and alar cartilages, and/or elevation of nasal tip*, is reported when both bone and cartilage are reshaped.
- Code 30420, *Rhinoplasty, primary; including major septal repair*, is reported when the surgeon reshapes both the external and internal nose. A fractured or deformed nasal septum is reshaped in this procedure. Septal cartilage may be removed or grafted. Nasal bones are also repositioned.

A **secondary rhinoplasty** is a revision of an original rhinoplasty to correct unfavorable results. Secondary rhinoplasty codes are separated into minor, intermediate, or major revisions as follows:

- Code 30430, *Rhinoplasty, secondary; minor revision (small amount of nasal tip work)*, is reported when the cartilages and nasal tip may be reduced by trimming or enlarged by grafting.

- Code 30435, *Rhinoplasty, secondary; intermediate revision (bony work with osteotomies)*, includes incision into bone (osteotomy). The nasal bones are repositioned in this procedure.
- Code 30450, *Rhinoplasty, secondary; major revision (nasal tip work and osteotomies)*, includes both the nasal tip work and osteotomies. Local bone grafts obtained from adjacent nasal bones are not reported separately.

Codes 30460 and 30462 are rhinoplasty procedures to correct deformities associated with a congenital cleft lip and/or palate condition.

EXAMPLE **11.2**

A 51-year-old female had an elective rhinoplasty and was unhappy with the results. She returned to her surgeon asking for a smaller nasal tip. The surgeon took her back to surgery and trimmed the cartilage and nasal tip. This secondary procedure is considered a minor revision since only nasal tip work was performed. Code 30430, *Rhinoplasty, secondary; minor revision*, is reported.

LET'S TRY ONE **11.1**

A 22-year-old female, an aspiring actress, was unhappy with the appearance of her nose. She requested a reduction in the wideness and elevation of the tip so she would resemble her favorite actress, Nicole Kidman. The plastic surgeon reshaped the cartilage after removing fat from the nose. Elevation of the nasal tip was performed.

What is the appropriate code for this procedure? _____

Accessory Sinuses (Codes 31000-31299)

The accessory sinuses or **paranasal sinuses** are air cavities within the cranial bone that open into the nasal cavity. There are 4 pairs of sinuses. As shown in Figure 11.2, the **maxillary sinuses** are in the maxillary bone located under the eyes. The **frontal sinuses** are in the frontal bone located just above the eyes. The **ethmoid sinuses** are between the nose and the eyes. The **sphenoid sinuses** are behind the nasal cavity at the base of the skull. The **septum** is a thin partition that separates the nostrils.

Figure 11.2 Paranasal Sinuses

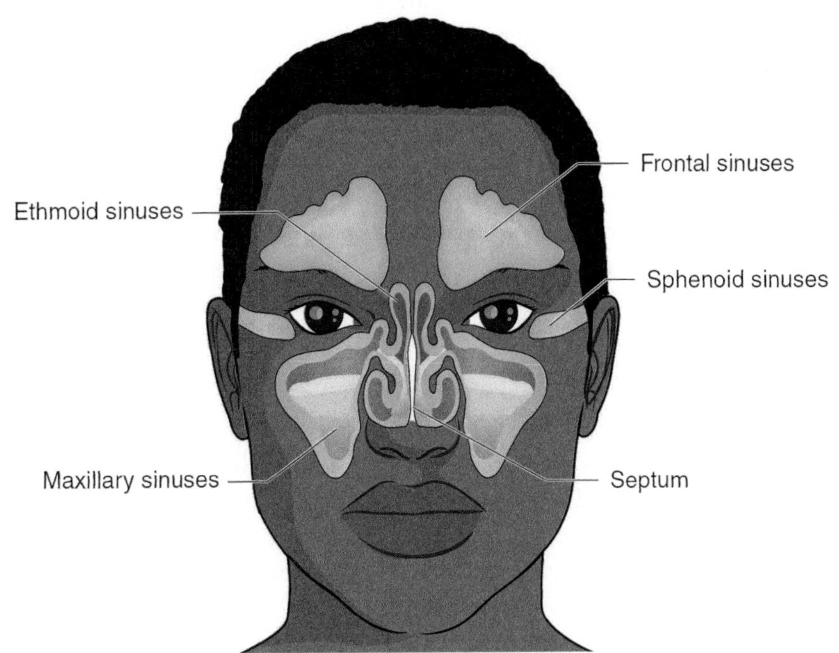

Categories and Procedures for the Accessory Sinuses

Procedures and their codes found under the Accessory Sinuses heading are organized by the categories listed in Table 11.5.

Table 11.5 Accessory Sinus Procedures and Codes

Codebook Category	Surgical Procedure(s)	Code(s)
Incision	Lavage	31000-31002
	Sinusotomy	31020-31032, 31050-31090
	Pterygomaxillary fossa surgery	31040
Excision	Ethmoidectomy	31200-31205
	Maxillectomy	31225-31230
Endoscopy	Diagnostic nasal/sinus endoscopy	31231-31235
	Surgical nasal/sinus endoscopy	31237-31298
Other Procedures	Unlisted procedure, accessory sinuses	31299

Coding Common Procedures of the Accessory Sinuses

The particular challenges of coding nasal/sinus endoscopies will be discussed in depth.

Nasal/Sinus Endoscopy

An **endoscopy** is an inspection of body organs or cavities using a lighted scope, placed through an existing opening or a small incision. Diagnostic and therapeutic nasal or sinus endoscopies are reported with codes 31231 through 31297. The surgical endoscopy codes are differentiated by the procedure accomplished, and multiple codes may be reported. The codes are assumed to be unilateral (on 1 side) unless otherwise specified. A surgical endoscopy always includes a diagnostic endoscopy.

Codes 31231 through 31235 are reported for diagnostic sinus endoscopies in which an endoscope is inserted through 1 of the nostrils to view the sinuses. An inspection of the nasal cavity, middle and superior meatus (opening), the turbinates (long, narrow, curled bone that directs airflow), and the spheno-ethmoid recess (small space where sphenoid sinus opens) are all included in these codes and are not reported separately. A diagnostic sinus endoscopy may be performed for a patient with chronic sinusitis for whom medical treatment has failed. Performing a diagnostic endoscopy will allow the physician to see all the structures and determine if any anatomical abnormalities or growths are present.

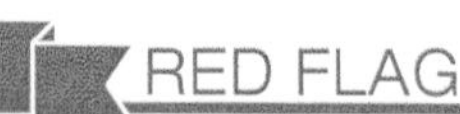

RED FLAG

In the codebook, you may see endoscopic "anterior and posterior ethmoidectomy" abbreviated as APE.

An endoscopy that corrects something is considered surgical. Codes 31237 through 31298 describe surgical endoscopies and include codes for biopsy, excision, hemorrhage control, repair, decompression, and dilation. Some of the surgical endoscopy codes include removal of polyps as indicated in parenthetic notes in the tabular, such as this note following code 31256:

> (For endoscopic anterior and posterior ethmoidectomy [APE], and frontal sinus exploration, with or without removal of polyp[s], use 31255 and 31276)

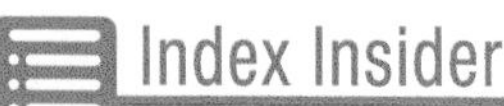

Index Insider

You can find codes for sinus endoscopies in the Index several ways: under the main entry *Endoscopy*, find the subterm *Nose* or *Sinuses*; under the main entry *Nose*, find the subterm, *Endoscopy*; and under the main entry *Sinus/Sinuses*, find the subterm *Endoscopy*. You will also find these codes indexed under the specific procedure accomplished, such as the main entries *Ethmoidectomy* or *Polypectomy*.

Carefully read the code descriptions and use the notes in the CPT® codebook as a guide to avoid unbundling and duplicate reporting.

Inside the OR

Codes 31254 and 31255 describe surgical endoscopy with ethmoidectomy. In this procedure, the surgeon places the endoscope in the nose and completes a thorough inspection of the internal nasal structures. A scalpel or biting forceps is inserted parallel to the scope and is used to remove any diseased tissue in the ethmoid sinus that may be blocking the sinus drainage. Polyps may be excised, which is included in the code. Electrocautery may be used to stop any bleeding. The nasal cavity may be packed with gauze and left in place for 24 to 48 hours. Code 31254 is reported for an anterior ethmoidectomy, and code 31255 is reported for a total ethmoidectomy (anterior and posterior).

LET'S TRY ONE **11.2**

Assign CPT® codes to each of the following procedures:

1. Endoscopy with anterior and posterior ethmoidectomy: _____
2. Simple nasal polypectomy, done in office: _____
3. Surgical endoscopy with maxillary antrostomy and removal of polyp: _____
4. Minor revision of rhinoplasty, nasal tip: _____
5. Removal of Lego from nose of 2 year old, done in office: _____

Larynx (Codes 31300-31599)

The larynx is a tube-shaped organ about 5 cm long, located between the pharynx and the trachea, and containing the vocal cords. The **vocal cords** are 2 bands of muscle that form a V shape inside the larynx. The larynx is also known as the *voice box*.

Categories and Procedures for the Larynx

Procedures and their codes found under the Larynx heading are organized by the categories listed in Table 11.6.

Table 11.6 Larynx Procedures and Codes

Codebook Category	Surgical Procedure(s)	Code(s)
Excision	Laryngotomy	31300
	Laryngectomy	31360-31382
	Pharyngolaryngectomy	31390-31395
	Arytenoidectomy or arytenoidopexy	31400
	Epiglottidectomy	31420
Introduction	Intubation	31500-31502
Endoscopy	Indirect laryngoscopy	31505-31513
	Direct laryngoscopy	31515-31571
	Fiberoptic laryngoscopy	31572-31579
Repair	Laryngoplasty	31580-31591
	Cricotracheal resection	31592
Destruction	Section, laryngeal nerve	31595
Other Procedures	Unlisted procedure, larynx	31599

Coding Common Procedures of the Larynx

Two procedures that present coding nuances are laryngectomy and laryngoscopy. Laryngectomy and laryngoscopy will be discussed in further detail in the following sections.

Laryngectomy

A **laryngectomy** is a removal of the larynx. This operation is performed in cases of cancer of the larynx, severe trauma to the larynx such as from a gunshot wound, or damage to the larynx from radiation treatment. Laryngectomy procedures are differentiated by the extent of the removal, neck dissection, and reconstruction. A radical neck dissection often includes the removal of the sternocleidomastoid muscle, the submandibular salivary gland, the internal jugular vein, and the lymph nodes in the neck that are under the chin as well as supraclavicular lymph nodes.

A total laryngectomy is reported with either 31360 or 31365: a surgeon removes the larynx in 31360 and the larynx and surrounding tissues in 31365, performing a radical neck dissection. A tracheostomy, the creation of an artificial opening in the trachea, is performed first in these procedures. Tracheostomy is integral to laryngectomy and therefore is not coded separately.

Subtotal supraglottic laryngectomy is reported with either 31367 or 31368: in 31367, the larynx is removed, and in 31368, the larynx and surrounding tissues are removed in a radical neck dissection. Any reconstruction is reported with a separate code.

Partial laryngectomies are reported with codes 31370 through 31382. Codes are differentiated by the area of resection and the incision.

- Code 31370 is reported for a horizontal partial laryngectomy, as shown in Figure 11.3.
- Code 31375 (laterovertical) is reported when the vocal cord and adjacent cartilage are removed.
- Code 31380 (anterovertical) involves making incisions into both halves of the thyroid cartilage, and then the anterior portion of the thyroid cartilage and the diseased part of both vocal cords are excised.
- Code 31382 (antero-latero-vertical) is reported when the resection also includes all or part of the **arytenoid** (cartilage where vocal cords are attached).

Inside the OR

In a horizontal partial laryngectomy, a tracheostomy is performed first to maintain the patient's airway (see Figure 11.3). The surgeon makes an incision into the neck and retracts the neck muscles. Then an incision is made to expose the larynx. A horizontal incision is made above or below the diseased area, and the diseased tissue is then removed. The patient's airway is then reconstructed. The pharynx and muscles are sutured closed. The incision is sutured in layers.

Figure 11.3 Horizontal Partial Laryngectomy

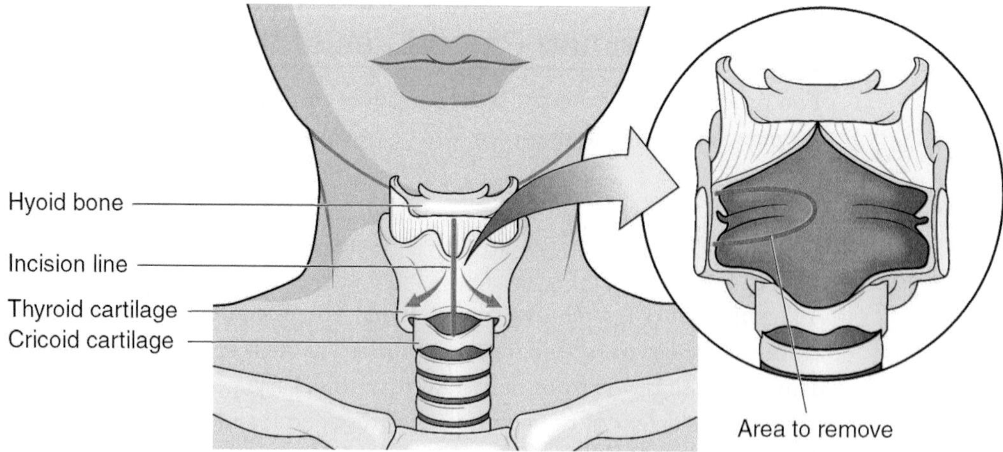

Laryngoscopy

As noted in the codebook at the beginning of the larynx Endoscopy category of codes, laryngoscopy includes examination of the tongue base, larynx, and hypopharynx (inferior portion of pharynx between the epiglottis and larynx). Various factors differentiate codes 31505 through 31579, the primary factor being the type of visualization—indirect or direct.

Indirect laryngoscopy, visualizing the larynx with a mirror held just below the back of the patient's throat, is being done less frequently because flexible laryngoscopes allow better visualization for the physician and more comfort for the patient. **Direct laryngoscopy**, visualizing the larynx with a rigid or flexible scope, allows the physician to see deeper into the throat. Laryngoscopy codes are further differentiated by the following criteria:

- whether the procedure is diagnostic or operative;
- the specific procedure performed: biopsy, dilation, removal of foreign body or lesion, insertion of an obturator, stripping of vocal cords and/or epiglottis, a therapeutic injection, or stroboscopy; and
- the use of an operating microscope.

EXAMPLE **11.3**

A 32-year-old male presented to the outpatient clinic, having had a hoarse voice for several months. The physician performed a diagnostic direct flexible laryngoscopy and noted a small vocal cord polyp. No other procedures were performed. This is reported with code 31575, *Laryngoscopy, flexible fiberoptic; diagnostic*.

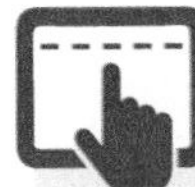

LET'S TRY ONE **11.3**

Read the operative report and answer the questions that follow.

PREOPERATIVE DIAGNOSIS: Chronic laryngitis

POSTOPERATIVE DIAGNOSIS: Hypertrophic vocal cords, bilateral

NAME OF OPERATION: Microlaryngoscopy

PROCEDURE
Under general endotracheal anesthesia, the patient was prepped and draped in the usual manner. A Dedo laryngoscope was used. The epiglottis, valleculae, pyriform sinuses, and post-cricoid area appeared normal. Under the operating microscope, the rest of the larynx was visualized. Both false cords, the ventricles, and the subglottic area also appeared normal. Both vocal cords appeared hypertrophic and dry. There was no abnormal swelling, mass, ulceration, or crusting. The vocal cords also appeared slightly hyperemic. A biopsy was performed. The patient tolerated the procedure well and was transferred to the postanesthesia care unit in satisfactory condition.

1. Was this a direct or indirect laryngoscopy? _____
2. Was an operating microscope used? _____
3. Was a biopsy performed? _____
4. What is the correct code for this procedure? _____

Trachea and Bronchi (Codes 31600-31899)

The trachea is the airway that connects the larynx to the bronchi, which are the tubes that conduct air into the lungs. The codes for the Trachea and Bronchi heading describe diagnostic and surgical procedures under the categories Incision; Endoscopy; Bronchial Thermoplasty; Introduction; and Excision, Repair.

Categories and Procedures for the Trachea and Bronchi

Procedures and their codes found under the Trachea and Bronchi heading are organized by the categories listed in Table 11.7.

Table 11.7 Trachea and Bronchi Procedures and Codes

Codebook Category	Surgical Procedure(s)	Code(s)
Incision	Tracheostomy	31600-31610
	Construction, tracheoesophageal fistula with prosthesis insertion	31611
	Tracheal puncture for aspiration/injection	31612
	Tracheostoma revision	31613-31614
Endoscopy	Tracheobronchoscopy	31615
	Bronchoscopy	31622-31651
	Endobronchial ultrasound	31652-31654
Bronchial Thermoplasty	Bronchoscopy	31660-31661
Introduction	Catheterization	31717
	Catheter aspiration	31720-31725
	Introduction, stent or tube for oxygen therapy	31730
Excision, Repair	Tracheoplasty	31750-31760
	Carinal reconstruction	31766
	Bronchoplasty	31770-31775
	Excision, tracheal stenosis/anastomosis, tumor, or carcinoma	31780-31786
	Suture, tracheal wound/injury	31800-31805
	Tracheostomy closure, scar revision	31820-31830
Other Procedures	Unlisted procedure, trachea and bronchi	31899

Coding Common Procedures of the Trachea and Bronchi

Most of the codes relate to tracheostomy and bronchoscopy procedures, which will be discussed in detail in the following sections.

Tracheostomy

A **tracheostomy** creates an opening in the neck to the trachea. The opening may be temporary or permanent. The physician first makes a horizontal neck incision and then dissects the muscles so the trachea is exposed, as shown in Figure 11.4. A tube is then inserted to maintain the patient's airway. Conditions that indicate a tracheostomy are neck cancer that is pressing on the airway affecting breathing, a severe neck or mouth injury, or paralysis of the muscles that affect swallowing. A tracheostomy is often included in a broader procedure such as laryngectomy, described above, if normal breathing and swallowing will be affected.

Figure 11.4 Tracheostomy Tube Placement

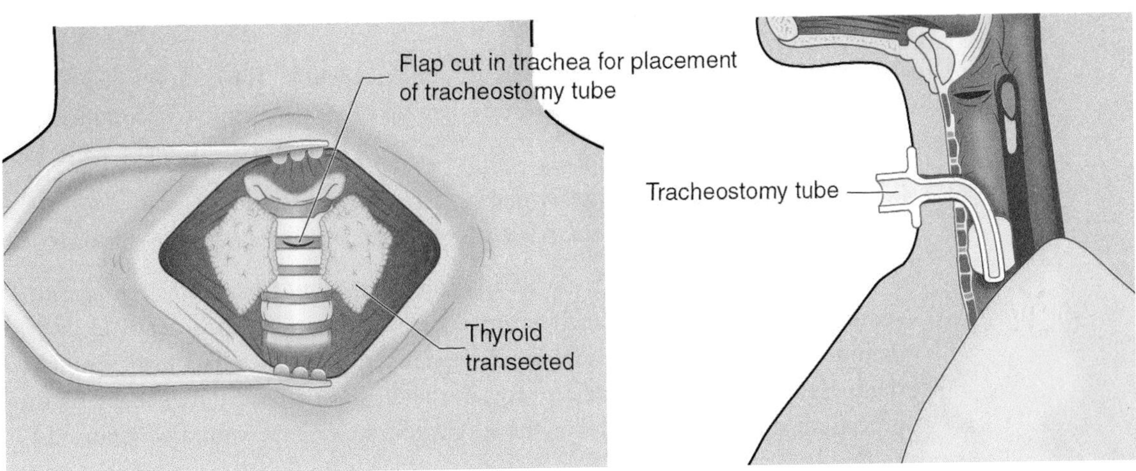

The codes in the codebook Incision category for standalone tracheostomies are differentiated by surgical conditions, age of patient, and structures affected:

- A planned tracheostomy on an adult is reported with code 31600, and on a patient younger than 2 years old, code 31601 is reported.
- An emergency tracheostomy is reported with code 31603 or 31605: 31603, *Tracheostomy, emergency procedure; transtracheal,* is reported when the physician punctures the trachea and inserts the tube; 31605, *Tracheostomy, emergency procedure; cricothyroid membrane,* is reported when the physician punctures the cricothyroid membrane just above the **cricoid** (the ring of cartilage around the trachea) and inserts the tube.
- Creation of a more permanent stoma is reported with code 31610, *Tracheostomy, fenestration procedure with skin flaps.*

CONCEPTS CHECKPOINT **11.2**

Answer true or false to each of the following statements.

1. _____ A planned tracheostomy may be reported as a separate procedure.
2. _____ Emergency tracheostomy codes depend on the technique for insertion of the tube.
3. _____ The age of the patient does not affect code assignment for a planned tracheostomy.

Bronchoscopy

Bronchoscopy is visual examination of the trachea, bronchi, and lungs using a rigid or flexible endoscope. This examination is indicated for patients with pulmonary symptoms such as persistent cough or wheezing, **hemoptysis** (spitting up blood), or abnormal x-ray results. During the bronchoscopy, the surgeon looks for abnormalities in the passages that might be the cause of symptoms. For a bronchoscopy, the patient's airway is anesthetized. The surgeon inserts the bronchoscope through either the nose or mouth and then advances the scope past the larynx to inspect the bronchus. All bronchoscopy procedures include fluoroscopic guidance. The only image guidance that can be coded separately is the add-on code 31627 that provides for computer-assisted, image-guided navigation. There are several add-on codes in this section with notes in the tabular list to explain their usage.

Bronchoscopy can be diagnostic, surgical, or therapeutic. The code for diagnostic bronchoscopy is 31622, reported only when no other procedure is accomplished during the bronchoscopy:

> 31622, *Bronchoscopy, rigid or flexible, including fluoroscopic guidance when performed; diagnostic, with cell washings, when performed (separate procedure)*

A diagnostic bronchoscopy is always bilateral, so modifier 50, *Bilateral procedure*, should not be applied to bronchoscopy codes. Diagnostic bronchoscopy is always included in a surgical bronchoscopy. For example, if during a diagnostic bronchoscopy the surgeon finds a lesion and removes it, the diagnostic procedure becomes a surgical procedure, and only the code for the surgical bronchoscopy would be reported.

Bronchoscopy codes 31623 through 31649 describe many procedures. Procedures that have important coding considerations are collection of tissue, needle aspiration biopsies, and placement of markers.

Collection of tissue: Code 31628 describes the collection of 1 or more tissue samples from a single lobe of the lung after a diagnostic bronchoscopy. One or more biopsies taken from additional lobes are reported with add-on code 31632, which is reported only once in addition to code 31628 no matter how many additional biopsies are taken from the lobe.

Needle aspiration biopsies: Code 31629 describes needle aspiration biopsies from the trachea and bronchus (main stem and/or lobar), reported once for multiple upper airway needle aspiration biopsies or multiple needle aspiration biopsies from a single lobe. Aspiration biopsies obtained from additional lobes are reported with add-on code 31633. Codes 31622, 31623, and 31624 describe cell washings, brushings, and lavage (rinsing) for obtaining cells for cytology and microbiology studies (to identify bacteria and other microbes); these procedures are not coded as biopsies.

Placement of markers: Code 31626 describes the placement of markers (gold fiducial markers, as shown in Figure 11.5) or dye that can be seen by radiograph directly on or near a tumor to mark the tumor's position for the surgeon. Code 31626 is a standalone code that is expected to be reported with other bronchoscopy codes.

Figure 11.5 Gold Fiducial Markers (Comparing Size to Match Head)

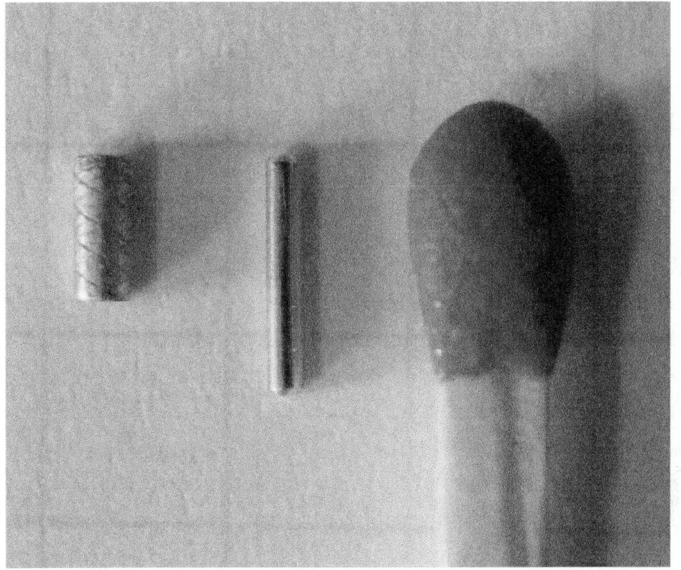

Index Insider

There are several ways to locate codes for bronchoscopy procedures in the Index. The main entries and subterms are the following:

- *Bronchi, Bronchoscopy;*
- *Bronchoscopy*, with subterms for the specific procedure;
- *Endoscopy, Bronchi*, and further subterms for the specific procedure; and
- *Lung, Biopsy.*

Multiple procedures may be accomplished during 1 bronchoscopy episode, and multiple codes may be reported. Keep in mind that 31622 (the separate procedure code for diagnostic bronchoscopy) is never reported with any of the other bronchoscopy codes. Some bronchoscopy code pairings may trigger a National Correct Coding Initiative (NCCI) edit. Multiple biopsies performed during 1 bronchoscopy on different anatomical sites and/or with different techniques may require the use of modifier 59, *Distinct Procedural Service*, to pass the NCCI edits.

CONCEPTS CHECKPOINT 11.3

Answer true or false to each of the following statements.

1. _____ Multiple bronchoscopy codes may be reported for 1 operative episode.
2. _____ Fluoroscopic guidance should be coded in addition to the bronchoscopy code(s).
3. _____ Diagnostic bronchoscopy is always bilateral.
4. _____ Diagnostic bronchoscopy is always included in surgical bronchoscopy.
5. _____ Diagnostic bronchoscopy codes may be reported with surgical bronchoscopy codes.

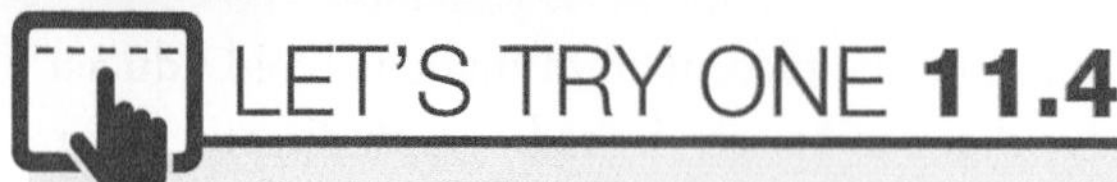

LET'S TRY ONE **11.4**

Read the operative report and answer the questions that follow.

BRONCHOSCOPY REPORT

PREOPERATIVE DIAGNOSIS: Probable bronchiectasis, right lower lobe, rule out unusual infections

POSTOPERATIVE DIAGNOSIS: Evidence of bronchitis, no other abnormality seen

NAME OF OPERATION: Fiberoptic bronchoscopy

PROCEDURE

The patient was taken to the bronchoscopy suite as an outpatient. The nose and hypopharynx were anesthetized with Pontocaine. Following satisfactory anesthesia, the fiberoptic bronchoscope was passed transnasally without difficulty. The hypopharynx, epiglottis, and cords were normal and moved normally. Trachea was normal without signs of deviation or compression. The carina was sharp and pulsatile. The tracheobronchial tree was inspected both right and left to the subsegmental level. There was some erythema and friability of the mucosa in the right middle and right lower lobe areas and mild mucopurulent secretions. Otherwise, the tracheobronchial tree was normal without evidence of neoplasm or bleeding. Specimens were obtained for cytology and microbiologic studies. The patient tolerated the procedure well without complications.

1. What procedure is described in this note? ______________
2. Was a biopsy done? _____
3. What is the correct code for this procedure? _____

Lungs and Pleura (Codes 32035-32999)

The lungs are 2 organs that bring oxygen to the blood and remove carbon dioxide from the body. The right lung has 3 lobes and the left lung has 2 lobes. The pleura is the double-folded membrane that covers each lung and lines the thoracic cavity.

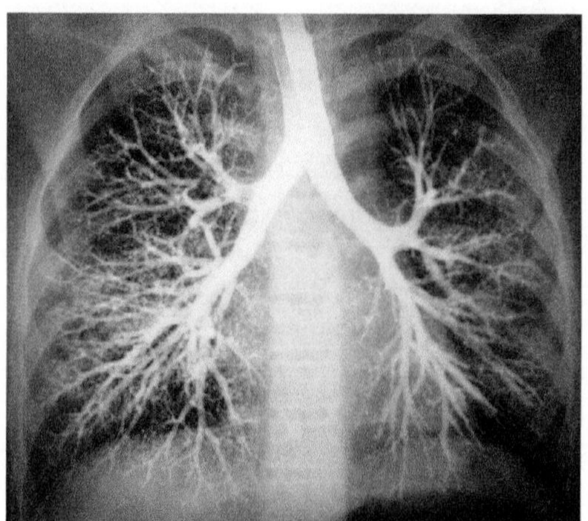

An x-ray of healthy lungs.

Categories and Procedures for the Lungs and Pleura

Procedures and their codes found under the Lungs and Pleura heading are organized by the categories listed in Table 11.8.

Table 11.8 Lungs and Pleura Procedures and Codes

Codebook Category	Surgical Procedure(s)	Code(s)
Incision	Thoracostomy	32035-32036
	Thoracotomy	32096-32160
	Pneumonostomy	32200
	Pleural scarification	32215
	Decortication, pulmonary	32220-32225
Excision/Resection	Pleurectomy	32310
	Decortication and pleurectomy	32320
	Biopsy	32400-32405
Removal	Removal of lung	32440-32491
	Resection/Repair of bronchus	32501
	Resection, lung tumor	32503-32504
	Thoracotomy	32505-32507
	Enucleation of empyema	32540
Introduction and Removal	Insertion and removal, catheter	32550, 32552
	Tube thoracostomy	32551
	Placement of device for radiation therapy	32553
	Thoracentesis	32554-32555
	Pleural drainage	32556-32557
Destruction	Instillation, agents for pleurodesis, fibrinolysis	32560-32562
Thoracoscopy (Video-assisted thoracic surgery [VATS])	Thoracoscopy, diagnostic	32601-32609
	Thoracoscopy, surgical	32650-32674
Stereotactic Radiation Therapy	Thoracic target delineation	32701
Repair	Lung hernia	32800
	Closure, chest wall	32810
	Closure, fistula	32815
	Reconstruction, chest wall	32820
Lung Transplantation	Donor pneumonectomy, preparation of donor lung	32850, 32855-32856
	Lung transplant	32851-32854
Surgical Collapse Therapy: Thoracoplasty	Resection of ribs	32900
	Thoracoplasty	32905-32906
	Pneumonolysis	32940
	Pneumothorax, therapeutic	32960
Other Procedures	Lung lavage	32997
	Ablation therapy	32998, 32994
	Unlisted procedure, lungs and pleura	32999

Coding Common Procedures of the Lungs and Pleura

Procedures on the lungs and pleura are reported with codes 32035 through 32999. These procedures include thoracostomy, biopsy of the lungs and pleura, surgical thoracoscopy, and removal of lung lesions. The guidelines for coding some of the more common procedures of the lungs and pleura are discussed in the following pages.

Biopsy of the Lungs and Pleura

Biopsy of the lungs or pleural cavity is indicated for patients with suspected lung mass, neoplasm, infection, tuberculosis, or other lung diseases. Codes for biopsies reflect the technique used, which is chosen based on the amount of tissue to be removed. The biopsy techniques include an open approach, a percutaneous needle puncture (as illustrated in Figure 11.6), wedge resection (in which a wedge-shaped sample of tissue is removed), and an endoscopic approach:

- codes 32096 through 32098, biopsy via thoracotomy (an open approach);
- codes 32400 through 32405, biopsy via percutaneous needle puncture;
- code 32507, diagnostic open wedge resection;
- codes 32604 through 32609, biopsy via thoracoscopy; and
- codes 32666 through 32668, diagnostic wedge resection via thoracoscopy.

Figure 11.6 Lung Tissue Biopsy

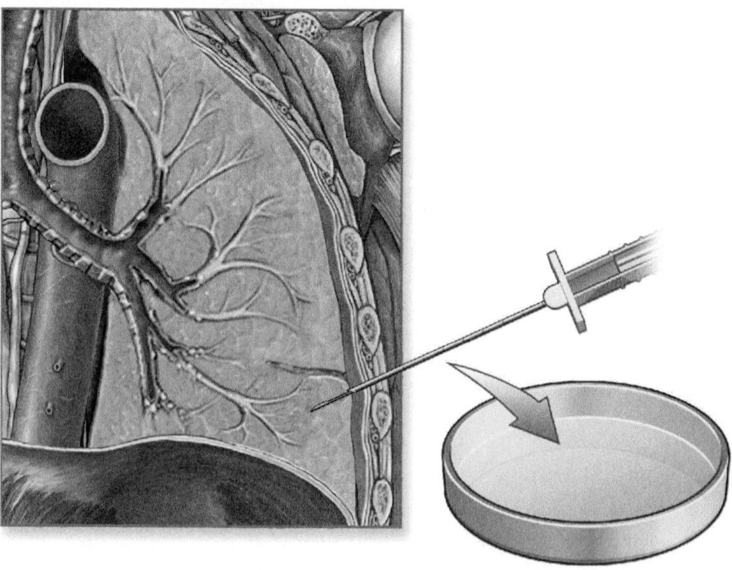

When a wedge resection is used for diagnostic purposes, it is important for the coder to distinguish between a *diagnostic* lung biopsy and a *therapeutic* lung resection, both of which may use a wedge technique, but the amount of tissue differs. A diagnostic wedge biopsy of the lung is obtained without attention to the surgical margins (area free from disease); a therapeutic wedge resection requires complete resection of the nodule or lesion plus disease-free margins. If during a wedge resection an intraoperative pathology consultation determines that a more extensive resection is needed at the same anatomical location, a *diagnostic* wedge resection is reported using codes 32507 (open) or 32668 (endoscopic), or add-on code 32668 (endoscopic) along with the appropriate thoracoscopy code. If the pathologist determines no more resection is needed, a *therapeutic* wedge resection would be reported with codes 32505 (open) or 32666 (endoscopic). More extensive lung resections include segmentectomy, lobectomy, bilobectomy, and pneumonectomy procedures, as shown in Figure 11.7. Therapeutic wedge resection codes are not reported with the more extensive lung procedure codes. Only the code for the most extensive procedure performed would be reported.

Figure 11.7 Lung Resections

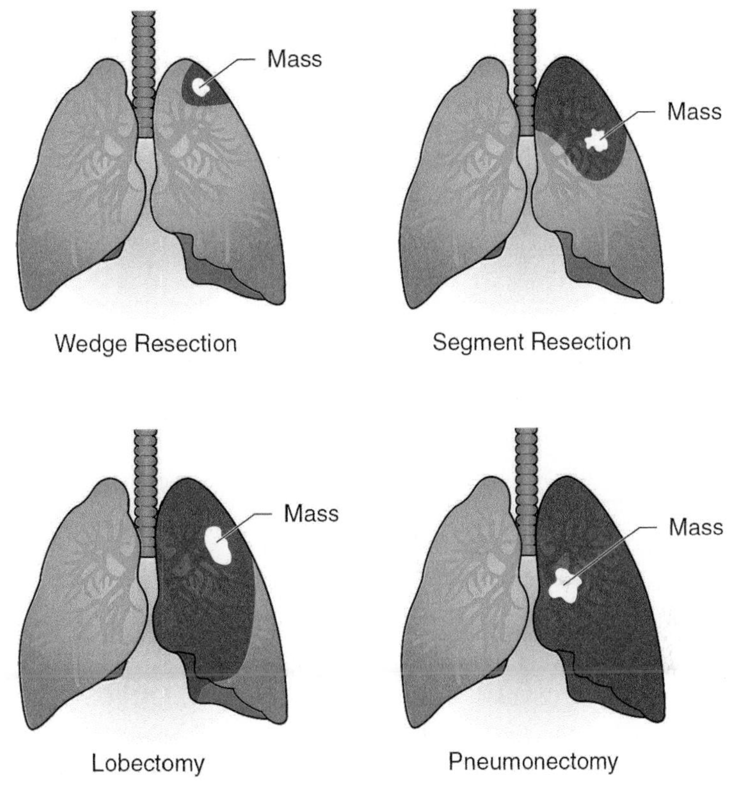

Lung Removal

Procedures to remove all or part of a lung are performed with an open approach using **thoracotomy** (surgical incision into chest cavity). The surgeon opens the chest cavity and the ribs are spread apart, or the sternum may be cut in half with a bone saw and spread apart to allow the surgeon access to the lungs and other structures.

The codes for lung removal are differentiated by the extent of the lung tissue removed. Removal of an entire lung is a **pneumonectomy**; removal of a single lung lobe is a **lobectomy**; removal of 2 lobes is a **bilobectomy**; and removal of a lung segment is a **segmentectomy**.

The codebook sequences the codes as follows:

- code 32440, removal of an entire lung;

- code 32442, removal of a lung and part of the trachea, which is sutured to the main bronchial tube of the lung that remains;
- code 32445, removal of a lung and the pleural membranes covering the lung and the chest cavity;
- code 32480, removal of a single lobe of a lung;
- code 32482, removal of 2 lobes of a lung; and
- code 32484, removal of a segment of a lung.

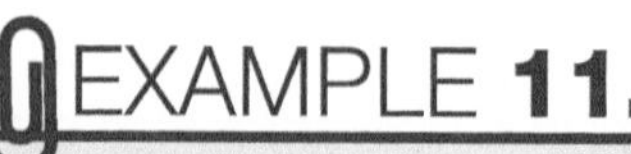

EXAMPLE 11.4

A 53-year-old male was found to have a mass on his lung in the left upper lobe that had been diagnosed as adenocarcinoma on a previous biopsy. The patient was taken to the OR for a segmental resection of the mass. This is reported with code 32484, *Removal of lung, other than pneumonectomy; single segment (segmentectomy).*

CONCEPTS CHECKPOINT 11.4

Answer true or false to each of the following statements.

1. _____ If a diagnostic wedge resection and lobectomy are performed on the same lung in the same operative episode, only the code for lobectomy is reported.
2. _____ A diagnostic wedge biopsy specimen may not have clear margins.
3. _____ A pneumonectomy is removal of the entire lung.
4. _____ A thoracotomy indicates an open procedure.

Tube Thoracostomy and Thoracentesis

The codebook Introduction and Removal category has codes for a tube thoracostomy and thoracentesis, both procedures to remove fluid from the chest cavity. However, in a thoracostomy, the chest tube stays in place, while in a thoracentesis, the tube or needle is removed at the end of the procedure.

A **thoracostomy** is a procedure to drain the space around the lungs when a disease causes pleural effusion (fluid buildup) or an injury causes blood or air to build up in the chest cavity. A tube thoracostomy is an open procedure in which the physician makes an incision and inserts a tube into the pleural space for drainage. The tube is sutured to the skin of the chest wall and may be connected to a suction machine. It is kept in place until most of the air or fluid has drained. Code 32551, *Tube thoracostomy, includes connection to drainage system (eg, water seal) when performed, open (separate procedure)*, is reported for this procedure. Chest tube insertion is inherent to many heart and lung surgeries and would not be reported separately if performed as part of a larger procedure.

Thoracentesis is puncture of the chest cavity to aspirate fluid, similar to a thoracostomy but done percutaneously. A physician may perform thoracentesis to remove a sample of fluid for diagnostic testing or to reduce the amount of fluid for a patient with pleural effusion to make the patient more comfortable. In a thoracentesis, the physician punctures through the space between the ribs with a hollow needle. By pulling back on the plunger of the syringe, the fluid is siphoned into the attached tube, as shown in Figure 11.8. The tube or needle is removed at the end of the procedure. Code 32554, *Thoracentesis, needle or catheter, aspiration of the pleural space; without imaging guidance*, is reported for the procedure described above. If the thoracentesis is performed with image guidance, code 32555 is reported. It is appropriate to use the RT (right) and LT (left) modifiers with these codes. If the procedure is completed on both sides during the same operative session, modifier 50, *Bilateral procedure*, may be reported.

Figure 11.8 Thoracentesis Showing Insertion Site and Plunger to Remove Fluid

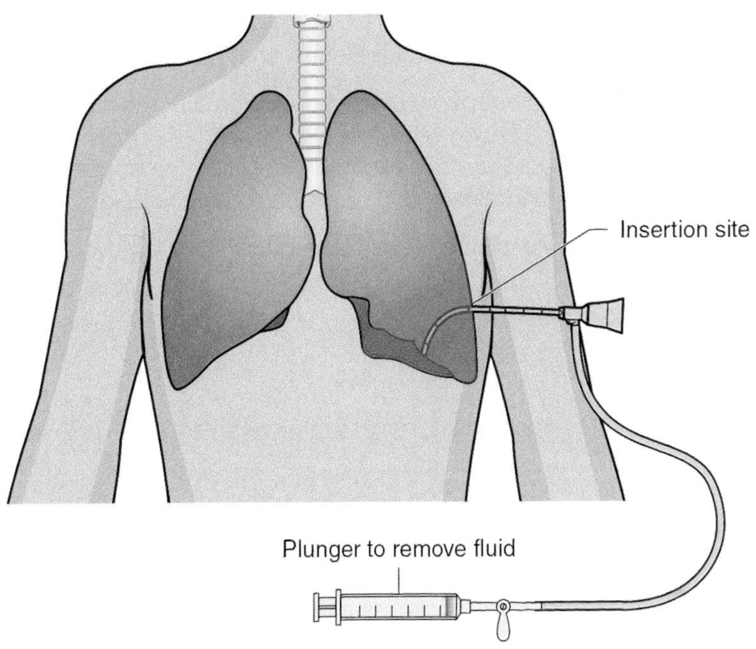

LET'S TRY ONE **11.5**

A 78-year-old man presents to the emergency department complaining of shortness of breath. A chest radiograph reveals a large left pleural effusion. The physician punctures the patient through the left side of his chest and performs an aspiration of the pleural fluid. The tube is then removed. No image guidance was used. The fluid is sent to pathology for diagnosis.

What is the correct procedure code? _____

Thoracoscopy Procedures

Thoracoscopy is the process of viewing the chest cavity using an endoscope. Surgical thoracoscopy is video-assisted thoracic surgery, which a health record may refer to as "VATS" or "VATS approach." The codes under the codebook category Thoracoscopy (Video-assisted thoracic surgery [VATS]) are differentiated by the procedures accomplished using this technique, including biopsies and resection procedures on the pleura, lung, pericardium, mediastinum, and other structures in the thoracic cavity. If multiple thoracoscopic procedures are accomplished during 1 operative episode, multiple codes may be reported. As with other endoscopic procedures, a surgical thoracoscopy always includes a diagnostic thoracoscopy.

Coders should read and be guided by the notes in the codebook following specific codes. For example, thoracoscopy with diagnostic lung or pleural biopsies are reported with codes 32607 through 32609. Parenthetic notes stipulate these codes are reported only once per lung even if multiple specimens are obtained. If the biopsy is followed by removal of the same lung (pneumonectomy), the biopsy code is not reported separately as it is considered part of the larger procedure.

LET'S TRY ONE **11.6**

Read the operative note and answer the questions that follow.

A 57-year-old female with a history of adenocarcinoma of the cecum was found to have a nodule on her right upper lung that has grown since the last CT scan. Using a VATS approach under general anesthesia, the lung was partially collapsed. The surgeon identified the nodule, and a biopsy was taken. A chest tube was inserted to allow for drainage and re-expansion of the lung.

1. What procedure was accomplished during this operative episode? ______________
2. What approach was used? ______________
3. How is this indexed? ______________
4. What is the correct code for this procedure? _____

CONCEPTS CHECKPOINT **11.5**

Choose the correct word(s) to fill in the blank in the following statements.

1. If a biopsy is followed by removal of the same lung, the biopsy code <u>is / is not</u> reported separately.
2. Multiple thoracoscopic procedure codes <u>may / may not</u> be reported for 1 operative episode.
3. Video-<u>accomplished / assisted</u> thoracic surgery is abbreviated as VATS.
4. Diagnostic thoracoscopy <u>is / is not</u> included in surgical thoracoscopy.

Chapter Summary

- Codes in the Respiratory System Surgery subsection are arranged by anatomical site from nose to lungs and then categorized by incision, excision, introduction, repair, destruction, and other procedures.
- Criteria for selecting rhinoplasty codes are the extent of work done and whether the operation is primary or secondary.
- Diagnostic endoscopy is always included in surgical endoscopy.
- Endoscopies may require multiple codes and are differentiated by the procedure accomplished.
- Some nasal surgical endoscopy codes include polyp removal.

- Laryngectomy procedures are differentiated by the extent of the removal, the involvement of neck dissection, and the performance of reconstruction.
- Tracheostomy is integral to laryngectomy and therefore is not coded separately.
- Indirect laryngoscopy utilizes a mirror to visualize the larynx, while direct laryngoscopy visualizes the larynx with a rigid or flexible scope.
- Tracheostomy procedures are coded based on whether they are planned or performed in an emergency.
- Tracheostomies may be temporary or permanent.
- Diagnostic bronchoscopies are always bilateral; modifier 50, *Bilateral procedure*, should not be used.
- The use of fluoroscopic guidance is included in bronchoscopy codes and not reported separately.
- Code 31622 for diagnostic bronchoscopy is never reported with other bronchoscopy codes because a diagnostic bronchoscopy is always included in a surgical bronchoscopy.
- Codes for removal of lung tissue are based on the amount of tissue removed.
- A diagnostic wedge resection is performed without attention to margins, whereas a therapeutic wedge resection would remove the entire nodule or lesion and margins would be clear.
- A tube thoracostomy and thoracentesis are similar procedures to remove fluid from the chest cavity. The chest tube stays in place in a thoracostomy and is removed at the end of the procedure in a thoracentesis.
- If a lung biopsy is followed by removal of the same lung during the same operative episode, the biopsy is not reported separately.

Navigator

Access interactive chapter review exercises, practice activities, flash cards, and study games.

Chapter 12

Surgery Coding: The Cardiovascular System

Fast Facts

- An adult's body contains more than 60,000 miles of blood vessels. If you attached them end-to-end, they could circle the globe about 2.5 times!
- The Ebers Papyrus, an ancient Egyptian medical document, described the connection between the heart and the lungs.
- While 38% of the US population is eligible to donate blood, only 10% does so each year. More than 41,000 blood donations are needed each day. The most common blood type, and the 1 most requested by hospitals, is Type O.

Sources: http://webmd.com/heart-disease.guide/how-heart-works, http://livescience.com, http://redcrossblood.org

Crack the Code

Review the sample operative report to find the correct cardiovascular system code. You may need to return to this exercise after reading the chapter content.

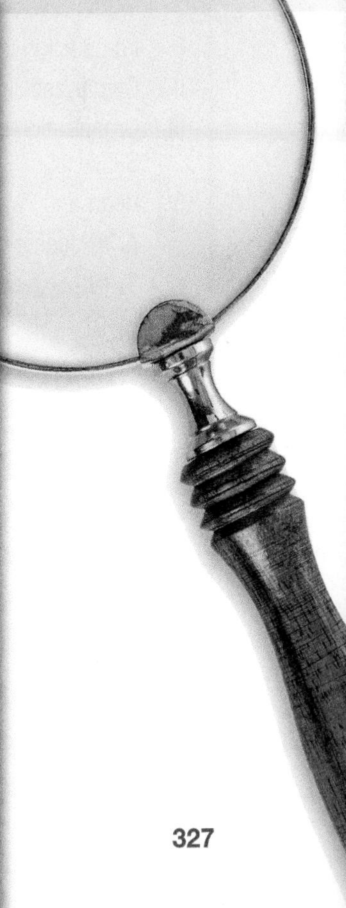

PROCEDURE: Placement of Port-a-Cath

INDICATIONS: The patient is a 70-year-old white female who has had a right modified mastectomy for breast cancer and, at the present time, has metastatic disease. She is receiving chemotherapy and desires placement of a Port-a-Cath. Because of the previous mastectomy on the right side, the Port-a-Cath is planned to be placed on the left side.

PROCEDURE: The patient was placed on the table in the supine position, and the anterior chest and neck area were prepped and draped in the usual sterile manner. There was an external jugular vein present approximately 2.5 cm above the clavicle on the left side. Using 0.5% local anesthesia, the skin was anesthetized, and the vein was dissected free using sharp and blunt dissection. It was ligated distally, and a loop of 2-0 silk was placed about it proximally. Following this an incision of approximately 2.5 cm was made at the sternal border on the left side at approximately the fourth interspace. A pocket was then fashioned in which the Port-a-Cath would be placed. Following this, a tunnel was made between the incision on the chest wall and the incision overlying the external jugular vein. The catheter of the Port-a-Cath was placed through this tunnel. A venotomy was performed, and the catheter was placed into the vein. Its position in the superior vena cava was assessed using fluoroscopy. The catheter was then tied in place. Then the 4 securing sutures were placed, and the catheter was cut to length and attached to the Port-a-Cath unit. The Port-a-Cath unit was then sutured in place in the pocket using the previously placed sutures. Following this, the subcutaneous tissue and the skin were closed superior to the Port-a-Cath unit. A Hubert needle was placed through the skin into the Port-a-Cath, and it was noted to aspirate and fill easily. Following the closure of the skin over the Port-a-Cath unit using 4-0 Vicryl, the same type of closure was performed over the entrance site of the catheter into the external jugular vein. Sterile dressings were applied. The Hubert needle was left in place with an extension tubing connection. The unit was filled with heparinized saline. The patient tolerated the procedure well, and blood loss was minimal and none was replaced.

answer: 36561

Learning Objectives

12.1 Describe the basic anatomy of the heart and coronary arteries.

12.2 Describe the arrangement of codes in the Cardiovascular System Surgery subsection and explain when this subsection is used.

12.3 Apply the use of symbols, guidelines, and instructional notes in coding cardiovascular procedures.

12.4 Apply appropriate CPT® modifiers when coding cardiovascular procedures and services.

12.5 Distinguish between various pacemaker systems when coding.

12.6 When coding coronary artery bypass grafting procedures, determine whether veins, arteries, or both are used.

12.7 Determine the type and use of catheters when coding catheterization procedures.

12.8 Distinguish between centrally inserted and peripherally inserted venous access catheters.

12.9 Assign codes for procedures on the heart and pericardium including pacemakers, defibrillators, and coronary artery bypass grafts.

12.10 Assign codes for procedures on arteries and veins including aneurysm repairs and bypass grafts.

12.11 Describe the arrangement of codes in the hemic and lymphatic subsection and explain when these codes are used.

12.12 Assign codes for procedures on the spleen, lymph nodes, and lymphatic channels.

12.13 Describe the arrangement of codes in the Mediastinum and Diaphragm subsection and explain when these codes are used.

Chapter Outline

Introduction to the Cardiovascular System

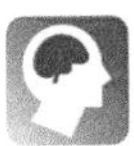

3-D
To explore the cardiovascular system in the BioDigital Human, go to: http://Coding.ParadigmEducation.com/BioDigital_Cardiovascular.

The **cardiovascular system**, which includes the heart and blood vessels, circulates blood throughout the body. The **arteries** carry blood away from the heart, bringing oxygen and nutrients to tissues. The **veins** bring blood back to the heart, carrying carbon dioxide and toxins. The exception to this division of labor is the **pulmonary artery**, which carries carbon dioxide and waste from the heart to the lungs, and the **pulmonary veins**, which carry oxygenated blood from the lungs to the heart.

Cardiovascular System Terminology

It is important for a coder to be familiar with the anatomical and medical terms used with the cardiovascular system in order to correctly report codes from the Cardiovascular System Surgery subsection. The terms in Table 12.1 include structures, devices, diagnoses, and procedures related to the cardiovascular system.

Table 12.1 Cardiovascular System Terminology

Term	Definition
aneurysm	Ballooning of a weakened portion of arterial wall
angioplasty	Surgical repair of blood vessel to dilate the opening
anomaly	Abnormality
aorta	The largest blood vessel in the body, arising from the left ventricle
arteriovenous fistula	Direct communication between an artery and a vein
artery	A vessel that carries oxygenated blood away from the heart to the body
atrium	Upper chamber of the heart
bypass	To go around (detour around blocked vessels)
cardiopulmonary	Refers to the heart and lungs
cardiopulmonary bypass	Heart/lung machine used during open heart surgery so blood bypasses the heart
cardioverter-defibrillator	Device that directs an electrical shock to the heart to restore normal rhythm
catheter	A tube placed in the body to put fluid in or take fluid out
electrode	A lead attached to a generator that carries electricity to the atrium or ventricle
embolism	Blood clot, air, or fat that moves into or through a blood vessel and causes a blockage
endarterectomy	Incision into an artery to remove the inner lining to eliminate disease or blockage
fistula	Abnormal opening from 1 area to another, inside or outside the body (can be surgically created or the result of injury or disease)
hematopoiesis	Formation of blood cells
infarction	Necrosis caused by obstruction of circulation to an area

Continues

Term	Definition
injection	Forcing fluid into a vessel or cavity
ischemia	Deficient blood supply due to obstruction of blood vessel
pacemaker	A surgically placed electrical device that controls the beating of the heart by electrical impulses A single chamber pacemaker has 1 electrode inserted in either an atrium or a ventricle; a dual chamber pacemaker has electrodes placed in both the atrium and ventricle
pericardium	Membranous sac enclosing the heart
phlebectomy	Excision of a vein
great saphenous vein	Longest vein in the body: extending from the foot to the groin
septal defect	Any anomaly in the separating wall
sinus of Valsalva	Aortic sinus: a dilatation in the aortic wall and valves
thrombosis	Presence or condition of a blood clot in a vessel
transluminal	Performed through the lumen or opening
truncus arteriosus	An arterial trunk: undivided short portion
valve	A membranous fold in a passage that prevents reflux
vein	A vessel that carries deoxygenated blood from the body to the heart
ventricle	Lower chamber of the heart

CONCEPTS CHECKPOINT **12.1**

Match the term in the first column to the definition in the second column.

1. _____ bypass
2. _____ pacemaker
3. _____ endarterectomy
4. _____ angioplasty
5. _____ catheter

a. Incision into an artery to remove the inner lining and disease or blockage
b. Surgical repair of a vessel to dilate the opening, used to treat atherosclerosis
c. To go around (detour around blocked vessels)
d. Surgically placed device that directs electrical pulses to the heart to maintain normal rhythm
e. A tube placed in the body to put fluid in or take fluid out

Organization of the Cardiovascular System Surgery Subsection

The Cardiovascular System Surgery subsection in the CPT® codebook includes codes for procedures on the heart, pericardium, arteries and veins, the hemic and lymphatic systems, mediastinum, and diaphragm. The codes are arranged by anatomical site headings and then by the specific procedures. The main headings for this subsection and the corresponding code numbers are listed in Tables 12.2 through 12.4. Consistent with the other surgical subsections in the CPT® codebook, many of the codes are differentiated by the specific anatomical site on which the procedure is performed.

Table 12.2 Headings Within the Cardiovascular System Surgery Subsection of the CPT® Codebook

Codebook Heading	Code Range
Heart and Pericardium	33010-33999
Arteries and Veins	34001-37799

Table 12.3 Headings Within the Hemic and Lymphatic System Subsection of the CPT® Codebook

Codebook Heading	Code Range
Spleen	38100-38200
General	38204-38232
Transplantation and Post-Transplantation Cellular Infusions	38240-38243
Lymph Nodes and Lymphatic Channels	38300-38999

Table 12.4 Headings Within the Mediastinum and Diaphragm Subsection of the CPT® Codebook

Codebook Heading	Code Range
Mediastinum	39000-39499
Diaphragm	39501-39599

Heart and Pericardium (Codes 33010-33999)

The **heart** is an organ with 4 **chambers**: the upper chambers are the **right atrium** and **left atrium**, and the lower chambers are the **right ventricle** and **left ventricle**. Figure 12.1 shows the anatomy of the heart and the coronary arteries.

Coronary arteries supply blood to the heart itself. These arteries can become blocked from disease, causing damage to the heart tissue, and a patient may suffer from a **myocardial infarction** (heart attack). **Cardiac catheterization** or **coronary artery bypass** surgery may be performed to restore blood flow to the heart. These and many other cardiovascular procedures will be reviewed in this chapter.

Figure 12.1 Structure of the Heart

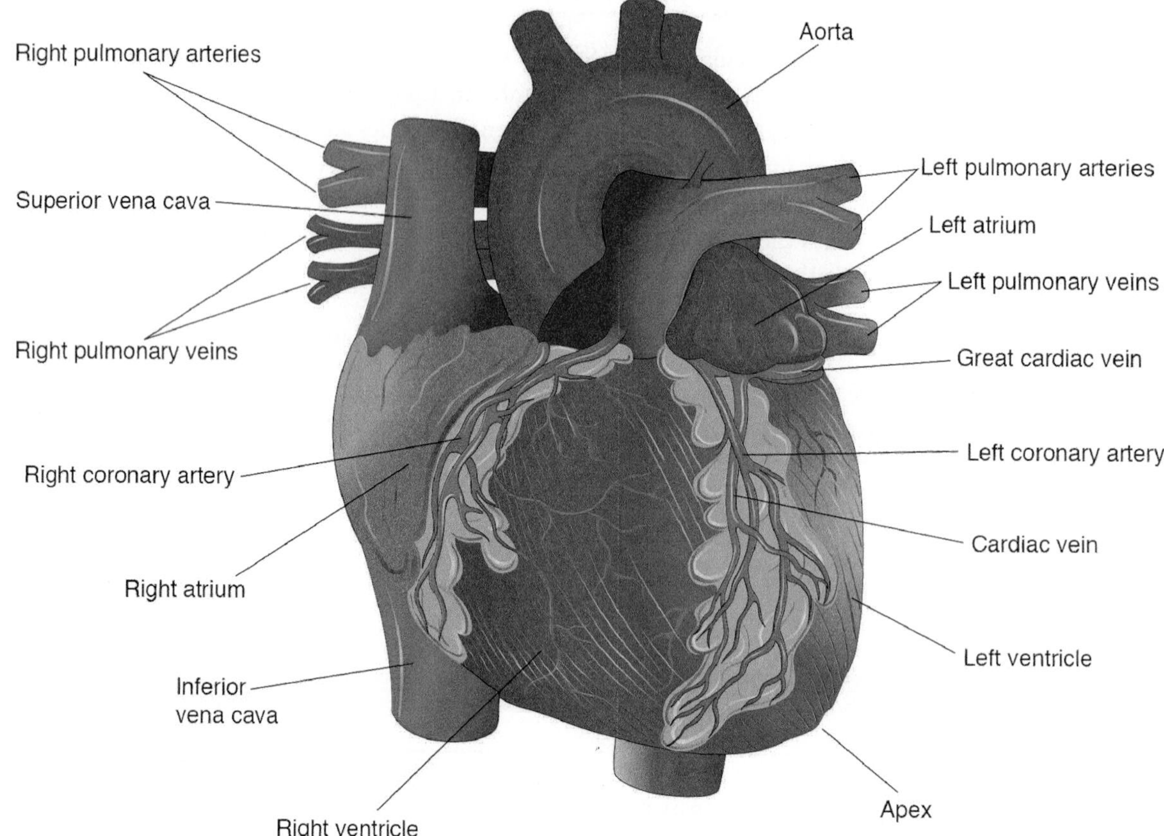

Surgeries on the heart and pericardium include insertion of devices to regulate heart rate, heart valve repair and replacement, coronary bypass procedures, and the correction of aneurysms. There are many instructional notes in the tabular list to guide the coder in assigning the correct code for procedures on the heart and its structures. Categories of codes that have notes are asterisked in the subsection table of contents.

Pacemaker or Implantable Defibrillator Codes

An **arrhythmia** is an irregular heart rate or rhythm. Cardiac specialists insert devices to control heartbeat based on the intervention needed.

Overview of Pacemaker and Implantable Defibrillator Systems

A **pacemaker** is an electrical device that controls the beating of the heart by electrical impulses. Pacemakers monitor the electrical activity of the heart, and the electrical impulses help the heart maintain normal rhythm. An **implantable defibrillator**, formerly known as a **pacing cardioverter-defibrillator**, is like a pacemaker in its use of low-energy pulses, but this device can also use high-energy pulses to treat life-threatening arrhythmia.

CPT® codes 33202 through 33273 describe the insertion and removal of pacemaker and defibrillator systems and components. The coder must consider several criteria when choosing codes for these procedures:

- the type of system inserted: pacemaker or implantable defibrillator;
- the approach for insertion: open by thoracotomy, endoscopic, subcutaneous, or transvenous;
- which component(s) of the system are placed or replaced; and
- where the component(s) are placed: epicardium, atrium, ventricle, or multiple chambers of the heart.

The CPT®codebook provides extensive notes on the devices and detailed graphics of a temporary pacemaker system, an implanted pacemaker system, and placement of biventricular pacing electrodes. The notes, graphics, and tabular material in the codebook should always be reviewed prior to assigning codes.

Components of Pacemaker and Implantable Defibrillator Systems

Pacemaker and implantable defibrillator systems both have basic hardware components that have procedures for placement, revision, relocation, and revision. These components are the following:

- the pulse generator, which contains the electronics and the battery, and
- the electrodes or leads, which transfer electricity.

A handy table in the codebook correlates the many procedures with the codes associated with the different components for a pacemaker system and an implantable defibrillator system. A **pulse generator** contains the electronics and the battery for the system. The generator is inserted and is placed in a subcutaneous skin pocket created either in a subclavicular site, axillary site, or below the ribs underneath the abdominal muscles. The **electrodes** are the leads that transfer electricity to the atrium and/or ventricle. They are inserted transvenously either through the subclavian or jugular vein, positioned under the skin overlying the heart, or placed directly on the heart's surface. If an electrode is placed **epicardially** (on the heart's surface), a thoracotomy may be required to open the chest to reach the epicardium. Electrodes may also be placed on the epicardium using a thoracoscopic approach. Epicardial placement of electrodes may be separately reported using codes 33202 (open) and 33203 (endoscopic). The coder must also separately report for insertion of a pulse generator if done at the time of epicardial placement of lead(s).

As shown in Figure 12.2, a **single chamber pacemaker system** includes a pulse generator and 1 electrode placed in either the atrium or ventricle. A **dual chamber pacemaker system** includes a pulse generator and 1 electrode in the right atrium and 1 electrode in the right ventricle. Sometimes an additional electrode is placed in the left ventricle to achieve the required pacing. This requires an additional code, 33224 or 33225 for transvenous placement, or 33202 or 33203 for epicardial placement.

Like a pacemaker, an **implantable defibrillator system** includes a pulse generator and electrodes. This type of system may require multiple leads even if a single chamber is

Figure 12.2 Single and Dual Chamber Pacemaker Systems

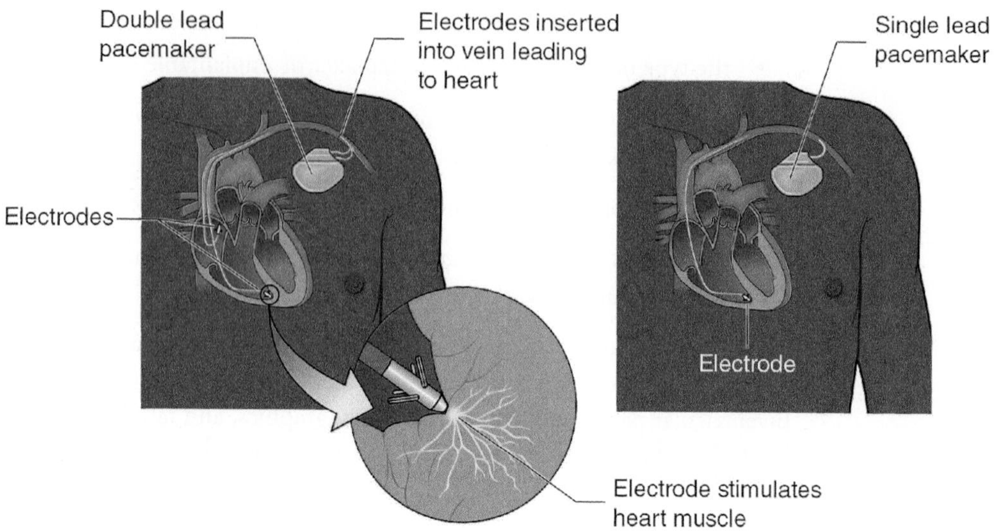

being paced. A single chamber system would have a lead in the ventricle, while a dual chamber system has leads in both the atrium and ventricle. The implantable defibrillator's pulse generator would be placed in a subcutaneous skin pocket in either the abdomen or the infraclavicular area.

The CPT® guidelines note the distinctions between single lead, dual leads, and multiple leads, to help in the application of codes 33206 through 33273. A **single lead** pacemaker or implantable defibrillator has pacing and sensing functions in either the atrium or the ventricle, but not both. The lead is in only 1 chamber of the heart. **Dual leads** refers to pacing and sensing functions in both 1 atrium and 1 ventricle. The leads are located in 2 chambers of the heart. **Multiple leads** refers to 3 or 4 leads with pacing and sensing functions in any combination of atrium and ventricle.

Codes 33206 through 33208 include the subcutaneous insertion of the pulse generator and the transvenous placement of the electrode(s). These codes, shown in Figure 12.3, are differentiated by the location of the electrodes.

Figure 12.3 Pacemaker System Insertion Codes

33206	Insertion of new or replacement of permanent pacemaker with transvenous electrode(s); atrial
33207	Insertion of new or replacement of permanent pacemaker with transvenous electrode(s); ventricular
33208	Insertion of new or replacement of permanent pacemaker with transvenous electrode(s); atrial and ventricular

In an emergency situation, a temporary pacemaker may be placed for a patient with a transient arrhythmic condition (such as symptomatic bradycardia) that is not considered to be an ongoing condition. A temporary pacemaker may also be placed if a permanent pacemaker is not necessary or available when needed. The generator is placed outside of the body instead of being implanted under the skin. A single chamber temporary pacemaker insertion or replacement is reported with code 33210, and a dual chamber temporary insertion or replacement with code 33211.

In a pacemaker or implantable defibrillator, the pulse generator is the power source or battery. There are times when the pulse generator must be removed or replaced due to a malfunction or dead battery. Pacemaker batteries last on average about 6 to 7 years. When the "battery" is changed, it is really the pulse generator that is changed. Separate codes exist for removal of a pulse generator only, removal with replacement, and removal with replacement of both pulse generator and electrodes. It is important for a coder to read operative notes carefully to determine the extent of the procedure performed.

The code for upgrading a single chamber system to a dual chamber system, as shown in Figure 12.4, includes removal of the previously placed pulse generator, testing of the existing lead, insertion and inspection of the new lead, and insertion of the new pulse generator. This code (33214) cannot be reported with the codes for removal and replacement of a pulse generator only (33227 through 33229).

Figure 12.4 Pacemaker Upgrade Code

33214	Upgrade of implanted pacemaker system, conversion of single chamber system to dual chamber system

A skin pocket is created to hold the pulse generator of a pacemaker or implantable defibrillator. The pocket may need to be relocated due to complications from the original placement of the generator, infection, or skin erosion at the original site. Revision of a skin pocket is included in codes 33206 through 33249 and 33262 through 33264. Relocation of a skin pocket for either a pacemaker (33222) or implantable defibrillator (33223) could be done alone or with a pulse generator and/or electrode insertion, replacement, or repositioning. When the relocation is done as part of a removal of an old pulse generator with placement of a new pulse generator, the pocket relocation can be coded separately. The pocket relocation codes shown in Figure 12.5 include any incision and drainage of a hematoma or abscess if performed, and the opening and closing of the site. These pocket relocation codes cannot be reported with the codes from the integumentary section for incision and drainage of hematomas or wound infections, the debridement codes, or wound repair codes (10140, 10180, 11042 through 11047, and 13100 through 13102).

Figure 12.5 Skin Pocket Relocation Codes

33222	Relocation of skin pocket for pacemaker
33223	Relocation of skin pocket for implantable defibrillator

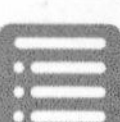

Index Insider

You can find pacemaker and implantable defibrillator procedure codes indexed under various main terms:

- *Pacemaker, Heart: Insertion* for electrodes, a pulse generator, or a temporary pacemaker; *Relocate Pocket, Replacement, Repositioning*; and *Upgrade* for a device change from a single chamber to a dual chamber device
- *Implantable Defibrillator*
- *Insertion*
- *Repositioning*, when electrode repositioning is to be reported.

EXAMPLE 12.1

A thin, 86-year-old female presented to her cardiologist's office complaining of skin erosion over her pacemaker implantation site. The cardiologist noted that her skin was intact and the hardware was not yet breaking through the skin. The pacemaker was functioning and not exposed. A revision of the pacemaker pocket was scheduled. The patient was brought to surgery, and the cardiologist successfully relocated the pocket 3 inches from the original site using the existing generator and electrodes. This is reported with code 33222, *Relocation of skin pocket for pacemaker*.

Before you can assign a code for a pacemaker procedure, you must know the answers to these questions:

- Is this a permanent or temporary pacemaker?
- Is this an initial placement or replacement?
- If this is a replacement, is a component of the device being replaced, or is the whole system being replaced?
- Is this a single or dual chamber device? (Where will the electrodes be placed?)
- Is this a transvenous, epicardial, or subcutaneous lead placement?

Once you have read the operative note and determined exactly what procedures were performed, you are ready to code.

LET'S TRY ONE 12.1

Code the following pacemaker procedures:

1. Mr. Smith, an otherwise healthy 55-year-old male, experienced episodes of dizziness and shortness of breath. He was also feeling fatigued, so he visited his physician. The physician did an electrocardiogram (ECG), which revealed a second-degree heart block. Mr. Smith was scheduled for an insertion of a pacemaker. A permanent pacemaker was implanted with a transvenous insertion of an electrode into the right ventricle. _____
2. A few days after Mr. Smith's initial pacemaker implantation, he felt very dizzy. His ECG showed some abnormalities, and his physician believed the pacemaker was malfunctioning. The pulse generator and lead were removed and replaced with a new pacemaker system. A permanent pacemaker was implanted with a transvenous insertion of an electrode into the right ventricle. _____
3. Mr. Smith continued to experience shortness of breath and fatigue. His physician decided to upgrade his single chamber ventricular pacemaker to a dual chamber device. The previously placed pulse generator and electrode were removed, and a new system was implanted. _____

Electrophysiologic Operative Procedures

Electrophysiologic operative procedures are used to treat cardiac arrhythmias. The procedures described with codes 33250 through 33266 include operative tissue ablation with and without cardiopulmonary bypass. In these procedures, the source of the

RED FLAG

Watch for the # in front of codes in the Cardiovascular System subsection. The # indicates the codes are out of numerical sequence. In the tabular list:

- 33227, 33228, and 33239 appear after code 33233;
- 33230 and 33231 appear after 33240;
- 33262, 33263, and 33264 appear after 33241 but before 33243.

arrhythmia is destroyed using electrical current, freezing, or cutting. Add-on codes 33257 through 33259 are reported when the tissue ablation is performed in conjunction with other cardiac procedures.

Heart (Including Valves) and Great Vessels

Procedures described in the heart and great vessels subsection (33300 through 33335) include exploration and repair of cardiac and great vessel wounds. Codes are differentiated by the use of cardiopulmonary bypass. Codes 33300 and 33305 describe the repair of cardiac wounds when penetrating trauma is suspected. Codes 33310 and 33315 describe exploratory cardiotomy and include removal of foreign bodies on the surface or within the heart. Codes 33220 through 33322 describe repair by suture of the aorta or great vessels. Codes 33330 and 33335 are reported when a graft is inserted in the aorta or great vessel.

Cardiac Valve Procedures

Valves in the heart allow blood to flow only in 1 direction. The 4 main valves are the mitral, tricuspid, aortic, and pulmonary. The tricuspid and pulmonary valves are in the right heart and the mitral and aortic valves in the left heart, as shown in Figure 12.6.

When heart valves do not work correctly because of valvular stenosis or insufficiency, surgery may be needed to repair or replace the damaged valves. Codes for procedures on cardiac valves are arranged first by anatomical site under the codebook categories

Figure 12.6 Heart Valves

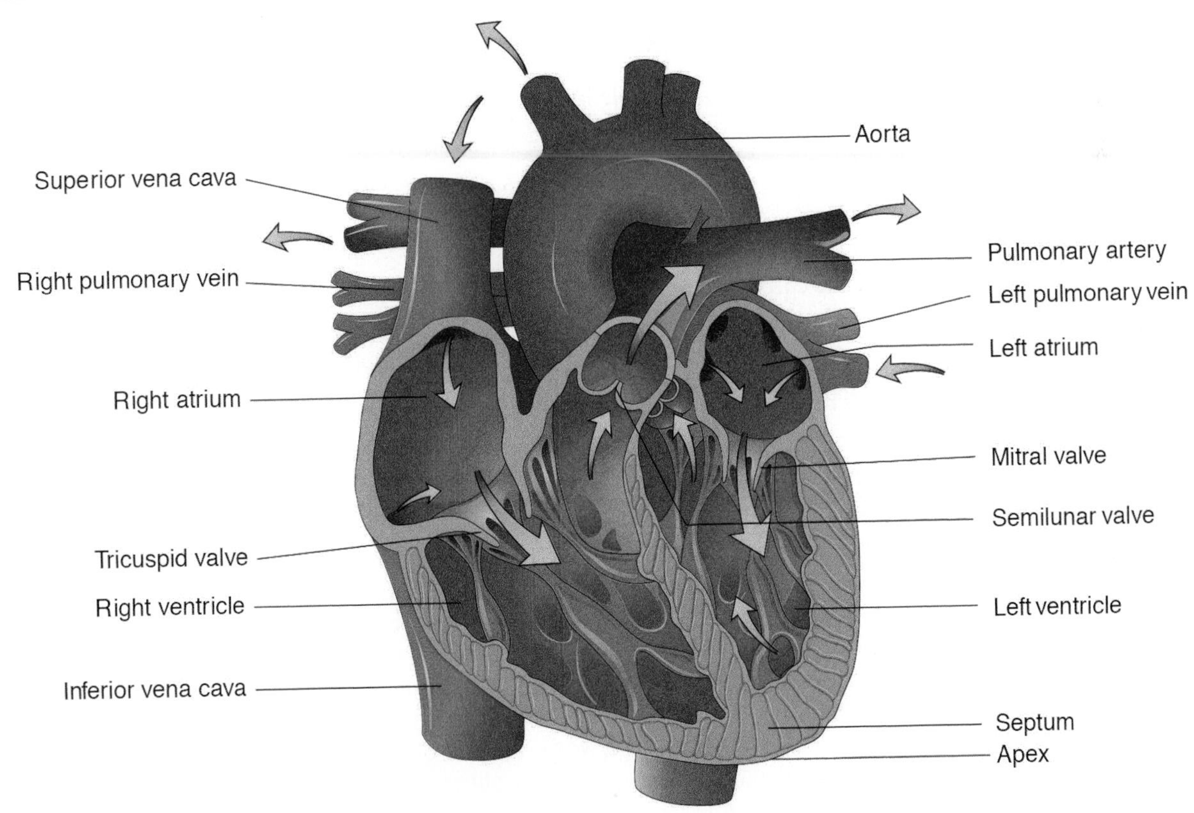

Aortic Valve, Mitral Valve, Tricuspid Valve, and Pulmonary Valve. Extensive notes provide guidance for reporting the Aortic Valve and Mitral Valve categories. Valve codes are further differentiated by the specific procedure and the anatomical approach. Multiple codes may be reported if multiple valve procedures are performed.

Transcatheter aortic valve replacement (TAVR) and **transcatheter aortic valve implantation (TAVI)** are reported with codes 33361 through 33366. **Transcatheter mitral valve repair (TMVR)** is reported with codes 33418 and 33419. These surgeries are performed on patients with **symptomatic aortic stenosis** (a narrowing of the valve that constricts normal blood flow), who are high risk and not candidates for the traditional open chest valve surgery technique due to their condition. These are minimally invasive procedures performed through smaller incisions than traditional heart valve surgery. The valves can be replaced with biological or mechanical valves. **Biological valves** could be bovine (cow), porcine (pig), or human tissue. **Mechanical valves** are made of metal or carbon parts and are more durable than the biological valves.

Aortic valve procedure codes include percutaneous, open arterial, and cardiac approaches. As noted in the CPT® guidelines, TAVR and TAVI codes include the constituent procedures of percutaneous access, placing the access sheath, balloon aortic valvuloplasty, advancing the valve delivery system into position, repositioning as needed, deploying the valve, inserting the temporary pacemaker, and closing the arteriotomy. The TMVR codes additionally include transseptal puncture. Angiography and radiological supervision and interpretation (imaging guidance) is included in these surgeries and not separately reported, with the exception of **diagnostic coronary angiography** (using x-ray imaging to see the coronary vessels), which may be separately reportable under some circumstances:

- No prior angiography study is available and a full diagnostic study is performed at the time of TAVR, TAVI, or TMVR.
- A prior study is available but the patient's condition with respect to the clinical indication for the procedure has changed.
- Inadequate visualization of the anatomy or pathology requires a new study.
- A clinical change during the procedure requires new evaluation.

Diagnostic coronary angiography that is performed on the same day or during the same operative episode as TAVR, TAVI, or TMVR should be reported with modifier 59, *Distinct procedural service*, or modifier XU, to indicate that it is a separate procedure. Depending on your specific circumstances, XU or 59 may be most appropriate.

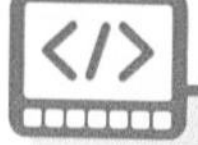

Coding for CMS

CMS has defined 4 HCPCS modifiers to use in place of modifier 59 under specific circumstances. These modifiers are referred to as X(ESPU). XE: *separate encounter*—a service that is distinct because it occurred during a separate encounter; XS: *separate structure*—a service that is distinct because it was performed on a separate organ/structure; XP: *separate practitioner*—a service that is distinct because it was performed by a different practitioner; XU: *unusual non-overlapping service*—the use of a service that is distinct because it does not overlap usual components of the main service.

Coronary Artery Bypass Grafting

When the coronary arteries become blocked, a **coronary artery bypass graft (CABG)** is performed to reestablish blood supply to the heart and prevent permanent damage to the heart itself. During a CABG procedure, a healthy artery or vein from another part of the patient's body is grafted to the blocked coronary artery. The graft bypasses the blocked coronary artery and establishes a new blood flow path.

The codes for CABG are assigned based on the type of vessel used to complete the bypass and the number of bypasses performed. The types of vessel include artery, vein, or both artery and vein. Coronary artery bypass graft codes are separated into 3 groups in the CPT® codebook: venous grafting only, combined arterial-venous grafting, and arterial grafting. It is important to distinguish between the number of bypasses completed using arteries and the number of bypasses completed using veins for correct code reporting.

EXAMPLE **12.2**

A 68-year-old male was found to have coronary artery disease in 3 vessels. A triple coronary artery bypass graft was performed. The left internal mammary artery was anastomosed to the left anterior descending artery and to the diagonal. A saphenous vein graft was used to bypass the right posterior descending artery. In this surgery, 2 arterial grafts and 1 venous graft were used to complete the bypasses. Codes 33534 (*2 arterial grafts*) and 33517 (*single vein graft*) are reported.

Venous Grafting Only

The exclusive use of venous grafts to complete CABG bypass(es) is reported with codes 33510 through 33516. Harvesting of the commonly used saphenous vein from the leg is included in these codes. However, sometimes the patient does not have a suitable lower extremity vein like the greater or lesser saphenous for use in the CABG. The surgeon may have to obtain a vein long enough to perform the bypass from an upper extremity, in which case add-on code 35500, *Harvest of upper extremity vein, 1 segment*, is reported in addition to the CABG code. If the femoropopliteal vein is used to complete the CABG, add-on code 35572, *Harvest of femoropopliteal vein, 1 segment,* is reported in addition to the CABG code. The CABG codes are selected depending on the number of bypasses completed, from code 33510 for 1 bypass to 35516 for 6 or more.

Combined Arterial-Venous Grafting

A CABG performed with a combination of arterial and venous grafts is reported with codes for each: the arterial graft is reported with a code from 33533 through 33536, and the venous graft is reported with an add-on code from 33517 through 33530. The add-on codes represent the number of grafts performed using veins and are reported with the primary procedure code for the specific bypass using arteries. The add-on codes represent the same procedures from the venous grafting only section but are used to report CABGs with both veins and arteries.

Arterial Grafting

The arterial grafting codes for coronary artery bypass, 33533 through 33536, are used alone when a CABG is performed with arterial grafts only, or are used in combination with the venous grafts add-on codes when a CABG is performed using both arteries and veins. The use of the internal mammary artery, gastroepiploic artery, epigastric artery, and radial artery are included in these codes. Arterial conduits from other sites are also included. When an upper extremity artery is harvested for the graft, the add-on code 35600, *Harvest of upper extremity artery, 1 segment, for coronary artery bypass procedure*, is reported in addition to the CABG code.

Inside the OR

In Figure 12.7, the patient's coronary artery is blocked. After a CABG is performed, blood flow to the heart is restored. A single vein graft like the 1 shown in Figure 12.7 is reported with code 33510, *Coronary artery bypass, vein only; single coronary venous graft*. In this open heart surgery, a sternotomy is performed, where the sternum is split in the middle with a bone saw. The surgeon cuts through the pericardium. The aorta is inspected. The saphenous vein is harvested from the leg, or a vein is taken from the arm or the back of the leg. A point is chosen beyond the area of diseased coronary artery. The vein is cut to fit and the end of the vein is sewn to the side of the coronary artery. (This is called an *end-to-side anastomosis*.) A hole is punched in the ascending aorta and the other end of the vein graft is sewn to that hole. The surgeon checks all sutures for leaks, and the site is irrigated. The sternum is closed with stainless steel wires. The fascia, subcutaneous tissues, and skin are closed in layers. The leg and/or arm incisions are closed in multiple layers. Drains are inserted as needed with separate incisions.

Figure 12.7 Preoperative and Postoperative Illustration of Coronary Artery Bypass Graft (CABG)

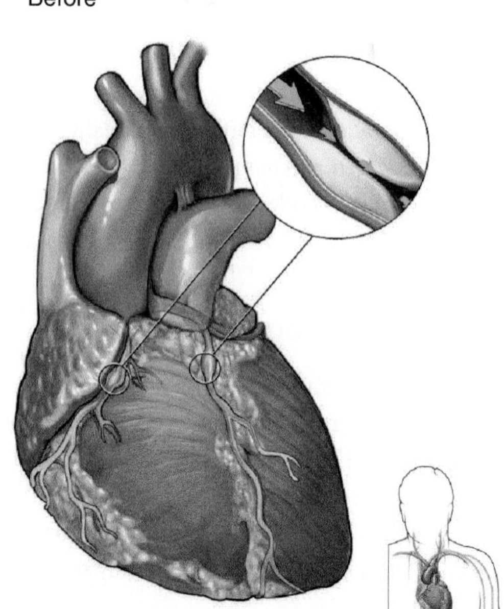

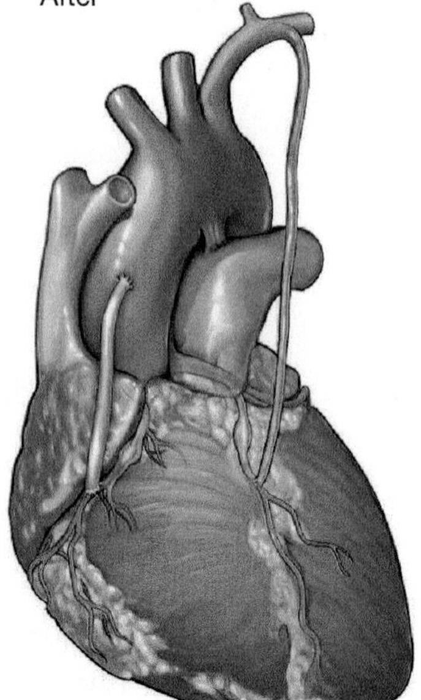

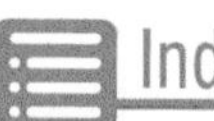

Index Insider

The most direct way to find CABG codes is under the main entry *Coronary Artery Bypass Graft (CABG)* with the subterm for the type of bypass. These codes are also indexed under the main entry *Coronary Artery*, subterm *Graft*, and either *Arterial Bypass*, *Venous Bypass*, or *Arterial-Venous Bypass*. CABG codes are not indexed under the main term *Heart*.

LET'S TRY ONE 12.2

Assign the correct code(s) for each of the following procedures.

1. A 62-year-old female was found to have severe narrowing of 2 coronary arteries due to atherosclerosis. Double coronary artery bypass grafting was completed using veins only. _____
2. An 81-year-old male complained of chest pain. A coronary angiogram revealed blockage of the left anterior descending and right coronary arteries. Coronary artery bypass was performed using 2 arterial grafts. _____
3. A 59-year-old male required a triple CABG due to blockage caused by coronary artery disease. A coronary artery bypass using 1 venous graft and 2 arterial grafts was performed. _____

CONCEPTS CHECKPOINT 12.2

Choose the most correct answer to complete the following statements.

1. A dual chamber pacemaker system has
   a. an electrode in the atrium only.
   b. an electrode in the ventricle only.
   c. 1 electrode in either the atrium or the ventricle.
   d. 1 electrode in the atrium and 1 in the ventricle.
2. Incision and drainage of a hematoma at the location of a pacemaker pocket
   a. can be reported as an additional code with the code for pocket relocation.
   b. is included in the code for relocation of pocket.
   c. is reported with a code from the integumentary section with the code for pocket relocation.
   d. is reported with a debridement code.
3. The codes for CABG procedures are dependent on
   a. the type of vessel used to complete the bypass.
   b. the number of bypasses performed.
   c. whether the patient has a pacemaker or not.
   d. both the type of vessel used and the number of bypasses performed.

Extracorporeal Membrane Oxygenation or Extracorporeal Life Support Services

Extracorporeal Membrane Oxygenation (ECMO) or Extracorporeal Life Support (ECLS) codes report the physician work involved in the provision of these labor-intensive services. Prolonged **Extracorporeal Membrane Oxygenation (ECMO)** or **Extracorporeal Life Support (ECLS)** is a procedure that provides support to the heart and/or lungs, allowing patients to rest and recover from sickness or injury. The ECMO/ECLS supports heart and lung function as it continuously pumps the blood out of the patient's body to an oxygenator and then returns the blood to the patient. The oxygenator is a medical device that adds oxygen and removes carbon dioxide from a patient's blood. The ECMO/ECLS can be done using 2 methods: veno-arterial or veno-venous. Veno-arterial ECMO/ECLS supports both the heart and lungs and requires the placement of 2 cannulas: 1 in a large vein and the other in a large artery.

Veno-venous ECMO/ECLS supports the lungs only and requires 1 or 2 cannulas, placed in a vein.

Placement of the cannula is a surgical procedure that can be done percutaneously (through the skin) or as an open procedure. Initial placement and repositioning of the cannula is included in the codes for ECMO/ECLS.

The initiation and daily management of patients receiving these services require physician oversight of the ECMO/ECLS circuit and parameters, including the monitoring of blood flow, oxygenation, carbon dioxide clearance, systemic response, anticoagulation and treatment of bleeding, cannula positioning, alarms, and safety of the patient. The daily overall patient management depends on the medical condition and may be reported with appropriate E/M codes in addition to the ECMO/ECLS codes.

Codes for ECMO/ECLS are dependent on several factors:

- veno-arterial versus veno-venous;
- initiation versus daily management;
- insertion versus repositioning;
- central versus peripheral;
- the age of the patient (birth through age 5 versus age 6 and older);
- removal of cannula.

Arteries and Veins (Codes 34001-37799)

Vascular procedures listed in this heading include excision, repairs, and bypass grafts on vessels other than coronary arteries. Notes at the beginning of the arteries and veins portion of the CPT® codebook describe the services included in primary vascular procedure codes that are not separately reportable: establishing inflow and outflow to the vessel by any technique or procedure; and an intraoperative arteriogram performed by the surgeon. The special instructions that appear before many of the vascular codes will be discussed in this chapter.

Endovascular Repair of Aortic Aneurysm

An **aortic aneurysm** is a bulge in a weakened part of the aortic wall caused by the pressure of the blood pumping. An aneurysm can expand and cause life-threatening conditions, such as a hemorrhage. Surgical treatment may be recommended when the physician determines that the aneurysm has grown to a critical size, based on its rate of growth and patient symptoms.

Endovascular repair of an aortic aneurysm requires the skill of both a vascular surgeon and a radiologist. The radiologist interprets images and provides guidance so the surgeon can locate the aneurysm more efficiently. Fluoroscopic guidance provided in conjunction with endovascular aneurysm repair is reported separately by the radiologist.

Codes for the repair of aortic aneurysms are differentiated by several criteria:

- location in the aorta (below the renal arteries or the visceral branches);
- extent of the surgical treatment (additional artery exposure or incisions); and
- whether the repair was for a rupture or for other than rupture.

Codes 34701 through 34706 describe procedures for abdominal aortic aneurysm repair. Codes 34841 through 34848 describe procedures for repair of the visceral aorta, which contains the celiac, superior mesenteric, and renal arteries. The location of these arteries can be seen in Figure 12.8.

Figure 12.8 Location of Abdominal Arteries

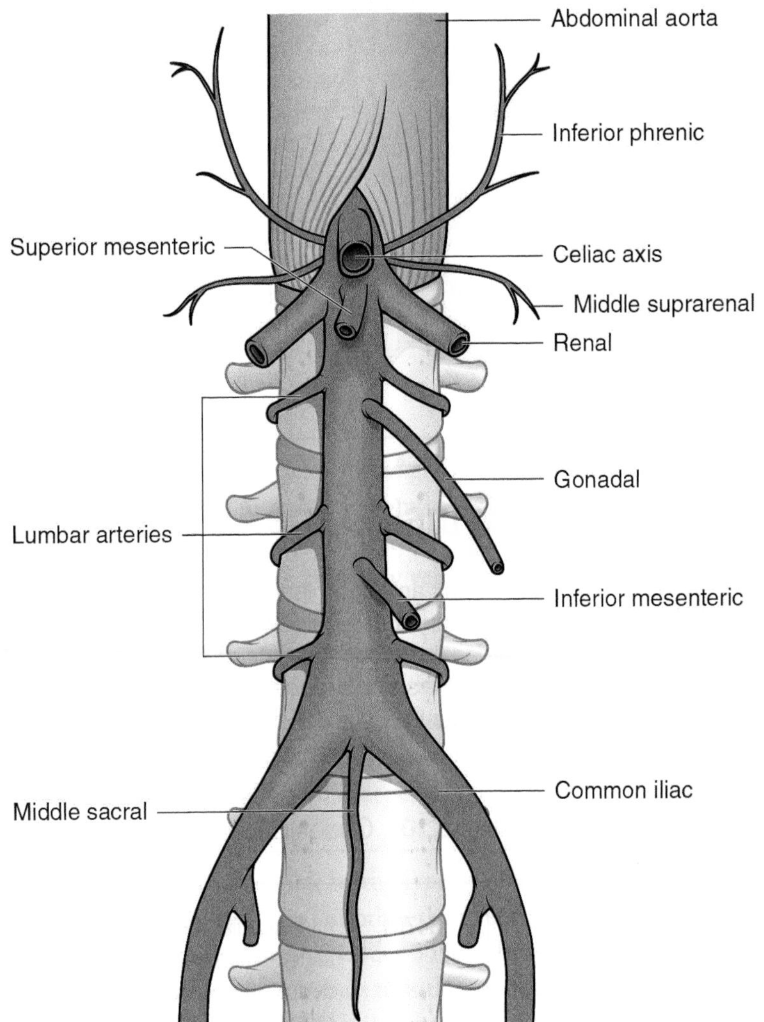

Codes 34701 through 34706 include exposing the femoral or iliac artery, manipulation of a stent or prosthesis, and closure of the arteriotomy site. Balloon angioplasty and stent deployment within the treatment zone are included and not reported separately. The introduction of guidewires and catheters is not included and can be reported separately. Figure 12.9 is a graphic representation of code 34701, *Endovascular repair of infrarenal aorta by deployment of an aorto-aortic tube endograft.* Figure 12.10 illustrates codes 34701 and 34702 and their full description from the codebook.

Bypass graft codes are further differentiated by the site of the bypass and arranged head to toe, from the carotid in the neck to the distal arteries in the legs. Each code describes the location of where the bypass graft starts and where it is connected. For example, 35516 *Bypass graft, vein; subclavian-axillary* describes a vein graft that extends from the subclavian artery to the axillary artery.

LET'S TRY ONE **12.4**

Assign codes for each of the following bypass procedures.

1. Femoral-popliteal bypass using the harvested saphenous vein: _____
2. Axillary-femoral bypass using a synthetic vein: _____
3. In-situ vein bypass, femoral-popliteal: _____

Vascular Injection Procedures

The procedures described by codes in the vascular injection subsection (36000 through 36598) include the introduction of needles and catheters, venipunctures, transfusions, apheresis, and other vascular injections. Interventional cardiovascular coding for procedures included in this subsection (and those cardiac catheterizations in the Medicine section) require specialization and a tremendous attention to detail. Some of the most common procedures in this subsection will be discussed in this chapter.

Central Venous Access Procedures

Coding Clicks

There are many different brands of central venous catheters and implanted ports. Do an Internet search to compare brands. Some of the common tunneled central venous catheters include Hickman, Broviac, Leonard, and Lifecath. Some of the common implanted ports include Port-a-Cath, BardPort, MediPort, and Infuse-a-Port.

A **central venous access device (VAD)** is a small, flexible tube placed in a large vein for a patient who needs long-term intravenous therapy like chemotherapy or antibiotics. A VAD remains in place for weeks or sometimes months, reducing anxiety and pain for the patient by avoiding needle sticks at each visit. A venous access device may have a subcutaneous port (placed just under the skin) or an external catheter. A subcutaneous pump may also be used to dispense medication.

Extensive codebook resources support the Central Venous Access Procedures category. Notes give the criteria that define a VAD: to qualify as a central venous catheter or device, the tip of the catheter must end in the subclavian, brachiocephalic (innominate) or iliac vein, the superior or inferior vena cava, or the right atrium. "The Central Venous Access Procedures Table" sorts the codes by the criteria that differentiate them:

- The codebook primarily groups the codes into 5 categories: insertion, repair, partial replacement, complete replacement, and removal.
- The placement procedures are either non-tunneled (fixed in place at the insertion site) or tunneled (passed under the skin from the insertion site to a separate exit site).
- The device is centrally or peripherally inserted.

- The placement is accompanied by ports or pumps.
- The age criteria of the patient is specified as younger than 5 years or 5 years or older; when unspecified, as any age.

As described in "The Central Venous Access Procedures Table," codes for central venous access procedures 36555 through 36590 are separated into 5 categories, which will be discussed in turn:

1. Insertion—placing a device through a new access site.
2. Repair—fixing the device without replacing any part of it.
3. Partial replacement—replacing the catheter component only.
4. Complete replacement of the entire device using the same access site.
5. Removal of the entire device.

Insertion Category of VAD Codes

Insertion VAD codes 36555 through 36571 are primarily differentiated by whether the placement is tunneled or non-tunneled. Next, the code specifies the type of insertion, either centrally or peripherally inserted. As shown in Figure 12.11, a **centrally inserted VAD** has an entry site of the jugular, subclavian, or femoral vein, or the inferior vena cava. A peripherally inserted VAD is inserted through a peripheral vein like the basilic or cephalic vein. A **peripherally inserted central catheter** is often referred to as a *PICC line*. Insertion codes then identify the presence of a port and/or pump. The final criterion is the age of the patient when specified: either younger than 5 years of age, or 5 years and older.

Figure 12.11 Centrally Inserted Vascular Access Device with Port

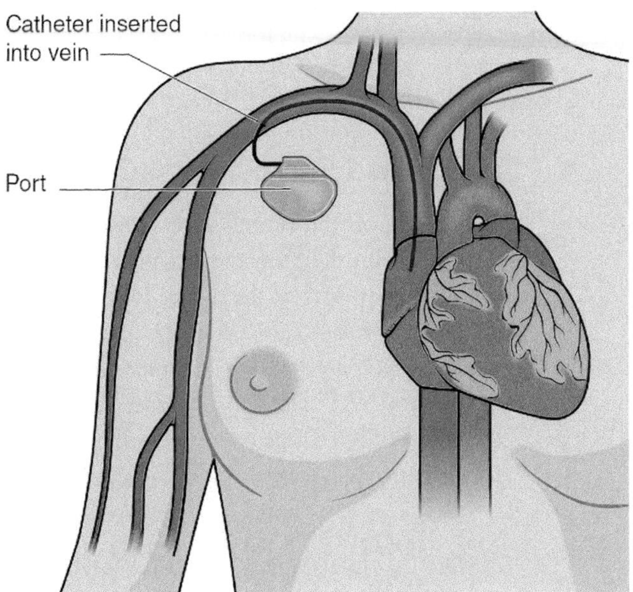

EXAMPLE **12.3**

A 4 year-old-boy requires long-term chemotherapy for treatment of leukemia. A Hickman catheter was inserted through the right subclavian vein, and a chest x-ray confirmed the tip terminated in the superior vena cava. The coder must answer the following questions to track the criteria for the correct code:

- Does the documentation show this was tunneled? No mention of tunneling.
- Was this device peripherally inserted or centrally inserted? Inserted through the subclavian so centrally inserted.
- Was a port or pump placed? No mention of port or pump placement.
- Is this patient 5 years of age or older? No, this patient is 4 years old.

The correct code for this procedure is 36555, *Insertion of non-tunnelled centrally inserted central venous catheter; younger than 5 years of age.*

LET'S TRY ONE **12.5**

A 45-year-old female requires long-term chemotherapy for her recurrent breast cancer. She was taken to the OR and a BardPort was inserted. The surgeon accessed the subclavian vein by cutdown. A guidewire was inserted. A subcutaneous tunnel was created. The catheter was passed over the guidewire through the tunnel and into the superior vena cava. The subcutaneous pocket for the port was created close to the midline. The catheter was connected to the port. Ultrasound confirmed the tip of the catheter terminated in the superior vena cava. The port was checked for leaks. The catheter and port were secured. The incision was sutured.

Read the procedure note above and answer the following questions.

1. Is this patient 5 years of age or older? _____
2. Was this device peripherally inserted or centrally inserted? _______________
3. Does the documentation show this was tunneled? _____
4. Was a port or pump placed? _____
5. What is the correct code for this procedure? _____

Repair and Replacement Categories of VAD Codes

Repair of a central venous access device is reported with codes 36575 or 36576, depending on the presence of a port or pump. As stated above, repair codes are to be used when no part of the device is replaced. Replacement of the catheter component is reported with 36578, *Replacement, catheter only, of central venous access device, with subcutaneous port or pump, central or peripheral insertion site.* Complete replacement of a central VAD through the same venous access site is reported with codes 36580 through 36585. These codes are differentiated by tunneling, the insertion site, and the presence of a port or pump.

Removal Category of VAD Codes

Removal of a non-tunneled VAD is not coded. These are simply pulled out by the physician or other healthcare provider at the patient's bedside or during an office visit. Removal of a tunneled VAD is coded with either 36589 or 36590 depending on the presence of a port or pump. Code 36589, *Removal of tunneled central venous catheter, without subcutaneous port or pump,* is reported for removal of a tunneled catheter where sutures securing the catheter are removed and the catheter is freed from the skin. This is usually done under local anesthesia. Code 36590, *Removal of tunneled central venous access device, with subcutaneous port or pump, central or peripheral insertion,* is reported when the physician makes an incision over the port or pump device and dissects it free. The catheter is disconnected and withdrawn. This may be done under local anesthesia. Code 36590 includes use of conscious (moderate) sedation.

EXAMPLE **12.4**

A 46-year-old female has completed her chemotherapy and presented for removal of her Port-a-Cath. She was taken to the sterile procedure room. Under local anesthesia, the surgeon made an incision and removed the port. The catheter was removed. The incision was closed and dressed. This removal would be reported with 36590, *Removal of tunneled central venous access device, with subcutaneous port or pump, central or peripheral insertion*.

EXAMPLE **12.5**

A 72-year-old female inpatient has completed her IV antibiotic treatment, which had been given through a PICC line. At the patient's bedside, the physician removed the PICC line without difficulty. Since the PICC line was not tunneled and was simply pulled out, no procedure code is reported for the removal.

CONCEPTS CHECKPOINT **12.3**

Choose the correct word or phrase to fill in the blank in each of the following statements.

1. A VAD inserted through the subclavian vein is peripherally/centrally inserted.
2. Codes for insertion of VADs are based on patient age in years, with age 5/6 as the determining age.
3. Fixing a VAD without adding or removing any component is repair/replacement.
4. Removal of a tunneled catheter is/is not coded.
5. The presence of a port or pump does/does not affect VAD code reporting.

Hemodialysis Access Procedures

Codes 36800 through 36870 are used to report procedures for hemodialysis access, intervascular cannulation for extracorporeal circulation, and shunt insertion. **Hemodialysis** is the extracorporeal (outside the body) removal of waste products that patients in end-stage renal disease (kidney failure) require to stay alive.

Hemodialysis requires access to the blood by an intravenous catheter, arteriovenous fistula, or synthetic graft. Central venous catheters are sometimes used for dialysis in patients who are in acute renal failure and expected to recover. For short-term access, a tube-shaped portal called a **cannula** can be inserted and left in place for several days. The cannula remains outside the body and can be used to remove blood from the vein, route it through the dialysis machine, and return it to the body.

The codes to report cannula insertions, revisions, and closures are the following:

- Codes 36800 and 36810 are for hemodialysis cannula insertion: code 36800 is reported for a vein-to-vein cannula and 36810 for an arteriovenous cannula.
- Code 36815 is reported for external revision or closure of the arteriovenous cannula.

For long-term hemodialysis, an **arteriovenous (AV) fistula** is created. An **arteriovenous anastomosis** (also known as an *AV fistual*) is a surgically created connective opening between an artery and a vein. This is created inside the body, often in the patient's non-dominant arm. An AV fistula creates extra blood flow into and pressure within the vein, making the vein larger and stronger. As the fistula heals (or matures), scar tissue builds up to strengthen the area even more. This provides easier access to blood vessels, making it easier to insert a needle for dialysis. An AV fistula can also be created using a method other than direct anastomosis, such as using a donor vein or a synthetic graft. Arteriovenous anastomosis codes 36818 through 36821 are differentiated by the anatomical site, as shown in the code descriptors in Figure 12.12.

Figure 12.12 Arteriovenous Anastomosis Codes

36818	Arteriovenous anastomosis, open; by upper arm cephalic vein transposition
36819	by upper arm basilic vein transposition
36820	by forearm vein transposition
36821	direct, any site (eg, Cimino type) (separate procedure)

Inside the OR

Code 36821 is reported for a direct AV anastomosis, also known as a *Cimino-type fistula*. In this procedure, a vein is divided and sutured to an opening created in a nearby artery. This allows blood to flow down the artery and into the vein, allowing an increased blood flow through the vein for hemodialysis.

As shown in Figure 12.13, 2 needles are inserted into the vein that has been widened by the fistula for hemodialysis. The patient's blood is drawn out through the arterial needle, moves through the hemodialysis machine, and is returned to the patient through the venous needle. Because capillaries are bypassed, blood flows rapidly, and dialysis is more effective.

Figure 12.13 AV Fistula

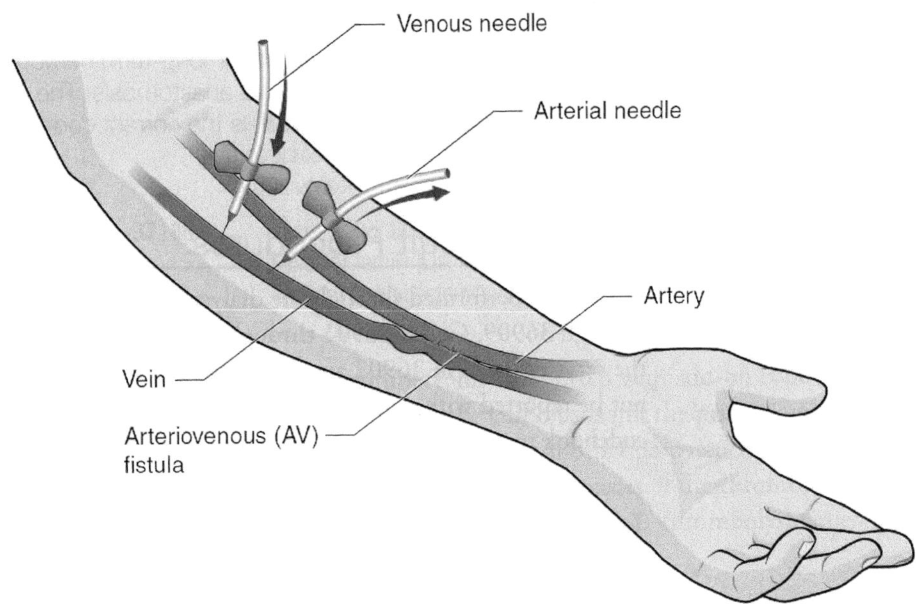

Coding for CMS

The Fistula First initiative is a quality-improvement project promoting the use of AV fistulas. Patients with AV fistulas have better survival rates and fewer complications when compared with patients using other hemodialysis access methods, so CMS has set a goal to increase the use of AV fistulas in dialysis patients.

Index Insider

Do not search the Index main entries *Fistula* or *Fistulization* for AV anastomosis codes, as they are not included under these main terms. The most direct way to find them is under the main entry *Anastomosis*, with the subterm *Arteriovenous Fistula*.

The creation of an AV fistula using a graft is coded with 36825 or 36830:

- When a vein harvested from the patient is used to create the fistula, report code 36825, *Creation of arteriovenous fistula by other than direct arteriovenous anastomosis; autogenous graft.*
- When a nonautogenous graft such as a biological collagen or thermoplastic graft (synthetic) is used, report code 36830, *Creation of arteriovenous fistula by other than direct arteriovenous anastomosis; nonautogenous graft (eg, biological collagen, thermoplastic graft).*

EXAMPLE **12.6**

A 42-year-old female patient with end-stage renal disease requires long-term dialysis while waiting for a kidney transplant. She was taken to surgery for a planned AV anastomosis. The surgeon dissected down to the basilic vein on the medial side of the patient's left upper arm. A subcutaneous tunnel was created on the anterior side of the arm and the vein was transposed to the tunnel. The basilic vein was then anastomosed to the brachial artery. This is reported with code 36819, *Arteriovenous anastomosis, open; by upper arm basilic vein transposition*.

Figure 12.15 Codes for Transcatheter Therapy for Thrombolysis

37211	Transcatheter therapy, arterial infusion for thrombolysis other than coronary or intracranial, any method, including radiological supervision and interpretation, initial treatment day
37212	Transcatheter therapy, venous infusion for thrombolysis, any method, including radiological supervision and interpretation, initial day
37213	Transcatheter therapy, arterial or venous infusion for thrombolysis other than coronary, any method, including radiological supervision and interpretation, continued treatment on subsequent day during course of thrombolytic therapy, including follow-up catheter contrast injection, position change, or exchange, when performed;

CONCEPTS CHECKPOINT **12.4**

Which of these procedures are included in the codes for percutaneous transluminal mechanical thrombectomy? (more than 1 answer may be correct) _____

a. fluoroscopic guidance
b. thrombolytic injection
c. transluminal stent placement
d. percutaneous angioplasty

Endovascular Revascularization (Open or Percutaneous, Transcatheter)

Endovascular revascularization codes (37220 through 37239) describe procedures on the iliac and lower extremity arteries that are done to revascularize occluded arteries. Only 1 code from each code family is reported for each lower extremity vessel treated because codes are arranged in a hierarchical manner. Less intensive services (with the lower code number in the code family) are included with the more intensive (higher code number). For example, code 37227, *Revascularization, endovascular, open or percutaneous, femoral, popliteal artery(s), unilateral; with transluminal stent placement(s), and atherectomy, includes angioplasty within the same vessel when performed*, includes all procedures described by codes 37224 through 37226. Coders should read the extensive instructional notes in this subsection to ensure appropriate codes are reported.

Ligation

Ligation is the tying off of veins and arteries. Codes 37565 through 37785 for ligation are found toward the end of the Cardiovascular System Surgery subsection and include procedures for biopsy of the temporal artery and division, excision, and stripping of veins. These codes are generally assigned by the anatomical site of the ligation and are arranged from head to toe (starting with the jugular vein and ending with a varicose vein in the leg). These procedures require incisions through the skin to access the vessel. Transcatheter procedures are not reported with these codes.

EXAMPLE 12.8

A 51-year-old woman had painful varicose veins on her right leg, requiring ligation and stripping. The surgeon made an incision through the skin to expose the long saphenous vein. Several more skin incisions were made along the vein. A wire was threaded through the length of the vein at the proximal end and brought out at the ankle. The vein was tied to the end of the wire, and the wire was pulled out with the vein attached. Each skin incision was closed in layered sutures. A pressure dressing was wrapped around the leg. This procedure would be reported with 37722 - RT.

Varicose veins are a common condition of the valves in the veins not functioning properly, allowing the veins to become filled with blood. This creates enlarged veins that appear blue and twisted under the skin. Varicose veins are often painful, especially after sitting or standing for lengthy periods. Many patients require surgery to ligate and strip (remove) the offending veins. Figure 12.16 shows codes 37718 and 37722, used to report the ligation, division, and stripping of the short and long saphenous veins in the leg. If identical procedures are performed on both legs, modifier 50, *Bilateral procedure*, is reported.

Figure 12.16 Codes for Vein Stripping

37718	Ligation, division, and stripping, short saphenous vein
37722	Ligation, division, and stripping, long (greater) saphenous veins from saphenofemoral junction to knee or below

Another technique to remove varicose veins is shown in Figure 12.17. **Stab phlebectomy** is a procedure in which tiny stab incisions are made over a varicose vein and a phlebectomy hook is used to grab the vein. The vein is then removed with a mosquito forceps. Stab phlebectomy is reported by the number of incisions made: use code 37765 to report 10 through 20 incisions; use code 37766 to report 21 or more incisions. If fewer than 10 incisions were made, use code 37799, *Unlisted procedure, vascular surgery.*

Figure 12.17 Stab Phlebectomy

37765	Stab phlebectomy of varicose veins, 1 extremity; 10-20 stab incisions (For less than 10 incisions, use 37799) (For more than 20 incisions, use 37766)
37766	more than 20 incisions

LET'S TRY ONE **12.7**

Assign the appropriate CPT® code for each of the following procedures.

1. Ligation and stripping of the short saphenous vein: _____
2. Ligation of the internal jugular vein: _____
3. Stab phlebectomy, right leg, 17 incisions: _____

Hemic and Lymphatic Systems (Codes 38100-38999)

Surgical codes for the hemic and lymphatic systems follow the Cardiovascular System Surgery subsection in the CPT® codebook. The hemic, lymphatic, and cardiovascular systems are vascular systems with related functions. The **hemic system** consists of the organs and processes involved in the production of blood, including the vessels and bone marrow. The **lymphatic system** consists of lymph nodes, lymph vessels, the spleen, and the thymus gland. The **lymph vessels** transport **lymph** (clear colorless tissue fluid) toward the heart, and it is drained in the cardiovascular system through the ducts in the chest. The Hemic and Lymphatic Systems Surgery subsection includes codes for open and laparoscopic surgical procedures on the spleen, bone marrow and stem cell harvesting, and open and laparoscopic surgical procedures on the lymph nodes.

Spleen Procedures

The Spleen heading in the codebook includes codes for excision, repair, laparoscopy, and introduction procedures. Indications for excision of the spleen or **splenectomy** include traumatic injury, hematological diseases, and Hodgkin's lymphoma. Iatrogenic spleen injury occurring during the performance of intraperitoneal procedures may necessitate a splenectomy. Figure 12.18 shows codes for total and partial splenectomies: 38100 for a total excision performed as a primary procedure, 38101 for a partial removal, add-on code 38102 for a total removal of the spleen performed at the time of another procedure (such as colectomy or other intraperitoneal surgery), and 38120 for a laparoscopic splenectomy.

Figure 12.18 Splenectomy Codes

Code	Description
38100	Splenectomy; total (separate procedure)
38101	partial (separate procedure)
38102	total, en bloc for extensive disease, in conjunction with other procedure (List in addition to code for primary procedure)
38120	Laparoscopy, surgical, spenectomy

General: Bone Marrow Stem Cell Transplantation

The General heading of the Hemic and Lymphatic Systems Surgery subsection presents codes for bone marrow and stem cell harvesting and preparation of cells for transplantation. Patients with diseases that affect the bone marrow and the immune system, such as leukemia or multiple myeloma, may benefit from stem cell transplants. The cells that are transplanted are **hematopoietic progenitor cells** (HPCs), produced in the bone marrow and able to replicate and differentiate for cellular functions.

Harvesting stem cells from bone marrow and preparing the cells for transplant are coded with 38207 through 38232:

- Codes 38207 through 38215 describe the steps necessary to prepare hematopoietic progenitor cells (bone marrow stem cells) prior to transplantation. These codes may be reported only once per day per CPT® guidelines.
- Codes 38230 and 38232 describe bone marrow harvesting and are specific to the source of the transplant, 38230 for an allogenic transplant (from a donor), and 38232 for an autologous transplant (the patient's own cells).

Harvested and prepared hematopoietic progenitor cells are injected into the recipient by intravenous (IV) infusion in a sterile environment. Codes 38240 through 38243 shown in Figure 12.19 describe the transplantation of these cells via injection:

- Code 38240 is reported once per donor for an allogenic transplantation.
- Code 38241 is reported for an autologous transplantation.
- Codes 38242 and 38243 are for infusions of hematopoietic progenitor cells (38243) or lymphocytes (38242) used to treat relapse, post-transplant cytopenia (reduction in number of blood cells), or lymphoproliferative (excessive lymphocytes) syndrome. These infusions may occur days, weeks, months, or even years after the initial transplantation.

Figure 12.19 Hematopoietic Progenitor Cell Transplantation Codes

38240	Hematopoietic progenitor cell (HPC); allogenic transplantation per donor
38241	autologous transplantation
38243	HPC boost
38242	Allogenic lymphocyte infusions

RED FLAG

Code 38243 (*HPC boost*) is out of numerical sequence and is found between 38241 and 38242 in the tabular portion of your CPT® codebook.

The physician must be present during the transplant, provide direct supervision of the clinical staff, and manage any uncomplicated adverse reactions such as nausea or urticaria, an itchy skin rash. Infusions of any medication that is related to the transplant and given concurrently cannot be reported separately. Infusion of medications unrelated to the transplant are separately reportable with use of modifier 59, *Distinct procedural service*, or modifier XU, depending on your specific circumstances. Management of adverse reactions considered complicated or severe (infection, bleeding, or anemia) may be reported with the appropriate evaluation and management code in addition to the transplant code.

CONCEPTS CHECKPOINT **12.5**

Answer true or false to each of the following statements.

1. _____ An autologous transplantation uses cells from a donor other than the patient.
2. _____ Management of severe adverse reactions cannot be reported in addition to the transplant code.
3. _____ Codes 38207 through 38215 may be reported only once per day.

Lymph Nodes and Lymphatic Channels Procedures

The Lymph Nodes and Lymphatic Channels heading contains codes for open and laparoscopic lymph node biopsy and removal, and for drainage and injection procedures of lymph nodes. Lymph node biopsies and removals are performed to diagnose infections or diseases such as cancer. Codes in the Incision category, 38300 through 38382, describe surgical drainage of the lymph that may be necessary if obstruction or lymphedema is present, preventing the normal circulation. Codes under the Excision category, 38500 through 38555, are assigned depending on the anatomical site for biopsy and/or removal of lymph nodes. The extent of procedures differentiate excisions from the Radical Lymphadenectomy category codes.

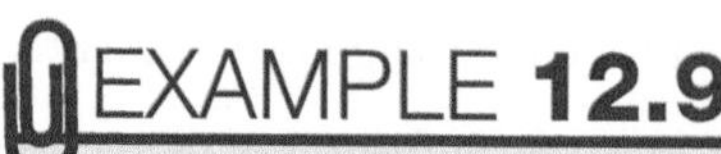

EXAMPLE **12.9**

Code 38510, *Biopsy or excision of lymph node(s); open, deep, cervical node(s),* is similar to 38720, *Cervical lymphadenectomy (complete)*, but the complete excision is a larger procedure. In the complete lymphadenectomy, neck tissue, lymph tissue, blood vessels, nerves, and muscles are removed. In the simpler excision of lymph nodes reported with 38510, a small piece of the lymph node or the entire lymph node and surrounding tissue may be removed but no other structures are involved.

There are 2 add-on codes in this subsection that describe a lymphadenectomy performed in addition to a primary procedure. The first add-on code 38746 describes a thoracic lymphadenectomy through a thoracotomy, removing mediastinal and regional nodes. A listing of codes that 38746 can be reported with follows the code description, as shown in Figure 12.20. The second add-on code 38747 describes an abdominal lymphadenectomy that includes the celiac, gastric, portal, and peripancreatic nodes, with or without para-aortic and vena caval nodes.

Figure 12.20 Add-on Code for Lymphadenectomy with Primary Procedure Code Listing

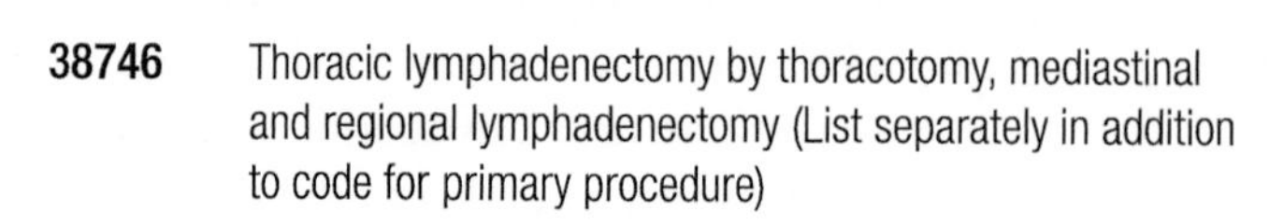

38746 Thoracic lymphadenectomy by thoracotomy, mediastinal and regional lymphadenectomy (List separately in addition to code for primary procedure)

LET'S TRY ONE **12.8**

A 12-year-old boy presented to the surgeon after a referral from his pediatrician. He has had an enlarged lymph node on his neck for several months that has not responded to antibiotic therapy. The patient was scheduled for a biopsy of the lymph node. The surgeon made a small incision through the skin over the superficial lymph node. A piece of the node was removed and sent for pathological evaluation. The skin incision was closed and dressed.

What is the appropriate code for this procedure? _____

Mediastinum and Diaphragm (Codes 39000-39599)

There are very few codes found in the Mediastinum and Diaphragm subsection. In fact, there are only 6 codes under the Mediastinum heading and 8 under the Diaphragm heading.

The **mediastinum** is the space in the chest between the lungs. Codes 39000 through 39499 include open exploration with drainage, removal of foreign body or biopsy, resection of cyst or tumor, and endoscopic biopsy.

The **diaphragm** is the sheet of muscle that separates the thoracic cavity from the abdominal cavity. Codes 39501 through 39599 include repair of lacerations, repair of diaphragmatic hernia, and resection of the diaphragm with simple (suture) or complex (prosthetic or muscle flap) repair.

Chapter Summary

- Pacemaker codes are determined by the system components and approach for placement.
- Cardiac valve procedures are differentiated by anatomical site, approach, and specific procedure. Multiple cardiac valve procedure codes may be assigned for 1 operative episode.
- Coronary artery bypass graft (CABG) procedures are assigned according to the type of graft used to complete the bypass: arteries only, veins only, or a combination of arterial and venous grafts. Codes are based on the number of grafts performed.
- Codes for repair of aortic aneurysms are differentiated by the location and extent of the aorta treated and the type and number of prostheses used.
- Bypass grafts other than coronary bypasses are differentiated by type of graft (vein, in-situ vein, or other than vein) and anatomical site.

- Central venous access procedure codes are differentiated by the insertion site, presence of a port or pump, the age of the patient, and whether the catheter was tunneled.
- Removal of non-tunneled VADs is not coded. Removal of a tunneled VAD is reported with codes differentiated by the presence of a port or pump.
- Codes for AV fistulas for hemodialysis are differentiated by the technique of creation: direct, donor vein, or synthetic graft.
- Percutaneous transluminal thrombectomy is reported per vascular family based on whether it is a primary or secondary procedure. Thrombolytic injections given during the operative episode are not reported separately.
- Ligation and vein stripping codes are differentiated by the anatomical site.
- Stab phlebectomy codes are assigned according to the number of incisions.
- Splenectomy codes are assigned according to technique and extent of removal.
- Codes describing the preparation of hematopoietic progenitor cells (HPC) are reported once per day.
- Codes for harvesting cells from bone marrow depend on whether the transplant is allogenic or autologous.
- Codes for the transplantation of HPC include management of uncomplicated adverse reactions.
- Codes for excision of lymph nodes are assigned according to technique and extent of removal.

Navigator

Access interactive chapter review exercises, practice activities, flash cards, and study games.

Chapter 13

Surgery Coding: Digestive System

Fast Facts

- Humans make 1 to 3 pints of saliva a day.
- In a lifetime, the human digestive system processes about 50 tons of food.
- The liver is the largest organ in the body.
- There are more than 400 distinct species of bacteria in the human colon.
- The mouth also contains a great deal of germs and bacteria. There are more germs in your mouth than there are people in Australia and Canada combined!

Sources: http://ncbi.nlm.nih.gov, http://science.education.nih.gov

Crack the Code

Review the sample operative report to find the correct digestive system code. You may need to return to this exercise after reading the chapter content.

DATE OF PROCEDURE: 05/20/2019

PROCEDURE PERFORMED: Insertion of peritoneal-venous shunt

SURGEON: Maurice Watson, MD

ANESTHESIA: General anesthesia

DESCRIPTION OF PROCEDURE:

The anterior and lateral aspects of left side of the body, from neck to pelvis, are prepped and draped in standard surgical sterile fashion. A small lateral incision is made in the upper abdomen. To enter the peritoneum, the incision is carried down to the abdominal wall layers. The peritoneal end of the catheter is inserted into the peritoneal cavity and secured with sutures. The catheter is maneuvered through a surgically created subcutaneous tunnel from the abdominal incision to the neck. The venous end of the catheter is inserted through a second incision in the neck over the internal jugular vein. The incision is sutured closed.

answer: 49425

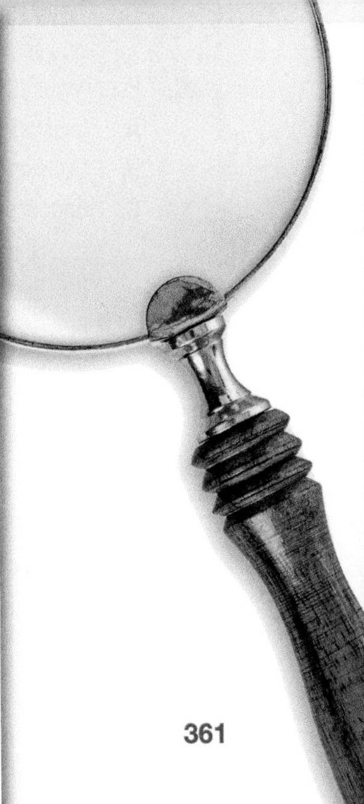

Learning Objectives

13.1 Identify the anatomy of the digestive system.

13.2 Describe the arrangement of codes in the Digestive System Surgery subsection and the surgical procedures specific to the digestive system.

13.3 Apply CPT® coding guidelines for reporting procedures of the digestive system.

13.4 Explain surgical endoscopic and laparoscopic procedures.

13.5 Discuss proper assignment of modifiers.

Chapter Outline

- **I.** Introduction to the Digestive System
- **II.** Digestive System Terminology
- **III.** Organization of the Digestive System Surgery Subsection
- **IV.** Lips (Codes 40490-40799)
  - **A.** Excision
  - **B.** Repair (Cheiloplasty)
- **V.** Vestibule of Mouth (Codes 40800-40899)
- **VI.** Tongue and Floor of Mouth (Codes 41000-41599)
- **VII.** Dentoalveolar Structures (Codes 41800-41899)
- **VIII.** Palate and Uvula (Codes 42000-42299)
- **IX.** Salivary Gland and Ducts (Codes 42300-42699)
- **X.** Pharynx, Adenoids, and Tonsils (Codes 42700-42999)
  - **A.** Excision of Adenoids and Tonsils
  - **B.** Repair of Pharynx
  - **C.** Other Procedures of the Pharynx, Adenoids, and Tonsils
- **XI.** Esophagus (Codes 43020-43499)
  - **A.** Incision
  - **B.** Excision
  - **C.** Endoscopy
    - **i.** Diagnostic and Therapeutic Endoscopies
    - **ii.** Esophagoscopy
    - **iii.** Esophagogastroduodenoscopy
    - **iv.** Endoscopic Retrograde Cholangiopancreatography
  - **D.** Laparoscopy
  - **E.** Repair
  - **F.** Manipulation
- **XII.** Stomach (Codes 43500-43999)
  - **A.** Bariatric Surgery
    - **i.** Gastric Bypass
    - **ii.** Adjustable Gastric Restrictive Device
    - **iii.** Longitudinal Gastrectomy
- **XIII.** Intestines (Except Rectum) (Codes 44005-44799)
  - **A.** Incision
  - **B.** Excision and Laparoscopy
  - **C.** Endoscopy, Small Intestine
  - **D.** Endoscopy, Stomal
- **XIV.** Meckel's Diverticulum and the Mesentery (Codes 44800-44899)
- **XV.** Appendix (Codes 44900-44979)
- **XVI.** Colon and Rectum (Codes 45000-45999)
  - **A.** Incision
  - **B.** Excision
  - **C.** Endoscopy
- **XVII.** Anus (Codes 46020-46999)
  - **A.** Anal Incision Procedures
  - **B.** Hemorrhoid Treatments
- **XVIII.** Liver (Codes 47000-47399)
  - **A.** Liver Transplantation
- **XIX.** Biliary Tract (Codes 47400-47999)
- **XX.** Pancreas (Codes 48000-48999)
- **XXI.** Abdomen, Peritoneum, and Omentum (Codes 49000-49999)
  - **A.** Laparoscopy
  - **B.** Introduction, Revision, Removal
  - **C.** Repair
- **XXII.** Chapter Summary

Introduction to the Digestive System

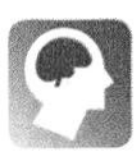

3-D
To explore the digestive system in the BioDigital Human, go to: http://Coding.ParadigmEducation.com/BioDigital_Digestive.

The purpose of the **digestive system**, also known as the *gastrointestinal tract*, is to ingest, process, absorb, and eliminate food. **Gastroenterology** is the medical specialty dedicated to the diagnosis and nonsurgical treatment of the digestive system. **Gastroenterologists** are physicians who diagnose and treat conditions of the digestive system.

Digestion begins by **ingesting** food into the oral cavity. In the **oral cavity**, the lips, mouth, tongue, and teeth break down the food mechanically, and the salivary glands break down the food chemically. The **salivary glands** produce saliva, which contains enzymes (proteins) that help to process food into smaller particles that can be passed from the mouth to the pharynx. The **pharynx** (throat) is a long muscular tube that passes food from the mouth to the esophagus. As the pharynx also passes air taken in through the nostrils (nose) to the trachea (windpipe), the **epiglottis** (cartilage flap at tongue's base) directs food from the pharynx into the esophagus during swallowing. The **esophagus** is a 9- to 10-inch muscular tube that connects to the stomach. A muscle at the top of the stomach, called the **lower esophageal sphincter**, contracts and relaxes, allowing food to enter the stomach and not return to the esophagus. Food is **digested** (broken down) as it travels from the mouth through the gastrointestinal tract.

The **gastrointestinal tract** comprises the esophagus, stomach, small intestine, large intestine, rectum, and anus. Food enters the stomach from the esophagus. The **stomach** is referred to in anatomical sections: the **fundus** (upper), the **body** (middle), and the **antrum** (lower). The stomach's lining contains mucous membranes that secrete digestive proteins called *pepsin enzymes* and *hydrochloric acid*, which continue the digestion process begun in the mouth, preparing food for the absorption process.

Below the antrum is the pylorus; the pyloric sphincter opens and closes the pyloric portion of the stomach. When ready, food is passed from the antrum to the **small intestine** (also called the **small bowel**) through the pyloric sphincter. The **pyloric sphincter** is the muscle that contracts (closing the opening) or relaxes (opening it) to allow broken-down food to pass from the stomach to the first section of the small intestine. The small intestine is about 20 feet long. The 3 sections of the small intestine are the **duodenum**, the **jejunum**, and the **ileum**. Millions of microscopic blood vessels (capillaries) that line the small intestine allow nutrients to pass from the small intestine into the bloodstream. Nutrients from digested food are absorbed in the small intestines into the blood and lymphatic system.

RED FLAG

Do not mix up the ileum of the small intestine with the ilium of the pelvic bone. Check the spelling and make sure you are certain you are referring to the correct structure. Misspelling can cause errors in coding and loss of points on certification exams.

Food materials that are not needed for nutrition are passed to the large intestine. The **large intestine** has 3 components: the **cecum**, the **colon**, and the **rectum**. At the lower end of the cecum, there is a small projection call the appendix. There is no biological function for the appendix. Materials from broken-down food that are not absorbed through the digestive system are referred to as **feces** (solid waste). Feces are eliminated from the body by moving from the small intestines to the large intestines to the anus and out of the body in a process called **defecation**.

The digestive system also includes the liver, gallbladder, and pancreas, which are essential to the digestive process. The **liver** is located in the upper right quadrant of the abdomen. Its primary purpose is to filter blood that passes from the capillaries of the small intestine, processing nutrients, chemicals, and drugs that enter the body.

The liver secretes a thick, yellowish-brown- to greenish-colored fluid called *bile*. **Bile** travels from the liver to the gallbladder. The **gallbladder** stores bile from the liver for use later to help food pass through the small intestine. Bile passes from the gallbladder to the duodenum through the **common bile duct**.

The pancreas is located behind the stomach. The **pancreas** helps with digestion by secreting digestive enzymes into the duodenum through the **pancreatic duct**. The pancreas also secretes insulin. **Insulin** is a hormone that regulates the absorption of glucose (sugar) and other nutrients.

Figure 13.1 illustrates organs and structures of the digestive system. Table 13.1 defines common medical terms used to describe anatomy and procedures of the digestive system.

Figure 13.1 The Digestive System

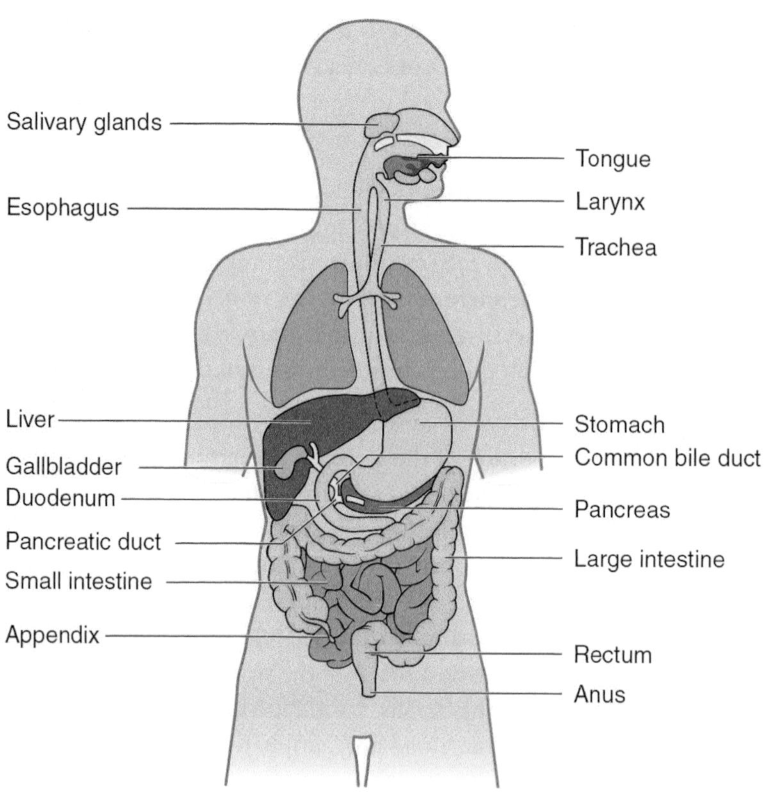

Digestive System Terminology

It is important for a coder to be familiar with the anatomical and medical terms used with the digestive system in order to correctly report codes from the Digestive System Surgery subsection. Table 13.1 presents common word parts used to describe structures, diagnoses, and procedures. Table 13.2 defines common terms relating to the digestive system surgical procedures.

Table 13.1 Word Parts Used in Digestive System Common Medical Terms

Word Part	Definition	Example
alveolo-	Alveolus (tooth socket)	Alveolitis—inflammation of a tooth socket
an/o	Anus/rectum	Anoscope—a short speculum for examining the anal canal and rectum
append/o, appendic/o	Appendix	Appendicitis—inflammation of the appendix
cheil/o	Lips of the mouth	Cheiloplasty—surgical repair of the lips
chol/e	Bile/Gall	Choledochectomy—removal of a portion of the common bile duct
cholecyst/o	Gallbladder	Cholecystogram—radiographic image of the gallbladder
col/o or colon/o	Colon/Large intestine	Colotomy—incision into the colon
dent/o	Teeth	Dentoalveolar—portion of alveolar bone around the teeth
duoden/o	Duodenum	Duodenotomy—incision into the duodenum
enter/o	Small intestine	Enterostomy—creation of an opening from the intestine to the outside of the body
esophag/o	Esophagus	Esophagoscopy—endoscopic inspection of the esophagus
gastro/o	Stomach	Gastrostomy—establishing a new opening into the stomach
gloss/o	Tongue	Glossectomy—resection or amputation of the tongue
hepat/o	Liver	Hepatotomy—incision into the liver
ile/o	Ileum	Ileostomy—establishment of an opening from the ileum to the outside of the body
labi/o	Lip	Labial frenum—membrane from gingiva to lip
lapar/o	Abdomen	Laparocele—abdominal hernia
lingu/o	Tongue	Sublingual—beneath the tongue
-lith/o	Stones	Sialolithotomy—incision into a salivary duct to remove a stone
-pepsia	Digest/Digestion	Dyspepsia—impairment of digestion
-pexy	Surgical fixation	Proctopexy—surgical fixation of a prolapsed rectum
-phagia	Eating/swallowing	Dysphagia—difficulty swallowing
-plasty	Surgical repair	Hernioplasty—repair of a hernia
proct/o	Anus/Rectum	Proctoscope—a rectal speculum
rect/o	Rectum/Straight	Rectocele—prolapse or herniation of the rectum
sigmoid/o	Sigmoid colon	Sigmoidoscopy—endoscopic inspection of the sigmoid colon
-stomy	Surgical opening, either natural or surgically	Tracheostomy—creation of an opening into the trachea
supra-	Above	Suprahyoid—above the hyoid bone
-tripsy	Surgical crushing	Lithotripsy—crushing of calculi

Table 13.2 Common Digestive System Terms

Term	Definition
calculus	An organic or inorganic concretion formed in any part of the body
colonoscopy	Endoscopic examination of the entire colon, from the rectum to the cecum
emesis	Vomiting
endoscopy	Examination of the inside of the body by using a lighted, flexible instrument called an *endoscope*
laparoscopic	Characteristic of procedures performed with a scope through small incisions in the abdominal cavity
lithiasis	Formation of a calculus
proctosigmoidoscopy	Endoscopic examination of the rectum that may include examination of a portion of the sigmoid colon
ptosis	Sinking down or prolapse of an organ
sigmoidoscopy	Endoscopic examination of the entire rectum and sigmoid colon, which may include a portion of the descending colon
sphincter	A muscle that opens and closes access to a duct, tube, or orifice

CONCEPTS CHECKPOINT **13.1**

Fill in the blanks to complete each of the following statements.

1. The purpose of the _____________, also known as the *gastrointestinal tract*, is to ingest, process, absorb, and eliminate food.
2. The _____________ consists of the mouth, lips, tongue, teeth, and salivary glands.
3. There are 3 sections of the _____________ intestines: the duodenum, the jejunum, and the ileum.
4. The _____________ intestine has 3 components: the cecum, the colon, and the rectum.

Organization of the Digestive System Surgery Subsection

The sequence of Digestive System surgery codes in the CPT® codebook follows the digestive process described in the Introduction to this chapter: general surgery codes are arranged under anatomical site headings in a roughly top-to-bottom progression starting with the lips and ending with the abdomen, peritoneum, and omentum. The peritoneum (membrane lining) and the omentum (protective, connective fat tissue) are accessory structures that help to support organs and other structures of the digestive system. Codes are further divided into procedural categories such as incision, excision, and repair. While not all of the digestive system procedures will be explained in detail in this chapter, some of the more common and more challenging codes you may be required to report are discussed in the upcoming sections. Table 13.3 illustrates the headings and code ranges in the Digestive System Surgery subsection of the CPT® codebook.

Table 13.3 Headings Within the Digestive System Surgery Subsection of the CPT® Codebook

Heading	Code Range
Lips	40490-40799
Vestibule of Mouth	40800-40899
Tongue and Floor of Mouth	41000-41599
Dentoalveolar Structures	41800-41899
Palate and Uvula	42000-42299
Salivary Gland and Ducts	42300-42699
Pharynx, Adenoids, and Tonsils	42700-42999
Esophagus	43020-43499
Stomach	43500-43999
Intestine (Except Rectum)	44005-44799
Meckel's Diverticulum and the Mesentery	44800-44899
Appendix	44900-44979
Colon and Rectum	45000-45999
Anus	46020-46999
Liver	47000-47399
Biliary Tract	47400-47999
Pancreas	48000-48999
Abdomen, Peritoneum, and Omentum	49000-49999

Lips (Codes 40490-40799)

Lips are the external part of the mouth, located in the lower center portion of the face, as shown in Figure 13.2. Lips serve as the opening to the oral cavity, used for the intake of food. The lips are also used for inhalation of air to the respiratory system, the creation of sound, and the articulation of speech. The 3 regions of the lips are the "wet" mucosa on the inside of the oral cavity; the **vermilion** or **vermilion border**, the red epithelium (thin surface tissue) that starts at the intraoral "moist line" and extends outward on the face; and a thin, pale zone of skin where the vermilion joins the facial skin. Procedures performed on the skin surrounding the lips are reported with codes from the Integumentary System Surgery subsection of the CPT® codebook. Procedures on the regions of the lips in the Digestive System Surgery subsection involve excision and repair.

Figure 13.2 External Portion of the Lips

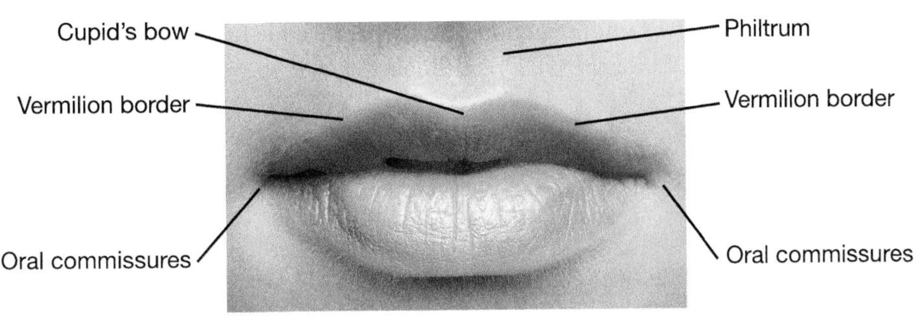

Figure 13.7 Partial Glossectomy

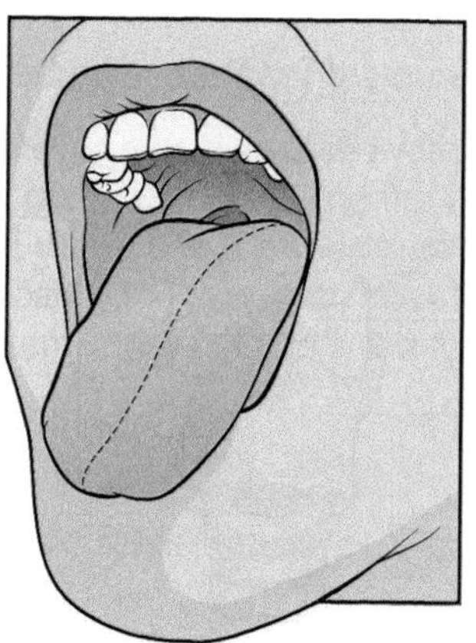

Incisions extended through the thickness of the tongue

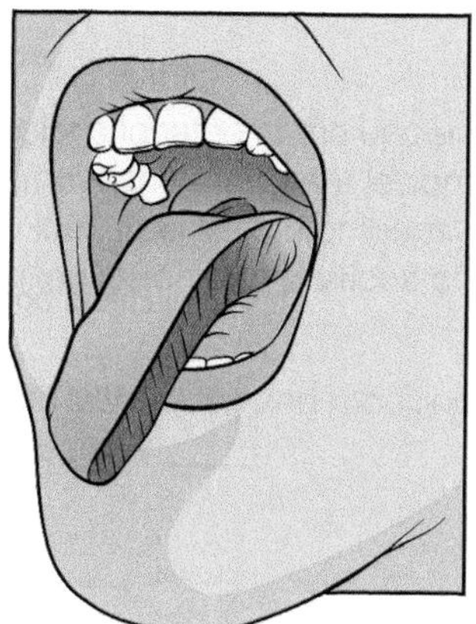

Half of the tongue or less may be removed

LET'S TRY ONE **13.3**

Choose the correct code for each of the following procedures.

1. A 25-year-old male patient with a personal history of cancer of the oral cavity was experiencing problems with swallowing and mastication. The problems caused the patient to lose 20 pounds since the last visit. The surgeon performed a complex vestibuloplasty with ridge extension and muscle repositioning. The procedure corrected the problem, and the patient began to gain weight. _____
2. A 19-year-old female patient presented to the emergency department (ED) after a car accident with a laceration to the floor of the mouth. The laceration was 3.1 cm and required a complex closure. After the repair, the patient was advised to follow up with her primary care physician. _____

Dentoalveolar Structures (Codes 41800-41899)

Dentoalveolar structures comprise the teeth and the bone structure that hold the teeth in place. In the oral cavity, the alveolus refers to the tooth socket. Procedures are organized under the categories of incision, excision and destruction, and other procedures. The incision category contains codes for drainage of abscesses, cysts, and hematomas and removal of a foreign body from either the bone or soft tissues of the dentoalveolar structures. Excision and destruction codes cover treatment of the gingiva, tissues around teeth and tooth sockets, and lesions. Other procedures include mucosal grafting, alveoloplasty, and gingivoplasty.

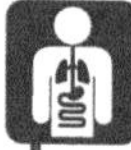

A&P Review

A quadrant in dentoalveolar codes refers to 1 of 4 areas of the teeth. Adult (permanent) dentition has 32 teeth, divided into 4 quadrants, each with 8 teeth.

Gingivectomy is the removal or trimming of overgrown gums, reported with code 41820, *Gingivectomy, excision gingiva, each quadrant.* **Gingivoplasty** is the surgical repair of the gums. Chronic inflammation of the periodontal tissues causes excessive plaque to form on teeth; when the condition cannot be treated by antibiotics, another

RED FLAG

Coders should be aware of differences between medical and dentistry billing. Dentists typically use HCPCS Level II codes to report procedures of the oral cavity; HCPCS dental codes (in Section D) are more descriptive than CPT® codes. Also, the claim form dentists use differs from that used by medical doctors. A third issue is that insurers may consider procedures of the oral cavity to be cosmetic and withhold coverage. Coders should review insurance payer policies regarding coding and billing for dental procedures prior to selection of the CPT® or HCPCS Level II codes.

option is gingivoplasty, reported with code 41872, *Gingivoplasty, each quadrant*. Codes 41820 and 41872 may be reported separately for each quadrant of the mouth where the removal or repair is performed. An **alveoloplasty** is the smoothing or recontouring of the alveolar ridge or tooth sockets, usually performed prior to fitting for dentures. Code 41874 is reported for each quadrant in which an alveoloplasty is performed.

Palate and Uvula (Codes 42000-42299)

The **palate** is the roof of the mouth, and the **uvula** is the tissue in the back of the throat. The codebook organizes procedures of the palate and uvula into categories of incision, excision and destruction, and other procedures. The surgical services include incision and drainage, biopsy, lesion removal, repairs, and reconstruction.

Treatment of lesions of the palate or uvula by excision may require a skin or mucosal graft. The skin graft is reported in addition to the excision code with the Integumentary System surgical codes 14040 through 14302; the mucosal graft is separately reported with code 40818.

A **cleft palate** is an opening in the hard palate or the soft palate, a congenital defect that results from the nonunion of the palate during gestation. **Palatoplasty** is the surgical repair of the palate. Palatoplasty for cleft palate is reported with codes 42200 through 42225. It is not uncommon for a baby to have both a cleft palate and a cleft lip. Cleft lip repairs were discussed earlier in this chapter. When the surgical repair of a cleft lip is performed with a palatoplasty for a cleft palate, you may report each code separately without the use of a modifier.

LET'S TRY ONE 13.4

Choose the correct code for each of the following procedures.

1. A 33-year-old patient with cancer of the uvula had a lesion removed. The procedure involved the excision of a small lesion and the creation of a local flap closure. _____
2. An 8-month-old female had reconstructive surgery for a cleft palate. The surgeon repaired the developmental cleft opening of the palate and reconstructed the alveolar ridge of the maxilla. The procedure also involved the harvesting of bone from the hip and closure of the surgically created wound of the donor site. The harvested bone was placed in the alveolar cleft to reestablish normal contours of the maxilla. _____

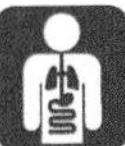

A&P Review

The palate is the roof of the mouth, the hard palate in the front and the soft palate in the back. The uvula, the hanging tissue structure in the throat, blocks food and liquid from entering the nasal cavity and assists with speech.

Salivary Glands and Ducts (Codes 42300-42699)

Salivary glands secrete enzymes that assist in digestion. The **parotid**, **submandibular**, and **sublingual glands** are salivary glands. The parotid gland is located near the ear and is the largest salivary gland. Saliva passes from salivary glands to the oral cavity through ducts. Procedures for the salivary glands and ducts are organized into the codebook categories of incision, excision, repair, and other procedures. Treatments include drainage of abscesses, lithotomies, biopsy, excision of lesions, duct repair, and injection for radiography. Codes are differentiated by the affected gland or ducts.

A **sialolithotomy** (codes 42330 through 42340) is an incisional treatment for a **salivary duct stone**, which is a concretion that blocks the passage of saliva to the oral cavity. A biopsy of a salivary gland is reported by the technique used to collect the specimen, code 42400 for a needle biopsy and code 42405 for an incisional biopsy.

A **sialography** is an x-ray image of the salivary glands. Dye may be injected to enhance the image, delivered through a small catheter that is inserted into the associated salivary duct. In this case, report code 42550, *Injection procedure for sialography*. For radiological supervision and interpretation of the sialography, separately report radiology code 70390, *Sialography, radiological supervision and interpretation*. Chapter 18 discusses the Radiology section of the CPT® codebook in detail.

LET'S TRY ONE **13.5**

Choose the correct code for the following procedure.

A patient with facial paralyses on the left side underwent bilateral parotid duct diversions to control drooling. The physician performed a Wilke type procedure, which involved an intraoral incision of the overlying parotid duct. The ducts were diverted and sutured to the mucosa so that the saliva into the duct was rerouted.

What is the correct code for this procedure? _____

Pharynx, Adenoids, and Tonsils (Codes 42700-42999)

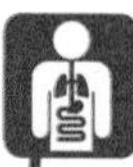

A&P Review

The adenoids and tonsils are a part of the lymphatic system. Adenoids, also known as the *pharyngeal tonsils*, are located in the back of the throat (pharynx) and up into the nasal cavity. Tonsils are located on the sides of the throat.

Surgical procedures of the pharynx, adenoids, and tonsils are categorized as incision, excision and destruction, repair, and other procedures. Incision and drainage codes 42700 through 42725 are selected based on the location of the abscess (peritonsillar, retropharyngeal, or parapharyngeal) and the approach (intraoral or external). Biopsy codes are selected based on the location of the lesion in the pharynx: oropharynx, if posterior to the mouth, and nasopharynx, if near the opening to the nasal cavity. When a laryngoscope is used to view the interior of the larynx for the collection of a biopsy, report the appropriate laryngoscopy biopsy code from the Respiratory System Surgery subsection of the CPT® codebook. The respiratory system is discussed in Chapter 11.

Excisions of Adenoids and Tonsils

Tonsils and adenoids defend the body against bacteria and viruses that enter through the mouth or nose. Sometimes tonsils and adenoids become infected. **Tonsillectomy** is removal of the tonsils, a viable treatment for chronic tonsillitis or for cancer of the tonsils. **Adenoidectomy** is the surgical removal of the **adenoids** (also known as the *pharyngeal tonsils*, located at the back of the throat). Chronic nasopharyngitis is a condition that is effectively treated by an adenoidectomy. A tonsillectomy and adenoidectomy may be performed during the same surgical session or independently. Codes are selected based on the age of the patient and if the tonsils and adenoids are removed during the same surgical session. Selection of adenoidectomy codes 42830 through 42836 requires the identification of the procedure as primary or secondary. A secondary adenoidectomy is performed when the primary excised tissue has grown back.

Repair of Pharynx

Throat cancer may damage the pharynx and require reconstruction surgery. A **pharyngoplasty** is the reconstruction of the pharynx. There are a variety of techniques that may be used for pharyngeal reconstruction, including skin grafts, tongue flaps, regional cutaneous flaps, and microvascular free-tissue transfers. When a pharyngeal flap is performed with a pharyngoplasty, report code 42225, *Palatoplasty for cleft palate; attachment pharyngeal flap*, in addition to the appropriate pharyngoplasty procedure code.

Other Procedures of the Pharynx, Adenoids, and Tonsils

A **pharyngostomy** is the surgical formation of an artificial opening into the pharynx. An esophagostomy tube may be inserted into the pharyngostomy for the purpose of feeding the patient when damage to the oral cavity prevents eating. To create a pharyngostomy, a horizontal incision is made below the jaw line to create a link between the **pharyngeal lumen** (opening to the throat) and the exterior of the neck. The incision is sutured to create an opening for placement of the external tube for feeding. The procedure is reported with code 42955, *Pharyngostomy (fistulization of pharynx, external for feeding)*.

The **oropharynx** is an area of the pharynx below the soft palate and above the epiglottis. The **nasopharynx** is the upper part of the pharynx, joining with the nasal cavity above the soft palate. Oropharyngeal (mouth and throat) or nasopharyngeal (nose and throat) hemorrhaging (bleeding) may occur as a complication of surgery performed on the pharynx, adenoids, and tonsils. Primary bleeding occurs within the first 24 hours after surgery, and secondary bleeding begins days after the procedure. Hemorrhaging may be controlled by such methods as removing a clot or packing the site with sponges, as shown in Figure 13.8. In this method, a catheter is inserted through the nose and nasal cavity and out of the mouth (A). A sponge is then attached to the catheter and pulled through the mouth to the back of the nasal cavity (B and C). The catheter is removed, and a gauze roll is placed in the nose (D). Another method to control hemorrhaging is through electrocautery. **Electrocautery** uses a probe heated by electricity to burn and/or remove tissue. Applying a vasoconstrictor solution such as silver nitrate and epinephrine may also be used to stop bleeding. Ligation of ethmoidal arteries using silver clips and/or electrocautery is another surgical method to stop oropharyngeal or nasopharyngeal bleeding.

Procedures to control bleeding of the oropharynx and nasopharynx are reported with codes 42960 through 42972. Code selection criteria are location of bleeding (oropharynx or nasopharynx) and the complexity of the procedure (simple, complicated, or requiring surgery).

If control of a hemorrhage is performed during the same operative session as the primary procedure (tonsillectomy or adenoidectomy), the code with the highest monetary value is listed first, and the other procedure is listed next with modifier 51, *Multiple procedures*, appended. If the control of oropharynx or nasopharynx hemorrhage procedure is performed after the initial surgical session, during the global period, append modifier 78, *Unplanned return to the operating room by the same physician or other qualified health care professional following initial procedure for a related procedure during the postoperative period.*

Figure 13.8 Nasal Packing for Hemorrhage Control

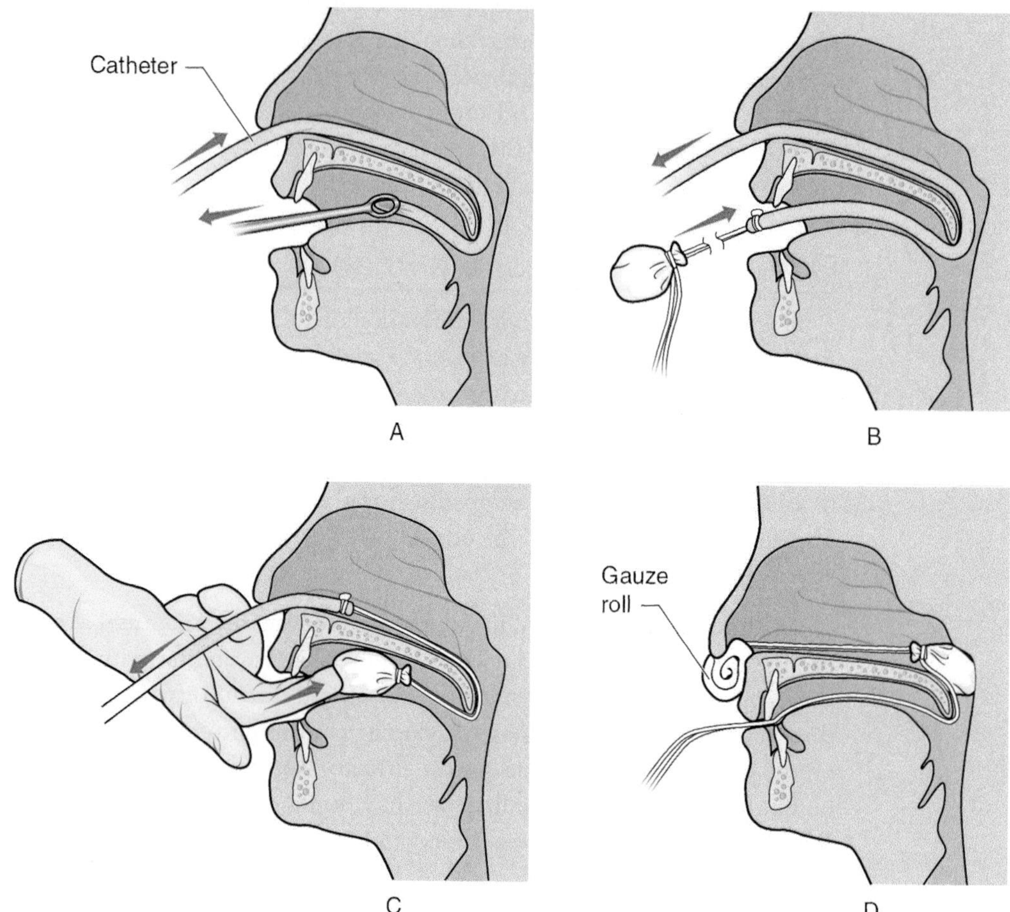

LET'S TRY ONE 13.6

Choose the correct code for each of the following procedures.

1. A 15-year-old female with chronic nasopharyngitis that did not respond to medication therapy underwent an adenoidectomy. _____
2. A 25-year-old male was diagnosed with multiple polyps (tags) on the left tonsil. The surgeon removed the 4 tags and sent the specimens to the pathologist. _____

Esophagus (Codes 43020-43499)

The esophagus is a muscular tube that connects the pharynx to the stomach. Food and liquid travel through the esophagus to the stomach. Associated structures referred to in code descriptors are the **cricopharyngeal muscle**, the part of the pharyngeal constrictor muscle near the cricoid cartilage at the top of the esophagus, and the **sphincter of Oddi**, a valve-like structure surrounding pancreatic and common bile ducts. Direction indicators used in the codes are *distal* (farthest from center) and *proximal* (nearest to center). Codes are categorized by types of procedures: incision, excision, endoscopy, laparoscopy, repair, and manipulation.

Incision

An **esophagotomy** is an incision into the esophagus. A **myotomy** is an incision into a muscle. An esophagotomy may be performed to remove foreign bodies lodged in the esophagus. Codes that report an esophagotomy to remove a foreign body are selected based on approach, either **cervical** (neck) or **thoracic** (chest). Report code 43020 for cervical approach and 43045 for thoracic approach. A cricopharyngeal myotomy may be performed to manage dysphagia, reported with code 43030.

Excision

An **esophagectomy** is the surgical removal of part or all of the esophagus. Esophagectomy is an effective treatment for cancer of the esophagus. Codes 43100 through 43135 represent a variety of different esophagectomy surgical techniques. Code selection is based on approach and partial versus total resection. Cervical, thoracic, or thoracic with abdominal incision are different approaches that may be used to access the esophagus.

When reconstruction is included in the procedure, select the appropriate esophagectomy code that includes reconstruction or interposition of the colon or small intestine. Interposition refers to using an excised portion of the intestine to replace the esophagus. If the physician uses a portion of the colon or small intestine to reconstruct the esophagus after an esophagectomy, an anastomosis is created to reconnect the affected intestines. The creation of a surgical connection between tubular structures, such as the intestines, is known as **anastomosis.** Mobilization of the intestine refers to detaching it from its support structures in preparation for resection or anastomosis. Figure 13.9 illustrates the different anastomosis connections: (A) end to end, (B) end to side, and (C) side to side.

Figure 13.9 Anastomosis Connections

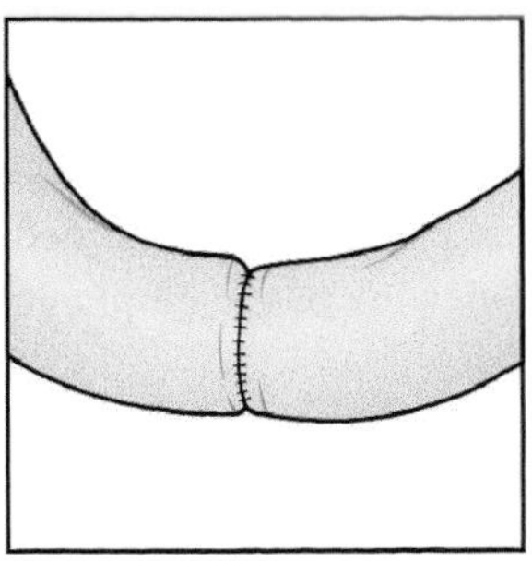
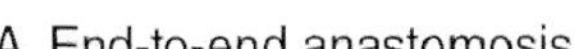

A. End-to-end anastomosis

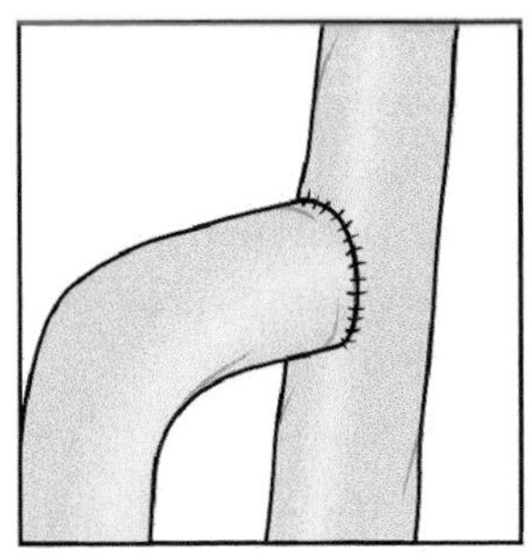

B. End-to-side anastomosis

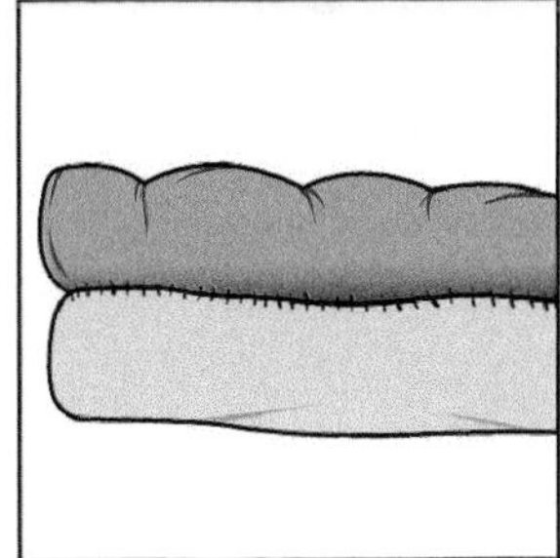

C. Side-to-side anastomosis

Codes 43100 and 43101 are used to report a lesion excision from the esophagus. They are selected based on approach—cervical, thoracic, or abdominal. Removal of a malignant lesion may include the removal of the cervical esophagus, a portion of the throat, or dissection of the neck. When selecting an esophagectomy code, coders must carefully read the operative report, the full CPT® code description, and associated parenthetic notes. For example, to report a laryngectomy, locate code 31360,

Laryngectomy; total, without radical neck dissection, in the Respiratory System Surgery subsection of the CPT® codebook. Codes 43107 through 43124 are excision codes that represent the removal of part or all of the esophagus; they are differentiated by the procedures on associated structures.

LET'S TRY ONE **13.7**

Read the description of the procedure and answer the questions that follow.

A 28-year-old male with cancer of the esophagus underwent a total esophagectomy with reconstruction. The procedure involved the removal of all the esophagus and the use of a portion of the colon to create a graft for reconstruction. Access to the esophagus was gained through 2 incisions: a slanted cervical incision and a horizontal upper midline abdominal incision. To create an esophagogastrostomy, the physician divided the esophagus at the cervical level. The esophagus was removed through the abdominal incision and divided from the stomach. A portion of the colon was excised and removed. The physician took care to preserve its major vascular supply. The distal and proximal bowel were reconnected. The excised portion of the colon was attached to the cervical esophagus and the stomach. An anastomosis created a usable esophagus. The incisions were repaired in sutured layers.

1. What was the surgical approach? ______________
2. Was a thoracotomy performed? ______________
3. Was an anastomosis created? ______________
4. Did the procedure include intestine mobilization? ______________
5. What code should be reported? _____

Endoscopy

Endoscopy is a very common procedure used to diagnose and treat conditions of the digestive system. As discussed in previous chapters, an **endoscopy** is a procedure that allows the physician to view inside the body by use of an instrument called an *endoscope*. An **endoscope** is a long, thin tube with a mini video camera on the end. During an endoscopy, the physician inserts the endoscope into an opening in the body and moves the scope through the body's passageway. The physician views the images in real time on a video monitor. Endoscopic procedures are named after the anatomical site viewed, for example, *esophagoscopy* (viewing of the esophagus) and *colonoscopy* (viewing of the colon).

Diagnostic and Therapeutic Endoscopies

Endoscopies are either diagnostic or therapeutic. A **diagnostic endoscopy** is performed to identify abnormal conditions of the structure or organ viewed. An endoscopy is considered therapeutic when an endoscope is used in surgical procedures, such as collecting a biopsy or inserting medical devices for therapeutic purposes. If bleeding occurs as a result of an endoscopy, the procedure to control the bleeding is not billed separately. During the course of a diagnostic endoscopy, a physician may identify a condition that should be treated or a lesion that should be biopsied. If the physician treats the condition or biopsies the lesion during the same operative session, the endoscopy is no longer considered diagnostic and is now a therapeutic endoscopy. All therapeutic endoscopies include diagnostic endoscopy, so only the code for the therapeutic procedure is reported. If multiple procedures are performed during an endoscopy, each is coded with modifiers 51 or 59 (depending upon third-party payer preferences) appended to the second and any additional procedures.

EXAMPLE **13.1**

Mr. Young had been complaining of painful swallowing, so his physician decided to perform a diagnostic esophagoscopy. During the procedure, the physician viewed the esophagus via a rigid endoscope inserted through the patient's mouth and into the esophagus under general anesthesia. She identified a lesion in the wall of the esophagus and decided to collect a specimen for biopsy. A specimen was removed with biopsy forceps. The endoscope was also removed. The specimen was sent to pathology for testing.

This example is considered a therapeutic endoscopy because a biopsy was collected. When selecting the appropriate code, report only the appropriate therapeutic endoscopy code. The diagnostic endoscopy is considered a fundamental part of the service and may not be reported separately.

Esophagoscopy

An **esophagoscopy** is the visualization of the esophagus by the use of an endoscope. Esophagoscopy codes 43180 through 43232 are used to report diagnostic and therapeutic endoscopic procedures. Examination of the upper esophageal sphincter along with the gastroesophageal junction is included in the code definitions. To view the proximal region of stomach, the endoscope enters the esophageal sphincter and is rotated backward. This procedure is known as a *retroflexion examination.* Retroflexion examination of the proximal region of the stomach is included in esophagoscopy codes and may not be billed separately.

Two basic criteria differentiate esophagoscopy codes: the type of scope used (flexible or rigid) and the approach (transoral or transnasal). A rigid esophagoscope enters the body through the oral cavity (transorally); a flexible esophagoscope can enter through the oral cavity (transorally) or the nasal cavity (transnasally). Rigid transoral esophagoscopy procedures are typically performed in a hospital under general anesthesia. Flexible transnasal esophagoscopy procedures are usually performed in physician offices, with patients in an upright position and topical anesthesia applied to decrease discomfort in the nasal cavity. Flexible transoral procedures are typically performed under moderate (conscious) sedation. Moderate (conscious) sedation administered by the same physician performing the medical or surgical procedure is reported with the appropriate moderate (conscious) sedation code from code range (99151-99153). Chapter 20 discusses assigning moderate sedation codes in greater detail. Table 13.4 shows the codes associated with each esophagoscopy.

Table 13.4 Esophagoscopy Codes

Type of Scope, Approach	Codes
Rigid, transoral	43180-43196
Flexible, transoral	43200-43232
Flexible, transnasal	43197-43198

RED FLAG

The "separate procedure" designation is used throughout the CPT® codebook to indicate a service or procedure that is normally an integral component of a total service or procedure. A separate procedure code cannot be reported in addition to the code for the total service or procedure of which it is considered an integral part. It is appropriately reported only when performed independently from other procedures.

Esophagoscopy codes are organized into "families," with the type of scope and approach being the parent or base code and specific diagnostic or therapeutic procedures being the child codes. Each code descriptor indented below a parent code is a different procedure or service performed at the same operative session as the parent code. The child codes include the base procedures of the parent code; therefore, the parent code may not be reported in addition to the child codes listed under it. Within a family of codes, diagnostic esophagoscopy codes are the first listed codes and may not be reported in addition to the other codes in the series. Figure 13.10 illustrates how a "family" of parent and child codes appears in the CPT® codebook. There are many resequenced codes in the esophagoscopy section. Resequenced codes may not appear within the associated code family but appear at the end of the section or within a different subsection. The CPT® codebook provides cross-references to direct coders to the location of the resequenced codes. A pound symbol (#) appears before the resequenced code.

Figure 13.10 Example of Esophagoscopy Parent and Child Codes

43191	Esophagoscopy, rigid, transoral; diagnostic, including collection of specimen(s) by brushing or washing when performed (separate procedure)
43192	with directed submucosal injection(s), any substance
43193	with biopsy, single or multiple

After determining the type of scope and point of entry, the codes are further differentiated by the services performed, which are the child codes. The types of procedures represented in the esophagoscopy codes include:

- submucosal and other injection;
- biopsy;
- removal of foreign body;
- dilation; insertion of guide wire with dilation;
- band ligation;
- removal of lesions;
- placement of stent;
- control of bleeding.

Some of the procedures will be discussed in more detail below. Child code numbers will be followed by the type of esophagoscopy specified in their parent codes—rigid, transoral; flexible, transoral; or flexible, transnasal.

Esophagoscopy With Submucosal Injection Esophagoscopy with submucosal injection(s), any substance, is reported by codes 43192 (rigid, transoral) and 43201 (flexible, transoral). For example, if 1 unit of incobotulinumtoxinA is injected during a flexible transoral esophagoscopy, report CPT® code 43201, *Esophagoscopy, flexible, transoral; with directed submucosal injection(s), any substance,* and HCPCS code J0588, *Injection, incobotulinumtoxinA, 1 unit.* Coders must read the parenthetic notes prior to assigning code 43201. The notes provide instructions for codes that may not be reported with code 43201.

Esophagoscopy With Biopsy Esophagoscopy with single or multiple biopsies is reported with codes 43193 (rigid, transoral), 43198 (flexible, transnasal), or 43202 (flexible, transoral).

Esophagoscopy With Removal of Foreign Body Esophagoscopies with removal of a foreign body are reported with codes 43194 (rigid, transoral) or 43215 (flexible, transoral). If fluoroscopic guidance is used during the procedure, report the separate procedure radiology code 76000 in addition to the esophagoscopy code. Append modifier 26, *Professional component,* to code 76000 if the procedure was performed in an inpatient setting.

Esophagoscopy With Dilation **Esophageal dilation** is a procedure that widens a narrowed area of the esophagus. Be careful to read the entire code description and parenthetic notes prior to selection, as some of these codes allow for the separate reporting of radiologic guidance, and some do not:

- Codes 43195, 43196, and 43220 do not include image guidance; separately report radiology code 74360.
- Codes 43213 and 43214 include image guidance; do not report a separate radiology code.

As a reminder, parenthetic notes instruct the coder not to report imaging codes in addition to codes 43213 or 43214. Figure 13.11 illustrates the guide wire technique and balloon dilation, as described by codes 43213 and 43214.

Figure 13.11 Esophagoscopy Guide Wire Technique and Balloon Dilation

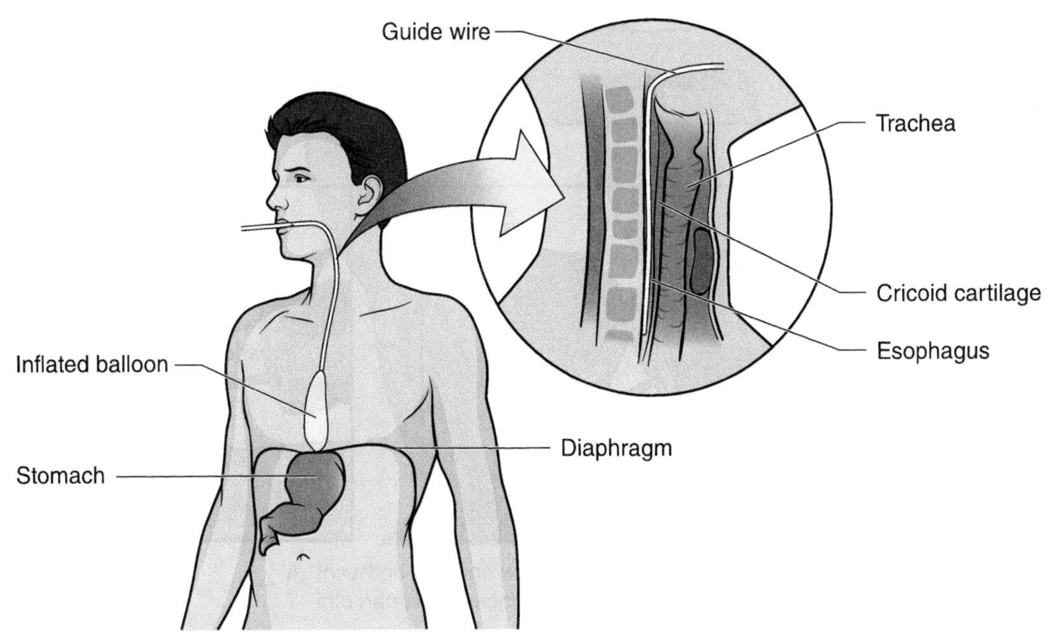

LET'S TRY ONE **13.9**

After reviewing the operative report below, select the appropriate code.

PROCEDURE PERFORMED: EGD with biopsy and check for *Helicobacter pylori*

DESCRIPTION OF PROCEDURE: The patient was brought to the endoscopy procedure room where an IV was started. She was then placed in the left lateral decubitus position with the mouth exposed. The patient was given 3 mg of Versed and 50 mg of Demerol IV push in increments. Her mouth was sprayed with numbing medication. A bite block was placed between her teeth.

The flexible endoscope was easily passed into the superior esophagus with a single swallow, and the esophagus showed no evidence of esophagitis. Examination of the stomach showed what seemed to be very mild gastritis in the bottom portion of the stomach. This area was biopsied by use of hot biopsy forceps and also checked for *H pylori*. The scope was then easily passed into the duodenum, which appeared completely normal. The scope was then carefully brought back into the stomach and reversed in direction for a reinspection of the esophago-gastric junction. This appeared normal, other than a small hiatal hernia. The scope was then straightened and easily removed. The patient tolerated the procedure well and was moved to the recovery room.

What code should be reported? _____

Endoscopic Retrograde Cholangiopancreatography

Endoscopic retrograde cholangiopancreatography (ERCP) is an examination that combines the use of a flexible endoscope with x-ray imaging to examine the biliary ducts that drain the liver, gallbladder, and pancreas to the duodenum. An endoscope is inserted through the mouth and moved through the esophagus and the stomach until it reaches the area of the duodenum where the biliary ducts drain. Conditions such as gallstones and pancreatitis are diagnosed with ERCP.

An ERCP is considered complete if 1 or more ductal system is visualized. The ductal systems are:

- pancreas: major and minor ducts;
- biliary tree: common bile duct, right hepatic duct, left hepatic duct, cystic duct, and gallbladder.

ERCP is reported with codes 43260 through 43278. Radiological supervision and interpretation is not included in ERCP codes and may be reported separately: report code 74328 for the biliary ductal system, 74329 for the pancreatic ductal system, or 74330 for both biliary and pancreatic ductal systems.

Cannulation is the insertion of a metal tube into the body to draw off fluid or to introduce medication. When a cannulation is attempted, but 1 or more biliary duct is not accessible because of the patient's condition, report the appropriate EGD codes 43235 through 43259, 43266, or 43270.

The parent code for the ERCP series of codes is 43260, *Endoscopic retrograde cholangiopancreatography (ERCP); diagnostic, including collection of specimen(s) by brushing or washing, when performed (separate procedure)*. Code 43260 is reported for diagnostic ERCP and is not reported in addition to other ERCP codes.

Therapeutic ERCP codes (43261 through 43278) are selected based on the procedure: biopsy, incisions, studies, destruction of calculi, placement of stents, removal of a foreign body, dilation, and ablation of tumors. Coders must read the section guidelines at the beginning of the ERCP section prior to code selection. The ERCP subcategory also includes extensive parenthetic notes to assist in accurate code reporting. Coders should review the entire section of codes prior to selection, because several codes in the ERCP section are out of numerical order.

CONCEPTS CHECKPOINT **13.4**

Identify if each of the following statements is true or false.

1. _____ Diagnostic ERCP codes are not reported in addition to other ERCP codes.
2. _____ ERCP codes include use of guide wire passage when performed.
3. _____ Radiological examination is not included in ERCP codes and may be reported separately.
4. _____ An ERCP is considered complete if 1 or more ductal system is visualized.
5. _____ Therapeutic ERCP codes are selected based on the procedure.

LET'S TRY ONE **13.10**

Choose the correct code for each of the following scenarios.

1. A 46-year-old female underwent an ERCP to remove a biliary stent. _____
2. A 58-year-old male patient with a history of alcoholism underwent a diagnostic ERCP. _____

Laparoscopy

Laparoscopy is the viewing of the abdominal organs or female reproductive organs through a laparoscope. A **laparoscope** is a small, flexible tube with a tiny camera on the tip. A laparoscopic procedure is performed under general anesthesia. During the procedure, a tube is inserted into a small incision below the navel. For better viewing or treatment, carbon dioxide is pumped into the abdomen, causing it to expand. The laparoscope is then inserted through the tube, allowing the abdominal organs to be viewed. After the exam, the gas, laparoscope, and any other instruments inserted during the procedure are removed, and the incision is closed.

A diagnostic laparoscopy is reported with code 49320, *Laparoscopy, abdomen, peritoneum, and omentum, diagnostic, with or without collection of specimen(s) by brushing or washing (separate procedure).* Codes 43279 through 43286 report surgical esophageal laparoscopic procedures, selected according to the purpose of the procedure:

- esophagomyotomy;
- fundoplasty (suturing of lower esophagus and upper stomach);
- esophageal lengthening.

Esophagectomy with laparoscopic mobilization of the abdominal and mediastinal esophagus and proximal gastrectomy is reported with codes 43286 through 43288. Code selection is based on the amount of esophagus removed and secondary procedure performed. Use code 43286 for total or near total esphagectomy with open cervical pharyngogastrostomy or esophagogastrostomy. Code 43287 reports removal of the distal two-thirds of the esophagus with separate thoracoscopic mobilization of the middle and upper mediastinal esophagus and thoracic esophagogastrostomy. Total or near total esophagectomy of the upper, middle, and lower mediastinal esophagus, with open cervical pharyngogastrostomy or esophagogastrostomy, is reported with code 43288.

Repair

Repair of the esophagus and other accessory structures is reported with codes 43300 through 43425, and a variety of open procedures is included:

- esophagoplasty—surgical repair or reconstruction of the esophagus;
- esophagogastrostomy—anastomosis of the esophagus to the stomach;
- esophagogastric fundoplasty—suturing of the upper stomach to the lower esophagus;
- esophagomyotomy—division of the muscle layers of the esophagus;
- hiatal hernia repair—correction of the protrusion of the stomach into the lower portion of the esophagus;
- esophagostomy, esophagojejunostomy—formation of an opening from the esophagus to other structures;
- lesion, fistula, and wound repair;
- esophageal lengthening.

These codes are generally differentiated by approach, indicated by the terms *abdominal, cervical, thoracic, laparotomy, thoracotomy, transthoracic,* and *transabdominal.* Figure 13.16 shows an example of the approach criteria.

Figure 13.16 Example of Repair Code Approach Criteria

43410	Suture of esophageal wound or injury; cervical approach
43415	transthoracic or transabdominal approach

Manipulation

Manipulation is the therapeutic manual adjustment of an anatomical site. CPT® lists 3 esophageal manipulation codes, as shown in Figure 13.17.

Radiologic supervision and interpretation associated with the dilation procedures (codes 43450 and 43453) separately report code 74360, *Intraluminal dilation of strictures and/or obstructions (eg, esophagus), radiological supervision and interpretation.*

Figure 13.17 Esophageal Manipulation Codes

43450	Dilation of esophagus, by unguided sound or bougie, single or multiple passes
43453	Dilation of esophagus, over guide wire
43460	Esophagogastric tamponade, with balloon (Sengstaken type)

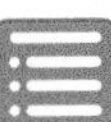

Index Insider

A physician may describe the procedure by its procedure name, such as esophagomyotomy with fundic patch, or by an eponym, such as the Thal-Nissen procedure. When using the Index, look under the eponym first; if you are unable to locate the code by the eponym, try the procedure name.

Thal-Nissen Procedure 43325

Or

Fundoplasty

Esophagogastric 43325

Esophagogastroduodenoscopic. 43210

  Laparoscopic . . .43279, 43280, 43283

  Laparotomy 43327

  Thoracotomy 43328

Esophagomyotomy

  Laparoscopic 43279

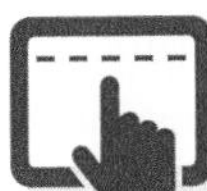

LET'S TRY ONE **13.11**

Choose the correct code for the following procedure.

A 25-year-old female patient with achalasia underwent a laparoscopic esophagomyotomy, also referred to as a *Heller myotomy*. Several small incisions were made in the abdominal wall so that a video camera and laparoscopic instrument could be inserted. An incision of the esophageal muscle was also made. To prevent reflux, a part of the fundus was wrapped around the lower portion of the esophagus, and the placement was secured with sutures. All instruments were removed, and the incision wounds were closed.

What code is reported? _____

Stomach (Codes 43500-43999)

Codes under the Stomach heading describe procedures on the body of the stomach, the antrum, the pylorus, and the vagus nerve. Surgical procedures of the stomach are subdivided by the categories of incision, excision, laparoscopy, introduction, bariatric surgery, and other procedures. For stomach diagnostic procedures, the codebook notes instruct the use of the laparoscopic code 49320 located under the Abdomen, Peritoneum, and Omentum heading. The therapeutic procedures include bariatric surgery that may involve the stomach, duodenum, jejunum, and/or ileum.

In the incision and excision categories, the parent codes are gastrotomy, pyloromyotomy, biopsy, excision of ulcers and tumors, gastrectomy, and vagotomy procedures. **Gastrotomy** (incisions in the stomach) codes are selected based on the purpose of the procedure. For example, code 43501, *Gastrotomy; with suture repair of bleeding ulcer*, is for a procedure whose purpose is to stop bleeding. Pyloromyotomy is an intervention to treat pyloric stenosis. Vagotomy is division of the vagus nerve. **Gastrectomy** is the surgical removal of all or part of the stomach and is used as treatment for morbid obesity in bariatric surgery. The laparoscopy category of codes includes gastric bypass and restriction procedures, placement of neurostimulator electrodes, and treatments for the vagus nerves.

Bariatric Surgery

Bariatric surgeries include the various open and laparoscopic gastric restriction techniques used to treat morbid obesity. Gastric restrictive procedures reduce the size of the stomach, limiting the amount of food the stomach can hold. Restrictive procedures include open and laparoscopic gastric bypass, the laparoscopic adjustable gastric restrictive device (gastric band or Lap-Band), laparoscopic vertical sleeve gastrectomy (stomach stapling), and open vertical-banded gastroplasty (stomach stapling and banding).

Gastric Bypass

A gastric bypass is performed in 2 steps:

1. The stomach is made smaller by surgically dividing it into a small upper section, referred to as a *pouch*, and a larger bottom section. The pouch is where the food enters the stomach from the esophagus.
2. The pouch is connected to the jejunum, the middle part of the small intestine. This allows food that enters the pouch to eventually exit into the small intestine, completely bypassing the larger, separated portion of the stomach and the first part of the small intestine (duodenum).

Roux-en-Y gastric bypass is 1 of the most common gastric bypass procedures. Figure 13.18 shows the results of a Roux-en-Y gastric bypass procedure. Gastric bypass codes used to report open Roux-en-Y gastric bypass procedures are 43621 and 43633 in the Excision category and 43846 in the Other Procedures category. Report code 43621 for a total gastrectomy with Roux-en-Y reconstruction, code 43633 for a partial removal of the lower (distal) stomach, and code 43846 with a short limb gastroenterostomy (150 cm or less). Code 43644 reports a laparoscopic Roux-en-Y gastric bypass.

Figure 13.18 Roux-en-Y Gastric Bypass

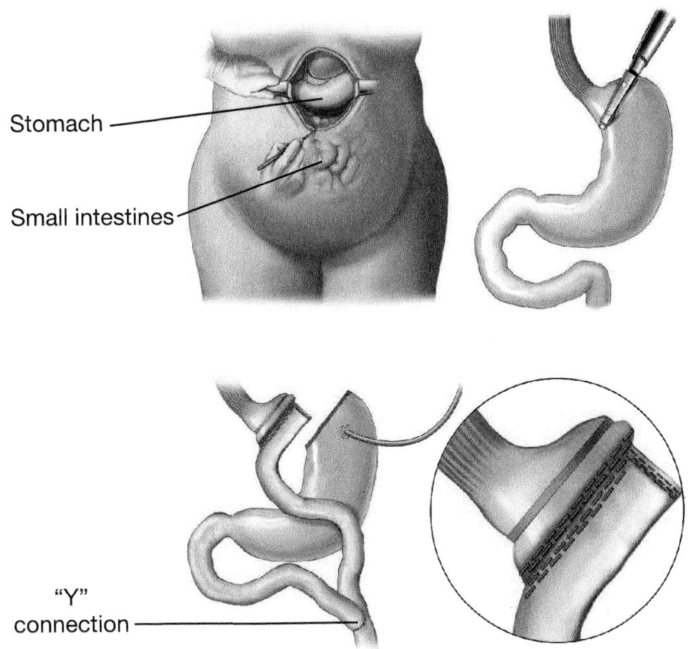

Adjustable Gastric Restrictive Device

Surgery for placement of an adjustable gastric restrictive device (known by the brand name Lap-Band) is performed by attaching an inflatable band around the top portion of the stomach. The surgeon tightens the band, creating a smaller upper stomach. The physician may adjust the size of the stomach by adding or removing saline solution to the band through a port placed under the skin. Figure 13.19 illustrates the gastric band procedure. Codes 43770 through 43774 report laparoscopic gastric restrictive procedures, revisions, removals, and adjustments.

Figure 13.19 Adjustable Gastric Band

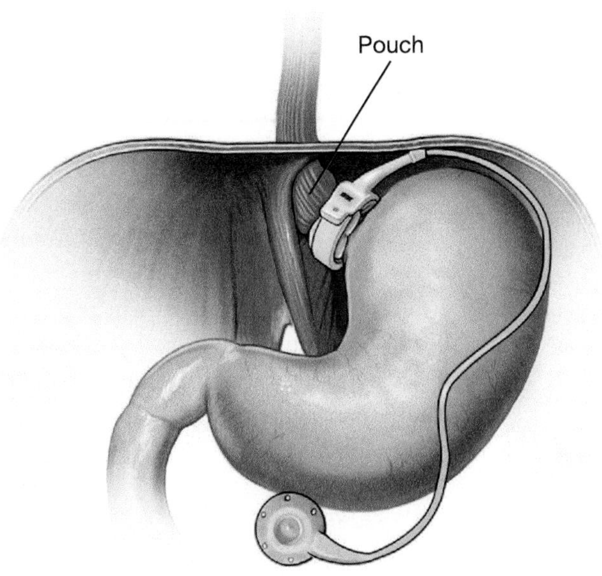

Longitudinal Gastrectomy

Coding Clicks

To view an animated video of a gastric band surgery, visit http://Coding.ParadigmEducation.com/Lap-Band.

A **longitudinal gastrectomy** (also known as a **vertical sleeve gastrectomy**) removes a portion of the stomach and uses staples to create a smaller elongated, sleeve-shaped stomach. Typically, a gastric sleeve is the first stage of a 2-part bariatric treatment for extremely morbidly obese patients. The second surgery, a Roux-en-Y gastric bypass, is performed after the patient has lost a significant amount of weight and is healthy enough to undergo the second surgical procedure. Patients who receive a longitudinal gastrectomy are typically more obese than patients who receive only a gastric band or a single-stage bariatric surgery. Code 43775 describes laparoscopic gastric restriction by means of a gastrectomy sleeve. An open gastric restrictive procedure for morbid obesity without gastric bypass is reported with code 43842. Report code 43843 for open gastric restrictive procedures that place staples to restrict food from access to other parts of the stomach.

CONCEPTS CHECKPOINT 13.5

Using information from the previous section, match the medical term in the first column to the correct description in the second column.

1. _____ bariatric surgeries
2. _____ gastrectomy
3. _____ gastric bypass
4. _____ gastric band surgery
5. _____ longitudinal gastrectomy

a. The surgical removal of all or part of the stomach
b. A gastrectomy procedure used as a treatment for morbid obesity
c. Various gastric restriction techniques used to treat morbid obesity
d. A procedure performed by attaching an inflatable band around the top portion of the stomach, creating a smaller upper stomach
e. A procedure that removes a portion of the stomach and staples the stomach to create a smaller elongated, sleeve-shaped stomach

Intestines (Except Rectum) (Codes 44005-44799)

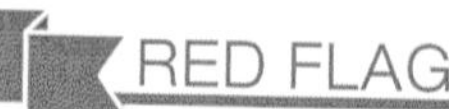

Although the appendix is connected to the cecum, codes to report surgical procedures of the appendix are located separately under the Appendix heading.

The duodenum, jejunum, and ileum are the 3 sections of the small intestine. The cecum, colon, and rectum are the sections of the large intestine. Codes 44005 through 44799 report surgical procedures on small and large intestine structures except for the rectum; rectal procedure codes are under the heading Colon and Rectum. The codes are arranged in the categories incision, excision, laparoscopy, enterostomy—external fistulization, endoscopy, introduction, repair, and other procedures. Watch for parenthetic notes indicating that an open-approach surgical procedure has a laparoscopic counterpart and vice versa. Open and laparoscopic procedure codes are not interchangeable.

Incision

The Incision category contains codes for enterolysis (freeing of adhesions), exploration, biopsy, foreign body removal, enteral alimentation, decompression, and reduction of volvulus (twisting of the intestine). **Enterotomy** is incision of the small intestine. **Colotomy** is incision of the colon (large intestine). Enterotomy and colotomy procedures are used for exploration, biopsies, and foreign body removal.

Excision and Laparoscopy

Open and laparoscopic procedures of the intestine include **enterectomy** (removal of the small intestine), **enterostomy** (artificial opening or fistulization of the small intestine), and **colectomy** (removal of the colon/large intestine). Intestinal cancer may damage the small and large intestines, treated by enterectomy, enterostomy, or colectomy. It is important for the coder to review the operative report carefully to identify if the procedure is open or laparoscopic.

Many enterectomies and colectomies require the removal of associated anatomical sites or the creation of an anastomosis to connect a passage from the separated sections of the intestine or colon. For example, base code 44126 describes a single resection and a single anastomosis: *Enterectomy, resection of small intestine for congenital atresia, single resection and anastomosis of proximal segment of intestine; without tapering.* If additional segments of the small intestine require resection and anastomosis, add-on code 44128 should be reported for each additional segment: *Enterectomy, resection of small intestine for congenital atresia, single resection and anastomosis of proximal segment of intestine; each additional resection and anastomosis (List separately in addition to code for primary procedure).*

Endoscopy, Small Intestine

Surgical endoscopy of the small intestine is termed *enteroscopy.* The codebook characterizes enteroscopy as a transoral antegrade approach, that is, in the direction of normal movement from the oral cavity down. A retrograde approach would be in the other direction, from the rectum up. This orientation defines the procedure by the most distal segment of the small intestine examined, that is, the structure farthest from the scope point of entry. For the purpose of defining enteroscopies, the antegrade sequence of structures is esophagus, pylorus, duodenum, jejunum, and ileum.

Surgical enteroscopy procedures include biopsy, removal of foreign body, dilations, removal or ablation of lesions, stent and tube placement, and control of bleeding. Enteroscopy procedures beyond the second portion of duodenum for the purpose of tumor(s), polyp(s), or other lesion(s) removal by hot biopsy forceps or bipolar cautery are selected based on whether the ileum was examined. **Bipolar cautery** is the same shape as tweezers, as illustrated in Figure 13.20. The bipolar cautery is connected to a hub that generates electricity. When connected, an electric current runs from tip to tip of the bipolar cautery. The heated cautery is used to cauterize and remove the lesion or polyp.

Figure 13.20 Bipolar Cautery

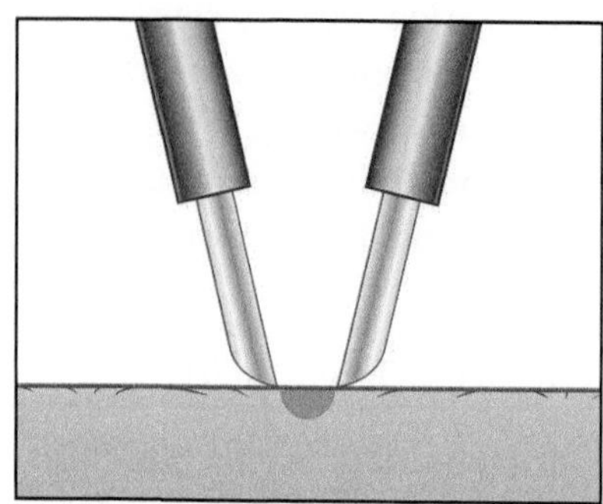

Control of bleeding is not reported separately when bleeding is due to the surgical endoscopy. Codes are selected according the section of the small intestine examined and therapeutic procedures performed. The parent code for each series of codes is used to report the diagnostic procedure, which may not be reported with any of the child codes for the surgical endoscopic procedures in the series. For example, code 44360, *Small intestinal endoscopy, enteroscopy beyond second portion of duodenum, not including ileum; diagnostic, with or without collection of specimen(s) by brushing or washing (separate procedure)*, is used to report an endoscopy of the small intestine beyond the second portion of duodenum but does not include the ileum. Figures 13.21 and 13.22 illustrate code 44360. The inclusion of "separate procedure" in the code description indicates that the procedure may not be reported with other codes in the series.

Figure 13.21 Small Intestinal Endoscopy

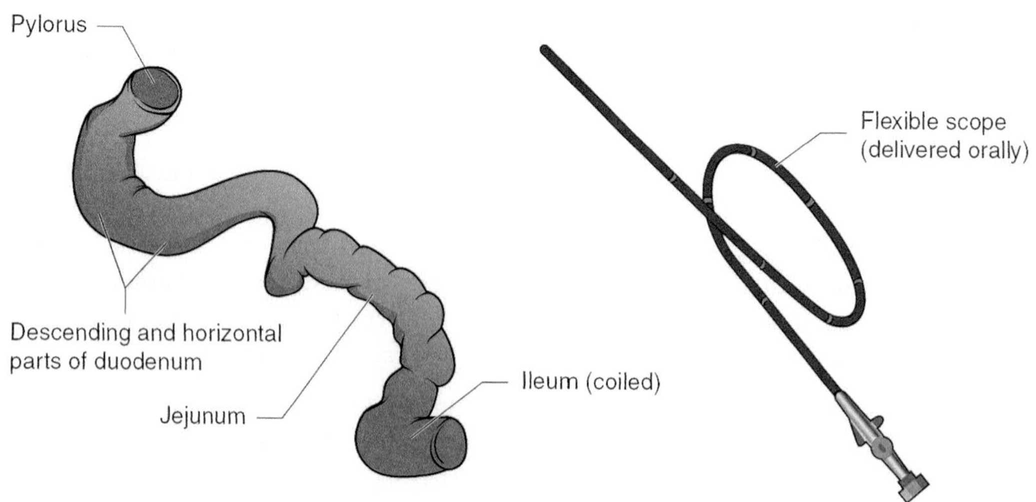

Figure 13.22 Small Intestinal Endoscopy Code

44360	Small intestinal endoscopy, enteroscopy beyond second portion of duodenum, not including ileum; diagnostic, with or without collection of specimen(s) by brushing or washing (separate procedure)

RED FLAG

Do not add modifiers to add-on codes. CPT® identifies add-on codes in 2 ways: by the statement "List separately in addition to code for primary procedure" at the end of the code description and by a plus (+) sign in front of the code.

Endoscopy, Stomal

An enterostomy is the creation of an artificial opening in the intestine through the abdominal wall to the outside of the body that allows fecal matter to be drained. Enterostomies for fecal drainage may be performed as a last resort when the intestines are unable to move fecal matter through the intestinal tract and out of the body due to disease or injury. Enterostomies are often named according to the section of the small intestine where the **stoma** (surgical opening) is created. For example, a surgical opening in the ileum of the small intestine is an **ileostomy** and of the colon is a **colostomy**.

Stomal endoscopy procedures are colonoscopies that visualize the colon–small intestine or the cecum by maneuvering the endoscope through an established stoma or an anastomosis. The procedures may also include an examination of the terminal ileum or small intestine proximal to an anastomosis. Ileoscopy through a stoma is reported with codes 44380 through 44384. Colonoscopy through a stoma is reported with codes 44388 through 44408.

</> Coding for CMS

When performing a colonoscopy through stoma on a Medicare beneficiary, use the appropriate HCPCS code, G6019 or G6020.

The codebook contains notes for circumstances when an endoscopy cannot be completed. When a total colonoscopy is scheduled and the patient is prepared for the procedure, but circumstances arise such that the physician is unable to advance the colonoscope to the splenic flexure via the stoma or the colon–small intestine anastomosis (such as blockage), report code 45378, *Colonoscopy, flexible; diagnostic, including collection of specimen(s) by brushing or washing, when performed (separate procedure).* If documentation supports a discontinued stomal endoscopy, report code 44388, *Colonoscopy through stoma; diagnostic, including collection of specimen(s) by brushing or washing, when performed (separate procedure).* Append modifier 53, *Discontinued procedure,* and be prepared to submit the appropriate documentation to the insurance payer.

CONCEPTS CHECKPOINT **13.6**

Match the medical procedure in the first column with the correct definition in the second column.

1. _____ colectomy
2. _____ colotomy
3. _____ stomal endoscopy procedure
4. _____ enterectomy
5. _____ enterostomy
6. _____ enterotomy

a. Incision of the small intestine
b. Incision of the large intestine
c. Removal of the small intestine
d. Removal of the large intestine
e. Creation of an artificial opening in the intestine through the abdominal wall, to allow for fecal matter to be drained to the outside of the body
f. Colonoscopy that visualizes the colon–small intestine or the cecum by maneuvering the endoscope through the stoma or an anastomosis

LET'S TRY ONE **13.12**

Choose the correct code for the following procedure.

A 45-year-old male underwent a diagnostic, small intestinal endoscopy. The endoscope was placed through the mouth and advanced into the small intestine. Four polyps were identified in the bowel lumen. All 4 polyps were removed with hot biopsy forceps placed through the endoscope.

What code is reported? _____

Meckel's Diverticulum and the Mesentery (Codes 44800-44899)

A **Meckel's diverticulum** is a pouch on the wall of the lower part of the intestine, as shown in Figure 13.23. Waste may collect in the pouches, causing the intestine to become inflamed. The tissues of the diverticulum may be the same as the stomach or pancreas. Although this is a congenital condition, it may not be diagnosed until adulthood. Mesentery is the double fold of membrane that attaches the intestine to the abdominal cavity. Procedures include excision of a Meckel's diverticulum and suture and removal of lesions from the mesentery.

Figure 13.23 Meckel's Diverticulum Repair

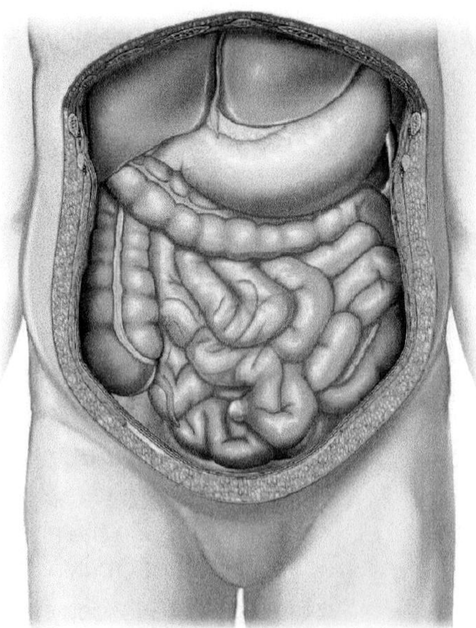

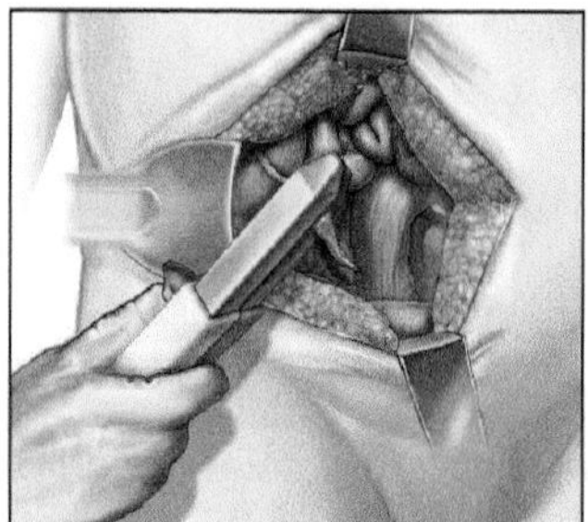

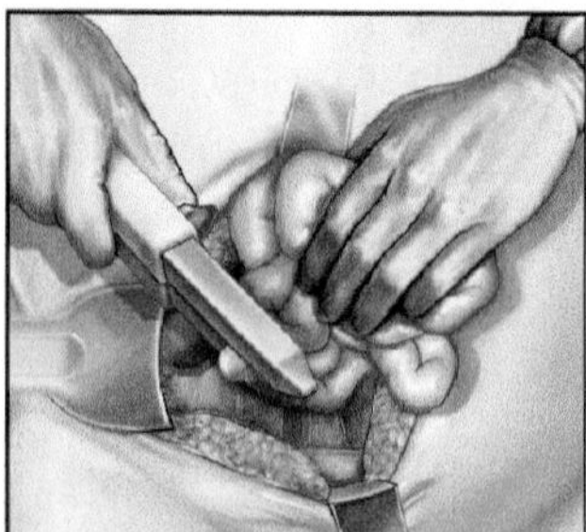

LET'S TRY ONE **13.13**

Choose the correct code for the following procedure.

The physician excised a lesion in the mesentery. She made an abdominal incision and then identified the lesion. The lesion was removed by carving it out of the mesentery. The incision was closed.

What code is reported? _____

Appendix (Codes 44900-44979)

The **appendix** is located in the lower right abdominal quadrant, on the cecum near the ileocecal junction. The appendix is a tube-shaped structure that is about 11 cm (4 in.) long, as illustrated in Figure 13.24. The function of the appendix is not clear. However, because of its location and shape, the appendix may become inflamed and/or infected, and it may even rupture. A ruptured appendix is life threatening, as it allows waste from the digestive system to enter the abdominal cavity. This may poison the blood system and infect other visceral organs.

Codes 44900 through 44979 are used to report incision and drainage or removal of the appendix (appendectomy). Appendectomies may be open or laparoscopic: an open appendectomy is reported with code 44950, or 44960 if the appendix has ruptured, and a laparoscopic appendectomy with code 44970. If an open appendectomy is performed at the time of another major procedure, report add-on code 44955 with the primary procedure.

Figure 13.24 Appendix

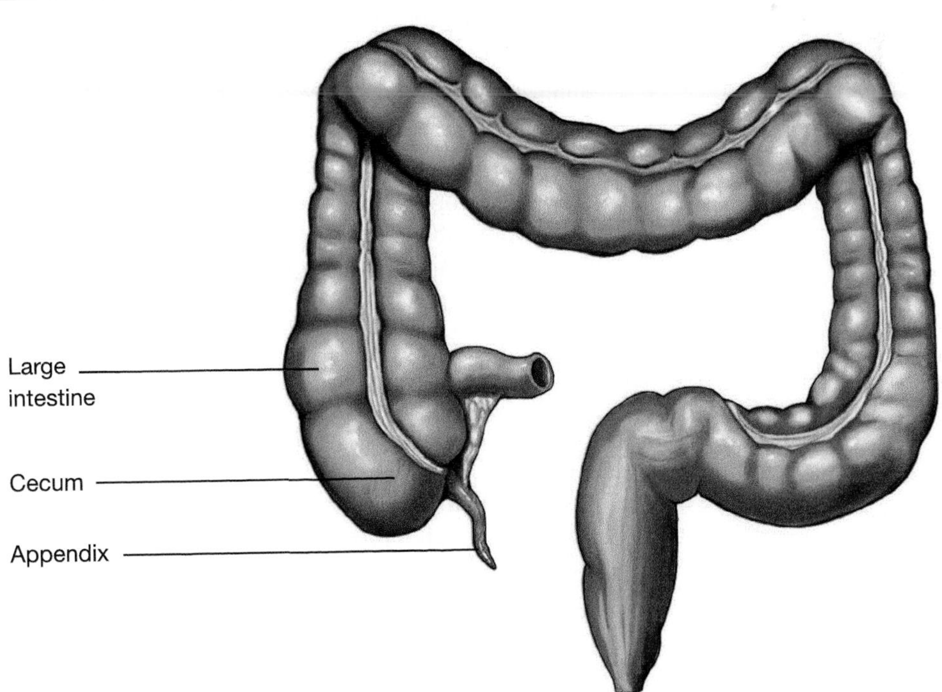

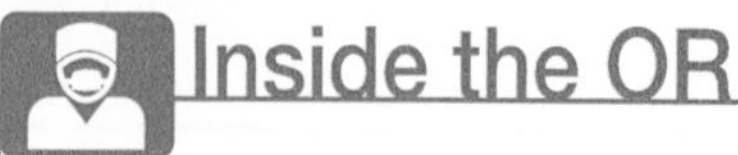

Inside the OR

PROCEDURE PERFORMED: Appendectomy

ANESTHESIA: General endotracheal

PROCEDURE: After informed consent was obtained, the patient was brought to the operative suite and placed supine on the operating table. General endotracheal anesthesia was induced without incident. The patient was prepped and draped in the usual sterile manner.

A transverse right lower quadrant incision was made directly over the point of maximal abdominal tenderness. Sharp dissection utilizing a Bovie electrocautery was used to expose the external and the internal oblique fascia. The fascia of the external and internal oblique was incised in the direction of the fibers, and the muscle was spread with a clamp. The transversus abdominis muscle, transversalis fascia, and peritoneum were incised gaining entrance into the abdominal cavity without incident.

The cecum was grasped along the taenia by use of a moist gauze sponge and mobilized into the wound. The appendix was then fully visualized, and the mesentery was divided between Kelly clamps and ligated with 2-0 Vicryl ties. The base of the appendix was crushed with a clamp, and then the clamp was reapplied proximally on the appendix. The base was ligated with 2-0 Vicryl tie over the crushed area and the appendix amputated along the clamp. The stump of the appendix was cauterized, and the cecum was returned to the abdomen.

The peritoneum was irrigated with warm sterile saline. The mesoappendix and cecum hemostasis was confirmed. The wound was closed in layers using 2-0 Vicryl for the peritoneum and 0 Vicryl for the internal oblique and external oblique layers. The skin incision was approximated with 4-0 Monocryl in a subcuticular fashion. The skin was prepped with benzoin, and Steri-Strips were applied. A dressing was placed on the wound. All surgical counts were reported as correct. The patient tolerated the procedure well.

The operative report documents an open procedure. Code 44970 reports a laparoscopic appendectomy, which is not supported by documentation. The correct code is 44950, *Appendectomy*.

Colon and Rectum (Codes 45000-45999)

The rectum is the final segment of the large intestine where it terminates in the anus. Codes 45000 through 45999 report procedures of the rectum and adjacent structures. Codes are categorized by incision, excision, destruction, endoscopy, laparoscopy, repair, manipulation, and other procedures.

Incision

Incision and drainage of abscess codes are selected based on the location of the abscess. Coders should read the operative report closely to determine the anatomical site: a pelvic abscess drained transrectally (45000); submucosal (45005); or supralevator, pelvirectal, or retrorectal (45020).

Excision

A common procedure to treat rectal cancer is a **proctectomy**, the surgical removal of the rectum. In the Excision category, proctectomy codes are open procedures; selection criteria are the approach (anal, abdominal, sacral, perineal, coccygeal) and/or the extent of the removal (partial or complete). It is important for coders to read the operative report carefully to identify all associated procedures and involved anatomical sites. Then the coder must read the rectal procedure code descriptions to identify the most accurate code. Proctectomies are complex procedures that may require the removal of surrounding organs and structures or the creation of enterostomies.

For example, the descriptor for base code 45126 includes the removal of several anatomical structures:

> *Pelvic exenteration for colorectal malignancy, with proctectomy (with or without colostomy), with removal of bladder and ureteral transplantations, and/or hysterectomy, or cervicectomy, with or without removal of tube(s), with or without removal of ovary(s), or any combination thereof*

The code description identifies the reason for the procedure—colorectal malignancy—and lists the possible associated procedures—proctectomy, colostomy, removal of bladder, removal of ureteral transplantations, hysterectomy, cervicectomy, removal of tubes, and removal of ovaries. The associated procedures may not be reported separately because they are included in code 45126.

Be aware of the distinctions between open and laparoscopic proctectomies. Watch for parenthetic notes indicating that an open-approach surgical procedure has a laparoscopic counterpart and vice versa. Open and laparoscopic procedure codes are not interchangeable.

Endoscopy

Rectal endoscopic procedures are performed by inserting a rigid or flexible endoscope into the rectum and advancing the scope to the area of the colon to be examined. Proctosigmoidoscopy, sigmoidoscopy, and colonoscopy are rectal endoscopic procedures. A **proctosigmoidoscopy** is an endoscopic exam of the rectum and sigmoid colon, using a rigid proctoscope. If a flexible instrument is used during a proctosigmoidoscopy, it is reported as a flexible sigmoidoscopy. A **sigmoidoscopy** is an endoscopic exam that includes the entire rectum and the sigmoid colon and may include examination of a part of the descending colon. A **colonoscopy** is an endoscopic exam, using a flexible colonoscope, of the rectum to the cecum, and may include examination of the terminal ileum. Colonoscopy procedures may be performed by insertion of a colonoscope through a colostomy, a colotomy, or the rectum.

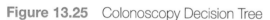

Coding for CMS

When performing a colorectal cancer screening on a Medicare beneficiary, select the appropriate HCPCS code from Section G (code ranges G0104 through G0106 or G0120 through G0122). If a biopsy or removal of a lesion is performed during the procedure, the procedure is no longer a screening colonoscopy. Report the appropriate HCPCS colonoscopy code from the Section G Intestinal codes. If the HCPCS colonoscopy codes do not completely describe the colonoscopy procedure, then select the appropriate CPT® colonoscopy code.

Codes 45300 through 45398 are used to report proctosigmoidoscopy, sigmoidoscopy, and colonoscopy procedures. The parent codes determine the particular type of endoscopy and are the diagnostic procedures (codes 45300, 45330, and 45378). Diagnostic endoscopies are not reported with surgical endoscopies of the same code series (the child codes). However, diagnostic endoscopy can be reported separately when performed at the same surgical session as another endoscopic procedure. For example, a diagnostic endoscopy of the duodenum (44360) may be reported with a diagnostic sigmoidoscopy (45330).

Diagnostic proctosigmoidoscopy (45300) and diagnostic sigmoidoscopy (45330) include collection of specimen(s) by brushing or washing. Diagnostic colonoscopy (45378) includes collection of specimen(s) by brushing or washing and colon decompression. **Colon decompression** is the removal of air from the colon, reducing possible future tears. When a patient is scheduled for a total colonoscopy, but due to extenuating circumstances the endoscope is unable to extend past the splenic flexure, report the appropriate colonoscopy code with modifier 53, *Discontinued procedure.* Codebooks may contain a colonoscopy decision tree to assist coders to accurately select colonoscopy codes and appropriately append modifiers. Figure 13.25 is a Colonoscopy Decision Tree including HCPCS Colonoscopy codes reported for Medicare patients that may not appear in your CPT® codebook.

Figure 13.25 Colonoscopy Decision Tree

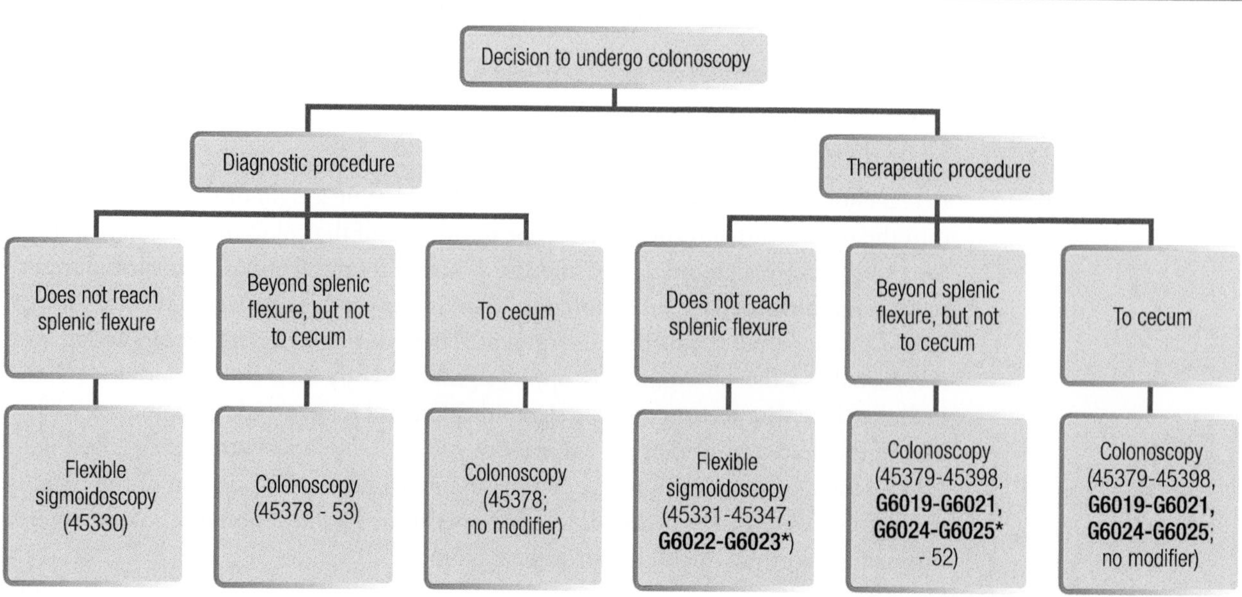

Adapted from "Colonoscopy Decision Tree," American Medical Association, 2014, *CPT 2015*, p. 284, Chicago: American Medical Association.

</> Coding for CMS

Evaluation and management (E/M) services performed on the same date of a diagnostic endoscopy may not be reimbursed, unless the documentation supports the medical necessity of the E/M service. Diagnostic endoscopies with global periods of 0 to 10 days include evaluation and management of the affected area. If the provider determines that a more detailed examination of the affected area is warranted, report the appropriate E/M code with modifier 25, *Significant, separately identifiable evaluation and management service by the same physician or other qualified health care professional on the same day of the procedure or other service*. During the postoperative period, if the E/M code is related to a different problem with a different diagnosis code, append modifier 24, *Unrelated evaluation and management service by the same physician or other qualified health care professional during a postoperative period*.

Once you have chosen the parent code, choice of the child code involves careful analysis of the patient's health record and careful review of the code descriptors, as described in Example 13.2.

EXAMPLE **13.2**

A surgeon injects saline solution into the colon prior to a lesion removal or biopsy. The parent code for a flexible colonoscopy is 45378. The child code descriptors show that code 45381 reports an injection of any substance directly into the submucosa. When submucosal injection is performed at the same time of lesion removal, both the injection and the lesion removal procedures are reported separately. Code 45381 is reported only once, regardless of the number of injections performed. Do not confuse code 45381 with 45382. Code 45382 is also an injection into the colon; however, the purpose is to control bleeding. If bleeding occurs as a result of the endoscopic procedure, and an injection is required to control the bleeding, neither code 45381 nor 45382 is reported. Control of bleeding as a result of an endoscopic procedure is not reported.

Endoscopic biopsies are reported when a portion of a lesion is removed and the specimen is sent for testing. If the entire lesion is removed, even if the specimen is from the same lesion that is sent for a biopsy, the appropriate endoscopic lesion removal code is reported. Coders must read the full code descriptors prior to selection of lesion removal codes. Colonoscopy lesion removal codes 45384, 45385, and 45388 are alike in that they all describe lesion removal, but they are different in the techniques used: code 45384 by hot biopsy forceps, code 45385 by snare technique, and code 45383 by ablation. When a biopsy and a lesion removal are performed for different lesions, both the biopsy and lesion codes are reportable. Modifier 59, *Distinct procedural service*, is appended to the biopsy code.

CONCEPTS CHECKPOINT 13.7

Identify if each of the following statements is true or false.

1. _____ Proctectomy codes are selected based on approach and/or the extent of the removal, either partial or complete.
2. _____ Diagnostic endoscopies are reported with surgical endoscopies of the same code series.
3. _____ When a patient is scheduled for a total colonoscopy, but due to extenuating circumstances the endoscope is unable to reach the splenic flexure, report the appropriate colonoscopy code without a modifier.
4. _____ Control of bleeding as a result of an endoscopic procedure is not reported separately.
5. _____ Endoscopic biopsies are reported when a portion of a lesion is removed and the specimen is sent for testing.
6. _____ When a biopsy and a lesion removal are performed for different lesions, both the biopsy and lesion codes are reportable. Modifier 59 is appended to the biopsy code.

Anus (Codes 46020-46999)

Procedures of the anus are reported with codes 46020 through 46999. Anatomical structures referenced besides the anus are the ischium (the portion of the hip bone near the spine), rectum, anal septum, anal sphincter, and levator muscle. Codes are arranged by incision, excision, introduction, endoscopy, repair, and destruction.

Hemorrhoids are a common condition of the anal canal. There are 2 types of hemorrhoids, internal and external. **Internal hemorrhoids** are small, swollen veins in the wall of the anal canal that may become very large, causing veins to expand and protrude out of the anus. **External hemorrhoids** are located beneath the skin, just outside of the anus. External hemorrhoids may result in **thrombosis (clotted) hemorrhoids**. Hemorrhoid location is documented according to its position in the anus: right posterior, right anterior, and left lateral, as shown in Figure 13.26. These 3 positions represent a column/group in the anus.

Figure 13.26 Hemorrhoid Locations

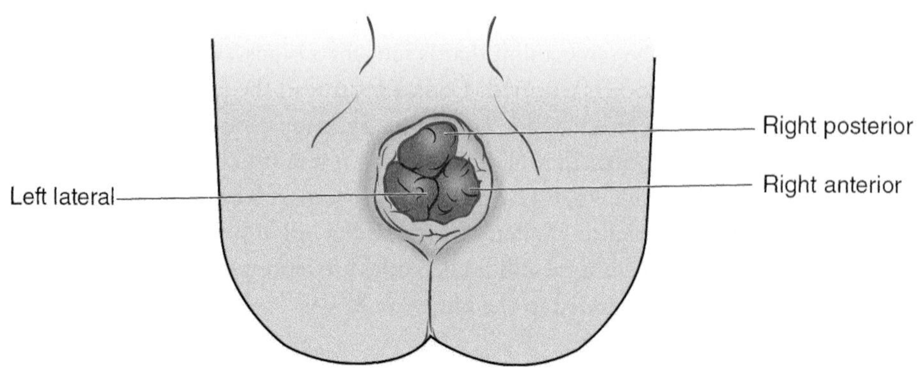

Anal Incision Procedures

Incision procedure codes cover various surgical treatments. The placement and removal of an anal seton (codes 46020, 46030, and 46060) is involved in treating anal fistulas. Incision and drainage of abscesses codes (46040 through 46060) are differentiated by the location of the abscess: ischiorectal, perirectal, intramural, intramuscular, submucosal, or perianal. An **anal sphincterotomy** is the surgical incision or division of the sphincter muscle that controls the anus for defecation and is reported with code 46080, *Sphincterotomy, anal, division of sphincter (separate procedure)*.

Hemorrhoid Treatments

Excision of internal and external hemorrhoids (hemorrhoidectomy) is reported with codes 46250 through 46262 and 46320. Hemorrhoidectomy codes are selected based on the location of the hemorrhoids and the number of columns/groups affected—for example, code 46261, Hemorrhoidectomy, internal and external, 2 or more columns/groups; with fissurectomy. A **fissurectomy** is the removal of a portion of the anus that has been torn. **Anal fissures** may occur when muscles of the anal sphincter begin to spasm due to the passage of feces.

Hemorrhoid ligation is a treatment used to treat internal hemorrhoids. During the procedure, the physician ties a rubber band around the base of the hemorrhoid, cutting off blood supply. The hemorrhoid withers and falls off in 2 to 7 days. Hemorrhoid ligations are reported with codes 46221, 46945, and 46946, based on the ligation method and the number of hemorrhoids. (Note that codes 46945 and 46946 are listed in the Excision subsection, out of numerical sequence.) Additional hemorrhoid ligation codes are found under the Colon and Rectum codebook heading. When performed via a flexible sigmoidoscopy, report code 45350; when performed via a flexible colonoscopy, report code 45398. Never report codes 45350 or 45398 together or with codes 46221, 46945, or 46946.

Hemorrhoid sclerotherapy is another treatment, found in the codebook Introduction category. In this procedure, a sclerosing (hardening of tissue) therapeutic solution is injected into the bleeding internal hemorrhoids to control bleeding. The solution immediately shrinks the veins, which stops the bleeding. An injection is made at the base of the hemorrhoid, causing the affected vein to harden or shrivel away. Code 46500, *Injection of sclerosing solution, hemorrhoids*, is used to report hemorrhoid sclerotherapy.

Stapled hemorrhoidopexy is a procedure used for prolapsed (falling out) internal hemorrhoids. Prolapsed hemorrhoids are repositioned anoscopically and excised as needed. Then staples are applied to hold the repositioned hemorrhoids in place. Report the procedure with code 46947, *Hemorrhoidopexy (eg, for prolapsing internal hemorrhoids) by stapling*. Code 46930 reports the destruction of internal hemorrhoids by thermal energy, including infrared coagulation, cautery, and radiofrequency. Destruction of hemorrhoids by cryosurgery (the prefix *cryo-* means extreme cold) does not have a specific CPT® code, so report code 46999, *Unlisted procedure, anus*, when cryosurgery is performed, and be prepared to submit a special report.

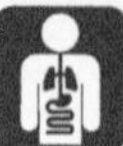

A&P Review

The liver's primary function is to produce bile, a substance that assists in breaking down fats so they may be absorbed in the small intestine. The liver filters the blood and stores vitamins, iron, and sugar. It destroys old red blood cells and converts ammonia into urine. The liver also breaks down hemoglobin, insulin, and hormones.

Liver (Codes 47000-47399)

The liver is the largest gland in the body and acts as a filter. Codes are arranged according to incision, excision, liver transplantation, repair, laparoscopy, and other procedures.

Liver biopsy codes are in both the incision and excision categories. Biopsies may be collected by open, laparoscopic, or percutaneous approach. Code 47000 reports a percutaneous liver biopsy by needle. If imaging guidance is used, it may be reported separately. Code 47001 is used to report needle biopsies when performed with other major procedures. Code 47100 reports an open wedge liver biopsy. During the procedure, the physician removes a wedge-shaped specimen from the liver that is sent to the pathology lab for testing.

Ablation of liver tumors may be performed as both open and laparoscopic procedures. Codes are located in the laparoscopy and other procedures categories.

Liver Transplantation

Conditions such as cirrhosis can cause irreversible damage to the liver, and patients may require a liver transplant. Liver allotransplantations (transplant from another human) include complex surgeries that involve harvesting a liver from a cadaver or living donor, preparing the recipient site, and implanting the liver. Liver transplants are performed by highly specialized physicians and surgery teams. To report the 3 components of a liver transplant, use codes 47133 through 47147. The following describes each component and the associated CPT® code(s):

1. The first component is donor **hepatectomy** (surgical removal of the liver), which includes harvesting the graft and cold preservation of the graft from the donor. Code 47133 reports donor hepatectomy from a cadaver. Codes 47140 through 47142 report living donor hepatectomy.
2. The second component is the backbench work that prepares the whole liver graft. Standard preparation includes 1 of the following procedures:
    - Cholecystectomy (gallbladder removal), if necessary, and dissection and removal of surrounding soft tissues to prepare vena cava, portal vein, hepatic artery, and common bile duct for implantation, reported with code 47143.
    - Trisegment split into 2 partial grafts, reported with code 47144.
    - Lobe split into 2 partial grafts, reported with code 47145.
3. The third component is the recipient liver allotransplantation, which includes recipient hepatectomy (partial or whole), transplantation of the allograft (partial or whole), and care of the recipient. The removal and replacement of the recipient liver with the donor liver is referred to as the *orthotopic approach*. The orthotopic approach is reported with code 47135. The heterotopic approach leaves the recipient liver in place while the donor liver is sewn in place. This procedure is rarely performed in the United States and is no longer listed in the CPT codebook. If the heterotopic procedure is performed, report code 47399, *Unlisted liver procedure*.

LET'S TRY ONE **13.14**

Choose the correct code for the following procedure.

A physician performed whole liver transplantation to the normal anatomical position of the liver in a 48-year-old male patient. The physician made an abdominal incision into the recipient of the liver. The diseased liver tissue was removed, hemostasis was achieved, and the liver bed was dried and prepared for the donor tissue. The donor liver from the cadaver was placed in the prepared liver bed. Anastomoses were created between the donor hepatic vessels and the appropriate recipient vessels. The donor bile duct was approximated to the recipient bile duct for drainage. Drains were placed, and the abdominal incision was closed.

What code is reported? ____

Biliary Tract (Codes 47400-47999)

The **biliary tract** contains the gallbladder, intrahepatic bile ducts, cystic duct (from the gallbladder to the common bile duct), and common bile duct (from liver and gallbladder to small intestine). These glands and ducts work together to deliver bile from the liver to the duodenum of the small intestine. Figure 13.27 illustrates the biliary tract glands and associated ducts. Codes 47400 through 47900 are used to report incisions, introduction, endoscopy, laparoscopy, excision, and repairs.

Cholangiography is the viewing of the bile ducts. Dye is injected into the bile ducts and viewed under fluoroscopic guidance. A cholangiography allows the physician to identify the site of biliary obstruction and determine what treatment is necessary to treat the obstruction. Obstructions in the biliary ducts interrupt the flow of bile produced by the liver into the intestines. Infections, changes in liver functions, and other serious complications may occur as a result of the obstructions. **Biliary percutaneous procedures** are performed by inserting a needle or tube into the skin between the ribs into the gallbladder or liver. Some percutaneous procedures may be performed via existing biliary catheters.

Code 47531 is used to report diagnostic cholangiography when performed through an existing catheter. Code 47532 is reported for diagnostic cholangiography by means of new access. Percutaneous placement, conversions, exchanges and removals of biliary catheters are reported with codes 47533 through 47540. Percutaneous placement of bile duct stent(s) procedures are selected based on access and if a separate biliary drainage catheter was also placed. New access to the biliary ducts through the small bowel to assist with an endoscopic biliary procedure is reported with code 47541. Therapeutic percutaneous biliary procedures, described by add-on codes 47542 through 47544, may be reported with selected primary percutaneous biliary procedure codes. Extensive parenthetical notes follow these add-on procedures to assist in appropriate reporting of therapeutic procedures.

Cholecystectomy is the surgical removal of the gallbladder. A cholecystectomy may be performed to treat **cholelithiasis**, commonly referred to as *gallstones*. **Gallstones** are bile crystals that have slowly accumulated in the gallbladder, causing inflammation, infection, and/or blockage in the associated biliary ducts. Cholecystectomy may be open or laparoscopic. Open cholecystectomy procedures are reported with codes 47600 through 47620. Laparoscopic procedures are reported with codes

Abdomen, Peritoneum, and Omentum (Codes 49000-49999)

The **abdomen** is the area of the body between the chest and the pelvis. The abdominal cavity contains the stomach, liver, gallbladder, spleen, pancreas, small intestine, kidneys, large intestine, and adrenal glands. The **peritoneum** is the membrane that lines the abdominal cavity and covers most of the abdominal organs. The **omentum** is a double layer of fatty tissue that covers and supports the intestines and abdominal organs.

Codes 49000 through 49999 are used to report procedures of the abdomen, peritoneum, and omentum.

There are extensive parenthetic notes to assist coders in selection of incision and excision categories. Because the codes in this section include 3 distinct anatomic sites, coders must carefully read the code descriptions to ensure they are selecting the correct code. Coders must also take time to read all associated parenthetic notes prior to selection of codes. Incision and drainage procedures are always open procedures, unless otherwise stated in the code description.

Laparoscopy

Code 49320 reports a diagnostic laparoscopy of the abdomen, peritoneum, and omentum, with or without collection of specimen by brushing or washing. Code 49320 may not be reported with surgical laparoscopic procedures, codes 49321 through 49325. If a diagnostic laparoscopy of the abdomen, peritoneum, and omentum is performed, and the physician identifies and addresses a condition during the same laparoscopic procedure, the procedure has changed from a diagnostic procedure to a surgical procedure. The appropriate surgical laparoscopic procedure code is reported.

Introduction, Revision, Removal

Conditions such as end-stage renal disease may require the insertion of a medical device to drain fluid from the abdominal cavity. Introduction, revision, conversion, replacement, and removal of medical devices in the abdomen, peritoneum, and omentum are reported with codes 49400 through 49465. This section contains many different types of procedures, many of which do not have parent codes. Because of this, coders must carefully read all associated guidelines and parenthetical notes prior to code selection. The following list groups related code sets in the Introduction, Revision, Removal subsection.

- Image-guided fluid collection drainage by catheter; codes 49405 through 49407
- Placement of interstitial device(s) for radiation therapy guidance; codes 49411 and 49412

- Tunneled intraperitoneal catheter; codes 49418 through 49422
- Peritoneal-venous shunt; codes 49425 through 49429
- Insertion of gastrointestinal tube, percutaneous, under fluoroscopic guidance including contrast injection(s), image documentation and report; codes 49440 through 49442
- Conversion, replacement, and removal of gastrointestinal tube, percutaneous, under fluoroscopic guidance including contrast injection(s), image documentation and report; codes 49446 through 49452

Insertion of gastrointestinal percutaneous tube under fluoroscopic guidance by use of contrast injection is reported with codes 49440 through 49442. Insertion codes are reported when a new gastrointestinal tube is inserted in a new percutaneous access site, after the removal of an old gastrointestinal percutaneous tube. Nasogastric (nasal and stomach) or orogastric (oral and stomach) tube placement to insufflate (blow air into) the stomach prior to a percutaneous gastrointestinal tube insertion is considered an integral part of the procedure and is not reported separately. Do not report codes 49440 through 49442 with code 43752, *Naso- or oro-gastric tube placement, requiring physician's skill and fluoroscopic guidance (includes fluoroscopy, image documentation and report).*

Repair

An **abdominal hernia** is a protrusion of the abdominal organs or structures through the front of the abdominal wall. Abdominal wall hernias are named according to the herniated area of the abdominal wall, such as the epigastric hernias and umbilical hernias.

Hernia repair codes are selected according to the type of hernia. Some hernia codes have additional criteria of "initial" or "recurrent," indicating if the hernia had been previously repaired. Surgical approach for hernia repairs may be open or laparoscopic. Additional code distinctions may include the age of the patient and condition of the hernia, such as reducible, incarcerated, or strangulated. **Reducible hernias** are corrected by manipulating the protruding organ or structure back into the abdominal cavity. **Incarcerated hernias** are not reducible, because the protruding organ or structure is stuck in the tear in the abdominal wall. Open surgical repair is typically the only treatment for an incarcerated hernia. A **strangulated hernia** is an incarcerated hernia that is losing or has lost blood supply. Strangulated hernias require immediate surgical repair. Figure 13.29 illustrates a strangulated hernia.

Figure 13.29 Strangulated Hernia

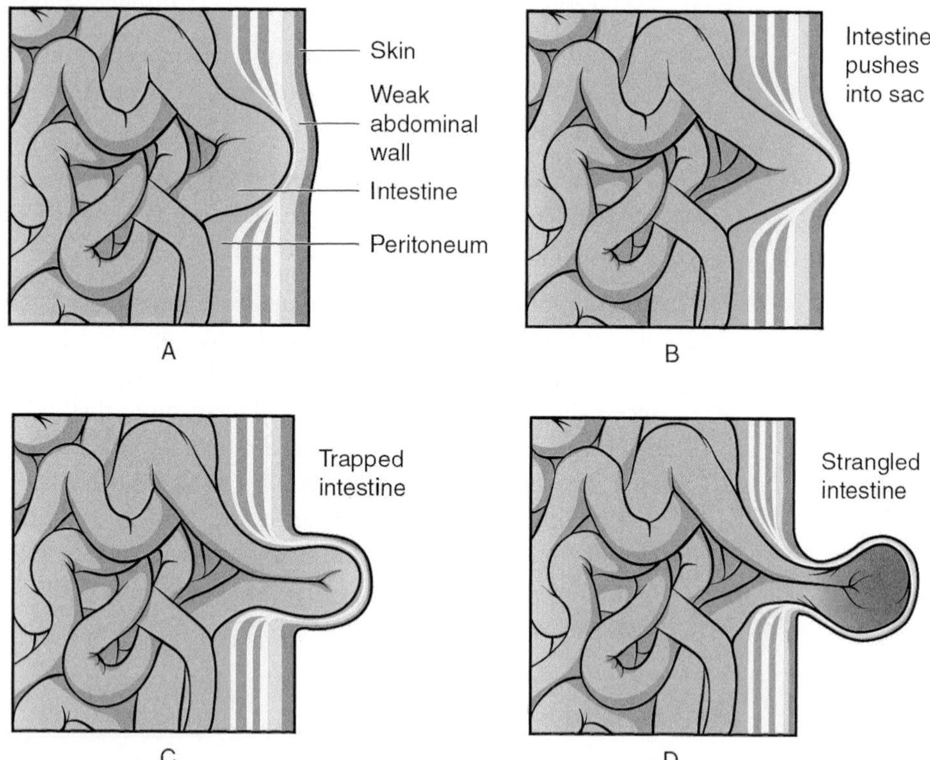

Chapter Summary

- The purpose of the digestive system, also known as the *gastrointestinal tract*, is to ingest, process, absorb, and eliminate food.
- The digestive system begins with the lips and ends with the anus.
- A flap graft is a piece of tissue that remains attached to the body by a major artery and vein or at the base until it is ready to be transferred to the recipient site on the body.
- A diagnostic endoscopy is performed to identify abnormal conditions of the structure or organ viewed.
- If bleeding occurs as a result of an endoscopy, the procedure to control the bleeding is not billed separately.
- All therapeutic endoscopies include diagnostic endoscopy; if a diagnostic endoscopy transitions to a therapeutic endoscopy during the operative session, only the code for the therapeutic procedure is reported.

- Endoscopic biopsies are reported when a portion of a lesion is removed and the specimen is sent for testing. If the entire lesion is removed, even if the specimen is sent for a biopsy, only the appropriate endoscopic lesion removal code is reported.
- When a biopsy and a lesion removal are performed for different lesions, both the biopsy and lesion codes are reportable. Modifier 59 is appended to the biopsy code.
- Laparoscopy is the viewing of the abdominal organs or female reproductive organs through a laparoscope. A laparoscope is a small flexible tube with a tiny camera on the tip.
- Open and laparoscopic surgery codes are not interchangeable.
- Bariatric surgeries are various open and laparoscopic gastric restriction techniques used to treat morbid obesity.
- Nasogastric or orogastric tube placement to insufflate the stomach, prior to a percutaneous gastrointestinal tube insertion, is considered an integral part of the procedure and is not reported separately.

Navigator

Access interactive chapter review exercises, practice activities, flash cards, and study games.

Chapter 14

Surgery Coding: The Urinary System

Fast Facts

- The bladder is a stretchy, balloon-like bag that swells when full and shrinks when empty. It has a urine-proof lining called *urothelium*.
- In the Middle Ages, alchemists tried to extract elements from urine. Alchemists thought they may be able to find gold, which they did not, but they did discover white phosphorous in urine.
- The average person passes 1.5 to 2 liters of urine in a day.
- Kidneys filter about 200 quarts of blood per day. That is more than 5 million quarts in a lifetime!

Source: http://livescience.com

Crack the Code

Review the sample operative report to find the correct urinary system code. You may need to return to this exercise after reading the chapter content.

DATE OF PROCEDURE: 07/01/2019

PROCEDURE PERFORMED: TUR bladder tumor

SURGEON: Raza Khan, MD

ANESTHESIA: General

PROCEDURE: After induction of general anesthesia, the patient was placed in the dorsolithotomy position. Genitalia were prepared and draped in the usual manner. External genitalia revealed phimosis. Urethra was prepared. A metallic Van Buren sounds up to 30 was passed by the urethra into the bladder without any difficulty. A #28 resectoscope was introduced, and a raw irregular area about 5.5 cm in the posterior left lateral wall and near the dome area was seen again. The rest of the bladder showed no tumor. Bladder mucosa was congested, hyperemic, and irritated, probably from the radiation. Ureteral orifices were normal. At this time the area of about 5.5 to 6 cm was completely resected, and dissection was done fairly deep. The base was thoroughly cauterized. The tissue was sent for pathological examination. Also urine cytology was obtained at the beginning of the procedure. No active bleeding was noticed. Bladder was emptied and resectoscope was removed. A #20 Foley catheter was introduced and left indwelling. Bimanual rectal examination was grossly unremarkable without any masses. The patient tolerated the procedure and general anesthesia well and left the OR in good condition.

answer: 52240

Urinary System Terminology

Familiarity with the word roots and suffixes related to the procedures on the urinary system will allow you to quickly recognize an organ and service. Table 14.1 lists common terms in the urinary system.

Table 14.1 Common Urinary System Terms

Word root or suffix	Definition(s)	Example
cyst/o	The bladder (organ); sac	Cystoscopy—viewing the bladder using a scope
lith/o	Stone, calculus	Nephrolithiasis—condition of stone in the kidney
nephr/o	The kidney (organ)	Nephrectomy—excision of kidney
-pexy	Surgical fixation	Nephropexy—surgical fixation of the kidney (putting back in place)
pyel/o	Renal pelvis, the structure within the kidney that collects urine	Pyeloplasty—surgical repair of the renal pelvis
ren/o	Kidney: structure, function, or procedure	Renal failure—loss of kidney function
-rrhaphy	Repair by suturing	Cystorrhaphy—repairing the bladder by suturing
-scopy	Visual examination using a scope	Cystourethroscopy, visual examination of the bladder and urethra
-tripsy	Surgical crushing	Lithotripsy—surgically crushing a stone
vesic/o	Urinary bladder	Vesicourethral suspension—suspension surgery of the bladder and urethra

CONCEPTS CHECKPOINT **14.1**

Fill in the blanks to complete each of the following sentences.

1. The term meaning repair of the bladder by suturing is ______________.
2. The 2 word roots meaning *bladder* are ______________ and ______________.
3. The term *nephrolithotripsy* can be defined as ______________.
4. The term *nephroscopy* can be defined as ______________.
5. A patient with a drooping kidney requires a surgical fixation of the kidney to tack it back into place. This procedure is termed ______________.
6. The organ that temporarily stores urine is the ______________.
7. The pair of tubes that lead from the kidneys to the bladder are the ______________.
8. The tube that passes urine to the outside of the body is the ______________.

Organization of the Urinary System Surgery Subsection

The codes in the Urinary System Surgery subsection are grouped by anatomical site in top-to-bottom sequence: kidney, ureter, bladder, and urethra. As with the other surgery subsections, the procedure codes are sequenced in the categories of incision, excision, introduction, repair, laparoscopy, endoscopy, and other procedures. There are a few categories that are specific to the urinary system, such as urodynamics, renal transplantation, and transurethral surgery. Table 14.2 presents a listing of the Urinary System Surgery subsection headings and corresponding code numbers.

Table 14.2 Headings Within the Urinary System Surgery Subsection of the CPT® Codebook

Heading	Code Range
Kidney	50010-50593
Ureter	50600-50980
Bladder	51020-52700
Urethra	53000-53899

Kidney (Codes 50010-50593)

The Kidney heading includes the code categories of incision, excision, renal transplantation, introduction, repair, laparoscopy, endoscopy, and other procedures. In the Incision category are codes for nephrotomy, nephrolithotomy, and pyelotomy. Excision procedures are kidney biopsy, nephrectomy, and lesion removal. Kidney transplants have a separate category, Renal Transplantation. The Introduction category describes catheterization, aspiration, and instillation procedures. Kidney repairs for abnormalities, injuries, and closures of fistulas are found under Repair. The Laparoscopy and Endoscopy categories contain codes for many of the preceding surgical procedures performed with scopes. Finally, Other Procedures has codes for tumor ablation and **extracorporeal shockwave lithotripsy (ESWL)**, a procedure that uses sound waves to break up kidney stones.

Nephrolithotomy

Many of the codes in the kidney section refer to surgical treatment of kidney stones. A **kidney calculus** or **stone** is a concretion of minerals and acid salts formed when urine becomes concentrated, allowing the minerals to crystalize. Kidney stones cause symptoms when they move around the urinary tract, and then they can become painful. Larger stones require surgical treatment if they are too large to pass or cause bleeding or damage to the kidney. **Nephrolithotomy**, the removal of calculus by making an incision into the kidney, is reported with codes 50060 through 50075, as shown in Figure 14.2.

Figure 14.2 Nephrolithotomy Codes

50060 Nephrolithotomy; removal of calculus

50065 secondary surgical operation for calculus

50070 complicated by congenital kidney abnormality

50075 removal of large staghorn calculus filling renal pelvis and calyces (including anatrophic pyelolithotomy)

Criteria to remember when reporting nephrolithotomy codes are as follows:

- Report code 50060 for a simple removal of calculus.
- Report code 50065 when the patient had a previous kidney surgery, which made the removal of the calculus more difficult for the surgeon.
- Report code 50070 when the patient has a congenital kidney abnormality characterized by obstructed or abnormally narrow calyces (chambers in the kidney), complicating the calculus removal.
- Report code 50075 for the removal of a **staghorn calculus**, a stone that fills the renal pelvis and calyces, requiring the surgeon to perform a **pyelotomy** (an incision in the renal pelvis) and **nephrotomy** (an incision in the kidney).

Inside the OR

To remove a staghorn calculus, the surgeon first makes an incision into the skin of the patient's flank. The incision is deepened through the muscles, fat, and fascia over the kidney. A portion of the patient's 12th rib may be removed. After locating the calculus, the surgeon makes an incision in the renal pelvis and may make an incision into the kidney. The calculus is removed through the incision. The area is irrigated. The surgeon inspects the kidney for defects. The incision on the kidney is closed, a drain is inserted, and the skin and subcutaneous tissue is closed in layers.

In a **percutaneous nephrostolithotomy**, the surgeon makes a small incision and, using radiological guidance, passes an instrument to either remove or crush the stone. Codes 50080 and 50081 are based on the size of the stone removed (less than or greater than 2 cm). Fluoroscopic guidance is reported in addition to the code for the lithotomy using codes 76000 and 76001 from the Radiology codebook section.

LET'S TRY ONE **14.1**

Read the description of the procedure in the Inside the OR feature. What is the appropriate code for this procedure? _____

Nephrectomy

Patients who have irreversible kidney damage may require a **nephrectomy**, the surgical removal of all or part of the kidney. Kidney damage may be caused by traumatic injury, chronic infection, nephrosclerosis (hardening of blood vessels in the kidney), and other conditions. Nephrectomy is also indicated for patients with renal cell carcinoma. Similar to the codes for surgical removal of other organs, nephrectomy codes are differentiated by the technique and the extent of the removal. Open nephrectomy is reported with codes 50220 through 50240, found in the Excision codebook category and shown in Figure 14.3. Nephrectomy performed laparoscopically is reported with codes 50543 and 50545 through 50548, found in the Laparoscopy codebook category.

RED FLAG

The kidneys are a pair of organs, so it is appropriate to use the RT (right) or LT (left) modifier to indicate which kidney was removed in a unilateral nephrectomy.

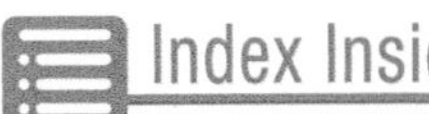

Visit http://Coding.ParadigmEducation.com/PartialNephrectomy to view a video of a laparoscopic partial nephrectomy. Because the link shows a surgery, viewer discretion is advised.

Index Insider

The main Index entry *Kidney*, subterm *Excision* includes the codes for nephrectomy; the subterm *Removal* is a dead end for finding nephrectomy codes. However, the fastest way to find nephrectomy codes in the Index is using the main term *Nephrectomy*, where you will find subterms for *Laparoscopic*, *Partial*, and *with Ureters*.

Figure 14.3 Open Nephrectomy Codes

50220	Nephrectomy, including partial ureterectomy, any open approach including rib resection;
50225	complicated because of previous surgery on same kidney
50230	radical, with regional lymphadenectomy and/or vena caval thrombectomy
	(When vena caval resection with reconstruction is necessary, use 37799)
50234	Nephrectomy with total ureterectomy and bladder cuff; through same incision
50236	through separate incision

Coding considerations for the open and laparoscopic nephrectomy procedures are as follows:

- If the nephrectomy also includes a partial ureterectomy, report an open approach with code 50220 and a laparoscopic approach with code 50546.
- If an open nephrectomy is complicated because of previous surgery on the same kidney, report code 50225.
- If the operation is a radical nephrectomy, which includes not only removal of the kidney but removal of the surrounding fat, fascia, adrenal gland, periaortic lymph nodes, and upper ureter: report an open approach with code 50230 and a laparoscopic approach with code 50545.
- If the open nephrectomy involves removal of the kidney, ureter, and small cuff of the bladder through 1 incision, report code 50234, and if through 2 separate incisions, with code 50236. In a similar procedure performed laparoscopically, nephrectomy with total ureterectomy, report code 50548.
- If the operation is a partial nephrectomy (removal of only a portion of the kidney), report an open approach with code 50240 and a laparoscopic approach with code 50543.

LET'S TRY ONE **14.2**

Report the appropriate code (and modifier as appropriate) for the following procedures.

1. A 35-year-old female was found to have a 2.5-cm mass on her right kidney. This appeared to be a renal cyst on the ultrasound, but due to the possibility of renal cell carcinoma, it was decided to remove this mass. The surgeon performed a laparoscopic partial nephrectomy. _____
2. A 45-year-old male was diagnosed with localized renal cell carcinoma of the right kidney. An open radical nephrectomy was performed. _____
3. A 57-year-old male with a long history of kidney stones was found to have severe scarring in the left kidney. After making an incision through the skin and down to the kidney, the surgeon removed the kidney and a portion of the ureter. _____

Kidney Transplantation

Many patients with **end-stage renal disease** (**ESRD**) (irreversible deterioration of kidney function) undergo a kidney transplant and are able to discontinue **dialysis**, a process that artificially filters waste products from the blood. Renal transplantation can be either **autogenic**, moving the patient's own kidney to a new site, or **allogenic**, receiving a kidney from a donor. The physician's work in **allogenic transplantation (allotransplantation)** involves 3 components that are separately reported.

Allotransplantation Component 1: Kidney Harvest and Preservation

The first component of kidney allotransplantation is the nephrectomy performed on either a cadaver or a living donor. A cadaver donor nephrectomy includes harvesting the kidney, preserving the organ by perfusing it (passing fluid on and through) with a cold preservation solution, and keeping it cold. A living donor nephrectomy includes harvesting the kidney, preserving the kidney by cold preservation solution perfusion and cold maintenance, and caring for the donor.

Coding considerations for kidney harvest and preparation in allotransplantation are as follows:

- Report a cadaver donor nephrectomy with code 50300.
- Report a donor nephrectomy based on the surgical approach: open with code 50320, *Donor nephrectomy (including cold preservation); open from living donor*, and laparoscopic with 50547, *Laparoscopy, surgical; donor nephrectomy (including cold preservation) from living donor.*
- Remember to include an RT or LT modifier to indicate which kidney was removed.

Allotransplantation Component 2: Kidney Backbench Work

The second component of allotransplantation is the backbench work reported with codes 50323 through 50329. **Backbench work** is the preparation of a donor organ for transplant, sometimes referred to as *back table prep*. Figure 14.4 presents the codes for these procedures.

Coding considerations for kidney backbench work on a donor kidney (renal allograft) are as follows:

- If a cadaver donor, report the standard preparation that includes all the constituents in the code descriptor with code 50323.
- If a living donor, report the standard preparation that includes all the constituents in the code descriptor with code 50325.
- If additional reconstruction is required such as venous, arterial, or ureteral anastomosis, report codes 50327 through 50329 in addition to the standard preparation codes.

Figure 14.4 Codes for Backbench Work

50323	Backbench standard preparation of cadaver donor renal allograft prior to transplantation, including dissection and removal of perinephric fat, diaphragmatic and retroperitoneal attachments, excision of adrenal gland, and preparation of ureter(s), renal vein(s), and renal artery(s), ligating branches, as necessary
	(Do not report 50323 in conjunction with 60540, 60545)
50325	Backbench standard preparation of living donor renal allograft (open or laparoscopic) prior to transplantation, including dissection and removal of perinephric fat and preparation of ureter(s), renal vein(s), and renal artery(s), ligating branches, as necessary
50327	Backbench reconstruction of cadaver or living donor renal allograft prior to transplantation; venous anastomosis, each
50328	arterial anastomosis, each
50329	ureteral anastomosis, each

Allotransplantation Component 3: Kidney Transplantation

The third component of renal allotransplantation is the transplantation of the donor kidney into the recipient. Poorly functioning kidneys that are not causing complications, such as high blood pressure or infection, are often left in place, as shown in Figure 14.5.

Figure 14.5 Kidney Transplant Without Recipient Nephrectomy

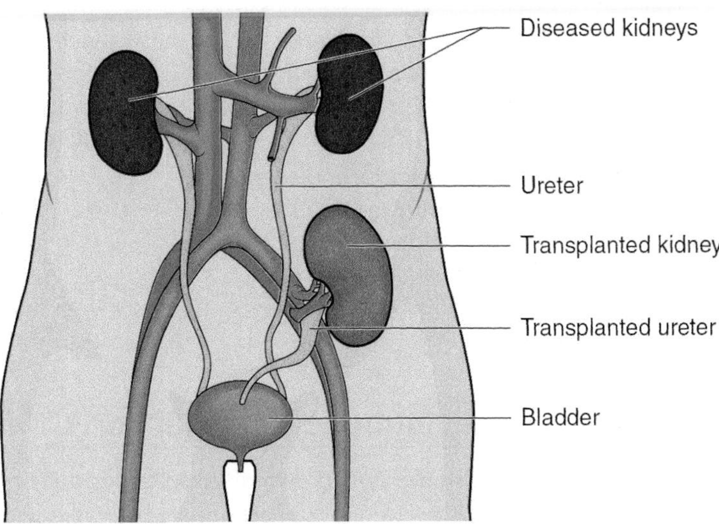

Coding considerations for transplantation of a donor kidney (renal allograft) are as follows:

- When an allotransplantation is performed without removing the recipient's diseased kidney, report code 50360, *Renal allotransplantation, implantation of graft; without recipient nephrectomy.*
- When a nephrectomy is performed on the recipient at the time of the allograft, report code 50365, *Renal allotransplantation, implantation of graft; with recipient nephrectomy.*
- When the recipient's own kidney is moved from its original anatomical site and reconnected to a new site, report code 50380, *Renal autotransplantation, reimplantation of kidney.*

CONCEPTS CHECKPOINT **14.2**

Fill in the blanks to complete each of the following sentences.

1. Harvesting a kidney from a deceased person is termed a ______________ nephrectomy.
2. Preparing the donor kidney for transplantation is known as ______________ work.
3. The procedure of placing a kidney from a living donor into the recipient is renal ______________.
4. The procedure of placing a kidney from a cadaver donor into the recipient is renal ______________.
5. The procedure of transplanting the patient's own kidney to a new site is renal ______________.

LET'S TRY ONE **14.3**

Assign the appropriate codes to the following procedures.

1. A 32-year-old obese female donated a kidney to her brother who was suffering from end-stage renal disease. The donor's nephrectomy was done as an open procedure due to the patient's obesity. _____
2. A 45-year-old male with renal vascular disease was scheduled for renal autotransplantation. His kidney was removed from its original anatomical site and revascularized by connecting the renal vessels to a new blood supply. _____
3. A 34-year-old male with end-stage renal disease was scheduled for an allograft using a kidney donated by his sister. The surgeon removed the diseased kidney and placed the donor kidney without complication. _____

Other Introduction (Injection/Change/Removal) Procedures

Codes in this urinary system subsection include percutaneous genitourinary procedures that are aspirations or injections, catheter placements, and catheter exchanges. Guidelines in the CPT® codebook describe services that are included when reporting these codes. For example, codes 50430 and 50431, *Injection procedures for nephrostogram or ureterogram*, describe the complete diagnostic procedure. Imaging guidance (such as ultrasound or fluoroscopy), which is a service needed to perform these procedures, is not separately reportable. Code 74425 for radiological supervision and interpretation is not to be used with these codes. A list of codes that may not be reported with codes from this subsection are included in the tabular list. Codes 50430 through 50435 are reported once for each renal collecting system/ureter accessed. The renal pelvis and its ureter are counted as 1 system. It should also be noted that codes 50430 through 50435 are out of numerical sequence and appear before code 50400 in the codebook.

</> Coding for CMS

Medicare pays for kidney transplantation and appropriate harvesting charges for both cadaver and living donors. Patients who qualify for Medicare only because of permanent kidney failure lose their coverage 36 months after the date of transplant. Coverage is extended for patients who need to go back on dialysis or require another transplant within 36 months.

Endoscopy

RED FLAG

Although the CPT® codebook lists codes for separate procedures, most are an integral part of another surgery and should not be reported separately unless it is clearly documented that it is a separate procedure. Modifier 59, *Distinct procedural service*, should be applied to indicate that services are appropriate to report together under the circumstances.

Renal endoscopy is indicated for patients with urinary symptoms who do not respond to medical treatment. In a **renal endoscopy**, the surgeon examines the renal and ureteric structures. Renal endoscopy codes are differentiated by 1 of 2 approaches. If through an established nephrostomy or pyelostomy (an artificial opening), codes 50551 through 50562 are reported, depending on the procedure. If through a small incision (nephrotomy or pyelotomy), codes 50570 through 50580 are reported, depending on the procedure. When performed as a separately identifiable service in conjunction with nephrotomy with exploration (50045) or pyelotomy with exploration (50120), a separate code for the renal endoscopy can also be reported from codes 50570 through 50580.

Ureter (Codes 50600-50980)

Many of the procedures performed on the ureters can be found under the Ureter anatomical heading, but some are found under other urinary system organs or under the Transurethral Surgery category (under the Bladder heading). For example, locate the code for transvesical ureterolithotomy (51060) under the Bladder heading and fragmentation of ureteral calculus with cystourethroscopy (52325) under the Transurethral Surgery heading. The Incision category describes codes for exploration, drainage, and insertion of stents. Ureterectomy is found under Excision. Injections, catheter changes, and manometric studies are under Introduction. The Repair codes include procedures for ureteroplasty, lysis, anastomosis, undiversion (surgical restoration of continuity), transplantation, closure, and deligation. The 2 categories Laparoscopy and Endoscopy provide codes for many of the preceding open surgical procedures performed with scopes.

Since there are 2 ureters, it may be appropriate to assign modifiers RT (right) or LT (left) to indicate the ureter on which the procedure was performed. Procedures done on both ureters should have modifier 50, *Bilateral procedure*, applied.

Ureterolithotomy

Stones that have developed in the kidney and have moved to the ureter are called **ureteroliths**. **Ureterolithotomy**, removal of calculus by making an incision into the ureter, is an open procedure reported with codes 50610 through 50630, as shown in Figure 14.6. These codes are differentiated by the location of the calculus removal—the upper, middle, or lower one-third of the ureter. Laparoscopic ureterolithotomy is reported with 50945 no matter where the calculus is located. The fourth parenthetic note below code 50630 in the codebook (see Figure 14.6) indicates 10 additional codes relating to endoscopic extraction or manipulation of ureteral stones.

Figure 14.6 Ureterolithotomy Codes

50610	Ureterolithotomy; upper one-third of ureter
50620	middle one-third of ureter
50630	lower one-third of ureter
	(For laparoscopic approach, use 50945)
	(For transvesical ureterolithotomy, use 51060)
	(For cystotomy with stone basket extraction of ureteral calculus, use 51065)
	(For endoscopic extraction or manipulation of ureteral calculus, see 50080, 50081, 50561, 50961, 50980, 52320-52330, 52352, 52353, 52356)

Endoscopy

Ureteral endoscopy codes are differentiated by the approach for the endoscopy, whether through an established **ureterostomy** (an opening) or through a **ureterotomy** (a small incision). Report endoscopy performed through ureterostomy with codes 50951 through 50961 and through ureterotomy with codes 50970 through 50980, depending on the specific procedure performed. When performed as a separately identifiable service in conjunction with ureterotomy with exploration (50600), you can report a separate code for the ureteral endoscopy from codes 50970 through 50980.

CONCEPTS CHECKPOINT **14.3**

Complete each of the following statements to show your understanding of ureteral codes.

1. Codes for removal of calculus from the ureter performed as an open procedure depend on
   a. the location of the stone in the ureter.
   b. the size of the stone.
   c. the type of anesthesia.
   d. the number of incisions.
2. Codes for a laparoscopic removal of calculus from the ureter
   a. depend on the location of the stone in the ureter.
   b. depend on the size of the stone.
   c. depend on the type of anesthesia.
   d. have no relation to location or size of the stone or type of anesthesia used.
3. Ureteral endoscopy codes
   a. depend on whether the approach was through an ureterostomy.
   b. depend on the specific procedure performed.
   c. may be reported with ureterotomy with exploration if a separate service.
   d. are characterized by all of these answers.

Bladder (Codes 51020-52700)

Like the other surgery sections, codes for bladder procedures are grouped in the codebook into categories of Incision, Removal, Excision, Introduction, Repair, Laparoscopy, and Endoscopy. The Incision category describes procedures for fulguration; insertions of catheters, stents, and radioactive materials; calculus extraction and fragmentation; and drainage. Removal codes describe aspiration. Excision procedures include hernia and ureterocele repair, cystectomy with associated lymph node excision, reimplantation and transplantation, diversion, anastomosis, and exenteration. Introduction codes cover injection procedures, catheter insertions, and irrigation. Repair codes involve cystoplasty and cystourethroplasty, fixation and suspension of structures, closure, and anastomosis. The Laparoscopy and Endoscopy categories provide codes for some of the preceding surgical procedures performed with scopes. The Bladder codebook section also contains additional categories related to the bladder—Urodynamics, Transurethral Surgery, and Vesical Neck and Prostate—which will be covered in detail in this chapter.

Urodynamics

Patients with lower urinary tract dysfunction such as urine leakage (incontinence), painful urination, problems emptying the bladder, and other symptoms may undergo diagnostic urodynamic testing. **Urodynamics** is the study of how well the bladder is holding and emptying urine, and it encompasses several tests: cystometrography, uroflowmetry, voiding pressure studies, measurement of post-voiding residual urine, and electromyography.

Urodynamics codes (51725-51798) can be used separately or in combinations if more than 1 urodynamic test is performed. Modifier 51, *Multiple procedures*, should be used if multiple tests are performed at the same session. All the urodynamic codes include the supplies and equipment needed for the test as well as the services of a physician or other qualified health professional and a technician. If a physician or other qualified health professional was involved only to interpret the test, thus providing a professional component, modifier 26, *Professional component*, should be applied. In the case of a test done in a hospital setting where the technicians are employed by the facility but the physician is not, the physician would provide only the professional component, and modifier 26 should be applied to the procedure code.

A **cystometrogram** is a study that can determine how much the bladder can hold, how much pressure builds up within the bladder, and how full the bladder is before the patient has the urge to urinate. The cystometrogram codes 51725 through 51729 shown in Figure 14.7 are assigned according to the complexity of the study and further differentiated by the additional studies that were performed.

Coding considerations for the cystometrogram codes are the following:

- Report code 51725 for a simple cystometrogram in which a pressure catheter is inserted into the bladder and connected to a manometer filled with fluid to measure the pressure and flow in the lower urinary tract.
- Report code 51726 for a complex cystometrogram when the bladder is filled by transurethral catheter while at the same time rectal pressure is measured.

Figure 14.7 Simple and Complex Cystometrogram Codes

51725	Simple cystometrogram (CMG) (eg, spinal manometer)
51726	Complex cystometrogram (ie, calibrated electronic equipment);
51727	with urethral pressure profile studies (ie, urethral closure pressure profile), any technique
51728	with voiding pressure studies (ie, bladder voiding pressure), any technique
51729	with voiding pressure studies (ie, bladder voiding pressure) and urethral pressure profile studies (ie, urethral closure pressure profile), any technique

- Report codes 51727 through 51729 for the performance of additional studies associated with complex cystometrograms: code 51727 for measuring urethral pressure; code 51728 for voiding pressure studies, in which the patient is urged to urinate when the bladder feels full and measurements are made of bladder pressure and volume at specific times; and code 51729 for a combination of urethral pressure studies and voiding pressure studies.

Uroflowmetry (UFR) measures urine speed and volume and is reported with codes 51736 (simple) or 51741 (complex). A simple uroflowmetry coded with 51736 measures the speed and volume of urine over time using a stopwatch to calculate the flow rate. A complex uroflowmetry coded with 51741 uses calibrated electronic equipment instead of a stopwatch to assess the rate of speed and volume in urine flow.

Electromyographic (EMG) studies of anal or urethral sphincter function measure the electrical signals that cause muscles to contract, allowing the physician to see if the muscle being measured is healthy or not. A **nonneedle EMG** (code 51784) uses an electrode placed on the skin's surface to measure the electrical signals. A **needle EMG** (code 51785) uses needle electrodes inserted through the skin and directly into the muscle.

Measurement of post-voiding residual urine involves using ultrasound to measure the residual urine or bladder capacity after the patient has urinated. The software in the ultrasound scanner calculates residual urine volume and bladder capacity based on the shape of the patient's bladder. Report this urodynamic test with code 51798.

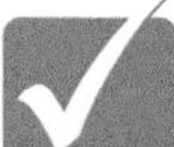

CONCEPTS CHECKPOINT **14.4**

Answer true or false to each of the following statements.

1. _____ Uroflowmetry measures rectal pressure.
2. _____ A simple cystometrogram measures pressure and flow in the lower urinary tract.
3. _____ Multiple urodynamic studies can be reported for the same session.
4. _____ Modifier 26 should be applied for multiple studies in the same session.
5. _____ If a cystometrogram and uroflowmetry are performed in the same session, only 1 can be reported.

LET'S TRY ONE **14.4**

A 41-year-old woman presented to the clinic with complaints of being unable to hold her urine. Neurogenic bladder was suspected, and an EMG was scheduled. A needle EMG of the urethral sphincter was performed. What is the appropriate code for this procedure? _____

Endoscopy and Transurethral Surgery

Procedures in the Endoscopy and Transurethral Surgery categories generally involve **cystourethroscopy**, the visual examination of the bladder and urethra using a scope. Code descriptions include many secondary procedures that are related to the main procedure, as shown in Figure 14.8.

Figure 14.8 Examples of Codes Containing Multiple Procedures

52285	Cystourethroscopy for treatment of the female urethral syndrome with any or all of the following: urethral meatotomy, urethral dilation, internal urethrotomy, lysis of urethrovaginal septal fibrosis, lateral incisions of the bladder neck, and fulguration of polyp(s) of urethra, bladder neck, and/or trigone
...	
52601	Transurethral electrosurgical resection of prostate, including control of postoperative bleeding, complete (vasectomy, meatotomy, cystourethroscopy, urethral calibration and/or dilation, and internal urethrotomy are included)

In an instance in which a secondary procedure included in the primary procedure code ends up requiring a significant amount of time and effort, modifier 22, *Increased procedural services*, should be used with the surgery code.

Endoscopy—Cystoscopy, Urethroscopy, and Cystourethroscopy

A diagnostic cystourethroscopy done as a separate procedure is reported with 52000. As you have learned, diagnostic endoscopy is always included in surgical endoscopy.

Transurethral Surgery

The term *transurethral* means "across or through the urethra" and describes an endoscopic approach. The Transurethral Surgery category is subdivided into codes for Urethra and Bladder and codes for Ureter and Pelvis, codebook groupings that indicate the anatomical sites for the procedures. Therapeutic procedures done endoscopically on the urethra and bladder are reported with codes 52204 through 52318 and include diagnostic cystourethroscopy. Codes for cystourethroscopy with fulguration (destroying lesion by laser or electric current) and/or resection of bladder lesions or tumors (52224 through 52240) are based on the size of the largest tumor(s), as shown in Figure 14.9.

Figure 14.9 Codes for Cystourethroscopy with Fulguration

52224	Cystourethroscopy, with fulguration (including cryosurgery or laser surgery) or treatment of MINOR (less than 0.5 cm) lesion(s) with or without biopsy
52234	Cystourethroscopy, with fulguration (including cryosurgery or laser surgery) and/or resection of; SMALL bladder tumor(s) (0.5 up to 2.0 cm)
52235	MEDIUM bladder tumor(s) (2.0 to 5.0 cm)
52240	LARGE bladder tumor(s)

The Ureter and Pelvis group of codes within the Transurethral Surgery category contains therapeutic procedure codes 52320 through 52356, which include any diagnostic procedures. The notes prior to the section carry some coding guidelines: for example, an exclusively diagnostic cystourethroscopy should be reported with code 52000. While the insertion and removal of a temporary ureteral catheter is included in all of these codes, the insertion of an indwelling ureteral stent is not included and may be reported separately with code 52332, as shown in Figure 14.10.

Figure 14.10 Code for Insertion of Indwelling Ureteral Stent

52332	Cystourethroscopy, with insertion of indwelling ureteral stent (eg, Gibbons or double-J type)

Report code 52332 for a unilateral stent insertion. If stents are inserted bilaterally, modifier 50, *Bilateral procedure*, is applied. Code a simple removal of the stent with 52310 and a complicated removal with 52315 when the procedure is more difficult due to previous surgery or the size or condition of the stent.

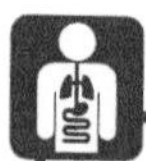

A&P Review

The vesical neck is the neck of the bladder where the urethra begins. The prostate is a walnut-sized gland located in front of the rectum, between the bladder and penis. The urethra runs through the prostate gland.

Vesical Neck and Prostate

Codes in the Vesical Neck and Prostate category (52400 through 52700) describe transurethral resection of the vesical (bladder) neck, transurethral resection of the prostate, and laser coagulation, vaporization, and enucleation of the prostate.

Vesical Neck Procedures

The endoscopic procedure described in code 52500, *Transurethral resection of bladder neck (separate procedure)*, is performed to relieve an obstruction of the bladder outlet. Report code 52500 only when this is performed as a separate procedure and not in conjunction with other transurethral procedures.

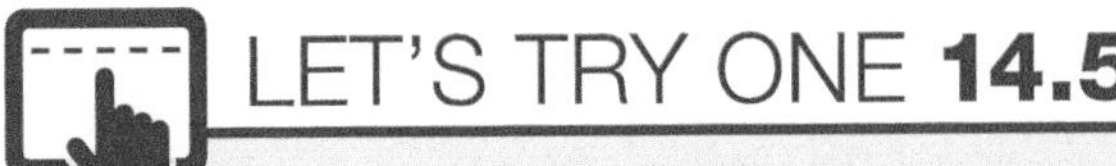

LET'S TRY ONE **14.5**

A report for a transurethral resection of a bladder tumor appears below.

DATE OF SURGERY 07-01-2019

PREOPERATIVE DIAGNOSES

1. Cancer of the bladder
2. Status post radiation and systemic chemotherapy

POSTOPERATIVE DIAGNOSES

1. Cancer of the bladder
2. Status post radiation and systemic chemotherapy

PROCEDURE PERFORMED Transurethral resection bladder tumor

SURGEON Raza Khan, MD

ANESTHESIA General

INDICATIONS

The patient has infiltrating CA of the bladder. The patient wanted to preserve his bladder, did not want to have a cystectomy, and was given systemic chemotherapy and radiation and a follow-up cystoscopy. The patient showed areas of tumor and was brought in for resection.

PROCEDURE

After induction of general anesthesia, the patient was placed in the dorsolithotomy position. Genitalia were prepared and draped in the usual manner. External genitalia revealed phimosis. The urethra was prepared. A metallic Van Buren sound up to 30 was passed by the urethra into the bladder without any difficulty. A #28 resectoscope was introduced, and a raw irregular area about 5.5 cm in the posterior left lateral wall, near the dome area, was seen. The rest of the bladder showed no tumor. Bladder mucosa was congested, hyperemic, and irritated, probably from the radiation. Ureteral orifices were normal. At this time, the area of about 5.5 to 6 cm was completely resected, and dissection was fairly deep. The base was thoroughly cauterized. The tissue was sent for pathological examination. Also, a urine cytology was obtained at the beginning of the procedure. No active bleeding was noticed. Bladder was emptied and resectoscope was removed. A #20 Foley catheter was introduced and left indwelling. Bimanual rectal examination was grossly unremarkable without any masses. The patient tolerated the procedure and general anesthesia well and left the OR in good condition.

After reading the operative report above, answer the following questions.

1. Why was this procedure done? ______________
2. What procedure was performed? ______________
3. What was the size of the tumor that was removed? ______________
4. What is the appropriate code for this procedure? ______________

Transurethral Resection of the Prostate

Patients with prostate cancer or benign prostatic hyperplasia (BPH) are often treated surgically with **transurethral resection of the prostate (TURP)**. Codes for TURP are shown in Figure 14.11: code 52601 for an initial resection and code 52630 for a resection of residual tissue or regrowth from a previous surgery.

Figure 14.11 Codes for Transurethral Resection of Prostate

52601	Transurethral electrosurgical resection of prostate, including control of postoperative bleeding, complete (vasectomy, meatotomy, cystourethroscopy, urethral calibration and/or dilation, and internal urethrotomy are included)
52630	Transurethral resection; residual or regrowth of obstructive prostate tissue including control of postoperative bleeding, complete (vasectomy, meatotomy, cystourethroscopy, urethral calibration and/or dilation, and internal urethrotomy are included)

Coding Clicks

View a 6-minute video illustration of the TURP surgical episode of care from preop to postop at http://Coding.ParadigmEducation.com/TURP.

If the resection of the regrowth of prostate tissue is performed within the postoperative period (defined as the global days as described in Chapter 8) by the same surgeon, report modifier 78, *Unplanned return to the operating/procedure room by the same physician or other qualified health care professional following initial procedure for a related procedure during the postoperative period.* Report an open resection of the prostate with codes 55801 through 55845, found in the Male Genital System Surgery subsection.

Laser Procedures of the Prostate

Patients with an enlarged prostate may require laser coagulation, vaporization, or enucleation of the prostate gland to remove tissue in the prostate. **Laser coagulation** heats the prostate tissue to a point that cells cannot survive. The tissue sloughs offs, and the body reabsorbs the tissue over a 2- to 3-month period. As illustrated in Figure 14.12, **laser vaporization** uses a green-light laser that emits energy that vaporizes (converts into gas) tissue. The laser tip is moved across the prostate surface, vaporizing the tissue bloodlessly and leaving a cavity where the tissue once was. Code 52648 describes contact laser vaporization. **Laser enucleation** is removal of the whole prostate organ (code 52649) and involves **morcellation,** in which tissue is divided and removed in small pieces. The entire prostate is treated in all 3 of these procedures, as shown in Figure 14.13.

Coding laser procedures of the prostate has the following considerations:

- Codes 52647 through 52649 include control of postoperative bleeding, vasectomy, meatotomy, cystourethroscopy, urethral calibration and/or dilation, internal urethrotomy, and transurethral resection.
- Report code 52647 for laser coagulation of prostate tissue. Code 52647 describes noncontact laser coagulation.

Figure 14.12 Laser Vaporization of Prostate

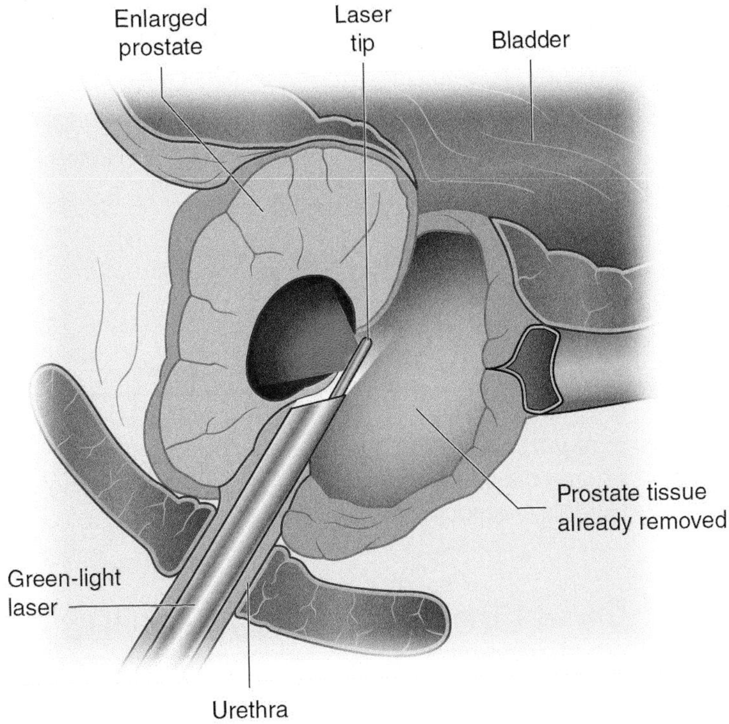

Figure 14.13 Codes for Laser Procedures of the Prostate

52647	Laser coagulation of prostate, including control of postoperative bleeding, complete (vasectomy, meatotomy, cystourethroscopy, urethral calibration and/or dilation, and internal urethrotomy are included if performed)
52648	Laser vaporization of prostate, including control of postoperative bleeding, complete (vasectomy, meatotomy, cystourethroscopy, urethral calibration and/or dilation, internal urethrotomy and transurethral resection of prostate are included if performed)
52649	Laser enucleation of the prostate with morcellation, including control of postoperative bleeding, complete (vasectomy, meatotomy, cystourethroscopy, urethral calibration and/or dilation, internal urethrotomy and transurethral resection of prostate are included if performed)

- Report code 52648 for laser vaporization of prostate tissue.
- Report code 52649 for complete removal of the prostate through enucleation.

Transurethral destruction of prostate tissue by microwave (53850) or radiofrequency thermotherapy (53852) is found under the Other Procedures subheading in the Urethra category.

CONCEPTS CHECKPOINT 14.5

Which 3 of the following procedures may be reported in addition to codes 52647 through 52649? _____, _____, and _____.

1. Insertion of ureteral stent
2. Vasectomy
3. Urethral calibration
4. Internal urethrotomy
5. Ureteroscopy with lithotripsy
6. Ureteral catheterization
7. Transurethral resection of prostate

LET'S TRY ONE 14.6

A 67-year-old male who had a TURP approximately 4 months ago returned with symptoms of obstruction. The surgeon performed a second transurethral resection and removed this residual tissue. What is the appropriate code for this procedure? _____

Urethra (Codes 53000-53899)

The codes in the Urethra section are categorized under Incision, Excision, Repair, Manipulation, and Other Procedures. Codes in the Incision category include drainage and meatotomy (a procedure to enlarge the urethral or ureteral opening). Codes in the Excision category include biopsy, excision of urethral polyps and carcinoma, urethrectomy, and excision of structures. The Repair codes include reconstruction and wound suturing. Note the codebook parenthetic guideline at the beginning of this category that codes for hypospadias repair (moving the urethra) are in the Male Genital System Surgery subsection. Manipulation procedures include dilation of stricture. The transurethral destruction of prostate tissue by thermotherapy is in Other Procedures. Some of the more common urethral surgical procedures will be discussed in this chapter.

Repair

Urethroplasy is the repair of a defect in the urethra, often performed on a patient with urethral stricture due to scarring. Urethroplasty is also performed to repair trauma or correct a prolapse. A **Johannsen type urethroplasty** is a complex procedure that is performed in 2 stages during 2 different operative episodes several months apart, and each stage is reported with unique codes:

- In the first stage (code 53400), the surgeon opens the area over the stricture and removes tissue. The damaged area of the urethra is left open with a diversion created from a strip of normal skin that covers the area of repair. A catheter is inserted, and the area is temporarily closed. The site takes at least 8 weeks to heal before the second stage is performed.
- In the second stage (code 53405), the surgeon closes the lateral skin edges, creating a new urethra, and permanently closes the site.

A 1-stage reconstruction of the male urethra is reported with code 53410 (anterior urethra) or 53415 (prostatic or membranous urethra). In a single-stage procedure, the stricture is removed and an end-to-end anastomosis is performed. Female urethroplasty with reconstruction is reported with code 53530.

Figure 14.14 shows codes for reporting suture repair of the urethra: 53502 is specific to female patients, and 53505 to male patients; 53510 is reported for male or female patients if the wound or injury is in the perineum; and 53515 is reported if the repair involves the prostate.

Figure 14.14 Codes for Female and Male Urethrorrhaphy

53502	Urethrorrhaphy, suture of urethral wound or injury, female
53505	Urethrorrhaphy, suture of urethral wound or injury; penile
53510	perineal
53515	prostatomembranous

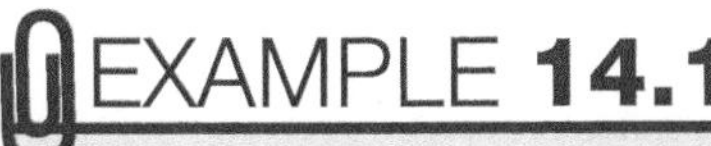

EXAMPLE **14.1**

A 72-year-old male patient underwent **urethrography** (x-ray imaging of the urethra), which showed a stricture approximately 1.5 cm in length. The patient was taken to surgery where the surgeon performed a 1-stage urethroplasty of the anterior urethra. This procedure would be reported with code 53410, *Urethroplasty, 1-stage reconstruction of male anterior urethra*.

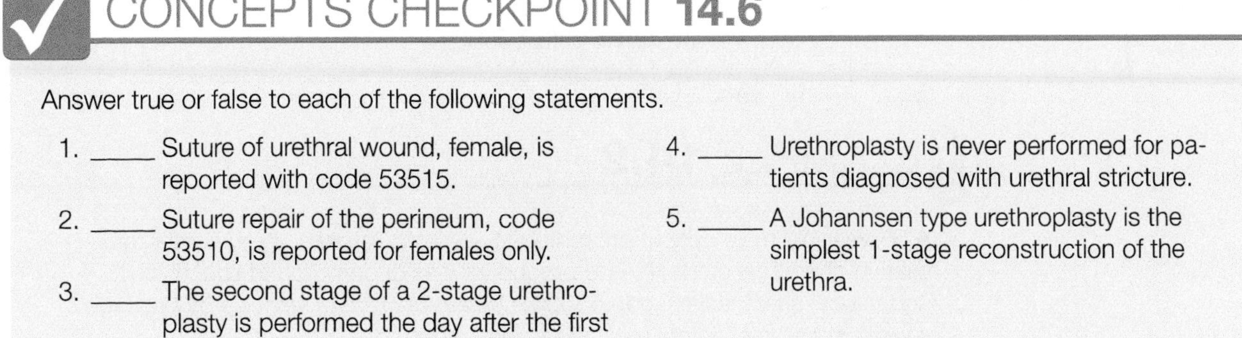

CONCEPTS CHECKPOINT **14.6**

Answer true or false to each of the following statements.

1. _____ Suture of urethral wound, female, is reported with code 53515.
2. _____ Suture repair of the perineum, code 53510, is reported for females only.
3. _____ The second stage of a 2-stage urethroplasty is performed the day after the first stage.
4. _____ Urethroplasty is never performed for patients diagnosed with urethral stricture.
5. _____ A Johannsen type urethroplasty is the simplest 1-stage reconstruction of the urethra.

Manipulation/Dilation

Codes in the Manipulation category (53600 through 53665) describe dilation of urethral stricture and are shown in Figure 14.15. Three criteria differentiate these codes:

- whether the patient is male or female;
- whether the dilation is an initial or a subsequent procedure; and
- the type of anesthesia provided.

Note that for the criterion of type of anesthesia, procedures performed under local anesthesia are reported with codes 53600, 53601, 53620, and 53621 for male patients and 53660 and 53661 for female patients. Procedures performed under general or conduction (spinal) anesthesia are reported with code 53605 for male patients and 53665 for female patients.

Figure 14.15 Codes for Dilation of Urethra

53600	Dilation of urethral stricture by passage of sound or urethral dilator, male; initial
53601	subsequent
53605	Dilation of urethral stricture or vesical neck by passage of sound or urethral dilator, male, general or conduction (spinal) anesthesia
	(For dilation of urethral stricture, male, performed under local anesthesia, see 53600, 53601, 53620, 53621)
53620	Dilation of urethral stricture by passage of filiform and follower, male; initial
53621	subsequent
53660	Dilation of female urethra including suppository and/or instillation; initial
53661	subsequent
53665	Dilation of female urethra, general or conduction (spinal) anesthesia
	(For urethral catheterization, see 51701-51703)
	(For dilation of urethra performed under local anesthesia, female, see 53660, 53661)

EXAMPLE **14.2**

A 55-year-old male patient presented to the ambulatory surgery center for dilation of urethral stricture. The procedure was accomplished successfully under local anesthesia. Code 53600, *Dilation of urethral stricture by passage of sound or urethral dilator, male; initial,* was reported.

Two weeks later, his symptoms reappeared and another dilation was scheduled. Urethral dilation was again performed under local anesthesia. Code 53601, *Dilation of urethral stricture by passage of sound or urethral dilator, male; subsequent,* was reported.

LET'S TRY ONE **14.7**

A 58-year-old female patient with a recently diagnosed urethral stricture presented to the clinic for a repeat of urethral dilation. This procedure was performed under local anesthesia without complications. What is the appropriate code for this procedure? _____

Chapter Summary

- Nephrectomy codes are differentiated by the technique (open or laparoscopic), the extent (partial or total) of removal of the kidney, and by donor nephrectomy.
- Allogenic renal transplants involve 3 components: harvesting of the kidney, backbench work (kidney preparation), and transplantation. Each component is reported separately.
- Renal allotransplantation and autotransplantation have separate codes.
- Ureterolithotomy codes are differentiated by the location of the calculus in the ureter.
- Urodynamic codes describe procedures that measure how well the bladder is holding and emptying urine.
- Multiple urodynamic codes may be applied for the same investigative session.
- Transurethral procedure codes are differentiated by the anatomical site and specific procedure performed.
- Transurethral resection of the prostate (TURP) code assignment is dependent on whether it is an initial resection or resection of a residual or regrowth of tissue.
- Destruction of prostate tissue can be accomplished by laser coagulation, vaporization, or enucleation.
- Urethroplasty can be performed in 1 or 2 stages.
- Codes for repair of urethral wounds are based on whether the patient is male or female.
- Codes for dilatation of urethral stricture have 3 criteria: gender of the patient, whether the dilation is initial or subsequent, and the type of anesthesia given.

Navigator

Access interactive chapter review exercises, practice activities, flash cards, and study games.

Chapter 15

Surgery Coding: Male and Female Genital Systems, Reproductive System Procedures, Intersex Surgery, Maternity Care and Delivery, and Endocrine System

Fast Facts

- Until the early 18th century, physicians held a "one-sex" reproductive model and thought that while there were obvious physical differences between males and females, the reproductive organs were homologous counterparts to one another.
- Inside the womb, a baby's body is covered in a thin layer of hair that disappears shortly after birth. This hair, called *lanugo*, may persist for weeks.
- The reproductive system contains the largest human cells (a female's ovum, at 120 micrometers in diameter) and the smallest human cells (a male's sperm, at 5 micrometers by 3 micrometers).
- The adrenal glands change size as you age. They begin around the size of the kidneys, and by old age they have shrunk so small they can barely be seen.
- Alcohol affects the endocrine system by raising blood sugar levels, interfering with certain hormones, reducing testosterone levels, and increasing the risk of osteoporosis by interfering with the calcium-regulating parathyroid hormone.

Sources: http://livescience.com, http://babycenter.com

Crack the Code

Review the sample operative report to find the correct female genital system code. You may need to return to this exercise after reading the chapter content.

DATE OF PROCEDURE: 02/11/2019

PROCEDURE PERFORMED: Laparoscopy with lysis of adhesions and right ovarian cystectomy

SURGEON: Alexander Burnett, MD

ANESTHESIA: General endotracheal anesthesia

DESCRIPTION OF PROCEDURE: Using the 3 port sites, hook, and Metzenbaum scissors with or without electrocautery, depending on adhesion, the adhesions were all taken down. Bowel was fully mobilized away from adnexa, and adnexa mobilized from pelvis sidewall. Right ovarian cystectomy was performed by incising tunica of ovary sharply, and then extending that bluntly, and shelling cyst the majority of the way out. There was a cyst rupture near end of dissection, and cyst wall was removed and sent to pathology.

answer: 58662-RT

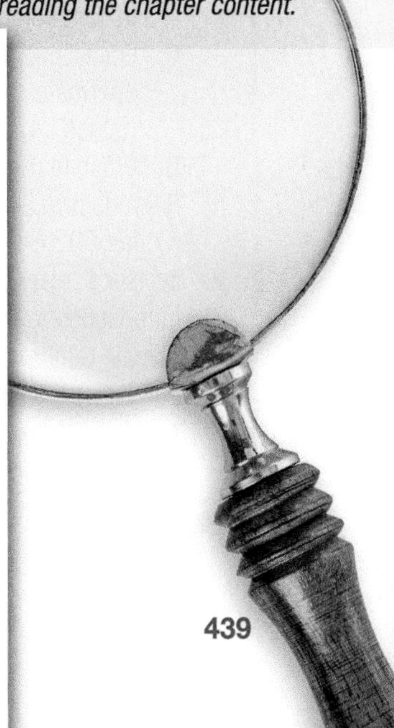

Learning Objectives

15.1 Identify the anatomical structures of the male genital system.

15.2 Describe the organization of the Male Genital System Surgery subsection of the CPT® codebook.

15.3 Apply codebook instructional notes when coding procedures of the male and female genital systems.

15.4 Report codes for procedures of the male genital system, including those of the penis, vas deferens, and prostate.

15.5 Describe the significance of the Reproductive System Procedures subsection of the CPT® codebook.

15.6 Explain the Intersex Surgery subsection of the CPT® codebook.

15.7 Identify the anatomical structures of the female genital system.

15.8 Describe the organization of the Female Genital System Surgery subsection of the CPT® codebook.

15.9 Report codes for procedures of the female genital system, including those of the uterus and ovaries.

15.10 Report appropriate modifiers when coding procedures of the male and female genital systems.

15.11 Identify the services included in maternity care and delivery codes.

15.12 Apply codebook instructional notes when coding maternity care and delivery procedures.

15.13 Report codes for procedures related to maternity care and delivery.

15.14 Identify the anatomical structures of the endocrine system.

15.15 Describe the organization of the Endocrine System Surgery subsection of the CPT® codebook.

15.16 Report codes for procedures related to the endocrine system, including those of the thyroid gland.

Chapter Outline

Introduction to the Male Genital System

3-D
To explore the male genital system in the BioDigital Human, go to: http://Coding.ParadigmEducation.com/BioDigital_MaleGenital.

The male genital (reproductive) system includes the external genitalia (the penis and scrotum) and the internal structures contained within them. The prostate gland is also a part of the male reproductive system, although there are surgical prostate procedures located in the Urinary System Surgery subsection because of the prostate's proximity to the urethra. The function of the male reproductive system is to produce and transport sperm and to secrete the hormone testosterone.

Male Genital System Terminology

Familiarity with the anatomy of the male genital system and its terminology will enable you to more easily report the proper codes for procedures described in this subsection of the codebook. Figure 15.1 illustrates the components of the male genital system, and Table 15.1 provides more information about each structure as well as common conditions.

Figure 15.1 Structures of the Male Genital System

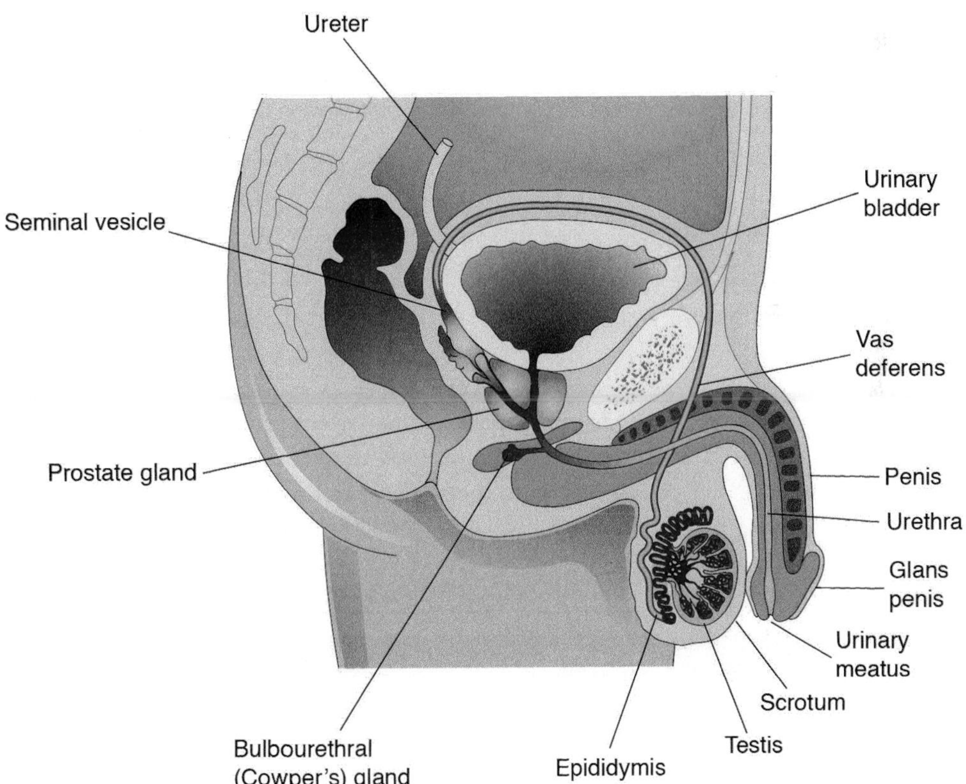

Table 15.1 Male Genital System Terms

Structure/Condition	Definition
corpus (pl., corpora) cavernosa	A column of tissue along the length of the penis that expands with blood during penile erection
epididymis	Tubes where sperm are stored
prepuce	Fold of skin covering the tip of the penis; also called the *foreskin*
hydrocele	A collection of serous fluid
penis	External part of urinary and reproductive system that serves as passageway for urine and semen
Peyronie disease	A disorder of the penis causing penile bending and pain on erection
prostate	Gland that surrounds the base of the urethra
scrotum	Pouch of skin that holds testes
seminal vesicles	Glands that produce fluid to mix with semen
spermatic cord	Cord that suspends the testes in the scrotum; contains the vas deferens, vessels, and nerves
testis	Male reproductive organ that produces sperm and testosterone
tunica vaginalis	Serous membrane that surrounds testes
vas deferens	Tube that transports sperm

CONCEPTS CHECKPOINT **15.1**

Match the structure in the first column with the description in the second column.

1. _____ vas deferens
2. _____ testis
3. _____ seminal vesicles
4. _____ epididymis
5. _____ prostate

a. Gland that surrounds the base of the urethra
b. Tubes where sperm is stored
c. Tube that transports sperm
d. Male organ that produces sperm
e. Glands that produce fluid to mix with semen

The names of male genital system procedures are much easier to understand when you know the word roots used to refer to the male genital organs. Table 15.2 lists the more common word roots related to the male genital system, their meanings, and examples of usages.

Table 15.2 Word Roots for the Male Genital System

Word root	Meaning	Example
balan/o	Glans penis (enlarged tip at end of penis)	Balanoplasty, repair of glans penis
epididym/o	Epididymis (coiled tube on top of testis)	Epididymitis, inflammation of epididymis
orchi/o, orchid/o, orch/o	Testis, testicle	Orchidopexy, surgical fixation of testis
test/o	Testis, testicle	Testicular cancer, cancer of the testis
prostat/o	Prostate gland	Prostatectomy, excision of prostate
vas/o	Vessel, duct	Vasectomy, excision of vas deferens Vasovasostomy, connection of vas to vas
vesicul/o	Seminal vesicle (glands that secrete fluid)	Vesiculectomy, excision of seminal vesicle

The Male Genital System Surgery Subsection

The headings in the Male Genital System Surgery subsection are organized by anatomical site. Each heading is further categorized by type of procedure, such as incision, excision, introduction, repair, manipulation, suture, and laparoscopy. Note that transurethral procedures related to the prostate appear in the Urinary System Surgery subsection (see Chapter 14). Table 15.3 provides a listing of the headings and corresponding code ranges within the Male Genital System Surgery subsection.

Table 15.3 Headings Within the Male Genital System Surgery Subsection of the CPT® Codebook

Heading	Code Range
Penis	54000-54450
Testis	54500-54699
Epididymis	54700-54901
Tunica Vaginalis	55000-55060
Scrotum	55100-55180
Vas Deferens	55200-55400
Spermatic Cord	55500-55559
Seminal Vesicles	55600-55680
Prostate	55700-55899

Penis (Codes 54000-54450)

The **penis** is the external part of the male urinary and reproductive systems that serves as a passageway for urine and semen. Within the Penis anatomical heading are several categories of codes. Incision procedures involve loosening the prepuce and draining abscesses or other conditions deeper than those in the skin and subcutaneous layers are reported with codes from the Integumentary System Surgery subsection. Destruction codes describe various methods of lesion removal specific to the penis. The Excision category contains codes for biopsy, excision of plaque, foreign body removal, amputation, circumcision, and frenulotomy. The Introduction codes include procedures for injection, irrigation, and various tests of penile function. Repair codes describe surgical treatments for chordee, hypospadias, angulation, epispadias, incontinence, priapism, and injury. Penile prosthetic procedures are also included. A final Manipulation code addresses treatment of foreskin adhesions.

Circumcision

One of the more common procedures performed on the penis is **circumcision**, which is the removal of the **foreskin**, a fold of skin covering the tip of the penis. The physician can remove the foreskin by different means. One procedure is clamping it with a plastic bell-shaped device (often the brand name Plastibell) while the patient is under regional dorsal penile block anesthesia or ring block anesthesia. Both dorsal penile block and ring block are types of local anesthesia: dorsal penile block involves injecting anesthetic agents into the dorsal penile nerves, while the term *ring block* is used when the anesthetic agent is circumferentially injected (in a ring around the penis). Circumcision can also be performed by a method other than clamp, device, or dorsal slit, as shown in Figure 15.2.

Figure 15.2 Steps in Circumcision

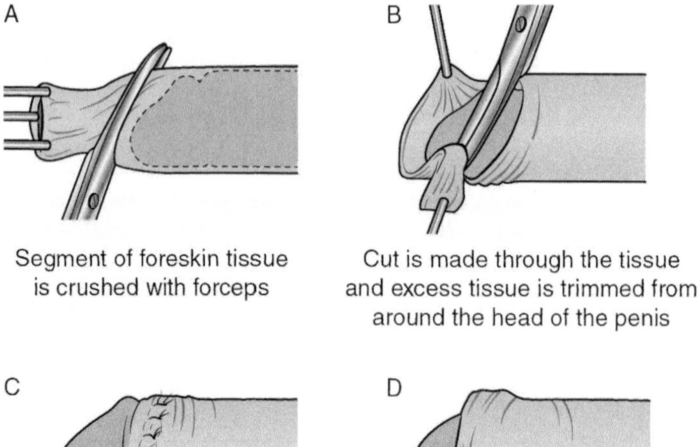
A
B
Segment of foreskin tissue is crushed with forceps
Cut is made through the tissue and excess tissue is trimmed from around the head of the penis

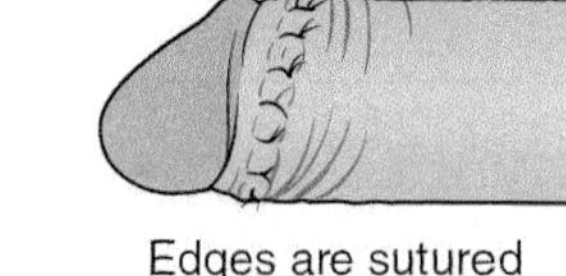
C

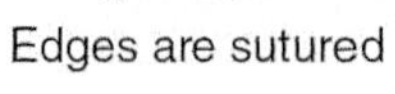
Edges are sutured

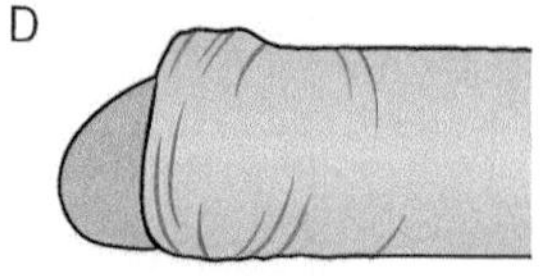
D

Final result after circumcision

Inside the OR

To perform a circumcision using a surgical excision method other than a clamp, device, or dorsal slit, the surgeon begins by using forceps to crush a segment of the foreskin (as shown in step A of Figure 15.2). The surgeon then makes an incision through this crushed tissue, dividing the foreskin (B). The surgeon then pulls the divided foreskin down and over the head of the penis and trims away the excess skin. Bleeding is controlled, and the new skin edges (where the foreskin was removed) are closed with absorbable sutures (C).

Circumcision is reported using codes 54150 through 54161, depending on technique used and age of the patient (neonate to 28 days or older). Report code 54150 when a device is used with anesthetic block. Modifier 52, *Reduced services,* is applied if the circumcision is performed without anesthesia. Report code 51460 for a circumcision performed on a neonate without a device. Modifier 63, *Procedures performed on infants less than 4 kg,* should not be applied to code 54160. A circumcision on a patient over 28 days is reported with code 54161 if done by a method other than clamp, device, or dorsal slit.

LET'S TRY ONE **15.1**

An 8-day-old male was brought to the clinic for circumcision. The circumcision was performed under local block anesthesia using a Plastibell device. The baby tolerated the procedure well. The penis was covered in petroleum jelly and wrapped in gauze. What is the appropriate code for this procedure? _____

Coding for CMS

Over the past decade, Medicaid funding for newborn circumcision has been discontinued in 18 states: Arizona, California, Colorado, Florida, Idaho, Louisiana, Maine, Minnesota, Mississippi, Missouri, Montana, Nevada, North Carolina, North Dakota, Oregon, South Carolina, Utah, and Washington. This change is due in part to declining circumcision rates as parents and pediatricians debate the medical necessity of circumcision and weigh the risks and benefits of the procedure.

Chordee and Hypospadias Repairs

Chordee is a congenital condition in which the penis curves downward. Chordee is often associated with **hypospadias**, another congenital condition in which the opening of the urethra is on the underside of the penis instead of at the tip. These conditions require surgical correction (urethroplasty), which can be performed at any age. Urethroplasty to correct chordee and hypospadias involves 4 tasks: straightening the shaft of the penis, creating the urinary channel, positioning the urinary meatus (opening) at the tip, and circumcising or reconstructing the foreskin. Urethroplasty may be done in stages, often with the straightening of the penis done in the first stage and the urethroplasty and reconstruction of the urinary channel in a separate surgery. A 1-stage repair would complete the urethroplasty during 1 surgical episode. The codes for urethroplasty for chordee and hypospadias repair (54300 through 54352) are assigned based on the stage, technique, and extent of the surgery required to correct the defect, as shown in Figure 15.3. Urethroplasty conducted for reasons other than to correct hypospadias or chordee are reported with urinary system codes 53400 through 53430, as noted under the Repair category in the codebook and discussed in Chapter 14.

Figure 15.3 Example of 1-Stage Hypospadias Repair Codes

54322	1-stage distal hypospadias repair (with or without chordee or circumcision); with simple meatal advancement (eg, Magpi, V-flap)
54324	with urethroplasty by local skin flaps (eg, flip-flap, prepucial flap)
54326	with urethroplasty by local skin flaps and mobilization of urethra
54328	with extensive dissection to correct chordee and urethroplasty with skin flaps, skin graft patch, and/or island flap

EXAMPLE 15.1

A 1-stage repair was performed on a 10-month-old boy with chordee and distal hypospadias. The chordee was corrected by excision of the fibrous band, and the hypospadias repair was completed by mobilizing the urethra and using a flap of skin from the foreskin for urethroplasty. This 1-stage procedure should be reported using code 54326, *1-stage distal hypospadias repair (with or without chordee or circumcision); with urethroplasty by local skin flaps and mobilization of urethra.*

LET'S TRY ONE 15.2

The first stage of a planned 2-stage hypospadias repair is completed on an 8-month-old infant. What is the appropriate code for this procedure? _____

Testis (Codes 54500-54699)

The term **testis** refers to each of the paired male reproductive organs that produce sperm and testosterone. Together, the organs are called **testes** or **testicles**. Note that the word roots *test/o*, *orchi/o*, and *orchid/o* may be used in the names of procedures related to the testes (eg, *testicular* prosthesis, *orchiectomy*, or *orchidotomy*).

Testis codes are grouped by several categories. The Excision codes include biopsy, lesion removal, and orchiectomy. Exploration codes describe procedures for undescended testicles. Repair codes describe surgical treatments for injury, testis torsion, contralateral testis, orchiopexy, insertion of a testicular prosthesis, and transplantation. The Laparoscopy category has endoscopic orchiectomy and orchiopexy procedure codes.

Orchiectomy

An **orchiectomy** is the surgical removal of a testis. An orchiectomy is often performed as a prophylactic measure for patients with prostate cancer to stop the production of testosterone, which can also arrest the growth of the tumor. An open orchiectomy is reported with codes 54520 through 54535, depending on the extent of the removal and the approach. A simple orchiectomy removes only the testis, while a radical orchiectomy removes en bloc the contents of half the scrotum. Code 54690 is reported for a laparoscopic orchiectomy. Orchiectomy codes are unilateral (involving 1 side); therefore, bilateral (two-sided) orchiectomies require the use of modifier 50, *Bilateral procedure*.

EXAMPLE 15.2

A 51-year-old male with adenocarcinoma of the prostate was scheduled for bilateral orchiectomies. A simple orchiectomy was performed through an incision in the scrotum. This is reported with code 54520 - 50, *Orchiectomy, simple (including subcapsular) with or without testicular prosthesis, scrotal or inguinal approach, bilateral procedure.*

LET'S TRY ONE **15.3**

A 49-year-old male with prostate cancer undergoes bilateral laparoscopic orchiectomies. What is the appropriate code for this procedure? _____

Orchiopexy

Orchiopexy, also known as **orchidopexy**, is the surgical fixation of the testis. This procedure is performed on patients with **cryptorchidism**, or undescended testicle(s). The undescended testis may be located in the scrotal, inguinal, or abdominal area, as shown in Figure 15.4. In an orchiopexy, the surgeon locates a testicle that has not descended into the scrotum and brings it down into the correct place within the scrotum. A patient suffering from cryptorchidism often also has an inguinal hernia, which may be repaired at the time of the orchiopexy, using a separate incision. If this happens, the hernia repair is reported separately with codes 49495 through 49525. Codes for orchiopexy are differentiated by the approach (the location from which the testis is moved) and whether the surgery was open or laparoscopic. Open orchiopexies are reported with codes from the Repair category: an orchiopexy performed by an inguinal approach is reported with code 54640, while an abdominal approach for an intra-abdominal testis is reported with code 54650. A laparoscopic orchiopexy for an intra-abdominal testis is reported with code 54692 from the Laparoscopy category. Orchipexy codes are assumed to be unilateral and require the use of modifier 50, *Bilateral procedure*, for bilateral procedures.

Figure 15.4 Illustration of Different Locations of Cryptorchidism

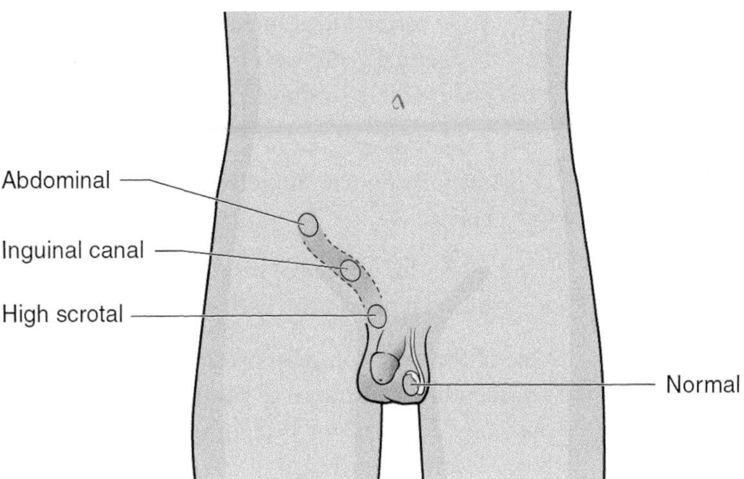

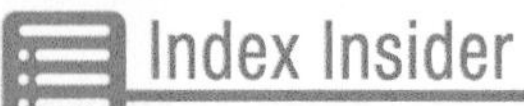

Index Insider

The CPT® codebook Index has main entries for both Orchiectomy and Orchiopexy.

EXAMPLE 15.3

A 9-month-old infant with undescended testicles underwent bilateral orchiopexies using an inguinal approach. This procedure is reported with code 54640 - 50, *Orchiopexy, inguinal approach, with or without hernia repair - bilateral procedure.*

LET'S TRY ONE 15.4

A 6-month-old infant with right cryptorchidism was brought in for an orchiopexy. The surgeon performed a laparoscopic orchiopexy, moving the testis from its previous intra-abdominal location into the scrotum. What is the appropriate code for this procedure? _____

Epididymis, Tunica Vaginalis, Scrotum, Vas Deferens, Spermatic Cord, and Seminal Vesicles (Codes 54700-55680)

The smaller genital structures of the epididymis, tunica vaginalis, scrotum, vas deferens, spermatic cord, and seminal vesicles each have limited codes in 6 categories. Incision codes describe drainage procedures for abscess, hematoma, and hydrocele conditions, as well as removal of a foreign body and cannulization. Excision codes cover procedures such as biopsy, lesion removal, and resections. The epididymis has an Exploration code. There is an Introduction code that covers various tests on the vas deferens. Repair and Suture categories include anastomosis, suturing, and hydrocele repair. Watch for instructional notes within the categories that provide helpful reminders:

- Refer to the Integumentary System Surgery subsection when coding debridement of external genitalia for necrotizing soft tissue infection, which is reported using codes 11004 through 11006.
- Codes for excision of skin lesions on the scrotum are also located in the Integumentary System Surgery subsection (see Chapter 9 for a discussion of these codes).
- Codes for vas deferens procedures assume the procedure is unilateral; report bilateral procedures with modifier 50, *Bilateral procedure*.

One of the most common procedures performed on the male reproductive system is a **vasectomy**, or removal of vas deferens, which is also known as the *male sterilization procedure*. A vasectomy is reported with code 55250, *Vasectomy, unilateral or bilateral.* Since *bilateral* is included in the description of code 55250, modifier 50, *Bilateral procedure*, cannot be applied to it. A **vasovasostomy**, or reversal of a vasectomy, involves anastomosing (reconnecting) the ends of the vas deferens so sperm can once again pass through. The code for vasovasostomy, code 55400, *Vasovasostomy, vasovasorrhapy*, is for a unilateral procedure. If bilateral vasovasostomies are performed, modifier 50, *Bilateral procedure*, should be applied.

CONCEPTS CHECKPOINT 15.2

Answer true or false to each of the following statements.

1. _____ Excision of a skin lesion of the scrotum should be reported with code 55150.
2. _____ When coding bilateral vasectomies, modifier 50 should be applied.
3. _____ When coding bilateral vasovasostomies, modifier 50 should be applied.

Prostate (Codes 55700-55899)

RED FLAG

Codes for transurethral removal or destruction of the prostate are found in the Urinary System Surgery subsection (under code ranges 52601 through 52640 and 53850 through 53852, respectively) rather than within the Male Genital System Surgery subsection.

The **prostate** is the gland that surrounds the base of the urethra. The prostate gland contains ducts that empty into the prostatic part of the urethra. The prostate secretes a fluid that mixes with semen when a male ejaculates.

Four categories organize the codes under the Prostate heading. The Incision codes cover biopsy and drainage procedures. The Excision category describes open **prostatectomy** (removal of prostate), and the Laparoscopy category describes laparoscopic prostatectomy. The category Other Procedures contains codes for electroejaculation, placement of therapeutic devices, and cryosurgical ablation of prostate tissue.

Like many other codes for surgical procedures, codes for prostatectomy are assigned based on the approach (perineal, suprapubic, or retropubic) and the extent of tissue removed. The range of codes relating to the extent of tissue removed in a prostatectomy with a perineal approach is shown in Figure 15.5.

Figure 15.5 Example of Prostatectomy Codes

55810	Prostatectomy, perineal radical;
55812	with lymph node biopsy(s) (limited pelvic lymphadenectomy)
55815	with bilateral pelvic lymphadenectomy, including external iliac, hypogastric and obturator nodes

Coding Clicks

For more information on the da Vinci Surgical System, visit http://Coding.ParadigmEducation.com/daVinci. This website contains clinical evidence, links to articles, information for patients, and videos of the system in action.

A subtotal prostatectomy is the removal of part or all of the prostate gland while preserving the seminal vesicles. A radical prostatectomy includes the removal of the entire prostate gland, the seminal vesicles, and the vas deferens. Laparoscopic radical prostatectomy is reported with code 55866, which includes the use of "robotic assistance." An example of such assistance is the **da Vinci surgical system**, a computer system that allows a surgeon to use external controls to manipulate miniaturized instruments placed inside the patient while viewing a highly magnified 3-D image of the surgical site. The da Vinci surgical system can be used for many types of surgeries.

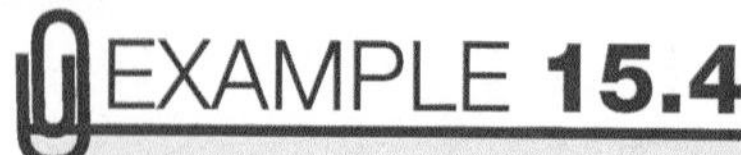

EXAMPLE 15.4

A 52-year-old male who was recently diagnosed with prostate adenocarcinoma was scheduled for a radical prostatectomy. He was taken to surgery, where the surgeon performed a retropubic prostatectomy. The pelvic lymph nodes were inspected and appeared to be free of tumors. Since no lymph nodes were biopsied or removed, this surgery is reported with code 55840, *Prostatectomy, retropubic radical, with or without nerve sparing.*

LET'S TRY ONE 15.5

A 61-year-old male with prostate cancer had a laparoscopic retropubic radical prostatectomy. What is the appropriate code for this procedure? _____

Reproductive System Procedures Surgery Subsection (Code 55920)

The single code found under the reproductive system procedures heading is 55920, reported for placement of needles or catheters. Code 55920 describes the placement of needles or catheters into pelvic organs or genitalia, excluding the prostate, for application of interstitial radioelements. The catheter or needle is used to place seeds (tiny glass, gold, or platinum capsules) containing radioactive isotopes, such as iodine-125 or palladium-103. The seeds are left in place to deliver radiation therapy over a period of several months. This method allows radiation delivery to the specific body area while normal tissue has minimal exposure. Code 55920 is for placement of the catheters only; placement of the radioactive isotopes are coded with brachytherapy codes from the Radiology section.

Intersex Surgery Subsection (Codes 55970 and 55980)

Intersex surgery, also known as **sex reassignment surgery**, is an operation to change genitalia from male to female or female to male. Intersex surgery may be indicated for transgender patients and those patients born with ambiguous genitalia. Intersex surgery is performed in a series of complicated staged procedures: code 55970 is reported for male-to-female intersex surgery, and code 55980 is reported for female-to-male intersex surgery. Two related procedures are also found among the Female Genital System codes: code 56805 for a clitoroplasty (in the Vulva, Perineum, and Introitus category) and code 57335 for a vaginoplasty (in the Vagina category).

Coding for CMS

CMS recently changed its benefit policies to include sex reassignment surgery for transgender people. Prior to 2014, CMS considered intersex surgery to be experimental. Coverage decisions are now based on the beneficiary's medical need, similar to other services covered by Medicare.

Introduction to the Female Genital System

The female genital (reproductive) system is made up of both internal organs (vagina, uterus, and ovaries) and external organs (vulva). The **ovaries** are responsible for producing the hormones estrogen and progesterone that support female health as well as for storing and developing **oocytes**, female reproductive cells. The **oviducts**, or **fallopian tubes**, serve as a passageway for the mature oocytes or ova to move from the ovary to the uterus. The **uterus** is an organ involved with the functions of menstruation, pregnancy, and labor.

Female Genital System Terminology

Familiarity with the anatomy of the female genital system and terminology pertaining to it will enable you to more easily report codes for procedures. Figure 15.6 illustrates the components of the female genital system, and Table 15.4 provides more information about each structure.

3-D
To explore the female genital system in the BioDigital Human, go to: http://Coding.ParadigmEducation.com/BioDigital_FemaleGenital.

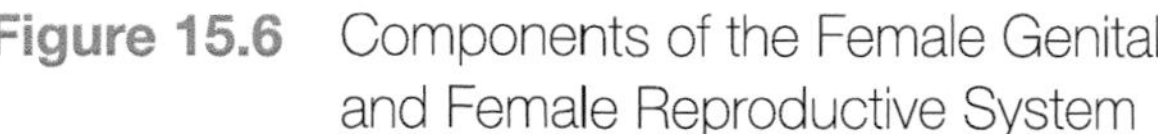

Figure 15.6 Components of the Female Genital and Female Reproductive System

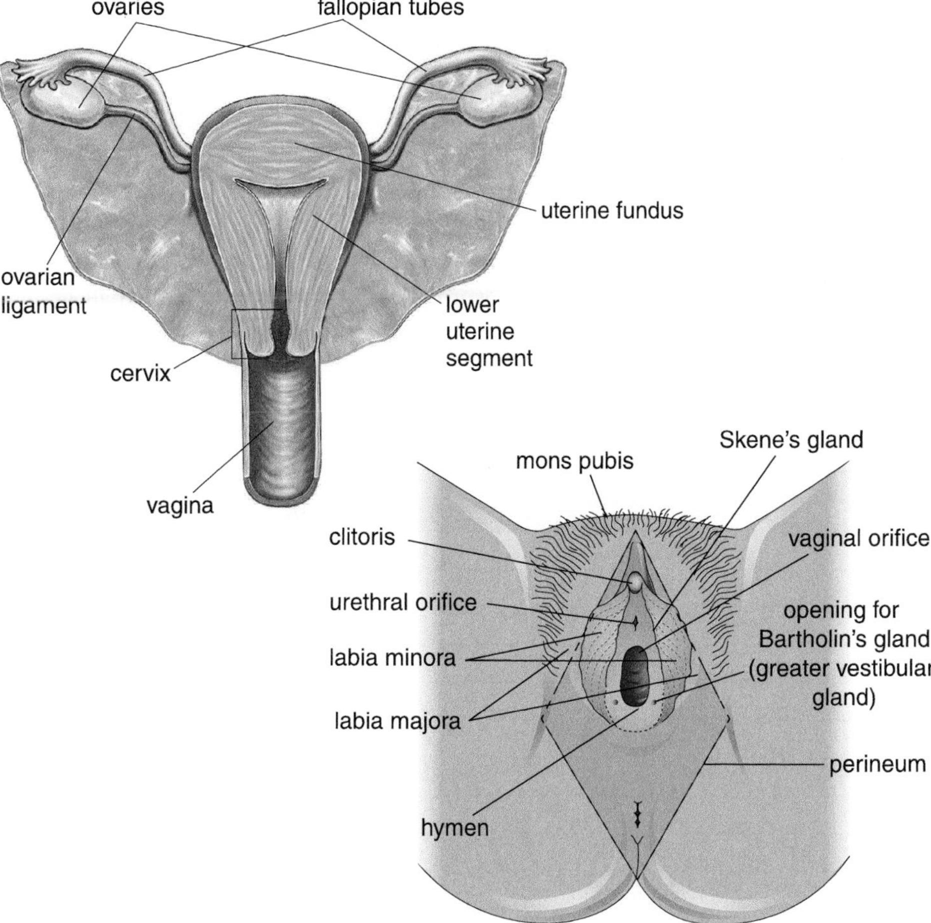

Table 15.4 Female Genital System Anatomical and Surgical Terms

Structure	Definition
anastomosis	Surgical connection between 2 normally distinct structures
Bartholin's glands	Pair of mucus-producing glands located on each side above the vaginal opening
cervix uteri	Narrow lower portion of uterus
clitoris	Highly erogenous erectile body located anterior to the urethra
conization	Excision of a cone of tissue
corpus uteri	Body of the uterus, large central portion
curettage	A scraping of the interior of a cavity
embryo	Unborn offspring in the stage of development from implantation of the zygote to the second month of pregnancy
fimbrioplasty	Repair of ovarian fimbria
gamete	A mature sex cell, sperm, or ovum
hymen	Fold of membrane found near the opening of the vagina
introitus	Entrance to the vagina
labium (pl., labia)	Fold at the margin of the vulva
marsupialization	Surgical alteration of a cyst or similar enclosed cavity by making an incision and suturing the flaps to the adjacent tissue, creating a pouch
oocyte	An immature female reproductive cell prior to maturation into an ovum capable of fertilization by sperm
oviduct	Fallopian tube, or uterine tube, that allows ova (female reproductive cells) to move from ovary to uterus
ovary	Pair of organs where oocytes are stored and developed
Pereyra procedure	A surgical technique for the correction of stress incontinence
perineum	Pelvic floor between the vaginal opening and anus
vagina	Tube that connects the uterus to the outside of the body
vulva	External genitalia that surrounds the vagina
zygote	Cell formed by the union of the sperm and the ovum

The names of female genital system procedures are much easier to understand when you know the word roots used to refer to the female genital organs. Table 15.5 gives the more common word roots related to the female genital system, their definitions, and examples of usages.

Table 15.5 Female Genital System Word Roots and Definitions

Word Root	Definition	Example
colp/o	Vagina	Colposcopy, viewing of the vagina
cervic/o	Cervix	Cervicectomy, excision of the cervix uteri
episi/o	Vulva	Episiotomy, incision into vulva
hymen/o	Hymen	Hymenectomy, excision of the hymen
hyster/o, metr/o	Uterus	Hysterectomy, removal of uterus
oophor/o	Ovary	Oophorectomy, removal of ovary
perine/o	Perineum	Perineoplasty, repair of the perineum
salping/o	Oviduct, fallopian tube	Salpingectomy, removal of oviduct
trachel/o	Neck	Trachelorrhaphy, repair by suture of the cervix uteri
vagin/o	Vagina	Vaginectomy, removal of vaginal wall
vulv/o	Vulva	Vulvectomy, removal of the vulva

CONCEPTS CHECKPOINT **15.3**

Match the term or word root in the first column to the definition in the second column.

1. _____ *perineum*
2. _____ *episi/o*
3. _____ *hyster/o*
4. _____ *oviduct*
5. _____ *oophor/o*

a. ovary
b. uterus
c. pelvic floor
d. vulva
e. fallopian tube

The Female Genital System Surgery Subsection

Table 15.6 Headings Within the Female Genital System Subsection of the CPT® Codebook

Heading	Code Range
Vulva, Perineum, and Introitus	56405-56821
Vagina	57000-57426
Cervix Uteri	57452-57800
Corpus Uteri	58100-58579
Oviduct /Ovary	58600-58770
Ovary	58800-58960
In Vitro Fertilization	58970-58999

The headings in the Female Genital System Surgery subsection are organized by anatomical site. Table 15.6 lists the headings and corresponding code numbers.

Each heading is further categorized by type of procedure, such as Incision, Excision, Introduction, Repair, Destruction, Manipulation, Endoscopy, and Laparoscopy. While not all the female genital system procedures will be explained in detail in this chapter, some of the more common and challenging codes you may be required to report are discussed in the upcoming sections.

Vulva, Perineum, and Introitus (Codes 56405-56821)

The **vulva** is the external genitalia that surrounds the vagina, the **perineum** is the area of the pelvic floor between the vaginal opening and anus, and the **introitus** is the entrance to the vagina. The Incision category contains procedures for treating abscesses, cysts, and adhesions. Codes in the Destruction category involve removal of lesions. The Excision codes describe biopsy; excision of the vulva, hymen, or Bartholin's gland; and excision of cysts. The Repair codes cover plastic repair of the introitus, clitoroplasty for intersex state, and nonobstetrical perineoplasty. The Endoscopy category has 2 codes for colposcopy of the vulva.

Other codes for excision of lesions, skin grafts, and repair of wounds on the female genitalia are located in the Integumentary subsection. Patients with malignant or premalignant lesions on the vulva may require a **vulvectomy**, or an excision of the vulva. Vulvectomies are reported with codes 56620 through 56640, depending on the extent of the tissue removed and the extent of lymph node removed.

Instructional notes immediately under the Vulva, Perineum, and Introitus heading provide the following definitions for procedural terms used in vulvectomy codes:

- Simple: describes the removal of skin and superficial subcutaneous tissues of the vulva;
- Radical: describes the removal of skin and deep subcutaneous tissues of the vulva;
- Partial: describes the removal of less than 80% of the vulvar area;
- Complete: describes the removal of greater than 80% of the vulvar area.

EXAMPLE 15.5

A 46-year-old female with carcinoma of the vulva required a simple complete vulvectomy. The surgeon removed the labia majora, labia minora, and clitoris. This procedure is reported with code 56620, *Vulvectomy, simple; complete.*

Vagina (Codes 57000-57426)

The **vagina** is the tube that connects the uterus to the outside of the body. Codes under the Incision category include colpotomy, colpocentesis, and drainage of hematoma. The Destruction category has treatments for vaginal lesions. The Excision category has procedures for biopsy, vaginectomy, colpocleisis, and excisions of septum, cysts, and tumors. Introduction codes cover vaginal irrigation and insertions of devices for therapeutic radiation treatment, birth-control diaphragms, and packs to control hemorrhage. The Repair category has extensive codes for colporrhaphy that will be discussed in this section, as well as colpopexy, closure of fistulas, graft implantation, sling operation for stress incontinence, and vaginoplasty for the intersex state. Manipulation codes describe vaginal dilation, removal of foreign bodies, and pelvic examination under general anesthesia. The Endoscopy/Laparoscopy category includes colposcopy procedures that will be discussed, as well as colpopexy and revision of vaginal grafts.

Vaginal Repair Codes

Colporrhaphy is repair by suturing. Colporrhaphy codes 57200 and 57210 are assigned for repair of nonobstetrical injuries to the vagina or perineum (as opposed to the obstetrical repairs involved in deliveries). There are a variety of codes for repair of a cystocele, rectocele, and enterocele. A **cystocele** is a herniation of the bladder located against the anterior vaginal wall, causing the wall to bulge. A **rectocele** is a protrusion of the rectum that causes the posterior vaginal wall to bulge. An **enterocele** is a herniation of the small intestine that protrudes into the tissues between the bladder and vagina or the rectum and the vagina. Figure 15.7 gives an example of colporrhaphy codes for herniations and shows the criteria for reporting the procedures. Codes for repairing these conditions are assigned based on the approach: anterior (code 57240), posterior (code 57250), vaginal (codes 52768 and 57285), or abdominal (codes 57270 and 57284); the codes are further differentiated by the type(s) of herniation repaired (cystocele, rectocele, enterocele, or multiple). A combination of approaches and herniations is described by code 57265, *Combined anterioposterior colporrhaphy; with enterocele repair*, which is reported for repair of cystocele, rectocele, and enterocele. Insertion of mesh or other prosthesis is not an included part of the primary colporrhaphy. Code 57267, *Insertion of mesh or other prosthesis for repair of pelvic floor defect, each site*, should be reported in addition to the code for repair and should be reported once for each site requiring insertion of mesh or other implant.

Figure 15.7 Colporrhaphy Codes

57240	Anterior colporrhaphy, repair of cystocele with or without repair of urethrocele, including cystourethroscopy, when performed
57250	Posterior colporrhaphy, repair of rectocele with or without perineorrhaphy

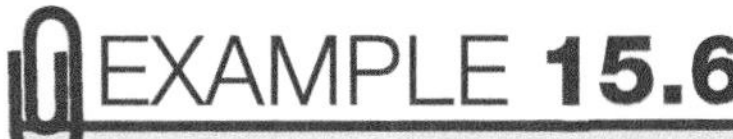

EXAMPLE **15.6**

A 44-year-old female presented for repair of both a cystocele and a rectocele. To repair the cystocele, the surgeon performed an anterior repair using mesh, and to repair the rectocele, he performed a posterior repair using mesh. This procedure is reported with codes 57260, *Combined anteroposterior colporrhaphy*, and 57267, *Insertion of mesh or other prosthesis for repair of pelvic floor defect, each site.* (Code 57267 is reported twice since mesh was used in 2 different sites.)

Vaginal Endoscopy/Laparoscopy Codes

Colposcopies are endoscopies that use a **colposcope**—a binocular lighted microscope—to directly visualize the vagina, cervix, and other structures. Codes 56820 and 56821 are reported for colposcopy of the vulva, codes 57420 and 57421 for colposcopy of the vagina, and codes 57452 through 57461 for colposcopy of the cervix. When multiple sites are examined, multiple codes should be reported. In this case, modifier 51, *Multiple procedures*, should be applied to the secondary procedure code(s) to indicate multiple procedures were performed during the same episode.

EXAMPLE **15.7**

A gynecologist performed a colposcopy with biopsy of the vulva and a colposcopy of the vagina with biopsy of the cervix. Two codes should be reported: code 56821, *Colposcopy of the vulva with biopsy*, and code 57421 -51, *Colposcopy of the entire vagina with biopsy of the vagina/cervix - multiple procedures*. Both colposcopies should be reported since they were performed at different anatomical sites.

CONCEPTS CHECKPOINT **15.4**

Choose the most correct code(s) for the following procedures.

1. Repair of cystocele with anterior colporrhaphy
   a. 57240
   b. 57260
   c. 57200
   d. 57210
2. Repair of rectocele with posterior colporrhaphy and mesh implant
   a. 57250
   b. 57250, 57267
   c. 57260
   d. 57260, 57267
3. Colporrhaphy for injury of vagina
   a. 57000
   b. 57020
   c. 57200
   d. 57210
4. Colposcopy of vagina with biopsy
   a. 57420
   b. 57421
   c. 57425
   d. 57410
5. Colposcopy of the vagina with biopsy of cervix and colposcopy of the vulva
   a. 56820
   b. 57421
   c. 57421, 56820 - 51
   d. 57425, 56820 - 51

Cervix Uteri (Codes 57452-57800)

The **cervix uteri**, also known as the **cervix**, is located at the base of the **corpus uteri**, the body of the uterus. Excision procedures include biopsy, curettage, lesion removal, trachelectomy, and excision of cervical stump. The Repair category of codes covers nonobstetric cerclage (as opposed to obstetric cerclage for pregnancy) and other trachelorrhaphy procedures. A Manipulation code provides for dilation of the cervical canal. The Endoscopy category of codes will be discussed in this section.

Cervical Endoscopy Codes

Colposcopy of the cervix may be required for patients who have abnormal Pap smears. In this case, the procedure usually includes obtaining a sample for biopsy, which may be accomplished in 1 of several ways. In a **loop electrosurgical excision procedure (LEEP)**, a thin wire and an electrical current are used to cut away tissue from the cervix for biopsy. A colposcopy of the cervix with loop electrode biopsy is reported with code 57460. A LEEP **conization**, or cone biopsy, removes a cone-shaped wedge of tissue for biopsy and is reported with code 57461. **Endocervical curettage** is a procedure in which the surgeon uses a narrow spoon-shaped instrument called a **curette** to scrape the lining of the endocervical canal to obtain the specimen. Colposcopy with endocervical curettage is reported with code 57456. Note that codes 57461 and 57456 may not be reported together, as they are both endocervical biopsies. Another way to obtain a cervical specimen is using a cold knife or laser instrument technique. A **cold knife** technique uses a scalpel or other sharp instrument to cut away a tissue specimen. A laser may also be used to cut away a tissue specimen. Biopsy and conization performed by cold knife or laser without using a colposcope are reported with codes 57520 through 57522 in the Excision category.

EXAMPLE **15.8**

A 44-year-old patient with an abnormal Pap smear presented to her gynecologist's office for a LEEP. A colposcopy with LEEP conization of the cervix was performed. This procedure is reported with code 57461, *Colposcopy of the cervix including upper/adjacent vagina; with loop electrode conization of the cervix.*

LET'S TRY ONE **15.6**

A 32-year-old female with a history of cervical carcinoma in situ presented for a cold knife cone cervical biopsy. She was taken to the OR and placed under general anesthesia. The surgeon obtained a cervical cone specimen from the cervical bed using Mayo scissors. What is the appropriate code for this procedure? _____

Corpus Uteri (Codes 58100-58579)

The corpus uteri is the large central portion of the uterus above the cervix and below the openings of the fallopian tubes. The cavity is lined with endometrium, and the functions of the organ are menstruation, pregnancy, and labor. In the CPT® codebook, the procedural codes are organized into 4 categories. The Excision category contains codes on endometrial sampling, dilation and curettage, hysterectomy, and myomectomy (excision of a myoma). The Introduction category of codes includes procedures for insertion and removal of an intrauterine device (IUD), artificial insemination, radiography, insertion of brachytherapy devices, endometrial surgery, catheterization, and chromotubation. Repair codes involve uterine suspension and treatment of rupture and anomaly. In the Laparoscopy/Hysteroscopy category, procedures represented are laparoscopic techniques for hysterectomy, myomectomy, biopsy, removal of foreign body, fallopian tube occlusion, and diagnostic hysteroscopy.

Hysterectomy

A **hysterectomy** is a procedure to remove the uterus. Codes for open hysterectomies (58150 through 58294) are found in the Hysterectomy Procedures subcategory in the Excision category. Laparoscopic hysterectomy codes (58541-58554) are located in the Laparoscopy/Hysterectomy category. Criteria for determining hysterectomy codes are:

1. The approach—abdominal or vaginal (for open procedures);
2. The weight of the uterus—250 g or less, or greater than 250 g;
3. The extent of the procedure—total, subtotal, or radical; and
4. The additional structures removed.

An example of criteria 2 and 4 in laparoscopic hysterectomy codes is shown in Figure 15.8.

Figure 15.8 Laparoscopic Hysterectomy Codes

58550	Laparoscopy, surgical, with vaginal hysterectomy, for uterus 250 g or less;
58552	with removal of tube(s) and/or ovary(s)
58553	Laparoscopy, surgical, with vaginal hysterectomy, for uterus greater than 250 g;
58554	with removal of tube(s) and/or ovary(s)

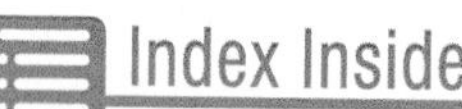

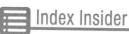

Index Insider

Hysterectomy codes can be found in the Index under the main entry *Hysterectomy*, organized by approach, extent of removal, and other procedures performed. Hysterectomy codes are also indexed under the main term *Uterus* and subterm *excision*.

Additional hysterectomy codes are located in the Urinary System Surgery subsection (51925) and the Maternity Care and Delivery Surgery subsection (59525).

EXAMPLE **15.9**

A 45-year-old patient with metromenorrhagia presented for a hysterectomy. She was taken to the OR and placed under general anesthesia. The surgeon performed a transvaginal hysterectomy. The specimen removed included the uterus and cervix, which weighed approximately 225 g immediately postoperative. This procedure is reported with code 58260, *Vaginal hysterectomy, for uterus 250 g or less*.

LET'S TRY ONE **15.7**

A 46-year-old female with symptomatic fibroid uterus desired a hysterectomy. She was taken to the da Vinci surgical suite where a laparoscopic vaginal hysterectomy with bilateral salpingectomies and right oophorectomy were completed. The uterus, fallopian tubes, and ovary weighed approximately 245 g. What is the appropriate code for this procedure? _____

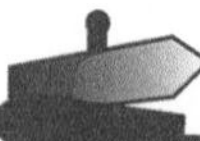

Learn Your Way

Historical background can help some learners concretize information, particularly sensing learners who deal well with facts. In the 1800s, female hysteria was considered a valid medical diagnosis. The term *hysteria* is formed from *hyster*, the word root meaning *uterus*, and *-ia*, the suffix meaning *abnormal condition*. Symptoms of female hysteria included fainting, nervousness, insomnia, fluid retention, and sexual desire. As many as 25% of women in the mid-1800s were considered to be suffering from female hysteria. As the diagnostic capabilities of the medical profession grew, the diagnosis of female hysteria was replaced by more specific medical conditions.

Oviduct/Ovary (Codes 58600-58770)

The **oviducts** (also called the *fallopian tubes* or **uterine tubes**) allow **ova** (egg cells) to move from the ovaries to the uterus. The 4 categories of codes—Incision, Laparoscopy, Excision, and Repair—describe procedures that are specific to the oviducts as well as procedures that overlap with the ovary. The Incision category provides codes for 1 of the most common procedures performed on the oviducts, tubal ligation for sterilization. The Laparoscopy category provides codes for lysis of adhesions, removal of all or part of the fallopian tubes or ovaries, treatments of lesions, occlusion of tubes, fimbrioplasty, and salpingostomy. Under Repair, procedures include lysis of adhesions, anastomosis, implantation, fimbrioplasty, and salpingostomy.

Ovary (Codes 58800-58960)

The ovaries are responsible for producing the hormones estrogen and progesterone that support female health, as well as for storing and developing oocytes, female reproductive cells. There are 2 categories of Ovary procedures, Incision and Excision. Drainage of ovarian cysts and abscesses and transposition of ovaries are described under Incision. Excision procedures include biopsy of ovary; open and laparoscopic procedures for excision of lesions on the ovary such as an ovarian cyst; oophorectomy; and staging procedures for malignancy.

Many of the codes found under the Ovary heading concern treatments specific for patients with malignant tumors. These procedures include initial resections, debulking for recurrent malignancy, and second-look surgeries for staging or restaging. Debulking is removing as much of the tumor as possible. How healthy a patient is and how far the cancer has spread help to determine how much surrounding tissue and organs are excised. Women of childbearing age with certain types of tumors and with early stage cancer may be able to beat the disease without needing to have their ovaries or uterus removed.

As shown in Figure 15.9, code 58943 is reported when a surgeon performs an **oophorectomy** (removes part or all of 1 or both ovaries) and also performs lymph node, peritoneum, and diaphragm biopsies. Code 58943 is reported for such a procedure whether or not it includes the performance of **salpingectomy** (removal of oviducts) and/or **omentectomy** (removal of omentum).

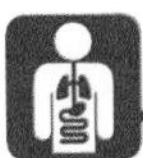

A&P Review

The peritoneum is a strong membrane with a smooth surface that lines the abdominal and pelvic walls. The omentum is a fold of the peritoneum that extends from the stomach to the transverse colon.

Figure 15.9 Oophorectomy Codes for Ovarian, Tubal, or Primary Peritoneal Malignancy

58940	Oophorectomy, partial or total, unilateral or bilateral; (For oophorectomy with concomitant debulking for ovarian malignancy, use 58952)
58943	for ovarian, tubal or primary peritoneal malignancy, with para-aortic and pelvic lymph node biopsies, peritoneal washings, peritoneal biopsies, diaphragmatic assessments, with or without salpingectomy(s), with or without omentectomy

Figure 15.10 shows codes for initial resection of malignancy that involves bilateral salpingo-oophorectomies and omentectomy. The base code for this procedure is 58950. When total abdominal hysterectomy and pelvic and para-aortic **lymphadenectomy** (removal of lymph nodes) are also performed at the same time, code 58951 is reported. When code 58950 is augmented with **radical debulking** (the reducing of the size of a tumor that has grown so large that it causes discomfort for the patient), code 58952 is reported.

Figure 15.10 Codes for Initial Resection of Ovarian, Tubal, or Primary Peritoneal Malignancy

58950	Resection (initial) of ovarian, tubal or primary peritoneal malignancy with bilateral salpingo-oophorectomy and omentectomy;
58951	with total abdominal hysterectomy, pelvic and limited para-aortic lymphadenectomy
58952	with radical dissection for debulking (ie, radical excision or destruction, intra-abdominal or retroperitoneal tumors)

Codes 58957 and 58958 are reported for resection of a recurrent malignancy (tumor). In addition to debulking a recurrent ovarian, uterine, tubal, or primary peritoneal malignancy, lysis of adhesions and excision of omentum are also included in code 58957. The surgeon may remove all visible tumors or simply reduce their size, depending on the structures involved. Code 58958 includes all of the procedures listed above, as well as pelvic and para-aortic lymphadenectomy. Code 58960 is reported for a laparotomy for staging or restaging of an ovarian, uterine, tubal, or primary peritoneal malignancy with or without omentectomy, lymphadenectomy, and/or biopsy of peritoneum. This is a **second-look operation** to check for recurrence of tumor(s).

EXAMPLE **15.10**

A 37-year-old female with recently diagnosed carcinoma of the ovary presented for removal of her right ovary. The surgeon performed a right total oophorectomy and biopsies of several lymph nodes. The surgeon also examined the diaphragm and peritoneum and performed peritoneal washing and biopsy. This procedure is reported with code 58943, *Oophorectomy, partial or total, unilateral or bilateral; for ovarian, tubal or primary peritoneal malignancy, with para-aortic and pelvic lymph node biopsies, peritoneal washings, peritoneal biopsies, diaphragmatic assessments, with or without salpingectomy, with or without omentectomy.*

LET'S TRY ONE **15.8**

A 42-year-old female with ovarian cancer was scheduled for an initial resection of a tumor. The surgical findings indicated widespread metastases. The surgeon performed a total abdominal hysterectomy, bilateral salpingo-oophorectomy, and omentectomy and removed lymph nodes from the pelvic and para-aortic area. What is the appropriate code for this procedure? _____

In Vitro Fertilization (Codes 58970-58999)

In vitro fertilization (IVF) is a series of procedures used to treat fertility problems. During IVF, mature oocytes are retrieved and fertilized by sperm in a lab. The embryo is then transferred to the uterus. This process is reported with codes 58970, 58974, or 58976.

Introduction to Maternity Care and Delivery

The Maternity Care and Delivery Surgery subsection immediately follows the Female Genital System Surgery subsection in the CPT® codebook. These surgical procedures encompass care for a mother during pregnancy, delivery, and the postpartum period, and for the fetus during the gestational period before birth.

Maternity Care and Delivery Terminology

Familiarity with maternity care terminology will help you understand the scope of the surgical services in the Maternity Care and Delivery Surgery subsection. Table 15.7 presents the terminology used in this subsection.

Table 15.7 Maternity Care and Delivery Terms

Term	Definition
abortion	Spontaneous or surgically assisted termination of a pregnancy
amniocentesis	Removal of fluid from the sac around the baby in the uterus
antepartum	Period of fetal gestation after confirmation of pregnancy until the beginning of labor, usually 36 weeks
cerclage of cervix	Suturing of the cervix to keep it closed during pregnancy
cesarean delivery	Extraction of a fetus from the uterus via abdominal incision
cordocentesis	Removal of a sample of the baby's blood from the umbilical cord
delivery	The process of passing the fetus and the placenta from the womb into the external world
ectopic pregnancy	Implantation of an embryo in a location other than the uterus, such as the fallopian tubes, usually requiring termination of the pregnancy
episiotomy	An incision made between the vagina and anus to facilitate delivery
external cephalic version	Procedure to turn a fetus from a side-lying or breech position to a head-down position
fetus	The gestational unborn child from the end of the eighth week to the moment of birth
hydatidiform mole	Abnormal mass of tissue that forms in the uterus at the beginning of a pregnancy
multifetal reduction (MPR)	Procedure used to reduce the number of fetuses carried to gestation
postpartum	The period after delivery of a baby that includes 6 weeks of care for the mother

The Maternity Care and Delivery Surgery Subsection

Unlike other surgery subsections, the organization of the Maternity Care and Delivery Surgery subsection does not use anatomical sites as headings with codes grouped in categories of procedures. Instead, the headings shown in Table 15.8 are a mix of care procedures that are sequenced to roughly correspond to the stages of maternity care, that is, antepartum care, delivery, and postpartum care.

Table 15.8 Headings Within the Maternity Care and Delivery Surgery Subsection of the CPT® Codebook

Heading	Code(s)
Antepartum and Fetal Invasive Services	59000-59076
Excision	59100-59160
Introduction	59200
Repair	59300-59350
Vaginal Delivery, Antepartum and Postpartum Care	59400-59430
Cesarean Delivery	59510-59525
Delivery After Previous Cesarean Delivery	59610-59622
Abortion	59812-59857
Other Procedures	59866-59899

Maternity Care and Delivery (Codes 59000-59899)

The first heading, Antepartum and Fetal Invasive Services, provides codes for fetal diagnostic and therapeutic procedures, from intrauterine sampling to stress tests to amniotic fluid treatments. The next heading, Excision, has codes for procedures to remove tissue or terminate an ectopic pregnancy. The Introduction and Repair codes describe cervical dilation, episiotomy, cervical cerclage, and suture of a ruptured uterus. At the end of the subsection, Abortion and Other Procedures codes cover treatment for spontaneous and assisted pregnancy termination. The 3 headings that organize the childbirth codes by type of delivery will be discussed in detail: Vaginal Delivery, Antepartum and Postpartum Care codes; Cesarean Delivery codes; and Delivery After Previous Cesarean Delivery codes (a listing that includes both vaginal and cesarean delivery results).

Maternity Care Guidelines and Global Package

The introductory material at the beginning of the Maternity Care and Delivery subsection of the codebook characterizes the stages of childbirth care and describes the services involved in each stage. Maternity care is a package of services that begin when a pregnancy has been confirmed and conclude when the postpartum period ends. The services in the CPT®-defined global package are appropriate for a pregnancy, delivery, and recovery without complications and which are rendered by a single physician or group practice.

Services Included in Global Obstetric Care It is important to first understand the services described as routine obstetric care in each of the 3 stages of maternity care: antepartum care, delivery, and postpartum care.

Antepartum care begins after the pregnancy is confirmed. In the maternity care package, antepartum care includes the following:

- the initial and subsequent prenatal history and physical examinations;
- recording of weights, blood pressures, and fetal heart tones;
- routine urinalysis;
- monthly visits up to 28 weeks' gestation; biweekly visits from 29 to 36 weeks' gestation; and weekly visits from 37 weeks' gestation until delivery.

Delivery services include the following:

- hospital admission;
- the admission history and physical examination;
- management of uncomplicated labor including fetal monitoring conducted by the attending physician;
- vaginal delivery (including episiotomy and/or forceps if needed) or cesarean delivery; the use of forceps, vacuum extraction, or rupture of membranes to assist delivery does not affect code assignment;
- initial evaluation and resuscitation of the newborn by the obstetrician;

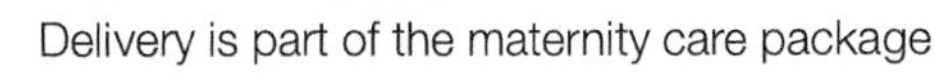

Delivery is part of the maternity care package.

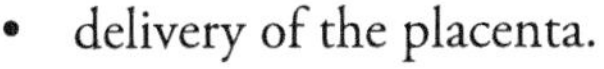

- delivery of the placenta.

Postpartum care services include the following:

- inpatient care related to the delivery;
- outpatient care related to the delivery for a period of 6 weeks.

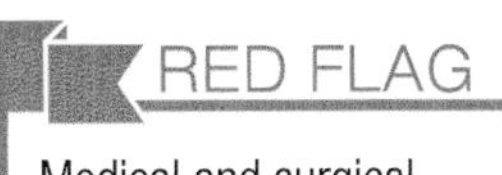

RED FLAG

Medical and surgical complications of pregnancy that require additional services should be coded separately.

Reporting Codes for Maternity Care and Delivery The code groupings for each type of delivery in the codebook give the package code first and then list constituent codes for nonroutine circumstances when (a) the whole package of services cannot be performed by the same healthcare provider; and/or (b) the services must be augmented. Table 15.9 shows how the global maternity care package codes and the separate constituents are reported for the different delivery methods.

Inside the OR

The patient was taken to the operating room where spinal anesthesia was obtained without difficulty. The patient was prepped and draped in the normal sterile fashion, in the dorsal supine position with a leftward tilt. A Pfannenstiel skin incision was made through the patient's previous skin incision and carried through to the underlying layer of fascia with the scalpel. The fascia was incised in the midline and the fascial incision extended laterally using Mayo scissors. The rectus muscles were separated in the midline and the parietal peritoneum identified tented upward and entered bluntly using the surgeon's fingers. The peritoneal incision was extended superiorly, inferiorly, and laterally in a blunt fashion. A bladder blade was then placed in the patient's pelvis deflecting the bladder downward, revealing the lower uterine segment. The vesicular uterine peritoneum of the lower uterine segment was incised using Metzenbaum scissors, and the vesicular uterine peritoneal incision was extended laterally using the same Metzenbaum scissors. The bladder flap was then created digitally using the surgeon's fingers. The blade was then replaced and the bladder flap deflected downward, revealing the lower uterine segment. The lower uterine segment was incised in a transverse fashion using the scalpel, and the lower uterine segment incision was extended bluntly using the surgeon's fingers. The infant's head was then delivered atraumatically. The nose and mouth were bulb suctioned. The remainder of the infant's body was then delivered atraumatically. The nose and mouth were again bulb suctioned and the cord was clamped and cut. The placenta was then delivered manually. The uterus was cleared of all clots and debris using dry laparotomy pads. All incisions were sutured.

Abortion and Miscarriage

The medical term *abortion* describes the premature expulsion from the uterus of the products of conception: the embryo or a nonviable fetus. An abortion may be categorized as either spontaneous (natural cause) or induced (deliberate). An induced abortion may be therapeutic (medically necessary) or elective (woman's choice).

Spontaneous Abortion (Miscarriage) A **spontaneous abortion** is the termination of pregnancy through miscarriage before 20 weeks, 0 days (gestational age of fetus). CPT® codes distinguish between types of spontaneous abortion, given below with descriptions of their characteristics and related CPT® codes:

- Complete abortion: the uterus is entirely emptied of its contents in any pregnancy trimester. This type is implied rather than described in a Maternity Care and Delivery code because no surgical intervention is necessary. Treatment is reported with appropriate E/M codes.
- Incomplete abortion: products of conception may remain in the uterus and require surgical intervention to completely remove. Report code 59812, *Treatment of incomplete abortion, any trimester, completed surgically.*

- Missed abortion: a fetus that has died remains in the uterus and requires intervention for removal. Report the code based on the trimester in which the procedure is performed: 59820 for the first trimester and 59821 for the second trimester.
- Septic abortion: the presence of intrauterine infection requires the evacuation of the products of conception and treatment of the infection. Report code 59830 for these services.

Induced Abortion An **induced abortion** is a medically assisted termination of a pregnancy. Coding is based on the technique used:

- Dilation and curettage: report code 59840.
- Dilation and evacuation: report code 59841.
- Intra-amniotic injection: report code 59850 for injection(s) and delivery of the fetus and associated material; report code 59851 if dilation and curettage and/or evacuation are required; and report 59852 if the injections fail and a hysterotomy is required.
- Vaginal suppository: report code 59855 for administration of the drug, cervical dilation, and delivery of the fetus and associated material; report code 59856 if dilation and curettage and/or evacuation are required; and report 59857 if the evacuation fails and a hysterotomy is required.

CONCEPTS CHECKPOINT **15.5**

Choose the best answer for the following multiple-choice questions.

1. Services related to medical complications of pregnancy
   a. may be reported separately.
   b. are included in the routine care codes.
   c. should be reported with code 59899.
   d. may not be reported for billing purposes.
2. If a provider sees a pregnant patient only once in the antepartum period and does not provide any other service,
   a. no code will be reported for billing purposes.
   b. evaluation and management code(s) are reported.
   c. the code reported depends on the type of delivery.
   d. a code for antepartum care only is reported.
3. The maternity care package for a patient delivering twins vaginally
   a. includes both deliveries.
   b. does not include both deliveries.
   c. includes services for all complications related to multiple gestation.
   d. includes a cesarean delivery.

Introduction to the Endocrine System

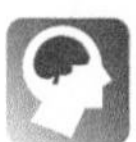

3-D
To explore the endocrine system in the BioDigital Human, go to: http://Coding.ParadigmEducation.com/BioDigital_Endocrine.

The **endocrine system** is made up of glands located throughout the body that release hormones into the blood, as shown in Figure 15.11. These hormones affect metabolism, growth, and development. The **thyroid**, located in the neck, is the largest endocrine gland. The thyroid secretes the hormones triiodothyronine (T3) and thyroxine (T4) necessary for body cell metabolism. The **parathyroid glands** are located on the posterior side of the thyroid gland and secrete the parathyroid hormone. The parathyroid hormone increases calcium levels in the blood by stimulating osteoclast activity. The **thymus gland** located above the heart produces T lymphocytes during early childhood. The **adrenal glands** sit on top of each kidney and secrete the hormones cortisol, aldosterone, epinephrine (adrenaline), and norepinephrine (noradrenaline). Hormones secreted by the adrenal glands help the body during stress by increasing glucose to provide energy and increasing blood pressure, heartbeat, and respirations. Aldosterone regulates electrolytes that are necessary for normal body function. The **pancreas** contains clusters of endocrine tissue that secrete hormones, including insulin. The pancreas also produces enzymes that help the digestive process, and codes for procedures on the pancreas are found in the Digestive System Surgery subsection.

Endocrine System Terminology

Familiarity with the endocrine system terminology will enable you to more easily report the proper codes for procedures described in this subsection of the codebook. Table 15.10 provides information about the function of anatomical structures and the definition of surgical procedures.

Table 15.10 Endocrine System Terms

Structure/Surgical Procedure	Function/Definition
adrenal gland	Secretes the hormones cortisol, aldosterone, epinephrine (adrenaline), and norepinephrine (noradrenaline)
adrenalectomy	Removal of the adrenal gland
carotid body	Small cluster of receptors located in the carotid artery
isthmus	A bridge of tissue
isthmusectomy	Excision of the isthmus (particularly the isthmus of the thyroid)
pancreas	Contains clusters of endocrine tissue, which secrete hormones, including insulin; also produces enzymes that help the digestive process
parathyroid gland	Secretes the parathyroid hormone, which increases calcium levels in the blood by stimulating osteoclast activity
parathyroidectomy	Removal of the parathyroid gland
thymectomy	Removal of the thymus gland
thymus glands	Produce T lymphocytes during early childhood
thyroid glands	Secrete the hormones triiodothyronine (T3) and thyroxine (T4) necessary for body cell metabolism
thyroidectomy	Removal of the thyroid gland

Figure 15.11 Locations of Endocrine Glands

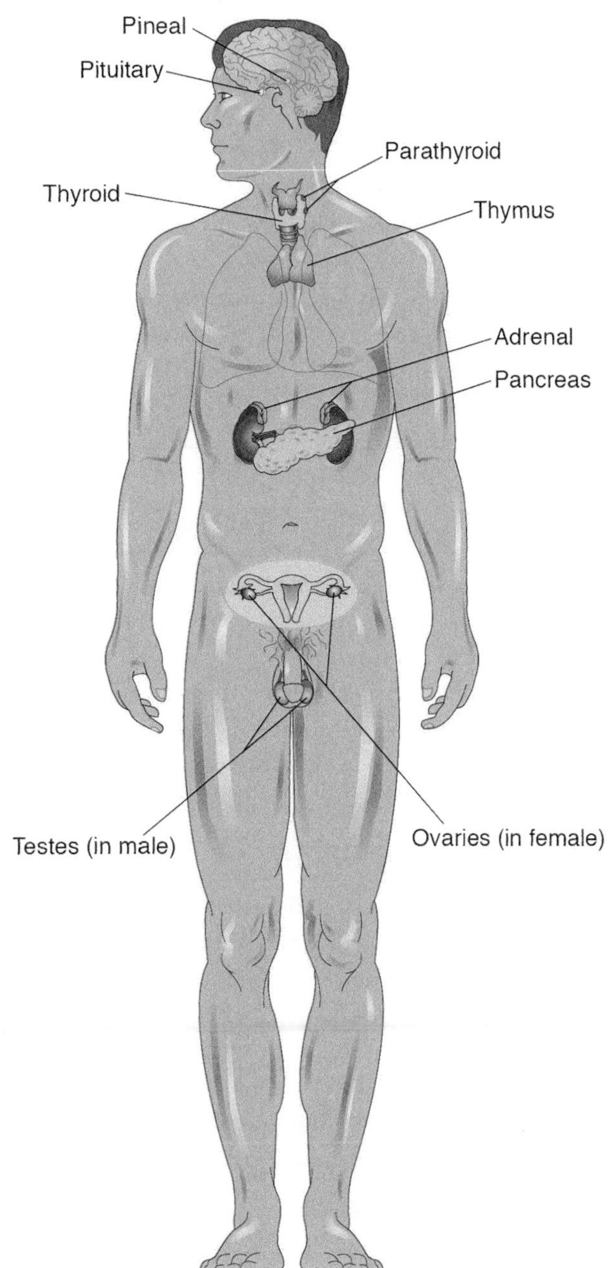

The Endocrine System Surgery Subsection

The headings in the Endocrine System Surgery subsection are organized by anatomical site. Each heading is further categorized by type of procedure, such as incision, excision, removal, and laparoscopy. A listing of the headings and corresponding codes within the Endocrine System Surgery subsection is provided in Table 15.11.

Table 15.11 Headings Within the Endocrine System Surgery Subsection of the CPT® Codebook

Heading	Codes
Thyroid Gland	60000-60300
Parathyroid, Thymus, Adrenal Glands, Pancreas, and Carotid Body	60500-60699

The Endocrine System Surgery subsection is located after the Maternity Care and Delivery Surgery subsection in the CPT® codebook. Common procedures of the endocrine system include thyroid biopsy, **thyroidectomy** (removal of the thyroid), **thymectomy** (removal of thymus gland), **adrenalectomy** (removal of the adrenal glands), and excision of carotid body tumors. Codes in the Endocrine System Surgery subsection are divided into 2 groups: (1) thyroid gland procedures, and (2) parathyroid, thymus, adrenal glands, pancreas, and carotid body procedures.

Thyroid Gland (Codes 60000-60300)

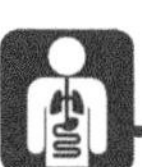

A&P Review

The thyroid is a butterfly-shaped gland at the base of the neck. It has a right and left lobe joined by the isthmus (a bridge of tissue). The platysma is a platelike muscle that originates from the fascia of the neck. The platysma acts to wrinkle the skin of the neck and depress the jaw.

The largest endocrine gland is the thyroid, a butterfly-shaped structure located in the neck that secretes hormones that affect cell metabolism. The CPT® codebook groups surgical procedures for the thyroid gland into 3 categories. The Incision code describes drainage of an infected thyroglossal duct cyst. Excision codes cover biopsy, excision of cyst and adenoma, thyroid lobectomy, thyroidectomy, and isthmusectomy. The Removal code describes aspiration and injection treatment of a cyst.

Thyroidectomy

When medical approaches are unsuccessful in treating **hyperthyroidism** (overactive thyroid), a full or partial thyroidectomy may be performed. The surgeon will select the most appropriate procedure based on patient's age, type of disease, and extent of disease. For example, patients with **goiters** (enlarged thyroid) or patients whose glands are pressing on the trachea may require a total or subtotal thyroidectomy, and patients with thyroid cancer in a single lobe may be treated by removing that lobe. Thyroid conditions are more common in females, and thyroidectomy is performed more often on females than males.

Thyroidectomy codes (60210 through 60271) are sequenced based on the amount of tissue removed, from least (a part of a lobe) to greatest (the entire thyroid gland):

- Partial thyroid lobectomy is reported with codes 60210 through 60212.
- Removal of an entire lobe of the thyroid is reported with code 60220 (unilateral) or 60225 (with contralateral subtotal lobectomy).
- Total or complete thyroidectomy is reported with code 60240.
- For patients with malignancy, total or subtotal thyroidectomy with neck dissection is reported with code 60252 (limited neck dissection) or 60254 (radical neck dissection).

- Thyroidectomy for a patient who had a partial thyroidectomy and is having the remaining thyroid tissue removed is reported with code 60260. Modifier 50, *Bilateral procedure*, should be applied to code 60260 if both lobes of the thyroid are removed.
- Thyroidectomy including the substernal thyroid gland is reported with code 60270 for a sternal split or transthoracic approach and code 60271 for a transverse cervical incision.

Inside the OR

A 45-year-old female with an apparently nonfunctioning goiter presented to the hospital for a thyroid lobectomy. Under general endotracheal anesthesia, the surgeon made a transverse cervical incision, as shown in Figure 15.12 (A). The platysma was divided and the muscles were separated (B). The right thyroid lobe was isolated and the blood vessels were ligated (C). The parathyroid glands were preserved to prevent hypoparathyroidism, the isthmus was severed, and the thyroid lobe was resected. The platysma was closed (D), the skin was closed, dressings were applied, and the patient was taken to the recovery room. This procedure is reported with code 60220, *Total thyroid lobectomy, unilateral; with or without isthmusectomy.*

Figure 15.12 Stages in a Thyroid Lobectomy

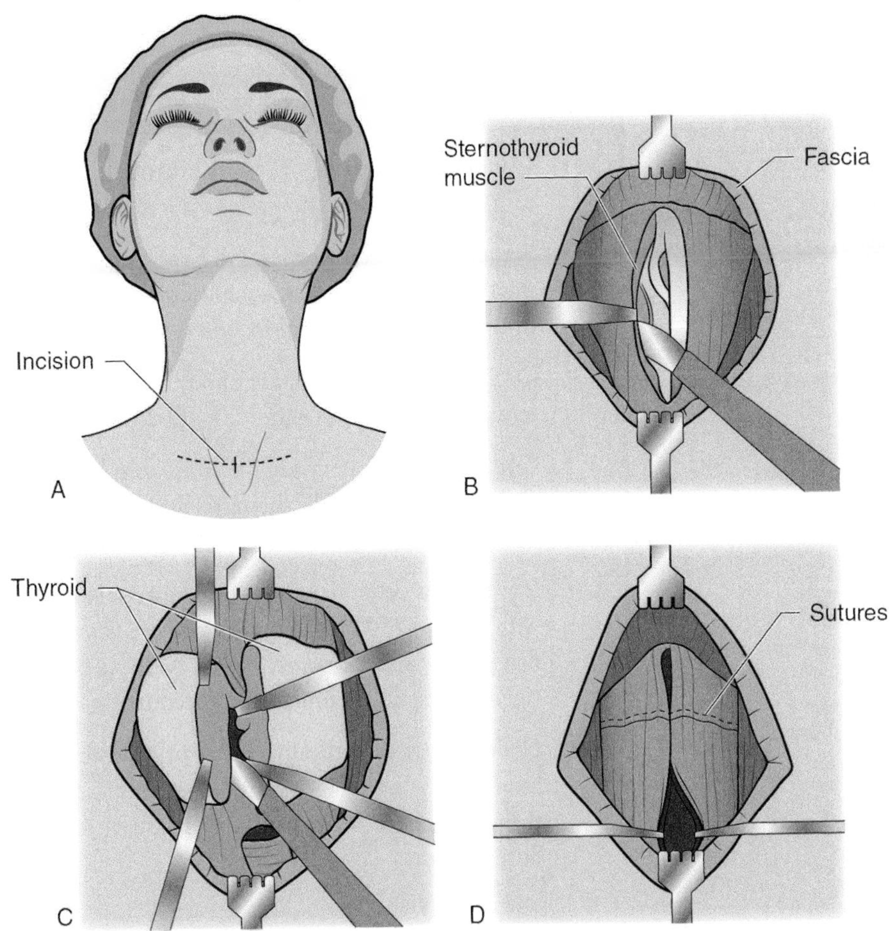

LET'S TRY ONE **15.9**

A 62-year-old female with known thyroid cancer was brought to the OR, where total thyroidectomy with radical neck dissection was performed under general anesthesia. What is the appropriate code for this procedure? _____

Parathyroid, Thymus, Adrenal Glands, Pancreas, and Carotid Body (Codes 60500-60699)

The remaining codes in the Endocrine System subsection (60500 through 60699) describe procedures on other endocrine system structures. The parathyroid glands are located beside the thyroid and regulate the amount of calcium in the blood and bones. The thymus is a bilobular lymphoid organ that is in the superior mediastinum. The thymus develops T cells, which are critical to the immune system. Adrenal glands are hormone-producing endocrine glands and are found on top of each kidney. The pancreas is a large, elongated gland situated behind the stomach between the spleen and the duodenum. The pancreas is responsible for producing insulin and glucagon as well as enzymes that aid digestion. The carotid body is a cluster of cells at the carotid artery (the main artery of the neck). The codebook categories of Excision and Laparoscopy comprise procedures for biopsy; exploration of the parathyroid gland, mediastinum, and adrenal gland; parathyroidectomy; adrenalectomy; mediastinal dissection; and excision of carotid body tumor.

Chapter Summary

- Codes for circumcision (54150 through 54161) are dependent on the technique and whether the patient is a neonate or over 28 days old.
- Surgery to correct chordee and hypospadias has 4 components: straightening the shaft of the penis, creating the urinary channel, positioning the urinary meatus (opening) at the tip, and circumcision or reconstruction of the foreskin.
- Orchiectomy codes are assumed to be unilateral. Bilateral orchiectomies require the use of modifier 50, *Bilateral procedure*.
- Codes for orchiopexy are differentiated by the original scrotal, inguinal, or abdominal location of the testis and whether the surgery was open or laparoscopic.
- Vas deferens codes may be either unilateral or bilateral: A vasectomy reported with code 55250 includes *unilateral or bilateral* in the code descriptor, so modifier 50, *Bilateral procedure*, cannot be applied; the code for a vasovasostomy (55400) describes a unilateral procedure, so modifier 50 should be applied.
- Codes for transurethral removal or destruction of prostate are found in the Urinary System Surgery subsection (52601 through 52640 and 53850 through 53852, respectively) and not with the male genital system procedure codes.

- The Maternity Care and Delivery codes appear after the female genital subsection and include codes for procedures done on patients who are currently pregnant or postpartum.
- A colposcopy is defined as an endoscopy of the vagina, but the term *colposcopy* may include a visual examination of other structures. Multiple colposcopy codes may be reported when multiple sites are examined.
- Both open and laparoscopic vaginal hysterectomy codes are differentiated first by the weight of the uterus (greater or less than 250 g) and then by the extent of the procedure.
- Many of the codes found under the Ovary heading concern treatment of malignancy, including procedures for initial resections, debulking for recurrent malignancy, and second-look surgeries for malignancy staging. These codes may be reported only for patients with malignant tumors.
- Maternity care is a package of services for patients without complications and is reported based on the type of delivery (vaginal, cesarean, VBAC, and attempted VBAC).
- Codes exist for each portion of the total maternity service (antepartum, delivery only, and postpartum) and should be used if 1 physician does not provide all of the services for the patient.
- Thyroidectomy codes (60210 through 60271) are based on the amount of tissue removed.

Navigator

Access interactive chapter review exercises, practice activities, flash cards, and study games.

Chapter 16

Surgery Coding: Nervous System

Fast Facts

- The human brain operates on the same electrical power as a 10-volt lamp.
- The brain has enormous storage capacity—scientists aren't exactly sure, but they estimate that the brain can hold around 2.5 petabytes (or a million gigabytes).
- Nerve impulse speeds vary, but the fastest 1 travels about 250 miles per hour, faster than a Formula 1 race car!

Sources: http://scientificamerican.com, http://sciencemuseum.org.uk

Crack the Code

Review the sample operative report to find the correct nervous system code. You may need to return to this exercise after reading the chapter content.

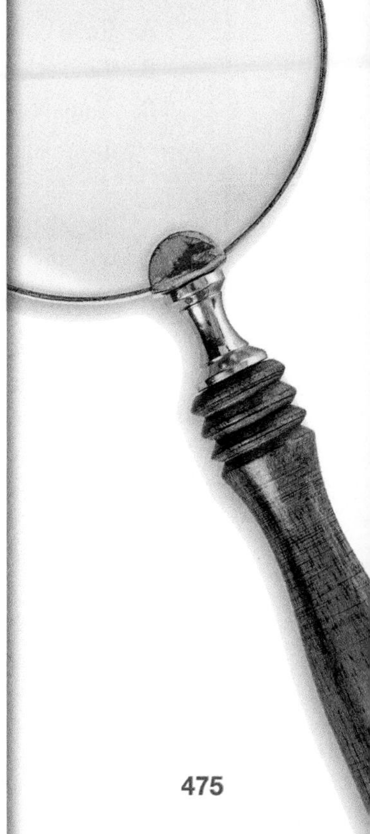

PREOPERATIVE DIAGNOSIS: L5-S1 herniated disc

POSTOPERATIVE DIAGNOSIS: Same

OPERATION: L5-S1 discectomy and L5 nerve root decompression

PROCEDURE: The patient was intubated and placed in prone position. An incision was marked on the lower back, and the back was prepped and draped in a sterile fashion. The incision was made with a #10 scalpel, Bovie coagulator, and down to the fascia. At this point, the fascia was incised with a #15 blade. A flap of fascia was then retracted with #2-0 Vicryl, and the muscle was gently dissected and retracted with a Taylor retractor. Under the microscope, a curette was placed between the L5-S1 interspace, and x-rays were obtained. The x-rays showed that the curette was between L5 and S1. Under the microscope with microdissection, and with the use of a Midas Rex, the lamina of L5 was partially drilled off, and yellow ligament was opened, removed, and then the L5 nerve root was identified. A large herniated disc was found, removed, and the L5 nerve root was completely decompressed. At this point, the interspace at L5-S1 was entered and the disc removed laterally, and then a complete decompression of the L5 into the foramen was accomplished. At this point, the area was irrigated with antibiotic solution, and a paste of Depo-Medrol, Amicar, and morphine was left in place. The fascia was closed with a #2-0 Vicryl, subcutaneous tissue with a #3-0 Vicryl, and the skin was closed with subcuticular #4-0 Vicryl.

answer: 63030

Learning Objectives

16.1 Describe the basic anatomy of the skull, meninges, brain, spine, and spinal cord.

16.2 Describe the organization of codes within the Nervous System surgery subsection.

16.3 Apply guidelines and instructional notes when coding nervous system procedures.

16.4 Apply appropriate HCPCS and/or CPT® modifiers when coding nervous system procedures.

16.5 Identify procedures within the Nervous System Surgery subsection that require separate radiological supervision and interpretation codes.

16.6 Describe the 3 procedures involved in a skull base operative session.

16.7 Describe laminectomy and corpectomy procedures.

16.8 Differentiate between anesthetic and neurolytic agents for nerve injections.

16.9 Code the following types of nervous system procedures: skull base surgery, spine and spinal cord procedures, and nerve destruction and repair.

Chapter Outline

- **I.** Introduction to the Nervous System
- **II.** Nervous System Terminology
- **III.** Organization of the Nervous System Surgery Subsection
- **IV.** Skull, Meninges, and Brain (Codes 61000-62258)
  - **A.** Twist Drill, Burr Hole(s), or Trephine Procedures
  - **B.** Craniectomy or Craniotomy Procedures
  - **C.** Surgery of Skull Base
    - **i.** Skull Base Surgery Approach Procedures
    - **ii.** Skull Base Surgery Definitive Procedures
    - **iii.** Skull Base Surgery Repair and/or Reconstruction Procedures
  - **D.** Cerebrospinal Fluid (CSF) Shunt Procedures
- **V.** Spine and Spinal Cord (Codes 62263-63746)
  - **A.** Spinal Injection, Drainage, or Aspiration Procedures
  - **B.** Laminotomy, Laminectomy, and Decompression
  - **C.** Extradural Exploration/Decompression: Corpectomy and Discectomy
- **VI.** Extracranial Nerves, Peripheral Nerves, and Autonomic Nervous System (Codes 64400-64999)
  - **A.** Introduction/Injection of Anesthetic Agent (Nerve Block), Diagnostic or Therapeutic
  - **B.** Neurostimulators (Peripheral Nerve)
  - **C.** Destruction by Neurolytic Agent (eg, Chemical, Thermal, Electrical, or Radiofrequency), Chemodenervation
  - **D.** Neuroplasty (Exploration, Neurolysis, or Nerve Decompression)
  - **E.** Neurorrhaphy
- **VII.** Chapter Summary

Introduction to the Nervous System

The **nervous system** coordinates and controls all of the body's activities. The nervous system is divided into the central nervous system and the peripheral nervous system. The **central nervous system** is made up of the brain and spinal cord, and the **peripheral nervous system** consists of the cranial nerves, spinal nerves, and all other

3-D
To explore the nervous system in the BioDigital Human, go to: http://Coding.ParadigmEducation.com/BioDigital_Nervous.

nerves outside the brain and spinal cord. The peripheral nervous system is further divided into the **somatic nervous system**, which deals with voluntary movement, and the **autonomic nervous system**, which controls involuntary automatic bodily functions such as heart rate, breathing, and digestion. The autonomic nervous system contains the sympathetic nervous system and the parasympathetic nervous system. The **sympathetic nervous system** activates the "fight or flight" response that prepares the body to react to a stressful situation by increasing the heart rate and slowing digestion. The **parasympathetic nervous system** controls rest, slows the heart rate, and stimulates digestion as it works in opposition to the sympathetic nervous system. The introductory notes in the Nervous System surgery subsection contain graphics of the nervous system with labels to point out the various parts of the brain and nerves. Certain instructional notes within the Nervous System surgery subsection are also accompanied by graphics that illustrate the anatomical sites of the different procedures. Figure 16.1 depicts the elements of the central nervous system.

Figure 16.1 Organs of the Nervous System

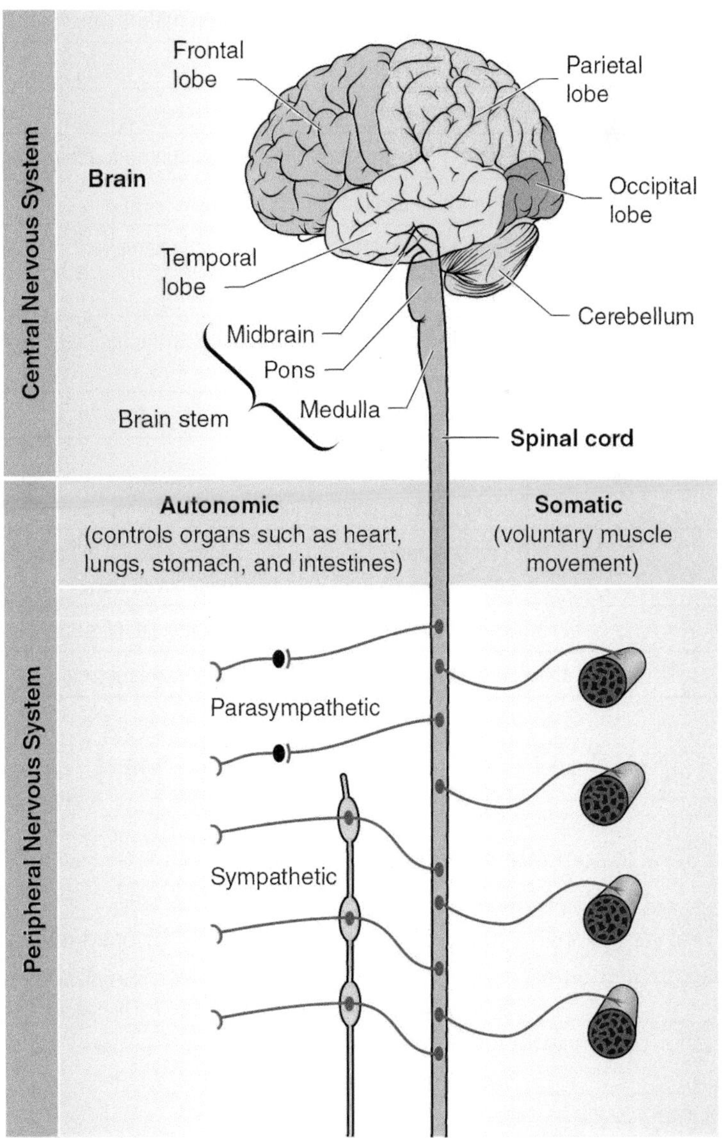

Nervous System Terminology

It is important for a coder to be familiar with the anatomical and medical terms used with the nervous system to correctly report codes from the Nervous System Surgery subsection. Table 16.1 provides more information about each organ or structure, as well as conditions and surgical terms unique to this body system.

Table 16.1 Nervous System Structures and Surgical Terminology

Term	Definition
cerebellum	Hindbrain, located under the posterior portion of cerebrum
cerebrospinal fluid (CSF)	Clear, colorless fluid that flows through the subarachnoid space around the brain and spinal cord
cerebrum	Largest portion of brain (encompassing the 4 lobes), divided into right and left hemispheres
corpectomy	Removal of the body of the vertebra
craniectomy	Removal of a portion of the skull
craniosynostosis	Congenital condition that causes premature closure of the sutures of the skull
craniotomy	Incision into the skull
decompression	Surgical operation for relief of pressure
epidural	Pertaining to the space located posterior to the dura mater
hemilaminectomy/laminotomy	Removal of a portion of the lamina
lamina	Portion of the vertebra that covers the nerve root
laminectomy	Removal of the lamina
meninges	The 3 layers of membranes that cover the brain and spinal cord: dura mater, arachnoid, and pia matter
neuroendoscopy	Examining the nervous system using an endoscope
neurorrhaphy	Repair of a nerve by suturing
radiosurgery	Using ionizing radiation to destroy tissue
spinal cord	A corded bundle of nerve fibers (protected by the spinal column, or vertebrae canal) that conducts nerve impulses from the brain to the lower body
stereotaxis	Using 3-dimensional imaging to locate site of surgery or radiation
ventricles	Spaces within the brain that contain cerebrospinal fluid

CONCEPTS CHECKPOINT **16.1**

Fill in the blank to complete the following statements.

1. The layers of membranes that cover the brain and spinal cord are called the ______________.
2. The ______________ is located under the posterior portion of the cerebrum.
3. The ______________ nervous system controls involuntary body functions.
4. The ______________ nervous system is composed of the brain and spinal cord.
5. The spaces within the brain that contain CSF are called ______________.

Organization of the Nervous System Surgery Subsection

The codes in the Nervous System Surgery subsection of the CPT® codebook fall under 3 headings based on anatomical site: Skull, Meninges, and Brain; Spine and Spinal Cord; and Extracranial Nerves, Peripheral Nerves, and Autonomic Nervous System. Table 16.2 provides all of the main headings within this subsection and the codes they include.

Table 16.2 Headings Within the Nervous System Subsection of the CPT® Codebook

Heading	Code Range
Skull, Meninges, and Brain	61000-62258
Spine and Spinal Cord	62263-63746
Extracranial Nerves, Peripheral Nerves, and Autonomic Nervous System	64400-64999

In addition to the anatomical site, procedure codes in the Nervous System Surgery subsection are further categorized by some basic criteria:

- the type of procedure: incision, drainage, excision, injection, endoscopy, repair, decompression (grafts are covered procedures);
- the approach: knowledge of the directional terms (such as anterior, posterior, and lateral) is required for correct code assignment;
- the specific stage of the procedure: skull base surgery codes distinguish between the approach, definitive, and reconstruction stages in 1 procedure; procedures may be performed for either diagnostic or therapeutic purposes.

Many procedures whose codes are located within the Nervous System Surgery subsection cannot be performed without radiological supervision and interpretation. Codes for radiological supervision and interpretation are reported with codes from the Radiology section of the CPT® codebook. When applicable, many of the instructional notes within the Nervous System Surgery subsection reference specific radiology codes to assist you in reporting them, as shown in Figure 16.2.

Figure 16.2 Example of an Instructional Note for Radiological Supervision and Interpretation

62268 Percutaneous aspiration, spinal cord cyst or syrinx

(For radiological supervision and interpretation, see 76942, 77002, 77012)

EXAMPLE **16.1**

A 45-year-old male patient underwent a percutaneous aspiration of a spinal cord cyst. Ultrasound was used to guide the needle to the exact anatomical location of the cyst. This procedure would be reported with codes 62268, *Percutaneous aspiration, spinal cord cyst*, and 76942, *Ultrasonic guidance for needle placement (eg, biopsy, aspiration, injection, localization device), imaging supervision and interpretation*.

Skull, Meninges, and Brain (Codes 61000-62258)

Figure 16.3 illustrates the skull, meninges, and brain structures. Surgical codes for the skull, meninges, and brain include the following CPT® codebook categories of procedures:

- Injection, Drainage, or Aspiration;
- Twist Drill, Burr Hole(s), or Trephine;
- Craniectomy or Craniotomy;
- Surgery of Skull Base;
- Endovascular Therapy;
- Surgery for Aneurysm, Arteriovenous Malformation, or Vascular Disease;
- Stereotaxis;
- Stereotactic Radiosurgery (Cranial);
- Neurostimulators (Intracranial);

Figure 16.3 Skull, Meninges, and Brain Structures

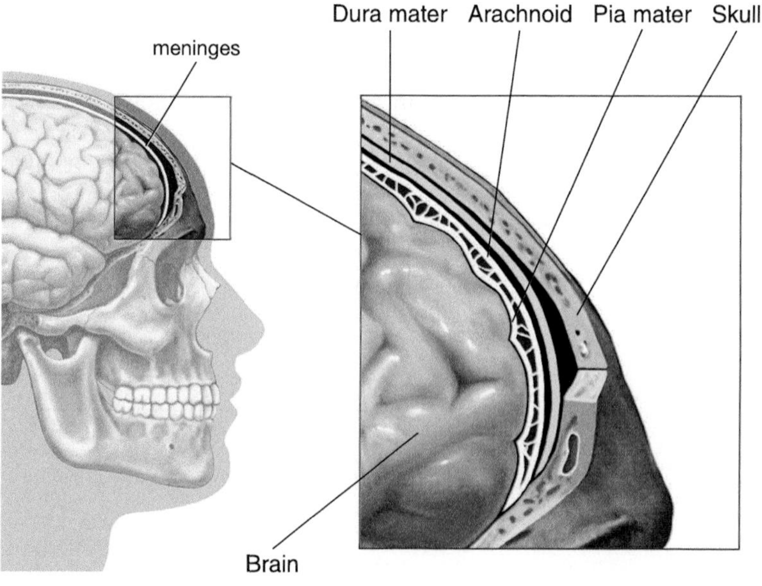

- Repair;
- Neuroendoscopy;
- Cerebrospinal Fluid (CSF) Shunt.

The procedures of accessing the brain through the skull, performing craniectomies and craniotomies, coordinating skull base surgeries, and shunting cerebrospinal fluid will be explained in detail in this chapter.

Twist Drill, Burr Hole(s), or Trephine Procedures

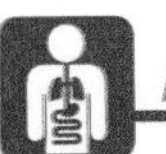

A&P Review

Subdural procedures are performed below the dura mater, the tough outer layer of meninges that covers the brain and spinal cord. Extradural procedures are performed outside the dura mater but within the skull. Epidural procedures are performed outside the dura mater or in the outermost part of the spinal canal.

Most procedures performed on the brain must begin with the creation of some sort of access point through the skull, which is too hard to be penetrated by a scalpel. Procedures such as the evacuation of a hematoma, the removal of a brain abscess, the biopsy of a tumor, and the clipping of a cerebral aneurysm all require a hole be drilled into the skull before they can be performed. CPT® codes describe several tools to open the skull, which involve drilling or trephining. A hole may be made using a **twist drill**, which is a manually operated drill. A **burr drill** is a special electric drill designed to stop drilling once the skull is penetrated. Holes created using burr drills are known as **burr holes**. A surgeon may "trephine" the skull to remove a circular section using a cylindrically shaped surgical saw called a **trephine**.

Some brain surgeries require only 1 hole for the operative approach, while others may require 2 holes that are then connected with a bone saw to allow a bigger portion of the skull to be removed, as in a craniotomy. If the hole in the skull is created in the same session as the craniotomy, only the code for the craniotomy should be reported.

The codes in the Twist Drill, Burr Hole(s), or Trephine category (61105 through 61253) may be performed for a variety of reasons, including to evacuate a hematoma, draw out fluid, or aspirate a cyst. Codes in this category are assigned based on the reason for the procedure (such as biopsy or drainage) and the location of the procedure (such as extradural or subdural), as shown in Figure 16.4.

Figure 16.4 Examples of Codes for Creation of a Burr Hole or Use of a Trephine

Code	Description
61140	Burr hole(s) or trephine; with biopsy of brain or intracranial lesion
61150	with drainage of brain abscess or cyst
61151	with subsequent tapping (aspiration) of intracranial abscess or cyst
61154	Burr hole(s) with evacuation and/or drainage of hematoma, extradural or subdural
	(For bilateral procedure, report 61154 with modifier 50)

EXAMPLE 16.2

A patient had an intracranial lesion that required a biopsy. To begin the procedure, the surgeon made an incision into the scalp and peeled it back. She then placed a burr drill over the area of the skull under which the lesion was located and used the drill to create a hole in the cranium. Once access to the brain was obtained, the surgeon located the lesion and used a forceps to obtain a piece for biopsy. She then sutured the scalp back into place over the burr hole, which will remain in the skull. This procedure should be reported with code 61140, *Burr hole(s) or trephine; with biopsy of brain or intracranial lesion*.

LET'S TRY ONE 16.1

A trauma patient with an extradural hematoma was brought to surgery. The surgeon created a single burr hole for evacuation of the hematoma. What is the appropriate code for this procedure? _____

Craniectomy or Craniotomy Procedures

When a larger portion of the skull beyond a burr hole or trephined hole needs to be removed for surgery access, a craniotomy or craniectomy is performed. In a **craniotomy**, a portion of the skull is temporarily removed and then replaced once the surgery has been completed. A **craniectomy** is similar to a craniotomy in that a portion of the skull is removed, but the piece of the skull is not immediately replaced. Craniectomies are usually performed to relieve swelling in the brain due to traumatic injury.

A&P Review

The tentorium cerebelli, a fold of dura mater over the posterior cranial fossa, covers the cerebellum. *Supratentorial* refers to a location above the tentorium cerebelli, while *infratentorial* means below this structure.

Like the codes for twist drill, burr hole, and trephine procedures, the codes for craniectomies and craniotomies (61304 through 61576) are assigned based on the purpose of the procedure and the anatomical site. A **cranial suture** is a fibrous joint where the skull bones meet. For a patient with craniosynostosis, the surgeon retracts the scalp over the fused suture lines, and the bones of the skull are cut and reshaped into a more anatomically correct position. While treatment of single or multiple cranial sutures can be reported using codes from the Craniectomy or Craniotomy category, if a full reconstruction of the defect to the skull created by the surgery is performed, it should be reported using cranioplasty codes from the Musculoskeletal System Surgery subsection. Instructional notes in the CPT® codebook will help you to remember this distinction, as shown in Figure 16.5.

Figure 16.5 Craniectomy Codes Followed by Instructional Notes for Reconstruction

61550	Craniectomy for craniosynostosis; single cranial suture
61552	multiple cranial sutures
	(For cranial reconstruction for orbital hypertelorism, see 21260-21263)
	(For reconstruction, see 21172-21180)

EXAMPLE 16.3

A trauma patient with a subdural hematoma (identified by CT scan) was taken to surgery for evacuation of the hematoma. A craniectomy was performed, and the infratentorial subdural hematoma was removed using suction. The dura mater was sutured closed, the skull pieces were screwed together, and the scalp was closed in layered sutures. This procedure was reported with code 61314, *Craniectomy or craniotomy for evacuation of hematoma, infratentorial; extradural or subdural*.

Surgery of Skull Base

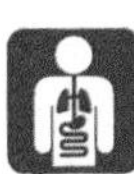

A&P Review

Fossa refers to any depression, hollow, or channel. Cranial (or cerebral) fossae are the depressions on the inside floor of the cranium.

The **skull base** is made up of the regions of the anterior, middle, and posterior cranial fossae, as shown in Figure 16.6. The CPT® codebook introduces this category with notes on 3 groupings of operations to remove lesions involving the skull base. These groups of codes correspond to the separate types of procedures that are typically performed during the same operative episode to minimize the risk of serious infections:

- the **approach procedure**: describes the method used to reach the lesion;
- the **definitive procedure**: describes the resection, excision, or other treatment of the lesion;
- the **repair/reconstruction procedure**: describes how the skull base is restored following the approach and definitive procedures.

Figure 16.6 Skull Base Surgeries Anatomical Sites

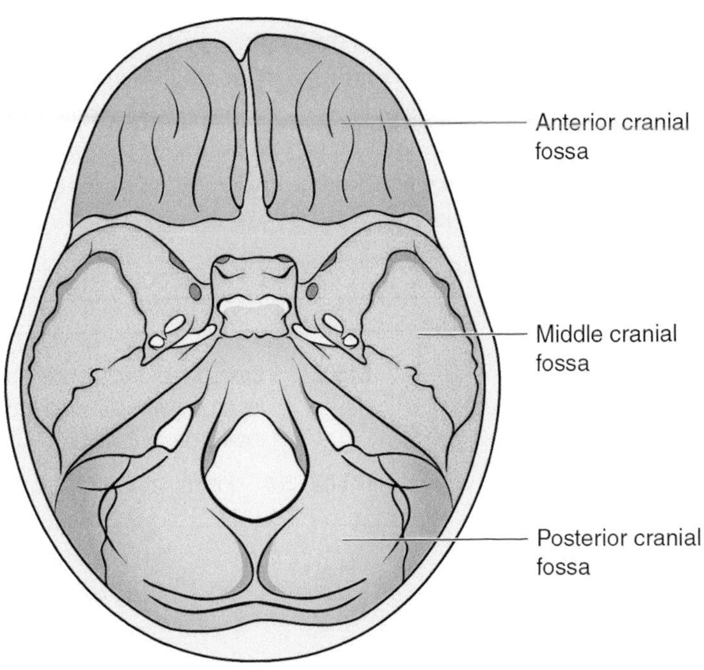

</> Coding for CMS

When both surgeons report the same surgery code with modifier 62, *Two surgeons*, CMS splits the reimbursement between them. When modifier 51, *Multiple procedures*, is used, the second procedure is reduced to 50% of the CMS allowable rate.

Surgeons often work together when performing skull base surgeries. For example, the first surgeon performs the approach procedure, while a second surgeon performs the definitive procedure of lesion removal, and a third surgeon performs the repair procedure. In this case, each surgeon would report 1 code for the portion of the skull base surgery for which he or she was responsible. A surgeon who performs more than a single procedure would report a separate code for each procedure. In this case, the surgeon would add modifier 51, *Multiple procedures*, to the end of the code for the secondary and any additional procedures. If both surgeons performed the same procedure, modifier 62, *Two surgeons*, would be applied to the surgery code.

Skull Base Surgery Approach Procedures

In the CPT® codebook, you will notice that the codes for skull base approach procedures are divided by anatomical site: anterior cranial fossa, middle cranial fossa, and posterior cranial fossa. Within each anatomical site, the codes are assigned according to the specific approach to the lesion or defect at the skull base. For example, code 61590 describes an infratemporal, pre-auricular approach. This means that the approach is located below the **temporal fossa** (on the skull just below the temporal lines) and in front of the patient's external ear. Code 61591 describes an infratemporal post-auricular approach, which is located below the temporal fossa but behind the external ear.

Skull Base Surgery Definitive Procedures

Definitive procedure codes cover the biopsy or removal of the lesion by resection or excision. Some tumors may extend along the carotid artery, requiring the surgeon to preserve this artery or manage aneurysms or malformations. The Definitive Procedures subcategory also includes add-on codes (61610 through 61612) for transection or ligation of the carotid artery, both with and without repair. Like the approach procedures, the definitive procedures are separated by anatomical site as follows: base of anterior cranial fossa, base of middle cranial fossa, and base of posterior cranial fossa. The codes are assigned according to the extradural or intradural location of the lesion. Codes for resection of intradural lesions include dural repair with or without graft, as shown in Figure 16.7.

Figure 16.7 Code for Resection of Intradural Lesion Including Dural Repair

61607	Resection or excision of neoplastic, vascular or infectious lesion of parasellar area, cavernous sinus, clivus or midline skull base; extradural
61608	intradural, including dural repair, with or without graft

EXAMPLE 16.4

A patient had an extradural lesion removed from the base of the middle cranial fossa (midline skull base). The surgeon used an infratemporal pre-auricular approach to the middle cranial fossa. The surgeon reports 2 codes:

- The approach procedure is reported with code 61590, *Infratemporal pre-auricular approach to middle cranial fossa (parapharyngeal space, infratemporal and midline skull base, nasopharynx), with or without disarticulation of the mandible, including parotidectomy, craniotomy, decompression and/or mobilization of the facial nerve and/or petrous carotid artery*.
- The definitive procedure of lesion removal is reported with code 61607, *Resection or excision of neoplastic, vascular or infectious lesion of parasellar area, cavernous sinus, clivus or midline skull base, extradural*.

Skull Base Surgery Repair and/or Reconstruction Procedures

The Repair and/or Reconstruction of Surgical Defects of Skull Base subcategory contains only 2 codes, 61618 and 61619, both to repair a cerebrospinal fluid leak. Code 61618 is reported when the surgeon uses a dural graft obtained from fascia; tensor fascia lata; adipose tissue; or pericranium, homologous, or synthetic grafts. Code 61619 is reported when the surgeon uses a vascularized pedicle graft or myocutaneous flap graft. If the defect that was created in removing the lesion needs to be repaired by extensive dural grafting, cranioplasty, or skin grafts, a separate code from the appropriate surgery subsection (such as the Integumentary System Surgery subsection for skin grafts) is reported instead of code 61618 or 61619.

CONCEPTS CHECKPOINT 16.2

Answer true or false to the following statements.

1. _____ If a burr hole is performed in the same operative session as a craniotomy, both procedure codes may be reported.
2. _____ Subdural procedures are performed above or outside of the dura mater.
3. _____ One surgeon may not report codes for both a skull base surgery approach procedure and a definitive skull base procedure on the same date of service.

Cerebrospinal Fluid (CSF) Shunt Procedures

Cerebrospinal fluid shunts are implanted in patients suffering from a condition known as **hydrocephalus**, which is literally translated as "water on the brain." In patients with hydrocephalus, an accumulation of **cerebrospinal fluid (CSF)** causes the ventricles in the brain to become enlarged. The pressure from the excess fluid inside the head can cause symptoms such as difficulty walking, mild dementia, or impaired bladder control. Once inserted, the cerebrospinal shunt drains the CSF from the brain into another part of the body, where it can be absorbed.

A cerebrospinal shunt is composed of 3 parts: the collection catheter, which is placed in the ventricles to collect the CSF; a one-way valve, which controls how much fluid flows out and does not allow for fluid to regurgitate back into the ventricle; and an exit catheter, which drains the CSF to another part of the body (often the peritoneal cavity). The codes in the CSF Shunt category are assigned according to the location of the exit catheter. Figure 16.8 shows a ventriculo-peritoneal shunt, so named because the fluid is drained from the ventricle via the exit catheter into the peritoneal cavity.

Figure 16.8 Ventriculo-Peritoneal Shunt

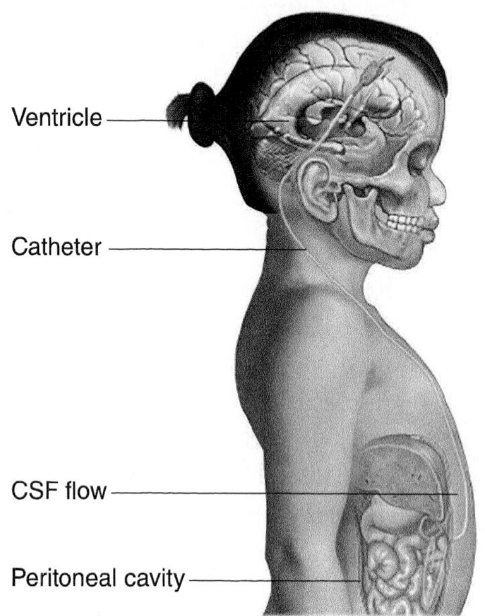

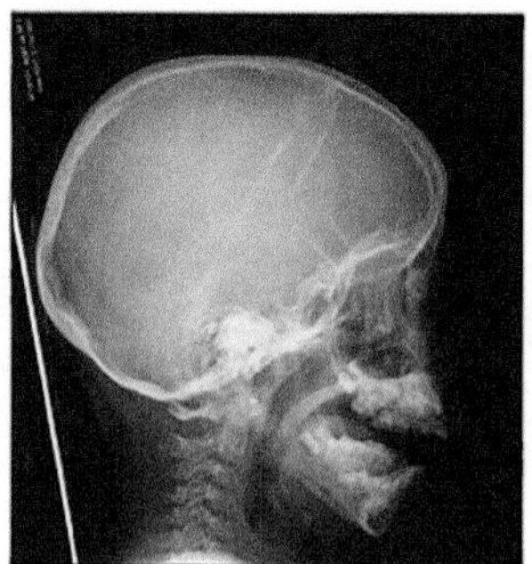

Inside the OR

To create a shunt to drain the CSF from the ventricles to the peritoneal cavity, the surgeon first makes an incision into the scalp and retracts it. A burr hole is drilled, and the first portion of the shunt is placed in the ventricles so that CSF begins to flow through it. The other end of the shunt is tunneled subcutaneously toward the peritoneal cavity. The end from the ventricle is connected to the end in the peritoneum, and the shunt is tested for patency. The dura is sutured closed, and then the scalp is replaced and sutured closed.

Spine and Spinal Cord (Codes 62263-63746)

The **spine**, also known as the **vertebral column**, is made up of a collection of small bones called vertebrae that extend from the skull to the lower back. The cervical, thoracic, and lumbar vertebrae are named according to the region and position on the vertebral column in which they are found, from top to bottom:

- cervical vertebrae are numbered C1 through C7;
- thoracic vertebrae are numbered T1 through T12;

- lumbar vertebrae are numbered L1 through L5;
- sacral vertebrae are numbered S1 through S5 and are fused together to form a triangular-shaped bone;
- the 4 coccyx vertebrae are fused together to form the tailbone.

Intervertebral disks are pads of cartilage that are found between the vertebrae. The spine provides a protective outer covering for the **spinal cord**, which is a band of nervous tissue that connects the brain to the rest of the body. Figure 16.9 provides an illustration of the vertebral column; the intervertebral disks are represented by the blue color that is visible between each pair of vertebrae.

Figure 16.9 Vertebral Column

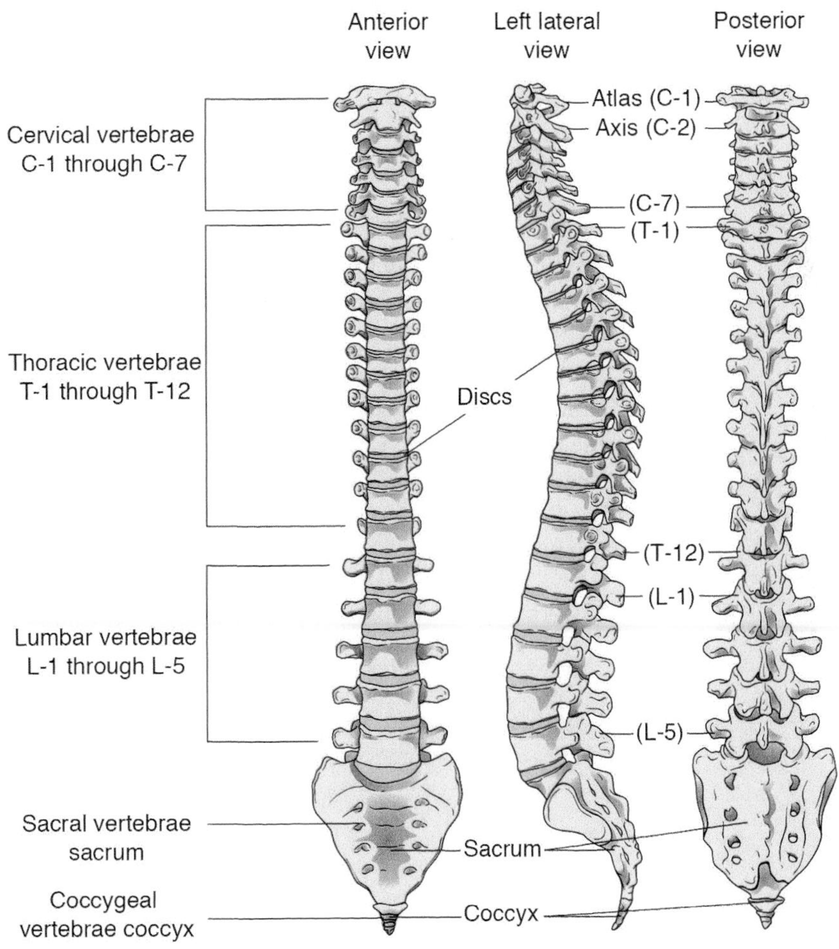

The Spine and Spinal Cord heading in the CPT® codebook includes the following categories of procedures:

- Injection, Drainage, or Aspiration;
- Catheter Implantation;
- Reservoir/Pump Implantation;

- Posterior Extradural Laminotomy, or Laminectomy for Exploration/Decompression of Neural Elements, or Excision of Herniated Intervertebral Discs;
- Transpedicular or Costovertebral Approach for Posterolateral Extradural Exploration/Decompression;
- Anterior or Anterolateral Approach for Extradural Exploration/Decompression;
- Lateral Extracavitary Approach for Extradural Exploration/Decompression;
- Incision;
- Excision by Laminectomy of Lesion Other Than Herniated Disc;
- Excision, Anterior or Anterolateral Approach, Intraspinal Lesion;
- Stereotaxis;
- Stereotactic Radiosurgery (Spinal);
- Neurostimulators (Spinal);
- Repair;
- Shunt, Spinal CSF.

This chapter will discuss codes for procedures such as spinal injections, catheter placement, laminectomy, corpectomy, and excision of spinal lesions. Codes are assigned based on the site of the procedure and/or the specific area of the vertebral column. Many procedures performed on the spine and spinal column may be performed with radiological supervision and interpretation of epidurography (imaging of the epidural space), which should be reported separately with code 72275 from the Radiology section. Fluoroscopic guidance should be reported with code 77003 from the Radiology section if it is not included in the CPT® code. This will be indicated by instructional notes within the tabular list, as shown in Figure 16.10.

Figure 16.10 Instructional Note for Fluoroscopic Imaging for Spinal Procedures

62267	Percutaneous aspiration within the nucleus pulposus, intervertebral disc, or paravertebral tissue for diagnostic purposes
	(For imaging, use 77003)
	(Do not report 62267 in conjunction with 10022, 20225, 62287, 62290, 62291)

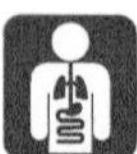

A&P Review

The subarachnoid space is the layer of meninges located between the arachnoid and the pia mater. The epidural space is located outside of the dura mater.

Spinal Injection, Drainage, or Aspiration Procedures

Many Spine and Spinal Cord codes report procedures for diagnostic and therapeutic injection and drainage. Injection to the spine and spinal cord of a **neurolytic substance**—a chemical such as phenol, alcohol, or glycerol that destroys nerve tissue or adhesions in an attempt to relieve pain—is reported with codes 62280 through 62282, depending on the site of the injection. Code 62280 is reported when the injection is administered at the subarachnoid level, as shown in Figure 16.11, while codes 62281 and 62282 are reported for injections at the epidural level. Code 62281 is reported for an epidural injection to the cervical or thoracic region, and code 62282 is reported for an epidural injection to the lumbar or sacral (caudal) region.

Figure 16.11 Illustration of Epidural and Subarachnoid Spaces for Injection

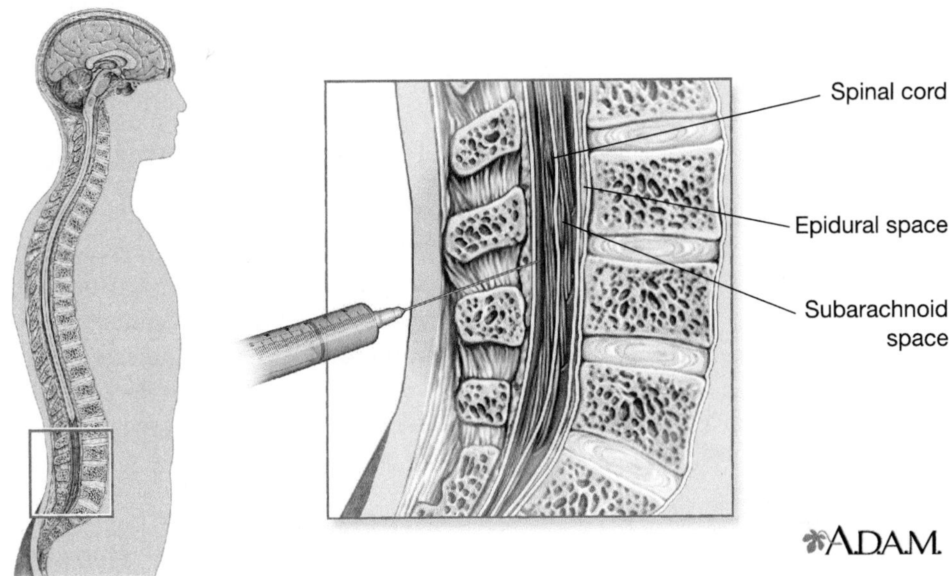

Spinal injections of substances other than neurolytics are reported with codes 62320 through 62323. These codes cover injections of anesthetics, antispasmodics, opioids, steroids, and other solutions used to relieve pain. Injection or catheter placement performed without imaging guidance in the subarachnoid or epidural space is reported with code 62320 for the cervical or thoracic region and code 62322 for the lumbar or sacral (caudal) region. If the injection is performed with imaging guidance, code 62321 or 62323 is reported, depending on the anatomical site.

Placement of a catheter to perform more than 1 injection on the same date of service is reported only once. If the catheter is left in place to be used for continuous infusion or intermittent injections over several days, codes 62324 through 62327 should be reported for the initial placement, depending on the anatomical site and the use of imaging guidance. Placement and management of catheters or pumps for longer-term drug administration are reported with codes 62350 through 62370. Daily management of continuous epidural or subarachnoid drug administration for a hospital patient should be reported with code 01996 from the Anesthesia section of the codebook.

LET'S TRY ONE **16.2**

A 55-year-old male complained of constant lower back pain. His condition did not respond to physical therapy or medication. To attempt to numb the pain, a surgeon performed an epidural anesthetic injection into the L4-L5 interspace of the patient's spine. What is the appropriate code for this procedure? _____

A **lumbar puncture**, also referred to as a **spinal puncture** or **spinal tap**, is a procedure in which a needle is inserted into the lumbar spine to obtain cerebrospinal fluid. Lumbar puncture can be performed for diagnostic or therapeutic purposes. A diagnostic lumbar puncture may be done to examine the CSF to rule out conditions like meningitis or subarachnoid hemorrhage and is reported using code 62270, *Spinal puncture, lumbar, diagnostic.* A therapeutic lumbar puncture is performed for drainage of CSF to lessen CSF pressure and is reported with code 62272, *Spinal puncture, therapeutic, for drainage of cerebrospinal fluid (by needle or catheter).*

Laminotomy, Laminectomy, and Decompression

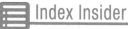

RED FLAG

Make sure to read the operative report carefully to determine whether a laminotomy or a laminectomy was performed.

Lamina is the portion of a vertebra that covers the nerve root. The lamina is a pair of plates that cover the vertebral arches and fuse together in the center to provide a base for the spinous process. A **laminectomy** is surgery performed to remove the lamina, thereby relieving pressure on the spinal cord and nerves. Relief of this pressure is called **decompression**. A **laminotomy** or **hemilaminectomy** is different from a laminectomy in that it involves the removal of only part of the lamina. Patients with spinal stenosis, spondylolisthesis (forward displacement of vertebra), or herniated discs who have not responded to medical treatment may require a decompression laminotomy or laminectomy to relieve pain.

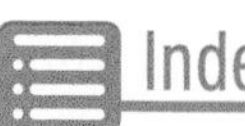

Index Insider

Laminotomy is not a main term in the alphabetic Index. The coder must go to the term *hemilaminectomy* to find the correct code range for the procedure performed.

Laminectomy, laminotomy, and decompression procedure codes are assigned based on the approach (posterior, anterior, lateral, or costovertebral); whether the site is extradural or intradural; and the vertebra involved (cervical, thoracic, lumbar, or sacral). A laminectomy (either unilateral or bilateral) is reported with codes 63045 through 63048. Laminectomy codes are reported based on how many vertebral segments were operated on, and add-on codes should be used for each additional segment after the first 1. A laminotomy or hemilaminectomy is reported with codes 63020 through 63044, and modifier 50, *Bilateral procedure*, should be used if the procedure was performed on both sides. Laminotomy and hemilaminectomy codes are reported based on how many vertebral interspaces were operated on, and add-on codes should be used for each additional interspace after the first 1, as shown in Figure 16.12.

Figure 16.12 Examples of Codes for Laminotomy and Hemilaminectomy

63020	Laminotomy (hemilaminectomy), with decompression of nerve root(s), including partial facetectomy, foraminotomy and/or excision of herniated intervertebral disc; 1 interspace, cervical
	(For bilateral procedure, report 63020 with modifier 50)
63030	1 interspace, lumbar
	(For bilateral procedure, report 63030 with modifier 50)
63035	each additional interspace, cervical or lumbar (List separately in addition to code for primary procedure)
	(Use 63035 in conjunction with 63020-63030)
	(For bilateral procedure, report 63035 with modifier 50)
	(For percutaneous endoscopic approach, see 0274T, 0275T)

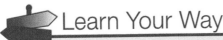

Learn Your Way

To understand the way spinal surgery is performed, the Felder-Silverman learning styles research indicates some students who are visual learners find it helpful to watch the procedure.

Visit the Spine-Health website at http://Coding.ParadigmEducation.com/SpinalSurgery to view an animated video of a laminectomy with narration explaining the procedure.

EXAMPLE 16.5

A surgeon performed a hemilaminectomy for a patient with spinal stenosis. The surgeon made an incision through the patient's back (a posterior approach) and removed part of the lamina and disc in 2 intervertebral spaces (interspaces), C3-C4 and C4-C5. This procedure is reported with 2 codes: 63020, *Laminotomy (hemilaminectomy), with decompression of nerve root(s), including partial facetectomy, foraminotomy and/or excision of herniated intervertebral disc; 1 interspace, cervical*; and add-on code 63035 for 1 additional interspace. Note that the excision of the herniated discs is included in these codes and therefore is not reported separately.

LET'S TRY ONE 16.3

A 49-year-old male with spondylolisthesis required decompression of the nerve root for pain control. Using a posterior approach, the surgeon performed a hemilaminectomy and decompression of nerve root with foraminotomy at L4-L5. What is the appropriate code for this procedure? _____

Extradural Exploration/Decompression: Corpectomy and Discectomy

Procedures under the Anterior or Anterolateral Approach for Extradural Exploration/Decompression heading (codes 63075 through 63091) include discectomy and vertebral corpectomy performed through the anterior approach. Figure 16.13 shows the anatomy associated with a **vertebral corpectomy**, which is the removal of part or all of the **vertebral body**, a thick segment of bone in each vertebra, and the intervertebral discs above and below the segment. This procedure is performed to relieve pressure on the spinal cord and nerve roots.

Figure 16.13 Anatomy of a Vertebra

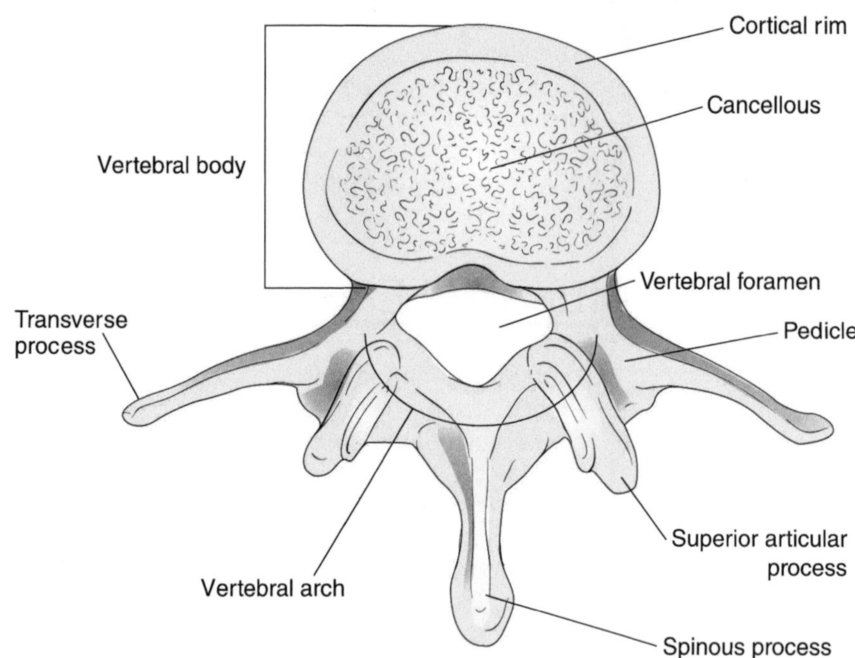

Coding Clicks

To view a video of a corpectomy, visit http://Coding.ParadigmEducation.com/Corpectomy.

Inside the OR

Made from stainless steel, tissue nippers are very sharp, compact cutting instruments. Nippers range in size from a blade length of 2 mm to 14 mm. Nippers may also be called *cutting forceps*.

Corpectomy codes are assigned according to the approach (anterior, transthoracic, thoracolumbar, or retroperitoneal) and the region from which the vertebral body was removed (cervical, thoracic, lumbar, or sacral). A separate codebook category contains 3 codes for the lateral extracavitary approach, 63101 through 63103. The codebook provides add-on codes to separately report each additional vertebral body removed after the first 1. However, when the discs above or below the vertebral segment are removed, no additional code is reported. Bone grafts, arthrodesis, and spinal instrumentation should be reported separately when performed in conjunction with a corpectomy.

EXAMPLE **16.6**

A vertebral corpectomy of T3 was performed using a transthoracic approach with decompression of nerve root and discectomy of T2-T3 and T3-T4. This procedure is reported with code 63085, *Vertebral corpectomy (vertebral body resection), partial or complete, transthoracic approach with decompression of spinal cord and/or nerve root(s); thoracic, single segment*. Since the discs that were removed are above (T2-T3) and below (T3-T4) the vertebral body (T3) that was removed, no additional code is reported for that portion of the procedure.

LET'S TRY ONE **16.4**

Vertebral corpectomy of L2 was performed using a retroperitoneal approach. Decompression of nerve root was completed. The surgeon removed the L1-L2 disc as well as the L2-L3 disc using nipper instruments. What is the appropriate code(s) for this procedure? _____

CONCEPTS CHECKPOINT **16.3**

Answer true or false to the following statements.

1. _____ A lumbar epidural injection of anesthetic or steroid is reported with code 62320.
2. _____ To accurately report a code for the injection of a neurolytic substance into the spine or spinal cord, you need to know whether the substance was injected into the epidural space or the subarachnoid space.
3. _____ A laminectomy is the surgical removal of a vertebral body.

Extracranial Nerves, Peripheral Nerves, and Autonomic Nervous System (Codes 64400-64999)

The Extracranial Nerves, Peripheral Nerves, and Autonomic Nervous System heading in the CPT® codebook includes the following categories of procedures:

- Introduction/Injection of Anesthetic Agent (Nerve Block), Diagnostic or Therapeutic;
- Neurostimulators (Peripheral Nerve);
- Destruction by Neurolytic Agent (eg, Chemical, Thermal, Electrical or Radiofrequency);
- Chemodenervation;
- Neuroplasty (Exploration, Neurolysis or Nerve Decompression);
- Transection or Avulsion;
- Excision;
- Neurorrhaphy;
- Neurorrhaphy with Nerve Graft, Vein Graft, or Conduit.

The codes cover procedures on the somatic nerves, autonomic nerves, paravertebral spinal nerves, sympathetic nerves, and peripheral nerves. This chapter will discuss procedures for pain management by nerve blocks and nerve destruction, as well as neurostimulators, neuroplasty, and neurorrhaphy.

Introduction/Injection of Anesthetic Agent (Nerve Block), Diagnostic or Therapeutic

The procedures in this category involve injections of anesthetic agents, steroids, and other diagnostic or therapeutic agents into nerves located in the spine and other anatomical sites. Nerves that cause pain to a patient can be numbed with an injection of anesthetic during a procedure called a **nerve block**. Nerve blocks can be administered

RED FLAG

Instructional notes in the tabular list state that anesthesia code 01996, *Daily hospital management of epidural or subarachnoid continuous drug administration*, may not be reported with the codes for continuous infusion of anesthetic agents found in the Introduction/Injection of Anesthetic Agent (Nerve Block), Diagnostic, or Therapeutic category.

Coding Clicks

To view a video of a patient undergoing a transforaminal epidural injection in the lumbar spine using fluoroscopic guidance and contrast, visit http://Coding.ParadigmEducation.com/Epidural.

Coding Clicks

To view an animation of a facet joint injection, visit http://Coding.ParadigmEducation.com/FacetJointInjection.

for therapeutic or diagnostic reasons. In a therapeutic nerve block, the anesthetic is injected simply to control pain, while in a diagnostic nerve block, an anesthetic with a specific duration is injected to determine the source of a patient's pain. The CPT® codebook groups procedures in this category by those for somatic nerves, paravertebral spinal nerves and branches, and autonomic nerves. Further anatomical criteria distinguish different types of injections and blocks.

Transforaminal injections are given through the **foramen**, the opening in the vertebra formed by the vertebral body and arch (see Figure 16.13). Epidural injections given using a transforaminal approach are reported with codes 64479 through 64484, depending upon the region of the spine into which the injection was administered (cervical, thoracic, lumbar, or sacral) and whether the injection was an initial or additional procedure. Imaging guidance and any contrast injections are included in these codes.

EXAMPLE **16.7**

A 44-year-old male presented to the pain clinic for an epidural injection to the L4 level. Using fluoroscopic guidance, the surgeon injected an anesthetic agent transforaminally into the epidural space. This procedure is reported with code 64483, *Injection(s), anesthetic agent and/or steroid, transforaminal epidural, with imaging guidance (fluoroscopy or CT); lumbar or sacral, single level.*

Facet joint injections are administered to **facet joints**, the bony surfaces between the vertebrae that articulate with each other. Injections to the facet joints are reported with codes 64490 through 64495, based on the region of the spine into which the injection was administered (cervical, thoracic, lumbar, or sacral) and the number of levels injected, as shown in Figure 16.14.

Figure 16.14 Example of Facet Joint Injection(s) and Add-on Codes With Instructional Notes

64490	Injection(s), diagnostic or therapeutic agent, paravertebral facet (zygapophyseal) joint (or nerves innervating that joint) with image guidance (fluoroscopy or CT), cervical or thoracic; single level
+ 64491	second level (List separately in addition to code for primary procedure)
	(Use 64491 in conjunction with 64490)
+ 64492	third and any additional level(s) (List separately in addition to code for primary procedure)
	(Do not report 64492 more than once per day)
	(Use 64992 in conjunction with 64990, 64991)

LET'S TRY ONE **16.5**

Assign procedure codes to each of the following.

1. A 49-year-old female patient with trigeminal neuralgia presented to the pain clinic for a trigeminal nerve block. The surgeon injected an anesthetic agent into the trigeminal nerve. _____
2. A 55-year-old male reported to the pain clinic for a facet injection to C4. The physician injected an anesthetic into the paravertebral facet joint at C4 using imaging guidance. _____
3. A 29-year-old female with sciatica agreed to a sciatic nerve injection for pain relief. The physician performed a single injection of an anesthetic into the sciatic nerve. _____

Neurostimulators (Peripheral Nerve)

A **neurostimulator** is a device that delivers mild electrical signals through thin wires called *electrodes* or *leads*. A **neurostimulation system** is made up of a generator that creates electrical impulses and the electrodes/leads that deliver the impulses to the nerves. In an implantable system, the generator is placed into a surgically created subcutaneous pocket and then connected to electrodes implanted through the skin and into the tissue to stimulate the target nerve. The electrical signals can block pain sensations in the area of the nerve or stimulate paralyzed muscles to prevent atrophy. **Peripheral neurostimulators** work to transmit impulses to nerves outside of the brain and spinal cord. **Gastric neurostimulators** are indicated for patients with gastroparesis (partial paralysis of the stomach muscles). Electronic analysis and programming of the pulse generators are reported with codes 95970 through 95975 in the Medicine codebook section.

When a neurostimulator system is implanted (as opposed to being surface applied), codes are provided to report insertion and removal of the system as well as the separate components of the system. There are also codes that describe application of neurostimulation. The coding division of labor follows:

- Codes 64550 and 64566 describe neurostimulation treatment: in 64550, a non-invasive surface neurostimulator is applied on top of the skin; in 64566, posterior tibial neurostimulation treatment includes programming.
- Codes 64553 through 64561 and 64575 through 64581 report the percutaneous implantation of neurostimulator electrodes, differentiated by nerve location: cranial nerves, peripheral motor or sensory nerves, sacral nerves, and neuromuscular nerves. Sacral nerve implants create impulses that cause the bladder muscle to contract so patients with conditions such as urinary urge incontinence, urgency-frequency syndrome, and urinary retention can void more normally. Neuromuscular placements stimulate a specific area of muscle.

- Codes 64568 through 64570 report the implantation, revision, replacement, and removal of neurostimulator electrodes and a pulse generator for a cranial nerve, such as the vagus nerve. In this procedure, the surgeon creates a pocket in the left chest for the pulse generator. The pulse generator is placed and connected to the previously placed electrode, which is attached to the vagus nerve in the left side of the neck, as shown in Figure 16.15. Indications for surgery for insertion of a vagal nerve stimulator include major depressive disorders, obsessive-compulsive disorder, epilepsy, atypical facial pain, and neck pain.
- Codes 64585, 64590, and 64595 report various procedures involved with revision, removal, insertion, or replacement of electrode arrays, pulse generators, or receivers. Code 64590 reports insertion or replacement of either peripheral or gastric neurostimulator pulse generators or receivers. Code 64595 is also reported if the device is malfunctioning and a new pulse generator is placed or if the device is removed because it is no longer needed.

</> Coding for CMS

CMS will provide benefits for insertion of a neurostimulation system for urinary urge incontinence, urgency-frequency syndrome, and urinary retention. Patients must have failed conventional therapy (behavioral and pharmacological) and be an appropriate candidate for surgery under anesthesia. (For more information, refer to the Medicare Claims Processing Manual Pub 100-4, 32.40.1, or visit http://Coding.ParadigmEducation.com/Neurostimulation.)

Figure 16.15 Implantation of Neurostimulator Electrodes and Pulse Generator for Vagus Nerve Stimulation

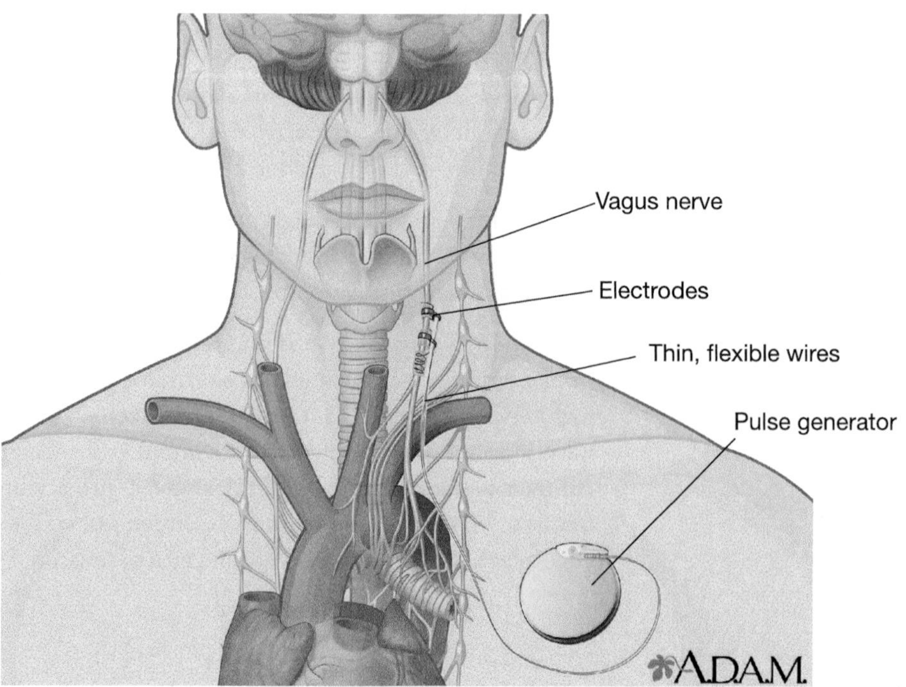

EXAMPLE 16.8

A 33-year-old female with obsessive-compulsive disorder (OCD) required a vagal neurostimulator implant. The surgeon inserted a cranial nerve neurostimulator electrode array attached to the vagus nerve. The pulse generator was placed in a subcutaneous pocket and attached to the electrodes in the left side of the neck. This procedure was reported with code 64568, *Incision for implantation of cranial nerve (eg, vagus nerve) neurostimulator electrode array and pulse generator*.

LET'S TRY ONE 16.6

A 33-year-old female with OCD required a removal of a vagal neurostimulator system that had been previously implanted. The surgeon made an incision over the unit and removed the cranial nerve neurostimulator electrode array and pulse generator. The skin incision was then closed with sutures. What is the appropriate code for this procedure? _____

Destruction by Neurolytic Agent (eg, Chemical, Thermal, Electrical, or Radiofrequency), Chemodenervation

Nerve destruction is performed by injecting a nerve with phenol or alcohol (a chemical neurolytic) to block pain or motor control to stop spasms or contractions. Nerve destruction can last from 3 to 12 months. **Chemodenervation** is performed by injecting a neurotoxin, such as botulinum toxin type A (best known under the brand name Botox), to paralyze dysfunctional muscle tissue by blocking the nerve signals. Chemodenervation usually lasts 3 to 4 months.

Destruction by neurolytic agents and chemodenervation are reported with codes 64600 through 64681, subcategorized into somatic nerves or sympathetic nerves. Figure 16.16 shows an example of codes assigned based on the site and number of injections: Chemodenervation of 1 extremity is reported with code 64642 when performed on 1 to 4 muscles and code 64644 when performed on 5 or more muscles. Add-on codes 64643 and 64645 are used to report additional sites. Codebook parenthetic instructions provide helpful reminders to use the add-on codes in conjunction with the base codes and report only 1 base code per session. One or more of the additional extremity codes (64643 or 64645) may be reported in addition to the base code. Chemodenervation of the trunk muscles (erector spinae, paraspinal muscles, rectus abdominous, and obliques) is reported with codes 64646 and 64647.

Figure 16.16 Chemodenervation Codes

64642	Chemodenervation of one extremity; 1-4 muscle(s)
+64643	each additional extremity, 1-4 muscle(s) (List separately in addition to code for primary procedure)
	(Use 64643 in conjunction with 64642, 64644)
64644	Chemodenervation of one extremity; 5 or more muscles
+64645	each additional extremity, 5 or more muscles (List separately in addition to code for primary procedure)
	(Use 64645 in conjunction with 64644)
64646	Chemodenervation of trunk muscle(s); 1-5 muscle(s)
64647	6 or more muscles
	(Report either 64646 or 64647 only once per session)

RED FLAG

Watch for codes out of sequence in the Destruction by Neurolytic Agent (eg, Chemical, Thermal, Electrical, or Radiofrequency), Chemodenervation category. Codes 64633 through 64636 are located between codes 64620 and 64630 in the tabular list.

EXAMPLE **16.9**

A 72-year-old female with a history of stroke was suffering from spasms in both lower limbs and underwent chemodenervation to correct the problem. The biceps femoris, rectus femoris, and tibialis anterior of her right lower limb were injected with a neurotoxin. The rectus femoris, vastus medialis, and vastus lateralis of her left lower limb were also injected. This procedure was reported with code 64642, *Chemodenervation of one extremity; 1-4 muscles*, and code 64643, *Chemodenervation of one extremity; each additional extremity, 1-4 muscle(s)*.

LET'S TRY ONE **16.7**

A 54-year-old male with multiple sclerosis suffered from spasms in both of his upper extremities. Chemodenervation of the left upper limb was performed, with injections to the biceps, triceps, and brachioradialis muscles. The biceps and brachioradialis muscles in the right upper extremity were also injected. What is the appropriate code(s) for this procedure? _____

CONCEPTS CHECKPOINT **16.4**

Answer true or false to the following statements.

1. _____ Botulinum toxin type A (Botox) is considered an anesthetic agent.
2. _____ Up to 4 injections to muscles of 1 extremity for chemodenervation should be reported with 1 code.
3. _____ Components of a neurostimulator system include corticosteroids, electrodes, and a pulse generator.
4. _____ Nerve destruction can be accomplished by injecting a nerve with alcohol.
5. _____ Two separate codes are required to report placement of a gastric neurostimulation system.

Neuroplasty (Exploration, Neurolysis, or Nerve Decompression)

Index Insider

There are several ways to locate the code for neuroplasty of the median nerve, and using the main term *Neuroplasty* is not the most efficient. Using the main terms *Neuroplasty* or *Decompression, Nerve* will provide you with a wide range of codes. Using the main term *Carpal Tunnel* or *Carpal Tunnel Syndrome* is a more direct route to the correct code. *Release, Carpal Tunnel* is another good way to locate the correct code for neuroplasty of the median nerve at the carpal tunnel.

Neuroplasty is a procedure to repair or restore a nerve by freeing it from scar tissue or adhesions. This is done by making an incision and dissecting the surrounding tissue away from the nerve. A common neuroplastic procedure is the release of the median nerve at the carpal tunnel to correct **carpal tunnel syndrome (CTS)**, an injury caused by repetitive motion of the wrist that commonly affects cashiers, office workers, and factory assembly-line workers. CTS is caused by the compression of the medial nerve as it passes under the transverse carpal ligament. Symptoms of CTS include numbness, tingling, weakness, and pain in the affected area. In a carpal tunnel release, the median nerve is decompressed by freeing the nerve inside of the carpal tunnel, restoring feeling to the hand. Like other surgical procedures, neuroplasty codes are assigned based on the anatomical site. In this example, carpal tunnel release performed as an open procedure is reported with code 64721, *Neuroplasty and/or transposition; median nerve at carpal tunnel.* Carpal tunnel release performed endoscopically is reported with code 29848 from the Musculoskeletal subsection, as instructed in the codebook parenthetic note. Laterality should be identified by using the RT (*Right side*) or LT (*Left side*) modifier.

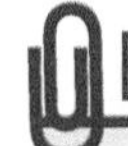

EXAMPLE 16.10

A 42-year-old female transcriptionist developed carpal tunnel syndrome of the right wrist. Her surgeon performed an open carpal tunnel release. The procedure is reported with code 64721 - RT, *Neuroplasty and/or transposition; median nerve at carpal tunnel - right side.*

LET'S TRY ONE 16.8

A 55-year-old male assembly-line worker developed carpal tunnel syndrome of the left wrist. The surgeon performed an open carpal tunnel release. How would this procedure be reported? _____

Neurorrhaphy

Neurorrhaphy is a procedure to repair a nerve by suturing. Neurorrhaphy is performed to restore sensation to a nerve that is damaged or partially severed by a traumatic injury. The damage at the ends of the nerve may be removed if necessary, and the undamaged nerve tissue is then sutured together (or a graft is placed).

Neurorrhaphy codes are determined by the site of the repair; whether or not a graft was used; and, if a graft was used, the type of graft (nerve or vein). Examples of codes for neurorrhaphy without grafting are 64831, reported for a suture of a single finger or toe nerve, and its associated add-on code, 64832, reported for each additional digital nerve repaired.

EXAMPLE 16.11

A 38-year-old construction worker lacerated her second and third fingers of the right hand with an electric saw. The wounds were deep and nerves were damaged, requiring neurorrhaphy. The surgeon sutured digital nerves on the second and third fingers. Reported for this procedure are 64831 - F6, *Suture of digital nerve, hand or foot; 1 nerve - right hand, second digit*, and 64832 - F7, *Suture of digital nerve, hand or foot; each additional nerve - right hand, third digit*. The HCPCS Level II modifiers may or may not be required by the payer and are added here to provide detail.

Code 64834 is reported for repair of common sensory nerves in the hand or foot, and 64835 is reported for repair of the median motor thenar nerve, which supplies motor innervation to the proximal thumb, as shown in Figure 16.17.

Figure 16.17 Illustration of Median Nerve

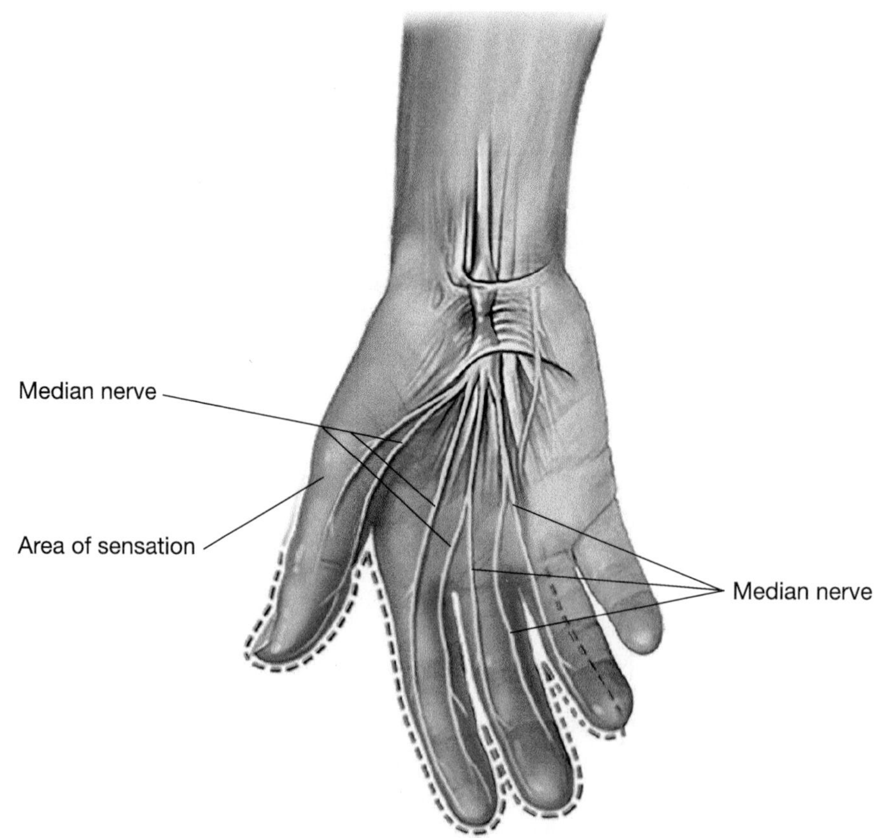

A nerve repair may have been delayed because the initial wound was contaminated. To report secondary or delayed suture, code 64872 is used with the primary procedure code. Repair requiring extensive mobilization or transposition of the nerve is reported with 64874 in addition to the primary procedure code. Repair requiring shortening of the bone of an extremity is reported with 64876 in addition to the primary procedure code.

EXAMPLE 16.12

A 65-year-old female was attacked by her cat and received numerous bites and deep lacerations. A wound in her temple area included damage to the facial nerve. The damaged nerve ends were removed, and the surgeon was able to suture the undamaged ends together without the use of a graft. This neurorrhaphy was reported with code 64865, *Suture of facial nerve; infratemporal, with or without grafting*.

LET'S TRY ONE 16.9

A 13-year-old boy was cutting a cantaloupe and sliced through the palm of his left hand near his thumb. The wound was cleaned, and the damage to the median motor thenar nerve was noted. A neurorrhaphy was performed, and the median motor thenar nerve was sutured. How would this procedure be reported?

____

RED FLAG

Neurorrhaphy procedures are often performed with an operating microscope, which should be coded with 69990, unless the code is listed as exempt from use in the notes above code 69990.

Codes for neurorrhaphy with nerve graft, vein graft, or conduit have their own category. In procedures described with codes 64885 through 64902, the surgeon removes the damaged nerve and replaces it with a nerve graft, which is sutured into place. Codes are assigned depending on the site and length of the graft. Codes 64905 through 64907 are used to report nerve repair using a pedicle from an intact nerve as a donor nerve, which is transferred to the recipient nerve. The first stage of the nerve pedicle transfer is reported with code 64905. The second stage is reported with code 64907 and involves resecting the donor nerve from the recipient nerve and reconnecting it to the original location. Nerve repair using synthetic conduit or vein graft is reported once for each graft. Code 64910 is reported for use of synthetic conduit and a vein allograft, and code 64911 is reported for use of an autogenous vein graft and includes the harvesting of the graft. Code 64912 is reported for nerve repair with nerve allograft, first strand, with add-on code 64913 reported for each additional strand. 64912 and 64913 are new codes for 2018.

Chapter Summary

- If a burr hole is drilled or trephine is performed in the same operative session as craniotomy, only the code for craniotomy is reported.
- Codes for craniectomy or craniotomy are based on the purpose of the procedure and the anatomical site.
- Codes for surgery to remove lesions of the skull base are separated into approach procedures, definitive procedures, and repair/reconstruction procedures. Surgeons involved in the operative session report the code(s) for the portion of the surgery that they performed.

- A cerebrospinal fluid shunt is composed of 3 parts: the collection catheter placed in the ventricles, a valve to control how much fluid flows out, and an exit catheter to drain the fluid to another part of the body. The codes are assigned by the location of the exit catheter.
- Codes for the injection of a neurolytic substance (to destroy nerve tissue or adhesion) are based on the site of the injection.
- Spinal injections of substances other than neurolytics include anesthetics, antispasmodics, opioids, steroids, and other solutions, and the codes are based on the site of the injection and the use of imaging guidance.
- Laminectomy and decompression procedure codes are based on the approach (posterior, anterior, lateral, and costovertebral), whether the site is extradural or intradural, and the vertebra involved (cervical, thoracic, lumbar, or sacral).
- Corpectomy codes are assigned according to approach (anterior, transthoracic, thoracolumbar, or retroperitoneal) and the region from which the vertebral body was removed (cervical, thoracic, lumbar, or sacral).
- Each additional corpectomy is assigned a separate add-on code. When the discs above or below the vertebral segment are removed, no additional code is reported.
- A neurostimulation system is composed of a generator that provides the impulses and electrodes that deliver the impulses to the nerves. The generator is placed into a surgically created subcutaneous pocket and connected to separately implanted electrodes.
- Destruction and chemodenervation codes are assigned based on the site of the injection.
- Neuroplasty is repairing or restoring a nerve by dissecting it free from scar tissue or adhesions that may be causing a compression.
- Neurorrhaphy codes are determined by the site of the repair and the use of a graft.

Navigator

Access interactive chapter review exercises, practice activities, flash cards, and study games.

Chapter 17

Surgery Coding: The Eye and Ocular Adnexa and the Auditory System

Fast Facts

- Your eyes heal very quickly. A corneal scratch will be feeling much better in only about 48 hours.
- An iris has 256 unique characteristics, compared with only 40 on a fingerprint. This is why retina scans are being used more frequently for security purposes.
- Ear infections are more common in children than adults because children's eustachian tubes are at a more horizontal angle.
- Sometimes those with ear damage will experience a change in how they perceive taste. Nerves called the *chorda tympani* go through the ear and connect the taste buds to the brain.

Sources: http://discoveryeye.org, http://hearinginstitute.ca

Crack the Code

Review the sample procedure note to find the correct auditory system code. You may need to return to this exercise after reading the chapter content.

PROCEDURE NOTE: Incision and drainage, infected cyst left external ear

This 28-year-old male developed a lump anterior to his left ear over the last week. It is painful to him. Denies fever or chills. Inspection of the ear area reveals a 2-cm size lump in the pre-auricular area of the external ear. It is tender to palpation; it is fluctuant. No cellulitis or erythema is present. Area is cleansed, local infiltration with 1% Xylocaine for anesthesia is performed. Area is incised with a #11 blade. A large amount of purulent material is expressed. Samples taken for culture and sensitivity. Loculations are broken up. Incision is irrigated, and Iodoform is packed. Band-Aid applied. Patient advised to return to have packing removed in 1 day.

answer: 69000-LT

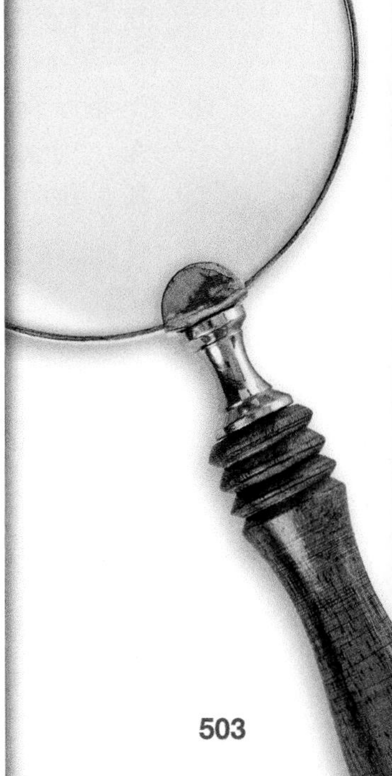

Learning Objectives

17.1 Identify the anatomical structures of the eye and ocular adnexa.

17.2 Discuss the arrangement of codes in the Eye and Ocular Adnexa Surgery codebook subsection.

17.3 Select eye and ocular adnexa codes based on coding guidelines.

17.4 Identify the anatomical structures of the auditory system.

17.5 Discuss the arrangement of codes in the Auditory System Surgery codebook subsection.

17.6 Select auditory system codes based on coding guidelines.

17.7 Discuss reporting guidelines for operating microscopes.

Chapter Outline

I. Introduction to the Eyes and Ocular Adnexa
II. Eye and Ocular Adnexa Terminology
III. Organization of the Eye and Ocular Adnexa Surgery Subsection
IV. Eyeball (Codes 65091-65290)
    A. Removal of the Eyeball
    B. Secondary Implant(s) Procedures
    C. Removal of Foreign Body
    D. Repair of Laceration
V. Anterior Segment (Codes 65400-66999)
    A. Cornea
    B. Anterior Chamber
    C. Anterior Sclera
    D. Iris, Ciliary Body
    E. Lens and Intraocular Lens Procedures
VI. Posterior Segment (Codes 67005-67299)
    A. Vitreous
    B. Retina or Choroid
        i. Retinal Detachment Repair
        ii. Retinal Detachment Prophylaxis
        iii. Retina or Choroid Destruction Procedures
VII. Ocular Adnexa (Codes 67311-67999)
    A. Extraocular Muscles
    B. Orbit
    C. Eyelids
VIII. Conjunctiva (Codes 68020-68899)
IX. Introduction to the Auditory System
X. Auditory System Terminology
XI. Organization of the Auditory System Subsection
XII. External Ear (Codes 69000-69399)
XIII. Middle Ear (Codes 69420-69799)
XIV. Inner Ear (Codes 69801-69949)
XV. Temporal Bone, Middle Fossa Approach (Codes 69950-69979)
XVI. Operating Microscope (Code 69990)
XVII. Chapter Summary

Introduction to the Eyes and Ocular Adnexa

Sight gives the ability to take in visual information from the world around us. The eyes collect information, and the brain interprets it. The eyes are like a personal camera, capturing images and live video and sending these images to the brain to be stored in the memory. The eyes not only collect information, but they can also provide information. **Ophthalmologists**, physicians who specialize in diseases of the eye, can detect conditions such as diabetes, high blood pressure, and high cholesterol during routine eye exams. They also perform medical and surgical procedures to correct vision. An **optometrist** is a healthcare professional who is qualified to examine the eyes and to prescribe and supply spectacles (glasses) and contact lenses. **Ophthalmology** is the field of medicine that specializes in the surgical and nonsurgical treatment of the eyes and related structures. Coding for ophthalmology requires knowledge of eye diseases and treatment and familiarity with terms not commonly used in other medical specialties.

Eye and Ocular Adnexa Terminology

Figure 17.1 identifies the anatomical structures of the eye. The **eyeball** has a slightly elongated globe shape and measures about 1 inch in diameter. The eyeball is securely set in a space in the bones of the face called the **orbit**. The **lacrimal bone** forms part of the medial (middle) wall of the orbit.

The **adnexa** of the eye refers to the eye's accessory structures, which include the lacrimal glands, extraocular muscles, eyelids, eyelashes, eyebrows, and the conjunctiva. The skin that covers the eye is the **eyelid**. The hairs that grow out of the eyelid are **eyelashes**. Eyelashes and eyelids protect the eye from dust and other debris. The **sclera** is the tough, white, outer coating of the eye. The anterior portion of the sclera and the inside of the eyelid are protected by the **conjunctiva**, a thin, clear membrane.

The anterior portion of the eye collects the light that will eventually be processed by the brain into images. Light enters the eye through the **pupil**, the black, circular opening in the center of the iris. The **iris** is the colored portion of the front of the eye. The pupil and the iris are covered by the **cornea**, a dome-shaped, transparent, fibrous tissue. The curved shape of the cornea creates a process called *refraction*. **Refraction** is the process of bending light rays, which allows light to be focused to the nerve receptors in the posterior part of the eye. Refraction also occurs at the lens and in the vitreous humor. The **lens** is a transparent, flexible layer of tissue behind the pupil. The **vitreous humor** is the clear gel that fills the inner core of the eye. The interior of the eye is lined by a thin, delicate nerve layer called the **retina**. The retina converts light into electrical impulses that send signals to and through the optic nerve, connected at the back of the eye. Optic nerves relay the signals to the cerebral cortex in the brain, which interprets those signals, allowing us to recognize what we see. The **macula** is a yellowish circular area within the retina that allows for central vision.

Table 17.1 lists word parts used in eye and ocular adnexa procedures. Table 17.2 defines common terms and abbreviations relating to the eye and ocular adnexa.

Figure 17.1 Anatomical Structures of the Eye

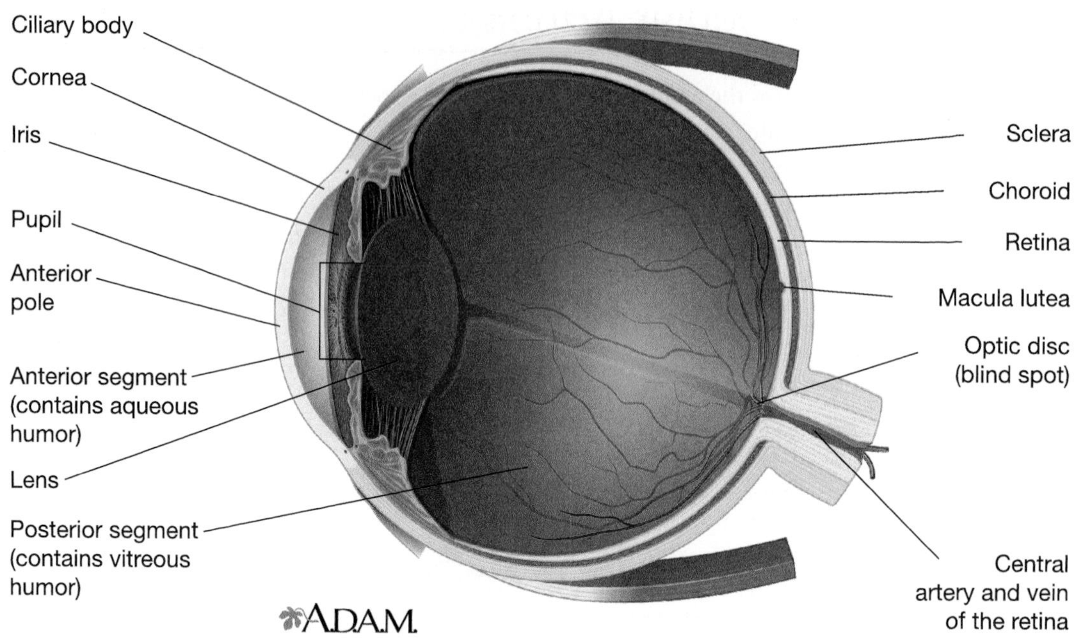

Table 17.1 Word Parts Used in Eye and Ocular Adnexa Procedures

Word Part	Definition	Example
blephar/o	Eyelid	Blepharotomy—incision into the eyelid
conjunctiv/o	Conjunctiva	Conjunctivoplasty—repair to the conjunctiva
core/ or pupill/o	Pupil	Coreoplasty—procedure to reshape the pupil
corne/ or kerat/o	Cornea	Corneoscleral—relating to the junction between the cornea and sclera
cycl/o	Ciliary body or muscle of eye	Cyclectomy—excision of the ciliary body
dacry/o or lacrim/o	Tears, tear duct	Dacryolith—stone in the tear duct
iri/o	Iris	Iridotomy—incision into the iris
ocul/o or ophthalm/o	Eye	Ocular implant—eye implant
opt/o or optic/o	Eye, vision	Optic nerve—nerve related to vision
palpebr/o	Eyelid	Palpebral conjunctiva—conjunctiva of the eyelid
papill/o	Optic disc, nipple-like	Papillitis—swelling of the optic disc
phac/o or phak/o	Lens of the eye	Phacoemulsification—method of emulsifying a cataract
retin/o	Retina	Retinopathy—disease of the retina
scler/o	Sclera (white of eye)	Sclerotomy—incision into the sclera
uve/o	Uvea, vascular layer of the eye (iris, ciliary body, and choroid)	Uveal tissue—coating of the eyeball pertaining to the iris, ciliary body, and choroid

Table 17.2 Common Eye and Ocular Adnexa Terms and Abbreviations

Term/Abbreviation	Definition
AC	Anterior chamber
adhesion	Inflammatory bands that connect opposing serous surfaces resulting from trauma or inflammation
adnexa	Conjoined, subordinate, or associated anatomical parts
anterior	Position located at the front relative to surrounding anatomical structures
CE	Cataract extraction
IOL	Intraocular lens
IOP	Intraocular pressure
LASIK	Laser-assisted in situ keratomileusis
OD	Right eye (from the Latin *oculus dexter*) *
OS	Left eye (from the Latin *oculus sinister*)*
OU	Both eyes (from the Latin *oculus uterque*, "each eye")*
PERLA	Pupils equal and reactive to light and accommodation
posterior	Position located at the back relative to surrounding anatomical structures
RD	Retinal detachment
VA	Visual acuity
VF or F	Visual field

**The Joint Commission, an association that rates hospitals, prohibits the use of abbreviations OD, OS, and OU to prevent confusion between the abbreviations. Its recommendation is to document laterality with the words right/left/both eye(s).*

CONCEPTS CHECKPOINT **17.1**

Select the correct answer for the following questions.

1. Physicians who specialize in diseases of the eye and perform medical and surgical procedures to correct vision are called
   a. optometrists.
   b. ophthalmology.
   c. ophthalmologists.
   d. None of the answers are correct.
2. The colored portion of the eye is called the
   a. iris.
   b. pupil.
   c. lens.
   d. sclera.
3. The white outer coating of the eye is called the
   a. iris.
   b. pupil.
   c. lens.
   d. sclera.
4. The black circular opening in the center of the eye where light enters is called the
   a. iris.
   b. pupil.
   c. lens.
   d. sclera.
5. The Latin abbreviation for "both eyes" is
   a. OD.
   b. OS.
   c. OU.
   d. AC.

Organization of the Eye and Ocular Adnexa Surgery Subsection

Surgical procedures of the eye and ocular adnexa are located in the CPT® code range 65091 through 68899. Table 17.3 lists the subsection headings and associated code ranges. Specific anatomical sites and structures further divide the codes. Procedure types such as incision, excision, removal, destruction, and repair categorize the codes. Nonsurgical ophthalmological services for diagnosis and treatment are reported with ophthalmological codes located in the Medicine section of the CPT® codebook, which will be discussed in Chapter 20.

Table 17.3 Headings Within the Eye and Ocular Adnexa Surgery Subsection of the CPT® Codebook

Heading	Code Range
Eyeball	65091-65290
Anterior Segment	65400-66999
Posterior Segment	67005-67299
Ocular Adnexa	67311-67999
Conjunctiva	68020-68899

Eyeball (Codes 65091-65290)

Codes used to report surgical procedures of the eyeball include removal of the eye with and without implantation, secondary implant(s) procedures, removal of a foreign body, and repair of lacerations. Parenthetic notes provide instructions regarding use of additional codes to accurately report surgical procedures of the eye.

Removal of the Eyeball

Removal of the eyeball may be performed by evisceration, enucleation, or exenteration. The distinctions between the procedures and their respective codes are as follows:

- **Evisceration** is the removal of the eyeball (globe) while leaving the sclera and extraocular muscles in place and is reported with code 65091.
- **Enucleation** is the removal of the whole eye from the orbit while leaving in place all other orbital structures. Enucleation without implantation of a prosthetic eye is reported with code 65101. Codes 65103 and 65105 report enucleation with implantation of prosthetic eye. If conjuctiva reconstruction is performed during an enucleation, report the appropriate conjunctivoplasty code separately.
- **Exenteration** removes the eye, adnexa, and part of the bony orbit. Codes 65110 through 65114 are used to report exenteration.

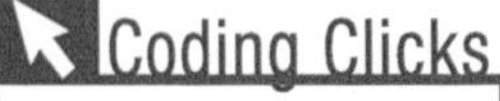

To have a better visual understanding of the enucleation procedure, visit http://Coding.ParadigmEducation.com/Enucleation.

The condition of the eye determines the extent of removal of the eyeball and associated structures. For example, evisceration and enucleation may be performed because of inflammation of the eye or other infections that are unresponsive to antibiotics. Enucleation is also an effective treatment for intraocular cancer and for relief of eye pain in an eye that has lost its vision. Exenteration of the eye is performed when the patient has large orbital tumors or intraocular tumors that have metastasized to the orbit of the eye.

Some patients have a prosthetic eye implanted into the orbit. A prosthetic eye (ocular prosthesis) is sometimes referred to as a *glass eye* or *fake eye*. There are 2 types of prosthetic eye implants, ocular and orbital. An **ocular implant** (artificial eye) is implanted inside the muscular cone of the eye, as shown in Figure 17.2. The ocular implant fills the space that was occupied by the natural eyeball. In order to make the ocular implant appear natural, ocular muscles may be attached to the ocular implant to enable movement. The ocular prosthesis is painted to look like the iris and the pupil of the other eye. An **orbital implant** is an implant outside the muscular cone. Orbital implant insertion, removal, and replacement codes are listed in the codebook in the Orbit category under the Ocular Adnexa heading.

Figure 17.2 Ocular Prosthesis and Ocular Implant

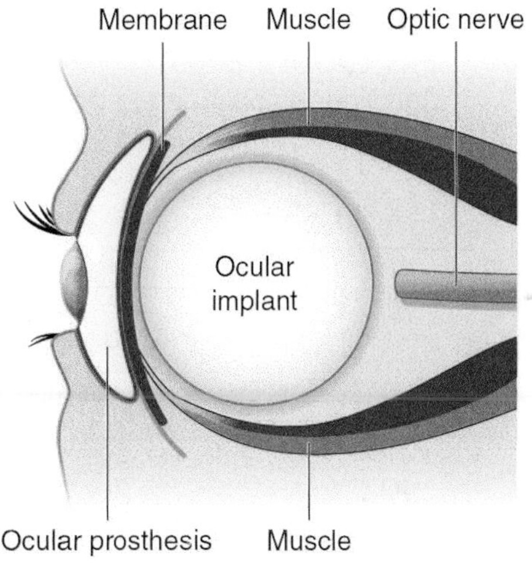

An ocular implant is always required after an evisceration. Typically a temporary implant is placed, and the patient is monitored until a permanent implant is placed. Code 65091 reports evisceration without an ocular implant or with insertion of a temporary ocular implant. When a permanent prosthetic eye is implanted during the initial procedure, report code 65093, *Evisceration of ocular contents; with implant.* Figure 17.3 illustrates these evisceration codes. Report code 65130, *Insertion of ocular implant secondary; after evisceration, in scleral shell,* for delayed ocular implants.

EXAMPLE 17.1

A 56-year-old male patient with absolute glaucoma underwent an evisceration of the left eye. Under general anesthesia, anesthetic with epinephrine was administered behind the globe of the left eye to reduce intraoperative bleeding and postoperative pain. The patient was appropriately prepared and draped in a sterile manner, and an eyelid speculum was placed in the left eye to hold the top and bottom eyelids open during the procedure. A strip of the conjunctiva was removed at the limbus before utilizing Westcott scissors to undermine the conjunctiva and Tenon's capsule in a careful anterior dissection. A full-thickness incision was then made at the limbus so that scissors could be introduced to excise the cornea in a circumferential manner. All intraocular contents of the eye were removed by use of an evisceration spoon. The intraocular content was sent to the pathologist for histopathologic identification and examination. Hemostasis of the nerve and vortex veins was achieved with cautery and direct pressure. A temporary ocular implant was placed. The eyelid speculum was removed. The patient tolerated the procedure well and was sent to recovery.

As noted above, an evisceration requires placement of an ocular implant, typically a temporary implant to allow monitoring of the patient before a permanent implant is placed. When a temporary implant is placed at the time of the initial procedure, report the code for evisceration without an implant (65091, *Evisceration of ocular contents; without implant*). If a permanent implant is inserted into the scleral shell at the time of an evisceration, code 65093, *Evisceration of ocular contents; with implant*, is reported. HCPCS modifier LT, *Left side*, is appended to the code to identify laterality of the eye.

Figure 17.3 Codes for Evisceration of Ocular Contents

65091	Evisceration of ocular contents; without implant
65093	with implant

Skin grafts are not included in the code descriptions and are reported separately, when performed. Skin grafts of the eyelids and orbits are reported with Integumentary System Surgery codes 15120, 15121, 15260, or 15261. When eyelid repair involves more than the skin, separately report code 67930, *Suture of recent wound, eyelid, involving lid margin, tarsus, and/or palpebral conjunctiva direct closure; partial thickness.*

LET'S TRY ONE 17.1

Read the description of the enucleation procedure and then answer the questions that follow.

The physician separated the right eyeball from the extraorbital muscles and optic nerve and removed it. After an ocular speculum was inserted, the physician dissected the conjunctiva free at the limbus (corneal-scleral juncture). The physician cut each extraocular muscle at its juncture to the eyeball and severed the optic nerve. The eyeball was removed, but the extraocular muscles remained attached at the back of the eye socket. A temporary spherical implant was placed in the eye socket. This implant was not attached to the extraocular muscles. The tissue was closed over the implant, and a bupivacaine solution was injected into the retrobulbar space to provide postoperative pain relief. Topical antibiotic ointment was applied to the conjunctiva and lid. The orbit was covered with a gentle pressure patch for at least 24 hours to lessen postoperative edema.

1. Was an artificial eye placed after enucleation? _____
2. Were extraocular muscles attached to an ocular implant? _____
3. What is the correct code and modifier for the procedure? _____

Secondary Implant(s) Procedures

A patient who had an enucleation in the past may experience infection or shifting of the implant. Removing or replacing the ocular implant requires a secondary ocular implant procedure, reported with codes 65125 through 65175. Prior to placement, the secondary ocular implant may require modification, which is integral to the procedure. Code 65125 provides for modifications as a separate procedure for the addition of screws or other alterations to the shape of the ocular implant. Code 65125 may not be reported with codes 65130 through 65175 for the same eye on the same date of service, because modification of the ocular implant is included in those codes. Figure 17.4 shows the criteria for coding secondary ocular implant insertion. Reinsertion of an ocular implant is reported with codes 65150 or 65155. Removal of an ocular implant is reported with code 65175.

Figure 17.4 Secondary Ocular Implant Insertion Codes

65130	Insertion of ocular implant secondary; after evisceration, in scleral shell
65135	after enucleation, muscles not attached to implant
65140	after enucleation, muscles attached to implant

Removal of Foreign Body

Foreign body removal from the external or intraocular eye is reported with codes 65205 through 65265. Codes are selected according to the location of the foreign body (external or intraocular) and the instrument used during the procedure. The **slit lamp** is an instrument that produces low-intensity light beams to provide an enlarged, 3-dimensional view of the front parts of the eye (the cornea, lens, iris, and

Figure 17.5 Slit Lamp

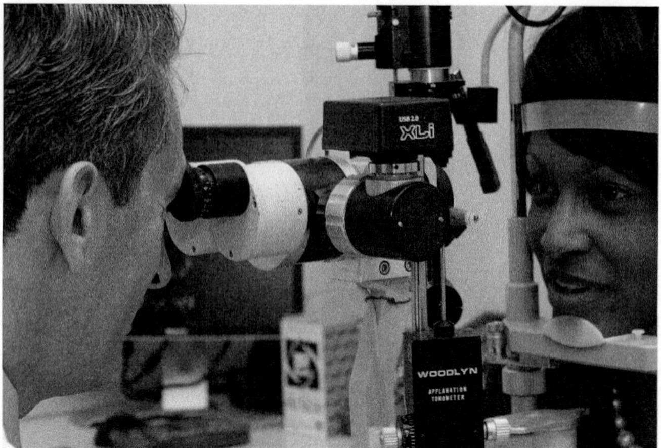

RED FLAG

The Removal of Foreign Body subcategory of "Eyeball" has extensive parenthetic notes prior to the listing of codes. Coders must read all of the notes prior to reporting any code listed in this subcategory.

vitreous gel). Figure 17.5 shows a slit lamp. Physicians may inject a **fluorescein dye** (orange organic dye) before a slit lamp examination to improve the detection of a foreign body. Code 65222 is used to report the removal of a foreign body from the external eye with the assistance of a slit lamp. When an electromagnetic or magnetic eye probe is used to extract a foreign body from the intraocular portion of the eye, code 65260 is used to report the procedure.

CONCEPTS CHECKPOINT **17.2**

Select the correct answer for the following multiple-choice questions.

1. What type of artificial eye is implanted inside the muscular cone of the eye?
   a. orbital implant
   b. ocular implant
   c. slit lamp
   d. None of the answers are correct.
2. A(n) _____ is an implant outside the muscular cone of the eye.
   a. orbital implant
   b. ocular implant
   c. slit lamp
   d. None of the answers are correct.
3. A(n) _____ provides a 3-dimensional view of the front parts of the eye.
   a. orbital implant
   b. ocular implant
   c. slit lamp
   d. None of the answers are correct.
4. Removal of the eye from the orbit while leaving in place all other orbital structures is
   a. enucleation.
   b. evisceration.
   c. exenteration.
   d. evacuation.
5. Removal of the eyeball (globe) while leaving the sclera and extraocular muscles in place is
   a. enucleation.
   b. evisceration.
   c. exenteration.
   d. evacuation.

Repair of Laceration

Codes for repair of laceration are arranged according to the location of the injury in the conjunctiva, cornea, and/or sclera. Lacerations of the conjunctiva codes are selected based on whether the patient requires hospitalization. See for example code 65273, *Repair of laceration; conjunctiva, by mobilization and rearrangement, with hospitalization.* During a mobilization and arrangement procedure, a flap of skin is created or a skin graft is sutured over the wound. A patch is placed over the eye to limit movement while the wound is healing. If the wound requires repair of the eyelid without reconstructive surgery and is limited to the skin layer, report the appropriate wound repair code from the Integumentary System Surgery subsection, in the Repair (Closure) category.

Anterior Segment (Codes 65400-66999)

The Anterior Segment heading covers procedures of the cornea, anterior chamber, anterior sclera, iris, ciliary body, and lens. Subcategories are arranged according to the procedure types, such as incision, excision, removal, introduction, and repair.

Cornea

The cornea is a dome-shaped transparent fibrous tissue that covers the pupil and the iris. The cornea's globular shape bends light as it enters the eye and travels to the retina, which allows for clear, sharp vision. Corneal surgical procedures include biopsy and lesion excision. Herpes zoster (shingles) is a virus that may cause corneal lesions. When medications such as steroids and antivirals are not effective in treating the lesions, a biopsy or excision of the lesion may be performed. Corneal biopsy is reported with code 65410. Excision of a corneal lesion, except pterygium, is reported with code 65400. **Pterygium** (surfer's eye) is a thin growth in the conjunctiva of the eye that spreads to cover the cornea, reducing its transparency and clouding vision. It is caused by prolonged exposure to ultraviolet light (UV) and outdoor elements such as dust and wind. Codes 65420 and 65426 are used to report excisions of pterygium.

Keratoplasty (corneal transplant) is the surgical repair of the cornea. Keratoplasty replaces a damaged cornea with a healthy cornea from an organ donor. Corneal degeneration, chemical injuries, and congenital disorders are just some of the conditions that may require keratoplasty. Transplant codes are categorized as penetrating, endothelial, or anterior lamellar (layered front microstructures):

- **Penetrating keratoplasty** replaces the full thickness of the cornea; codes 65730, 65750, and 65755 are selected based on the absence of the eye lens (aphakia) or the presence of an artificial lens (pseudophakia).
- **Endothelial keratoplasty** replaces the endothelial layer (inside posterior layer) of the cornea; code 65756 is used to report an endothelial keratoplasty that requires a graft; the preparation of the graft is reported with add-on code 65757.
- **Anterior lamellar keratoplasty** replaces the front part of the cornea, code 65710.

CONCEPTS CHECKPOINT 17.3

Using information from the above section, select the correct answer to the following questions.

1. Which keratoplasty procedure replaces the full thickness of the cornea?
   a. endothelial
   b. penetrating
   c. anterior lamellar
   d. None of the answers are correct.
2. Which keratoplasty procedure replaces the back layer of the cornea?
   a. endothelial
   b. penetrating
   c. anterior lamellar
   d. None of the answers are correct.
3. Which keratoplasty procedure replaces the front part of the cornea?
   a. endothelial
   b. penetrating
   c. anterior lamellar
   d. None of the answers are correct.
4. Pterygium is
   a. a heavy, thick growth in the conjunctiva of the eye that spreads to cover the cornea.
   b. a thin growth in the eyelid that spreads to cover the iris.
   c. a thin growth in the conjunctiva of the eye that spreads to cover the cornea.
   d. a thick growth in the conjunctiva of the eye that spreads to cover the iris.
5. Which of the following statements regarding the cornea is *not* true?
   a. The cornea is a dome-shaped, transparent, fibrous tissue that covers the pupil and the iris.
   b. The shape of the cornea has nothing to do with clear, sharp vision.
   c. The shape of the cornea bends light as it enters the eye.
   d. Herpes zoster (shingles) is a virus that may cause corneal lesions.

Anterior Chamber

A&P Review

Trabecular meshwork is a spongy tissue around the posterior of the cornea. The trabecular meshwork allows aqueous humor to drain from the anterior chamber into the blood system via a set of tubes called *Schlemm's canal.*

Procedures to correct conditions of the anterior chamber are reported with codes 65800 through 66030. The **anterior chamber** is the fluid-filled space inside the eye between the iris and the back side of the cornea. Like vitreous humor fills the inner core of the eyeball, **aqueous humor**, a fluid similar to plasma but with lower protein, fills the front chamber between the lens and cornea.

Hyphema and glaucoma are 2 conditions that affect the anterior chamber. **Hyphema** is caused by blood filling the anterior chamber, often because of a trauma. **Glaucoma** results from the inability of aqueous humor to drain from the eye through the **canal of Schlemm** into the bloodstream. The accumulation of aqueous humor causes increased intraocular pressure and eventually blindness.

Paracentesis is removal of bodily fluid with a needle. Paracentesis of the anterior chamber removes aqueous humor. During the procedure, anesthetic eyedrops are administered to numb the eye. After the eye is numb, a needle is inserted into the anterior chamber of the eye to withdraw a small amount of fluid. The withdrawal reduces the pressure inside the eye. In addition to relieving intraocular pressure, anterior chamber paracentesis helps to dislodge blockages or blood clots, allowing them to move to a different area of the eye that does not affect the retina. To remove any possible contaminates, the surgeon may irrigate (wash out) the eye with water or saline solution. Air may be injected into the eye after the removal of fluid to stabilize eye pressure.

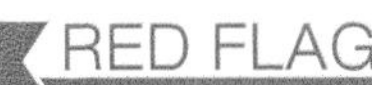

RED FLAG

Codes 65860 through 65865 are separate procedures and would not always be coded if another procedure is performed.

Coding Clicks

Watch a narrated video of a goniotomy and other surgical ophthalmological procedures at http://Coding.ParadigmEducation.com/Goniotomy. The site shows video of a surgery, so viewer discretion is advised.

Paracentesis of the anterior chamber is reported with incision codes 65800, 65810, and 65815. Codes are selected according to the extent of the procedure:

- code 65800—removal of aqueous (separate procedure);
- code 65810—removal of vitreous and/or discission of anterior hyaloid membrane, with or without irrigation and/or air injection;
- code 65815—removal of blood, with or without irrigation and/or air injection.

Goniotomy is a surgical procedure that lowers intraocular pressure, reported with incision code 65820. The procedure involves an incision through the trabecular meshwork to increase the outflow of aqueous humor into Schlemm's canal. Goniotomy is an effective treatment for conditions such as congenital glaucoma and aniridia. **Aniridia** is a disorder in which the patient does not have a visible iris. Patients with aniridia have a high probability of developing glaucoma. A goniotomy is a preventive measure for patients with aniridia. A parenthetic note following the code prohibits associating code 65820 with modifier 63, *Procedure performed on infants less than 4 kg.*

Adhesions or scars may form as the result of previous trauma to the eye. Codes 65860 through 65880 are used to report severing of adhesions or scar tissue from the anterior segment. Code 65860 reports the use of a laser technique, and codes 65865 through 65880 report incisional techniques. Incisional techniques are selected based on the location of the adhesions or scars. Adhesions of the iris to the cornea are called **anterior synechiae**. Adhesions of the iris to the lens are called **posterior synechiae**. Severing anterior synechiae is reported with code 65870. Severing posterior synechiae is reported with code 65875.

LET'S TRY ONE **17.2**

A 68-year-old female with anterior synechiae had adhesions removed from the anterior chamber. The physician applied a topical anesthetic to the affected eye. A special contact lens was placed on the affected eye to allow the physician to view the eye's angle structures and trabecular meshwork while using the laser. An yttrium-aluminum-garnet (YAG) laser was used to sever adhesions that were binding the iris to the cornea. The laser caused the adhesions to fall out of the visual field. What code is reported? _____

Anterior Sclera

The **anterior sclera** is the tough, white, outer coating of the eyeball in the front part of the eye. Codes 66130 through 66250 report excisions, aqueous shunts, and repairs/revisions of the anterior sclera.

Fistulization (creation of a passageway) of the sclera is an effective treatment for glaucoma. The creation of a fistula allows fluid to drain from the eye, decreasing intraocular pressure. Excision codes 66150 through 66172 (shown in Figure 17.6) report fistulization of sclera for glaucoma with iris removal. Codes are selected based on the procedure type:

- code 66150—a **trephination** technique, which uses a trephine (surgical instrument) to cut out circular sections of the iris and sclera;

- code 66155—thermocauterization by use of hot forceps;
- code 66160—**sclerectomy** (removal of the sclera) with punch or scissors;
- codes 66170 or 66172—ab externo trabeculectomy (AET), also known as *nonpenetrating trabeculectomy*; report code 66170 for an initial AET and 66172 when scarring from a previous ocular surgery or trauma is indicated.

EXAMPLE **17.2**

A 67-year-old male patient with chronic angle-closure glaucoma of the right eye underwent a fistulization of the sclera with an ab externo trabeculectomy. After sedation with general anesthesia, the patient was appropriately prepared and draped in a sterile manner. An ocular speculum was placed in the right eye. The anterior chamber was opened through an incision in the limbus. The surgeon removed a partial-thickness portion of the trabecular meshwork. An opening in the sclera remained for aqueous humor to flow through the fistula into the space between the conjunctiva and the sclera. The incision was closed by sutures. Water was injected into the right eye to restore intraocular pressure. The ocular speculum was removed. The patient tolerated the procedure well and was moved to recovery.

The above documentation states that the procedure was performed due to chronic angle-closure glaucoma. Documentation does not mention either a previous procedure or scarring from a previous procedure. The documentation identifies the creation of a fistula in addition to an ab externo trabeculectomy. Code 66170, *Fistulization of sclera for glaucoma; trabeculectomy ab externo in absence of previous surgery*, accurately reports the above operative session. HCPCS modifier RT, *Right side*, is appended to the CPT® code to report laterality.

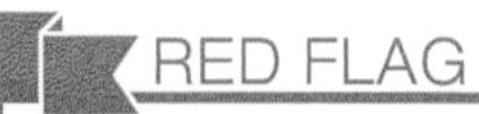

Report CPT® Category III code 0123T for *Fistulization of sclera for glaucoma, through ciliary body.*

Index Insider

To locate codes for fistulization of the anterior sclera in the Index, try looking under *Sclera* or *Incision*. Below are the relevant entries from the Index.

Sclera
  Fistulization
    for Glaucoma
    0123T
    Sclerectomy with Punch or Scissors with Iridectomy
    66160
Incision
  Sclera
    Fistulization
      Sclerectomy with Punch or Scissors with Iridectomy
      66160

Figure 17.6 Fistulization of Sclera Codes

Code	Description
66150	Fistulization of sclera for glaucoma; trephination with iridectomy
66155	thermocauterization with iridectomy
66160	sclerectomy with punch or scissors, with iridectomy
66170	trabeculectomy ab externo in absence of previous surgery
	(For trabeculotomy ab externo, use 65850)
	(For repair of operative of operative wound, use 66250)
66172	trabeculectomy ab externo with scarring from previous ocular surgery or trauma (includes injection of antifibrotic agents)

Iris, Ciliary Body

The function of the iris is to regulate the amount of light entering the eye with tiny muscles that control the pupil. The ciliary body lies directly behind the iris. Muscles of the ciliary body attach to the lens. The ciliary body's primary function is to produce aqueous humor. The ciliary body also contracts and relaxes to adjust the shape of the lens. When contracted, the lens thickens, allowing the eye to focus on items up close; when relaxed, the lens thins out to focus on items at a distance. Figure 17.7 illustrates the ciliary body.

Procedures of the iris and ciliary body are reported with codes 66500 through 66770. **Iridectomy** is removal of the iris and has various procedure codes. Excision codes 66600 through 66635 report iridectomy with corneal and corneoscleral sectioning (cutting of the cornea, or the cornea and sclera. The code selection is based on the procedure's purpose: code 66600 for lesion removal and code 66625 for glaucoma. Iridotomy or iridectomy by laser surgery for glaucoma is reported once per session with code 66761.

Ciliary photocoagulation is a method used to treat glaucoma. The procedure involves the delivery of pulses from a laser to a specialized lens placed on the sclera above the ciliary body. The pulses around the eye destroy affected areas of the ciliary body and create holes in the iris. The destruction of specific points on the ciliary body and iris reduces the intraocular pressure. Code 66762 reports iridoplasty by photocoagulation.

Figure 17.7 Ciliary Body of the Eye

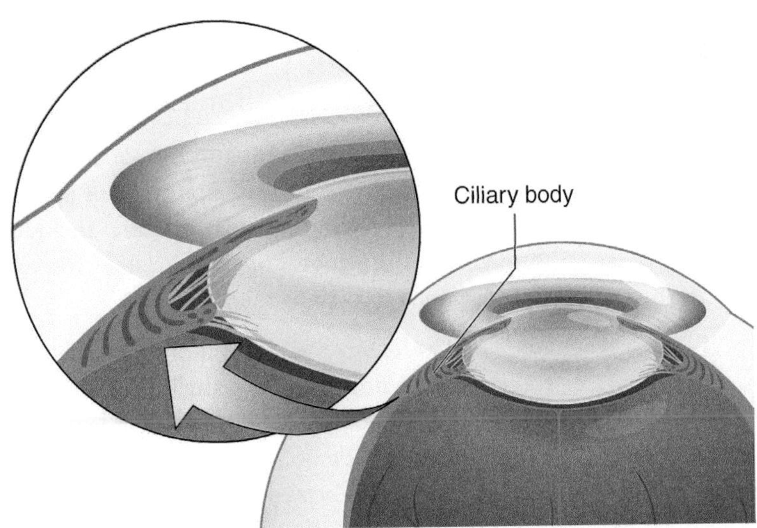

CONCEPTS CHECKPOINT **17.4**

Using information from the previous section, identify whether each of the following statements is true or false.

1. _____ Codes for paracentesis of the anterior chamber are selected according to the extent of the procedure.
2. _____ Codes for procedures of the iris and ciliary body are selected based on the purpose of the procedure.
3. _____ Fistulization is the creation of a passage-way.
4. _____ Codes for anterior segment procedures by incisional techniques are selected based on the location of the adhesions or scars.
5. _____ Goniotomy is a surgical procedure that increases intraocular pressure.

LET'S TRY ONE **17.3**

Assign the appropriate codes to the following procedures.

1. A 45-year-old male was diagnosed with cancer of the left eye. He agreed to undergo an iridectomy. During the procedure, the surgeon placed a contact lens on the patient's left eye to direct the argon laser beam. The laser was used to excise a full-thickness piece by chipping away the iris. Due to the damage to the eye, the surgeon decided to cut deeper down through the iris into the ciliary body. _____
2. A 70-year-old female with acute angle-closure glaucoma underwent cryotherapy to destroy the ciliary body. _____
3. A 58-year-old male with pupillary abnormalities agreed to undergo iridoplasty to improve vision. The surgeon uses photocoagulation to widen the anterior chamber angle. _____
4. A 72-year-old male patient with acute angle-closure glaucoma underwent an iridotomy to enhance the flow of fluids in the anterior chamber. The surgeon made an incision in the corneal-scleral juncture and then sliced through the iris bombe. Incisions were made in 2 areas of the iris bombe to allow outward flow of aqueous. Sutures were placed to close the incision site, and intraocular pressure was restored by an injection of saline. A pressure patch was applied. No tissue was removed during the procedure. _____

Lens and Intraocular Lens Procedures

Codes in the categories Lens and Intraocular Lens Procedures involve insertion, removal, and repositioning of lens and lens prostheses. Notes preceding the Lens "Removal" group describe the procedures included in the lens extraction codes (66830 through 66940): removal of all associated structures, use of pharmacological agents, and injections integral to the procedure.

Code 66830 reports the removal of a secondary membranous cataract after a previous surgery in which the posterior shell of the lens was not removed from the eye. Codes 66840 through 66940 report removal of lens materials and are selected based on procedure type (eg, code 66840, an aspiration technique) or purpose of the procedure (eg, code 66930, for dislocated lens).

Many of these codes describe treatments for cataracts. A **cataract** is the clouding of the lens caused by the accumulation of protein, which results in blurry vision. The elderly are especially susceptible to cataracts. However, cataracts may be congenital (present at birth) or may result from trauma, diabetes mellitus, or corticosteroid (cortisone) injections. Cataracts may be treated by **discission**, the breaking down of abnormal lens material, and extraction of the material. Codes are differentiated by technique, approach, and the use of implants.

Cataract extraction is listed under intraocular lens procedures. Extracapsular cataract extraction (ECCE) and intracapsular cataract extraction (ICCE) are the most common types of cataract extractions.

An **extracapsular cataract extraction (ECCE)** is the removal of the natural lens from its protective capsule. The back of the capsule is left intact. The most common ECCE is reported with code 66984, *Extracapsular cataract removal with insertion of intraocular lens prosthesis (1 stage procedure), manual or mechanical technique (eg, irrigation and aspiration* *or phacoemulsification).* Code 66982 reports a complex ECCE requiring devices or techniques not generally used in routine cataract surgery, which is rarely performed.

Inside the OR

ECCE can use a manual or a mechanical technique. The manual procedure requires an incision in the cornea or sclera for removal of the natural lens and placement of the intraocular lens (IOL) implant. The mechanical technique or phacoemulsification involves 2 incisions in the corneal-scleral juncture. A **phaco probe** is inserted into the eye and delivers ultrasound waves to break up the cataract and lens. The probe also aspirates (vacuums) the broken particles. An IOL implant is inserted, and the incision may be closed with a suture or allowed to heal without sutures.

Intracapsular cataract extraction (ICCE) is reported with code 66983, *Intracapsular cataract extraction with insertion of intraocular lens prosthesis (1 stage procedure).* In an ICCE procedure, the lens and the capsule that houses the lens are removed.

Not all cataract extractions require the implantation of an intraocular lens (IOL). If an IOL is not implanted, contacts or glasses are worn to correct vision.

Inside the OR

In an ICCE, a fairly large incision is made in the corneal-scleral juncture. Removal of the lens is accomplished with a cryoprobe, an instrument that delivers extreme cold to tissue during surgical procedures. The physician injects an air bubble into the anterior chamber to protect the cornea. An intraocular lens (IOL) is implanted to replace the clouded natural lens. The incision is closed with sutures. A saline solution is injected to restore intraocular pressure. A topical antibiotic or a pressure patch is applied.

LET'S TRY ONE **17.4**

Assign the appropriate codes to the following procedures.

1. A 28-year-old female had a posterior dislocation of the left lens. The surgeon performed an intracapsular removal of lens material due to a dislocated lens. _____
2. An 87-year-old male with a total senile cataract underwent a standard extracapsular cataract removal of the right eye, with insertion of an intraocular lens prosthesis. The cataract removal and insertion of the intraocular implant were performed in 1 procedure. _____

Posterior Segment (Codes 67005-67299)

The posterior segment of the eye includes the vitreous body, retina, choroid, and posterior sclera. Subcategories of the posterior segment are arranged by anatomical site. Codes are further divided into subcategories for the type, repair, prophylaxis, and destruction.

Table 17.4 Word Parts Used in the Auditory System

Word Part	Definition	Example
acou/o, audit/o	Hearing	Acousma—auditory hallucination
audi/o	Hearing; the sense of hearing	Audiometry—measurement of hearing
aur/o, auricul/o	Ear	Auricle—part of the external ear
cochle/o	Cochlea	Cochlear implant—amplification device inserted into cochlea
mastoid/o	Mastoid process	Mastoidectomy—hollowing out of the mastoid process
myring/o	Eardrum, tympanic membrane	Myringotomy—paracentesis of the tympanic membrane
ossicul/o	Ossicle	Ossicular chain—3 bones of middle ear that transmit sound
ot/o	Ear	Otopathy—disease of the ear
-otia	Ear condition	Melotia—Congenital displacement of the auricle of the ear
salping/o	Eustachian tube, auditory tube	Salpingitis—inflammation of the auditory tube
tympan/o	Eardrum, tympanic membrane	Tympanostomy—insertion of a tube in the tympanic membrane
vestibul/o	Vestibule	Vestibuloactive drug—agent that acts on structures of the vestibule

Table 17.5 Common Auditory System Terms and Abbreviations

Term/Abbreviation	Definition
AD	Right ear (from the Latin *auris dextra*)*
AOM	Acute otitis media
AS	Left ear (from the Latin *auris sinistra*)*
EENT	Eyes, ears, nose, and throat
ENG	Electronystagmography—test of the inner ear by assessing eye movement
ENT	Ears, nose, and throat
ETD	Eustachian tube dysfunction
HEENT	Head, eyes, ears, nose, and throat
PE tube	Pressure equalization tube
SOM	Serous otitis media

**The Joint Commission, an association that rates hospitals, prohibits the use of abbreviations AD and AS to prevent confusion between the abbreviations. Its recommendation is to document laterality with the words* right *or* left.

Organization of the Auditory System Surgery Subsection

Surgical procedures of the auditory system are organized by anatomical sites: external ear, middle ear, inner ear, and temporal bone, middle fossa approach. Table 17.6 lists the headings and associated code ranges. Categories are arranged by procedures of incision, excision, removal, repair, and introduction.

Table 17.6 Headings Within the Auditory System Surgery Subsection

Heading	Code Range
External Ear	69000-69399
Middle Ear	69420-69799
Inner Ear	69801-69949
Temporal Bone, Middle Fossa Approach	69950-69979

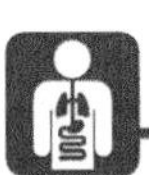

A&P Review

A **cauliflower ear** occurs primarily from trauma to the ear, when the cartilage is separated from the blood supply. Because of the lack of nutrients from the blood supply, fibrous tissues begin to form in the external ear, which cause the ear to swell. **Surfer's ear** is so named because it is most commonly found in individuals with extended exposure to cold water. The medical term is *exostosis*, the development of new bone on the surface of an existing bone in the external auditory canal.

RED FLAG

Do not report cerumen (earwax) removal code 69210 with any evaluation and management (E/M) code when the impacted cerumen is removed without an instrument. If an instrument is used, append modifier 25, *Significant, separately identifiable evaluation and management service by the same physician or other qualified health care professional on the same day of the procedure or other service*, to the E/M code, and report code 69210 separately.

External Ear (Codes 69000-69399)

Codes for surgical procedures of the external ear and external ear canal are categorized by incision, excision, removal, and repair.

Incision and drainage codes include treatment of an abscess or hematoma of the external ear. Codes 69000 and 69005 are selected based on the extent of the procedure (simple or complicated). Code 69020 reports treatment of an abscess in the external ear canal. Ear piercing is a cosmetic procedure coded with 69090.

Excision codes cover biopsies, simple repairs, amputations, and lesion treatment. A biopsy of the external ear is reported with code 69100 and of the external ear canal with code 69105. Excisions or amputations (total removal) of the external ear may be required to treat cancer of the ear or cauliflower ear. Code 69110 reports a partial or simple repair, and code 69120 reports complete amputation. An **exostosis**, referred to as *surfer's ear*, is the development of new bone on the surface of an existing bone in the external auditory canal. Removal of an exostosis is reported with code 69140, *Excision exostosis(es), external auditory canal.* If reconstruction of the ear is required after an exostosis excision, report the appropriate skin graft code from the Integumentary System Surgery subsection.

Removal codes describe treatment for all manner of foreign bodies that may become lodged in the external ear canal as well as impacted cerumen. Removal of foreign bodies is reported with codes 69200 and 69205 based on whether general anesthesia is administered. **Cerumen** (earwax) is a waxy substance found in the external ear canal that protects and lubricates the ear. The external auditory canal may become impacted with wax that does not naturally move to the external ear. Impacted cerumen decreases hearing and interferes with accurate assessment of auditory stimuli. Depending on the severity of the impaction, the provider may choose to irrigate (wash) the ear by spraying warm water and a mild liquid additive directly into the ear. The pressure of the water and the solution breaks down the wax buildup. See Figure 17.11. Removal of impacted cerumen using irrigation is reported with code 69209. For more severe impactions, an earpick curette, a steel instrument that resembles a tiny, long-handled spoon, is used to scoop out the impacted cerumen. See Figure 17.12. Code 69210 is reported for removal of impacted cerumen requiring use of instrumentation. Codes 69209 and 69210 are unilateral procedures; report modifier 50 for bilateral procedures. Do not report codes 69209 and 69210 together when performed on the same ear. Report only the code with the highest relative value unit (RVU).

Repair codes include otoplasty and reconstruction of the external auditory canal. **Otoplasty** is a surgical procedure to change the shape of the ear. Otoplasty is typically considered a cosmetic procedure not associated with trauma. Code 69300 is used to report otoplasty of a protruding ear, with or without size reduction. If moderate sedation is used, also report the appropriate moderate sedation code from code range 99151 through 99153 or 99155 through 99157.

Atresia is the absence of the external ear canal. Reconstruction of the external ear is an effective treatment for damage caused by stenosis (hardening) or congenital atresia.

Figure 17.11 Removal of Impacted Cerumen Using Irrigation/Lavage

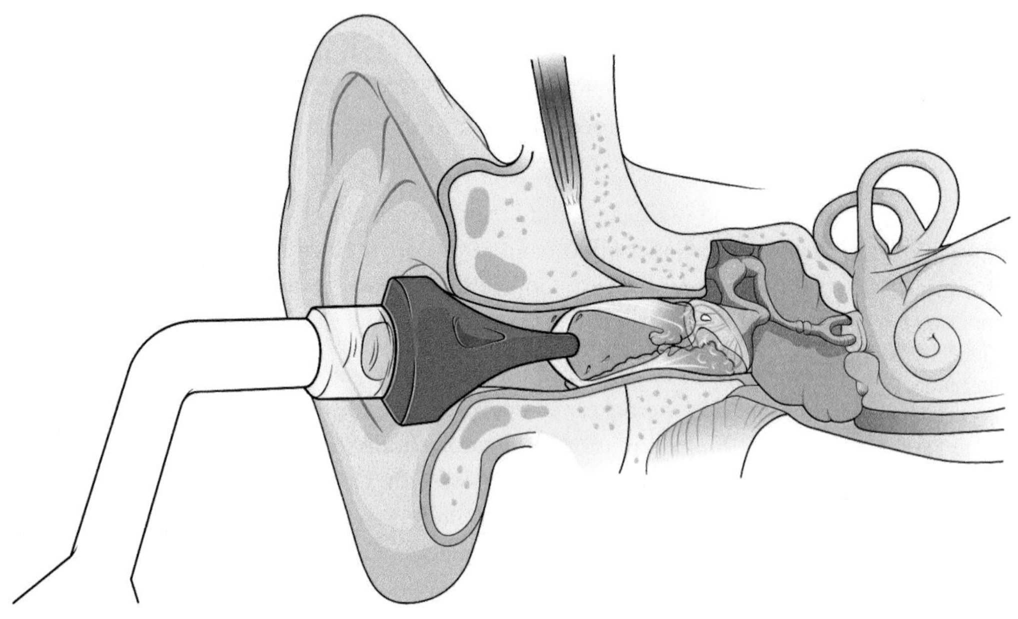

Figure 17.12 Removal of Impacted Cerumen Requiring Instrumentation

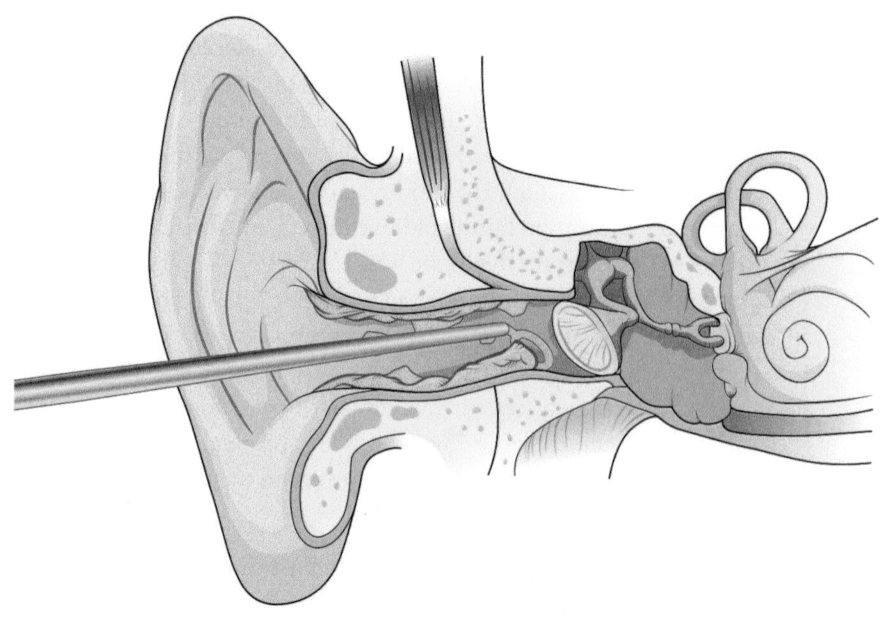

The reconstruction procedure involves drilling behind and above the temporomandibular joint to the ossicles, to create or enlarge the bony canal. The eardrum is reconstructed, and split-thickness skin grafts are used to line the new canal. Skin and soft tissues are removed to create a large canal opening. Code 69320 reports reconstruction of the external auditory canal for congenital atresia in a single stage.

CONCEPTS CHECKPOINT **17.6**

Using information from the previous section, match the medical term in the first column with the correct definition in the second column.

1. _____ atresia
2. _____ cauliflower ear
3. _____ cerumen
4. _____ exostosis
5. _____ otoplasty

a. Surgical procedure to change the shape of the ear
b. The absence of the external ear canal
c. Waxy substance found in the external ear canal
d. Cartilage of the ear is separated from the blood supply, causing swelling
e. Surfer's ear

LET'S TRY ONE **17.5**

Read the external ear procedure and answer the questions that follow.

A 15-year-old patient with a cauliflower deformity of the left ear underwent an external ear excision to remove the defect. During the procedure, the surgeon removed a full-thickness triangular wedge section of the external ear from the curved upper portion of the left ear. A small portion of normal tissue surrounding the defect was also removed. The surgeon then took a split-thickness skin graft from the patient's neck behind the left ear and placed the graft over the wound of the left ear. A graft of 4 sq cm was sutured onto the left ear.

1. Is the entire ear removed? _____
2. Is a graft performed? _____
3. What is the procedure code for the external ear excision? _____
4. If needed, what is the code for the graft? _____

Middle Ear (Codes 69420-69799)

Codes for surgical procedures of the middle ear are categorized by incision, excision, repair, and other procedures.

Incision codes describe procedures of the eustachian tube and tympanic membrane. The **eustachian tube** is a narrow passage leading from the pharynx (throat) to the cavity of the middle ear. The eustachian tube allows for equalization of pressure on each side of the eardrum and drainage of fluid into the throat. Allergies and infections may cause the eustachian tube to become inflamed or plugged, resulting in a condition called **eustachian tube dysfunction**. This condition blocks the drainage of fluid and disrupts the equalization of pressure in the middle ear. To correct the condition, the eustachian tube is surgically inflated with air forced through a catheter. The catheter is inserted through the nose and removed at the end of the procedure. Code 69799, *Unlisted procedure, middle ear*, is used to report transnasal eustachian tube inflation

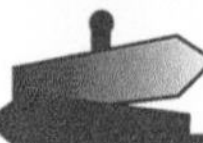

Learn Your Way

Do you learn by doing? If so, you have an active learning style according to the Felder-Silverman model. Use your learning style to remember the function of the eustachian tubes. How? Unpop your ears. You may have experienced blockage in the eustachian tubes brought on by sudden changes in pressure from flying or driving. You know they are blocked because of the uncomfortable sensation felt in the ear. This sensation is quickly alleviated by swallowing, chewing, or yawning. The popping feeling is the equalization of pressure returning to the eustachian tubes.

with catheterization. When a catheterization is not performed with a transnasal eustachian tube inflation, it is bundled into the reimbursement of the office visit, which is reported with the appropriate E/M code.

Myringotomy is an incision of the tympanic membrane. If reinflation of the eustachian tube is needed, a myringotomy with eustachian tube inflation may be performed. Code 69420 reports a myringotomy including aspiration and/or eustachian tube inflation. Code 69421 is reported if general anesthesia is used.

Tympanostomy is the insertion of plastic or metal ventilating tubes in the ear drum to allow fluid drainage. It is an effective treatment for conditions such as eustachian tube dysfunction and conductive hearing loss. Codes 69433 and 69436 report the insertion of

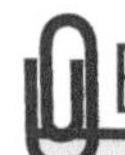

EXAMPLE **7.3**

A 1-year-old was not responding to medical management for a history of chronic and recurrent episodes of otitis media (ear infections) with persistent middle ear effusions (fluid collection). She underwent a tympanostomy. The young patient was brought to the operating room and placed in the supine position. Face-mask technique was used to administer general anesthesia. Once an acceptable level of anesthesia was achieved, the operating microscope was brought into position, and visualization was made of the left ear canal. A small amount of wax was removed with a loop. A 4-mm operating speculum was introduced. An anteroinferior-quadrant radial myringotomy was then performed. A large amount of mucoid middle ear effusion was aspirated from the middle ear cleft. A pressure equalization (PE) tube was inserted, followed by otic drops and a cotton ball in the external meatus. The head was then turned to the opposite side, where a similar procedure was performed on the right ear. Once again, the middle ear cleft had a mucoid effusion. A tube was inserted into an anteroinferior-quadrant radial myringotomy. Anesthesia was then reversed, and the patient was transported to the recovery room having tolerated the procedure well with stable vital signs.

The above procedure documents the insertion of a ventilating tube under general anesthetic. Since code 69433 is reported only for tympanostomy with a local or topical anesthetic, code 69436 fully and accurately describes the procedure. However, code 69436 is a unilateral code. The above scenario describes a bilateral procedure. Some payers require that the unilateral code be reported twice with modifier 50, *Bilateral procedure*, appended on the second code. Other payers require that the unilateral procedure is reported once with modifier 50 appended to the code. Coders must check the payer's policy prior to appending modifier 50.

RED FLAG

Modifier 50 reports bilateral services. Some payers allow the reporting of modifier 50, whereas some payers require that the same code be reported twice with the modifier on the second code. Review the payer billing policy prior to reporting modifier 50.

ventilating tubes under general anesthesia. Tubes may be permanent or temporary. Temporary tubes may fall out on their own or require surgical removal. Code 69424 reports surgical removal of a ventilating tube requiring general anesthesia. Figure 17.13 illustrates how tympanostomy codes 69433 and 69436 appear in the CPT® codebook.

Figure 17.13 Tympanostomy Codes

69433	Tympanostomy (requiring insertion of ventilating tube), local or topical anesthesia
	(For bilateral procedure, report 69433 with modifier 50)
69436	Tympanostomy (requiring insertion of ventilating tube), general anesthesia
	(For bilateral procedure, report 69433 with modifier 50)

Middle ear excision codes include procedures for mastoidectomies and treatments for polyps and tumors. A **mastoidectomy** is surgery to remove infected cells in the hollow, air-filled spaces in the mastoid bones around the canal and behind the ear, as shown in Figure 17.14. When antibiotics are not effective, mastoidectomy may be performed to treat **mastoiditis** (inflammation of the mastoid) and **meningitis** (swelling of the brain). Mastoidectomy codes are selected based on the extent of the procedure. The differences in the procedures and the associated codes are as follows:

- complete mastoidectomy—removes the infected air cells; code 69502;
- modified radical mastoidectomy—some middle ear bones are removed and the eardrum is reconstructed; code 69505;
- radical mastoidectomy—may include the removal of the eardrum and middle ear structures; skin grafting of the middle ear may be required; code 69511.

Figure 17.14 Mastoidectomy Procedure

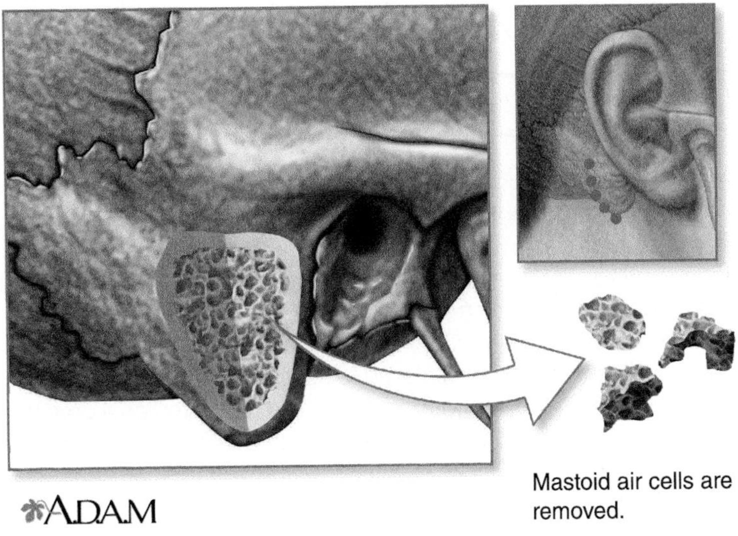
Mastoid air cells are removed.
ADAM

If a skin graft is performed, report the procedure separately with the appropriate skin graft code from the Integumentary System Surgery subsection. Mastoidectomies that include the removal of the mastoid (petrous) portion of the temporal bones are reported with code 69530, *Petrous apicectomy including radical mastoidectomy*.

The middle ear repair codes cover treatments of the mastoid, tympanic membrane, and ossicles. A **cholesteatoma** is a cyst that grows on the margins of the eardrum. A cholesteatoma can grow very rapidly and may quickly expand to the middle ear and mastoid. Mastoidectomy is a common procedure to remove cholesteatomas. Because they commonly grow back after a mastoidectomy, a recurrence of a cholesteatoma may require a second mastoidectomy in the same location as the previous procedure. The second mastoidectomy is referred to as a *mastoidectomy revision*. Mastoidectomy revisions are reported with codes 69601 through 69605. Codes are selected based on the result of the procedure. For example, code 69603 reports a revision mastoidectomy resulting in radical mastoidectomy, whereas code 69604 reports revision resulting in tympanoplasty.

Tympanoplasty is the surgical repair of a perforated (torn) tympanic membrane (eardrum) that doesn't heal on its own. Eardrum perforation may result from chronic middle ear infections or trauma. Tympanoplasty codes 69610 through 69646 are selected based on the extent of the procedures. Coders should read the operative report carefully to discern the parent code criteria. Parent code criteria include:

- Codes 69631 through 69633: tympanoplasty without mastoidectomy (includes canalplasty, atticotomy, and/or middle ear surgery);
- Codes 69635 through 69637: tympanoplasty with antrotomy or mastoidotomy (includes canalplasty, atticotomy, middle ear surgery, and/or tympanic membrane repair);
- Codes 69641 through 69646: Tympanoplasty with mastoidectomy (including canalplasty, middle ear surgery, tympanic membrane repair).

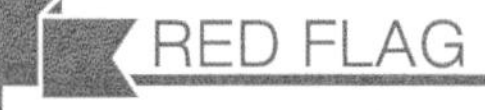

Ossicular codes that do not include prosthesis in their descriptions do not report prosthesis service procedures.

Ossicular chain reconstruction is the replacement of the malleus, or incus bone of the ear, with a prosthesis to improve or restore hearing, such as a partial ossicular replacement prosthesis (PORP) or total ossicular replacement prosthesis (TORP).

LET'S TRY ONE **17.6**

Read the description of the tympanoplasty procedure and answer the questions that follow.

Through a postauricular incision, the physician removed outer portions of the mastoid and drilled out some of the mastoid air cells to enter the mastoid antrum (air chamber). The edges of the tympanic membrane were coarsened. The physician moved the eardrum forward. The middle ear was explored, and lysis of adhesions was performed. Debris was removed, and the ossicular bones were inspected and palpated. The ossicular chain was reconstructed using a synthetic reconstructive prosthesis. A partial ossicular prosthesis (PORP) was used because the stapes suprastructure was present. A piece of cartilage was placed between the eardrum and prosthesis. Light packing was placed to support the reconstructed ossicle prior to positioning of the eardrum graft. Fascia from the temporalis muscle was harvested as a graft to repair the perforation. The graft was placed on top of the remaining eardrum. The canal skin was repositioned, and the canal was packed.

1. What structure(s) was removed? _____
2. Was there a prosthesis placed? _____
3. Was the ossicular chain reconstructed? _____
4. What is the code to report the above procedure? _____

Inner Ear (Codes 69801-69949)

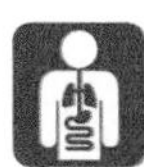

A&P Review

The **labyrinth** is the network of passages with bony walls lined with periosteum (fibrous membrane that covers bone) within the inner ear. The vestibule of the ear, the semicircular canals, and the cochlea are parts of the bony labyrinth. The labyrinth is lined with periosteum (a fibrous membrane), which holds in the endolymph fluid in a sac.

Codes for surgical procedures of the inner ear are categorized by incision/destruction, excision, and introduction and include treatments of the labyrinth, endolymph (labyrinth fluid), semicircular canal, vestibular nerve, and cochlea.

A **labyrinthotomy** is a surgical incision into the labyrinth, which can effectively treat conditions such as Meniere's disease. **Meniere's disease** is the buildup of endolymph in the inner ear. Left untreated, Meniere's disease can cause tinnitus (ringing in the ear) and hearing loss. A labyrinthotomy requires the placing of antibiotics or local anesthetics into the ear. In a transcanal approach, the physician makes a small incision into the anesthetized tympanic membrane, inserts a small catheter or needle into the middle ear, and injects the drug. Incision code 69801 reports a labyrinthotomy with perfusion of vestibuloactive drugs via a transcanal approach. Meniere's disease may also be treated by a **labyrinthectomy**, either removing all of the labyrinth or opening up the inner ear and destroying some of the soft tissue. This results in deafness. Code 69905 reports a labyrinthectomy by transcanal approach. When a mastoidectomy is also performed, report code 69910.

Coding Clicks

To watch an FDA video of a cochlear device implantation, visit http://Coding.ParadigmEducation.com/CochlearImplant.

Code 69930, *Cochlear device implantation, with or without mastoidectomy*, is the only code listed under the codebook Introduction category. A **cochlear device** is an electronic medical mechanism that receives sound, processes it, and sends small electric currents near the auditory nerve. Nerves within the inner ear send a signal to the brain. The brain learns to recognize this signal and processes the sound as "hearing." The device typically has 2 main components: an externally worn microphone, sound processor, and transmitter system; and the implanted receiver and electrode system.

Temporal Bone, Middle Fossa Approach (Codes 69950-69979)

Codes under the Temporal Bone, Middle Fossa Approach heading report procedures of the temporal bone using the middle fossa approach. The temporal bone is located at the base of the skull underneath the temple, as shown in Figure 17.15. The **middle fossa approach** involves an incision above the ear and a craniotomy (cranial incision) over the temporal lobe of the brain. The middle fossa approach is used to access the internal auditory canal for the removal of small acoustic tumors. Surgeons prefer this method because it allows for full viewing of the internal auditory canal, which increases the possibility of preserving hearing.

Coding Clicks

To view a video of a lateral temporal bone resection, visit http://Coding.ParadigmEducation.com/Resection.

Other procedures using the middle fossa approach are total facial nerve decompression (69955), decompression of the internal auditory canal (69960), and removal of temporal bone tumors. Code 69979 is reported for unlisted procedures of the temporal bone using the middle fossa approach.

Figure 17.15 Location of the Temporal Bone

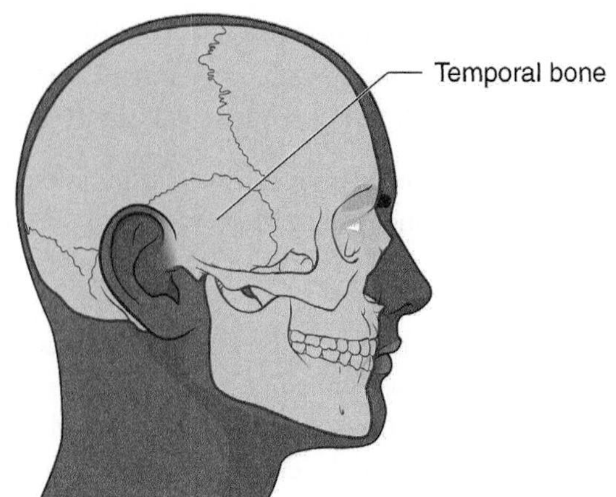

LET'S TRY ONE **17.7**

Select the correct code for the following procedure descriptions.

1. A 45-year-old female patient with vestibular Meniere's disease underwent a labyrinthotomy by transcanal approach. The procedure included insertion of corticosteroids through a small catheter into the middle ear. _____
2. A 29-year-old male was diagnosed with peripheral vertigo. To control the vertigo, a shunt was inserted into the endolymphatic sac of the left ear. _____
3. An 18-year-old female with Bell's palsy underwent a total facial nerve decompression. The approach was through the temporal bone via the middle fossa. The procedure included nerve and muscle grafts. _____
4. A 48-year-old male with cancer of the temporal bone had the tumor removed. _____

Operating Microscope (Code 69990)

An **operating microscope** is a tool used during delicate surgical procedures that require the magnification of anatomical sites such as the middle ear, eye, oral cavity, and nerves. Figure 17.16 illustrates an ENT operating microscope. Add-on code 69990 reports microsurgical techniques requiring the use of an operating microscope. Do not report code 69990 when the use of an operating microscope is an included component of the surgery. Parenthetical notes list procedure codes that may be reported with code 66990. When reported with codes for the primary procedure, modifier 51 is not appended.

Figure 17.16 Operating Microscope Used in Ears, Nose, and Throat Microsurgical Procedures

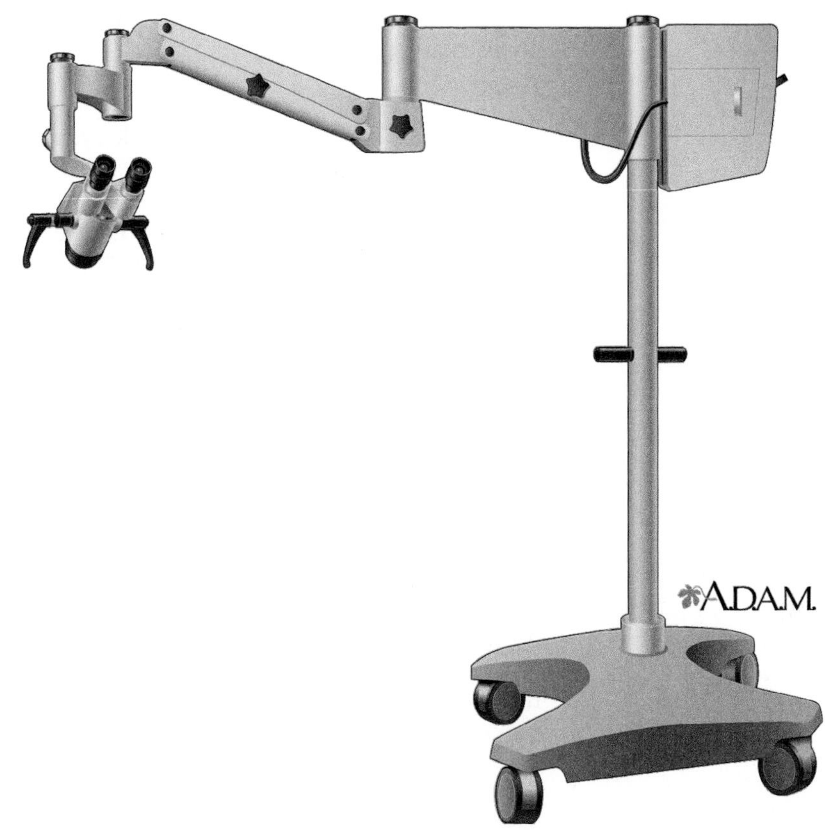

LET'S TRY ONE **17.8**

Use your CPT® codebook, encoder program, or NCCI edits to identify the codes that allow reporting of the operating microscope add-on code 69990. Place an *X* next to any code that does *not* allow reporting with code 69990.

1. _____ 61304
2. _____ 61548
3. _____ 63078
4. _____ 64840
5. _____ 68811

Chapter Summary

- Evisceration is the removal of the eyeball (globe) while leaving the sclera and extraocular muscles in place. An ocular implant is always placed after an evisceration.
- Enucleation is the removal of the whole eye from the orbit while leaving in place all other orbital structures.
- If reconstruction of the conjunctiva is performed during an enucleation, report the appropriate conjunctivoplasty code separately.
- Skin grafts are not included in the code's description and are reported separately when performed.
- Modification of a secondary ocular implant may not be reported for the same eye on the same date of service, because modification of the ocular implant is integral to secondary ocular implants.
- The Anterior Segment codes include procedures of the cornea, anterior chamber, anterior sclera, iris, ciliary body, and lens.
- Keratoplasty is the surgical repair of the cornea. Code selection is based on the type of procedure: penetrating, endothelial, or anterior lamellar.
- Intracapsular cataract extraction (ICCE) and extracapsular cataract extraction (ECCE) are the most common types of cataract extractions.
- Retinal detachment repair codes are selected based on the method or extent of the procedure.
- Ocular adnexa structures include the extraocular muscles, orbit, and eyelid. Codes are arranged by anatomical site and then further divided by procedure type.
- Orbital implant insertion, removal, and replacement codes are listed in the codebook in the Orbit category of the Ocular Adnexa codes.
- The ear has 3 parts: external, middle, and inner.
- The middle ear bones are the malleus, incus, and stapes.

- If reconstruction of the ear is required after an exostosis excision, report the appropriate skin graft code from the Integumentary System Surgery subsection.
- The eustachian tube is a narrow passage leading from the pharynx to the cavity of the middle ear.
- Ossicular chain reconstruction is the replacement of the malleus or incus bones of the ear with a prosthesis to improve or restore hearing.
- A labyrinthotomy is a surgical incision into the labyrinth of the inner ear.
- Do not report codes for an operating microscope when it is an included component of the surgery.

Navigator

Access interactive chapter review exercises, practice activities, flash cards, and study games.

Chapter 18

Radiology Coding

Fast Facts

- Wilhelm Roentgen accidentally discovered x-ray imaging while studying the path of electricity.
- Nikola Tesla's discovery of the rotating magnetic field led to the creation of magnetic resonance imaging (MRI).
- NASA used x-ray technology to take images of outer space for the first time in 1979.
- On average, 16 million mammograms are ordered or provided during physician office visits yearly.

Sources: http://encyclopedia.com, http://onlineradiologyschools.org, http://www.cdc.gov/nchs/fastats/mammography.htm

Crack the Code

Review the sample operative report to find the correct radiology code. You may need to return to this exercise after reading the chapter content.

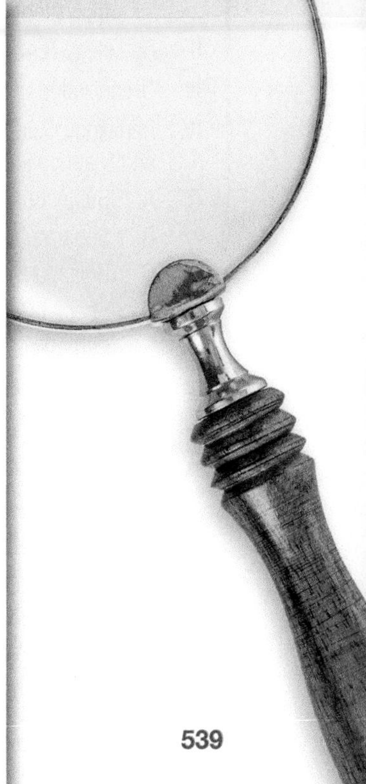

DATE OF PROCEDURE: June 15, 2019

RADIOLOGIST: Frances Vann, MD

PROCEDURE PERFORMED: Intraoperative Cholangiogram

FINDINGS: Intraoperative cholangiogram performed. Contrast was injected through the cystic duct remnant. There was slight dilatation of the common bile duct with unrestricted flow of contrast into the duodenum. However, there was a 5-mm filling deficiency in the proximal common bile duct, mostly due to a stone.

IMPRESSION: Common bile duct stone. A second set of plain x-rays was requested during the operative session to confirm. Dr. Vann interpreted the additional film during the operative session. Slight dilatation of the common bile duct.

answer: 74300 and 74301

Learning Objectives

18.1 Identify the different imaging services used in radiology.

18.2 Describe the radiologic global service and compare the technical and professional components.

18.3 Understand terms used in the Radiology section of the CPT® codebook.

18.4 Apply radiology reporting guidelines.

18.5 Discuss the use of modifiers 26, 52, 59, and TC in radiology coding.

18.6 Explain the arrangement of the Radiology section of the CPT® codebook.

18.7 Differentiate between computed tomography (CT) scans, magnetic resonance imaging (MRI), radiography, and ultrasound.

18.8 Describe the different radiology techniques for diagnostic studies.

18.9 Describe fluoroscopy and the codes associated with this technique.

18.10 Differentiate between screening and diagnostic mammograms and describe the reporting of mammography codes.

18.11 Identify the different types of bone and joint studies.

18.12 Define the different methods of radiation oncology.

18.13 Evaluate the reporting criteria for radiation treatment codes.

18.14 Describe nuclear medicine and differentiate between its uses for diagnostic and therapeutic purposes.

18.15 Define documentation requirements for selection of radiology codes.

Chapter Outline

I. Introduction to Radiology
- **A.** Radiology Code Components: Technical Component, Professional Component, and Global Services
  - **i.** Technical Component
  - **ii.** Professional Component
  - **iii.** Global Services

II. Radiology Terminology

III. Organization of the Radiology Section

IV. Radiology Guidelines (Including Nuclear Medicine and Diagnostic Ultrasound)
- **A.** Subject Listings
- **B.** Separate Procedure
- **C.** Unlisted Service or Procedure
- **D.** Special Report
- **E.** Supervision and Interpretation
- **F.** Administration of Contrast Material(s)
- **G.** Written Report(s)

V. Diagnostic Radiology (Codes 70010-76499)
- **A.** Radiologic Examinations
- **B.** Computed Tomography Scan
- **C.** Magnetic Resonance Imaging
- **D.** Angiography

VI. Diagnostic Ultrasound (Codes 76506-76999)
- **A.** Pelvic Ultrasound

VII. Radiologic Guidance (Codes 77001-77022)
- **A.** Fluoroscopic Guidance
- **B.** Computed Tomography Guidance
- **C.** Magnetic Resonance Guidance

VIII. Breast, Mammography (Codes 77053-77067)

IX. Bone/Joint Studies (Codes 77071-77086)

X. Radiation Oncology (Codes 77261-77799)
- **A.** Consultation: Clinical Management
- **B.** Clinical Treatment Planning
  - **i.** Therapeutic Radiology Treatment Plan
  - **ii.** Therapeutic Radiology Simulation
- **C.** Medical Radiation Physics, Dosimetry, Treatment Devices, and Special Services
- **D.** Radiation Treatment Delivery
- **E.** Stereotactic Radiation Treatment Delivery
- **F.** Neutron Beam Treatment Delivery
- **G.** Proton Beam Treatment Delivery
- **H.** Radiation Treatment Management
- **I.** Hyperthermia and Clinical Intracavitary Hyperthermia
- **J.** Clinical Brachytherapy

XI. Nuclear Medicine (Codes 78012-79999)

XII. Instructions for Reporting Radiology Codes

XIII. Chapter Summary

Introduction to Radiology

Radiology is the branch of medicine that uses imaging to treat and diagnose diseases. A **radiologist** is a medical doctor who specializes in the study of radiologic services. All medical specialties may use radiologic services, which include several imaging modalities or modes of delivery. **Radiography** is an imaging technique based on x-rays passing through tissue and emerging to "hit" film on the other side. **Ultrasound** uses sound waves to create images and is an example of a nonradiation radiology service. **Computed tomography (CT)** processes radiographic images through a computer to produce an image. **Magnetic resonance imaging (MRI)** produces images via electromagnetic fields and radio waves. **Radiation oncology** uses high-energy ionizing radiation to treat malignant and benign tumors. This chapter will discuss these various radiologic diagnostic and therapeutic tools.

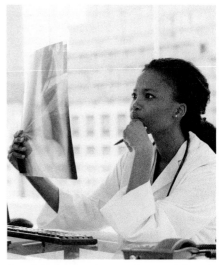

A radiologist is a doctor who specializes in the study of radiologic services.

Radiology Code Components: Technical Component, Professional Component, and Global Services

A radiology service is really 2 services bundled into 1 procedure, composed of a technical component and a professional component. The technical component is the technological performance of the diagnostic test. The professional component is the review, interpretation, and documentation of the image created. The following sections will explain how to report radiology services in different circumstances: when only the test was performed, when only the report was written, or when both services were performed together.

Technical Component

The **technical component** of a radiology code reports the deployment of equipment for the diagnostic test by the owner of the equipment. The technical component of a radiology code includes the following elements:

- the radiology technician;
- the equipment;
- film, film processing, and other nondurable supplies needed for the imaging;
- the facility costs (overhead) for supplying the services.

The technical component of a radiology service performed in a hospital is reported under the hospital outpatient prospective payment system (OPPS) for Medicare, which allows diagnostic services to be billed under Medicare Part B. OPPS billing guidelines are covered in detail in Chapter 21. Most other payers follow this same payment structure. When only the technical component of a radiology service is performed, append HCPCS modifier TC, *Technical component,* to the CPT® code.

EXAMPLE 18.1

A 25-year-old female patient who fell while riding her bike had a 2-view x-ray of the knee performed in the hospital. The physician reviewed the x-ray film, documented the findings in the health record, and discussed the diagnosis and treatment plan with the patient. Because the equipment, technician, and supplies are an expense to the facility, the x-ray is billed with HCPCS modifier TC to report only the technical component. Code 73560 - TC, *Radiologic examination, knee; 1 or 2 views - Technical component*, would be reported.

Professional Component

The **professional service component** of a radiologic service identifies the portion of the service provided by the physician. This includes interpretation of the film or digital image by the physician and the written report detailing the findings. The type of radiologic services performed will determine the extent of the written report. If a radiologic service is performed in a hospital setting using the facility's equipment, supplies, and personnel, the physician's professional service is reported by appending CPT® modifier 26, *Professional component,* to the CPT® code.

EXAMPLE 18.2

A physician referred a patient to have a chest x-ray at the Northstar Medical Center outpatient facility to determine why he has been having chest congestion for 2 weeks without any relief. The radiologist reviewed the x-ray film, wrote a written report that detailed the findings, and sent a copy of the report to the physician who requested the chest x-ray.

Because the services took place in the hospital outpatient facility, the technical component of the chest x-ray is reported by the hospital. The radiologist reports only the professional component by appending modifier 26, *Professional component*, to the CPT® code. Code 71046 - 26, *Radiologic examination, chest, 2 views, frontal and lateral - Professional component*, would be reported.

Global Services

Global services include both the technical and professional component of a service. Typically, global services take place in the physician's office, where the physician or medical group owns the equipment, employs the technician, supervises the procedure, and provides the interpretation and report. When a global service is performed, a modifier is not appended to the CPT® code.

EXAMPLE 18.3

While hiking, Janet fell and bumped her knee. She explained to the doctor that her knee had been hurting for 2 days. The physician's office owns digital x-ray equipment. The physician ordered a 2-view x-ray of Janet's knee. The digital image of the knee was sent to the doctor through the physician's office EHR system. The doctor reviewed the x-ray and documented the findings in the EHR system. The physician then discussed the results and treatment plan with Janet.

Because the physician's office is financially responsible for the technical component and performs the professional services of the x-ray, the physician reports the global service 73560, *Radiologic examination, knee; 1 or 2 views*, and a modifier is not required.

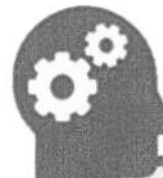

Think Like a Coder

Nyja is the coding manager in a cardiology office. She is reviewing some of the codes submitted by Jamie, a newly hired coder. Jamie is responsible for coding diagnostic studies performed in the Northstar Medical Center outpatient department that are later reviewed by a medical center staff cardiologist, who creates a written report. As Nyja reviews the records, she identifies a consistent error. The coder is not reporting diagnostic tests performed in the hospital's outpatient department correctly. It appears that Jamie is reporting global codes without appropriate modifiers. Why is reporting the global procedure code incorrect?

Radiology Terminology

A good understanding of vocabulary related to radiology, imaging equipment, and reporting guidelines is valuable in coding. Coders will need to know combining forms, prefixes, and suffixes related to radiology. Table 18.1 contains an overview of the word parts used in radiology terminology. Table 18.2 contains a list of commonly used medical terms in radiology.

Table 18.1 Word Parts Used in Radiology Terminology

Combining Forms, Prefixes, and Suffixes	Definition	Example
radi/o	Radiation, x-ray	Radiography—an imaging technique using x-rays
son/o	Sound, ultrasound	Sonohysterography—ultrasound of the uterus
-gram	A recording	Cephalogram—an x-ray recording of the head
-graphy	A process of recording	Arthrography—recording images of joints
-opaque	Impenetrable	Radiopaque—not transparent with radiation

Table 18.2 Radiology Commonly Used Terms

Medical Term	Definition
angiography	Visualization of blood vessels using radiography
anteroposterior (AP) projection	Direction of an x-ray beam from the patient's front (anterior) to back (posterior)
arthrography	Visualization of the inside of a joint by use of CT, MRI, or fluoroscopic imaging
bilateral	Relating to both sides of a 2-sided anatomical structure
biometry	The analysis of biological data using mathematical and statistical methods
complete	In radiology, *complete* indicates the maximum possible views taken
computed tomography (CT) scan	Computer processing of a series of x-ray views taken from many different angles to create cross-sectional images of bones and soft tissues
contrast or contrast material	A radiopaque (not transparent with radiation) substance used during an x-ray exam (or some MRI exams) to provide visual contrast in the pictures of different tissues and organs; the substance can be given orally or intravenously (by injection)
diagnostic	Relating to procedures performed to identify illness, diseases, or injuries indicated by a patient's current medical signs and/or symptoms
diagnostic order	A request with instructions for a diagnostic procedure
fluoroscopy	An imaging technique that uses x-rays transmitted to a monitor to display real-time, moving images of the internal structures of a patient
magnetic resonance angiography (MRA)	Use of magnetic resonance imaging equipment and contrast materials to better visualize blood vessels
magnetic resonance imaging (MRI)	A technique that uses a magnetic field and radio waves to create detailed images of the organs and tissues within the body
mammography	Radiographic visualization of the breast
oblique position	Body position at a slant or on a slope
positron emission tomography (PET)	Visualization of metabolic or body functions using radioactive tracers
posteroanterior (PA) projection	Direction of an x-ray beam from the patient's back (posterior) to front (anterior)
projection	Direction in which x-rays travel from the radiographic equipment through the subject to the image receptor
prone position	Patient positioned on stomach, face down
single photon emission computed tomography (SPECT)	Radioactive tracers used in combination with a CT scan to visualize blood flow to tissue and organs
supine position	Patient positioned on back, face up
therapeutic	Performed to treat illness, disease, or injuries
tomography	A radiographic technique that produces cross section images of tissue structures at a predetermined depth
unilateral	Relating to 1 side of a 2-sided anatomical structure
venography	Radiographic visualization of a vein
view	A radiographic image study described by an x-ray exposure of an anatomical site
x-ray	High-energy electromagnetic radiation with short wavelengths that are absorbed to different degrees by different materials; popularly, an image created by use of x-ray technology

CONCEPTS CHECKPOINT **18.1**

Using information found in Table 18.2, match the medical term in the first column with the correct definition in the second column.

1. _____ bilateral
2. _____ diagnostic order
3. _____ prone position
4. _____ supine position
5. _____ unilateral

a. Both sides of an anatomical structure
b. Lying on back, face up
c. Lying on stomach, face down
d. One side of an anatomical structure
e. Request and instructions to perform a diagnostic procedure

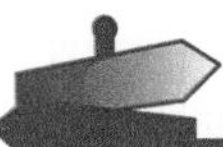

Learn Your Way

The word *prone* comes from the Latin *pronus*, meaning "bent forward, inclined to," and from the adverbial form of the prefix *pro-*, meaning "forward." *Supine* is derived from the Latin *supinus*, "bent backward, thrown backward." Verbal learners may particularly connect with language etymology and find that learning where words come from helps them remember the meaning of those words. Visual learners may learn terms better by seeking out photos and illustrations instead.

Organization of the Radiology Section

The CPT® codebook organizes radiology codes in schemes relevant to code selection. Diagnostic radiology and diagnostic ultrasound codes are arranged by anatomical site. Radiologic guidance and radiation oncology are subdivided by type of service. Nuclear medicine codes are divided based on diagnostic or therapeutic services. Radiology codes range from 70010 through 79999. Table 18.3 provides all the main headings within the Radiology section and the codes the headings include.

Table 18.3 Headings Within the Radiology Section of the CPT® Codebook

Subsection	Code Range
Diagnostic Radiology	70010-76499
Diagnostic Ultrasound	76506-76999
Radiologic Guidance	77001-77022
Breast, Mammography	77053-77067
Bone/Joint Studies	77071-77086
Radiation Oncology	77261-77799
Nuclear Medicine	78012-79999

Radiology Guidelines (Including Nuclear Medicine and Diagnostic Ultrasound)

The Radiology Guidelines are located at the beginning of the Radiology section of the CPT® codebook. They provide guidance for separate procedures, supervision and interpretation, written reports, and administration of contrast material(s). The guidelines should be reviewed prior to code selection, and their application will be discussed in depth.

Subject Listings

Subject listings (procedures) in the Radiology section apply only when services are performed by or under the responsible supervision of a physician or other qualified healthcare professional. Qualified healthcare professionals are those equipped to perform specified professional services because of their specialized education, training, or licensure and are usually subject to regulations. Training for nonphysician practitioners (NPPs) does not include radiology technician services; therefore, they are not permitted to supervise radiology technician services. If NPPs have specialized training and are licensed to perform radiology services, they may bill for radiology services they personally perform; however, they are still not qualified to supervise radiology technicians.

Separate Procedure

Many diagnostic and surgical procedures require the use of radiologic imaging. When imaging is an integral part of the procedure, the imaging code should not be reported independently of the procedure. A code that includes the designation **separate procedure** is the base or parent procedure that may be reported alone when the procedure is not an integral part of the primary procedure. When the separate procedure is bundled into the primary procedure, reporting the separate procedure in addition to the primary procedure is considered unbundling.

There will be circumstances in which the physician finds it necessary to perform the separate procedure independently of the primary procedure or as a distinct unrelated procedure. When the separate procedure is performed as part of another procedure, report the separate procedure code and append modifier 59, *Distinct procedural service*. When the separate procedure is performed by itself, a modifier is not required. A fluoroscopy is an example of a separate procedure. A **fluoroscopy** is an imaging technique that uses x-rays to obtain real-time moving images of the internal structures of a patient with a fluoroscope, a device that projects a radiographic image on a fluorescent screen for immediate viewing. Using the National Correct Coding Initiative (NCCI) edits and encoder programs will help coders identify separate codes that may be unbundled.

EXAMPLE 18.4

A patient with myocarditis had an endomyocardial biopsy. Prior to the procedure the patient was placed under general anesthesia. A local anesthetic was applied to an area of the neck, where a small incision was made. A catheter was inserted into the blood vessel. Fluoroscopy real-time imaging was used to guide the catheter through the blood vessels to the heart. Upon reaching the heart, a small specimen was collected and removed. The incision was closed, and the specimen was sent to the pathologist for testing. The procedure took less than 60 minutes.

Code 93505, *Endomyocardial biopsy*, is reported. Although the procedure documentation includes the use of fluoroscopic imaging, because it is an integral part of the procedure, it is not separately reported. If documentation supported that the fluoroscopic procedure was not related to the endomyocardial biopsy, code 76000, *Fluoroscopy (separate procedure), up to one hour physician or other qualified health care professional time*, would be reported with modifier 59, *Distinct procedural service*.

Unlisted Service or Procedure

Services or procedures that do not have a CPT® code listed are reported with the appropriate "unlisted" radiology codes. A special report, such as the health record or diagnostic study, describing the procedure and documentation of the medical necessity for the services or procedure, should be submitted with the insurance claim. Unlisted Radiology codes for all of the different radiologic modalities are itemized in the Radiology Guidelines.

Special Report

Special reports are submitted with insurance claims to provide insurance payers with details of services and procedures that are not typically performed. A physician prepares a special report to detail a procedure that may be beyond the description of the CPT® code or a new/experimental procedure. It is rare that special reports are submitted with radiology services. However, when they are required by the insurance payer, the special report should include the nature, extent, medical necessity, effort, and equipment used in the radiologic procedure. The length of time the procedure took to perform should also be documented.

CONCEPTS CHECKPOINT **18.2**

Using information from the previous section, select the correct statement.

1. Subject listings in the Radiology section apply only when services are performed by or under the supervision of
   a. the responsible physician.
   b. a qualified healthcare professional.
   c. a physician or a qualified healthcare professional.
   d. a medical assistant.
2. A separate procedure is not
   a. a parent procedure code.
   b. an integral part of procedures listed within a specific family of codes.
   c. sometimes bundled into other operative procedures.
   d. ever reported with another code from the same family of codes.
3. A separate procedure
   a. always requires the appending of modifier 59.
   b. does not require a modifier if it is the only procedure performed.
   c. does require modifier 25 if the procedure is not bundled into the primary procedure.
   d. may be unbundled with modifier 72.
4. Unlisted radiology codes are supplied for
   a. nuclear medicine and diagnostic ultrasound procedures.
   b. nuclear medicine and oncology procedures.
   c. diagnostic ultrasound and surgical procedures.
   d. diagnostic ultrasound, nuclear medicine, and cardiology procedures.
5. A special report should include information about a procedure's
   a. extent, image, effort, and equipment.
   b. nature, extent, medical necessity, effort, time, and equipment.
   c. nature, extent, medical necessity, and effort.
   d. nature, phase, medical necessity, effort, and equipment.

Supervision and Interpretation

In radiology, **supervision and interpretation** refers to the medical provider's use of imaging equipment during a surgical procedure or diagnostic study and the medical opinion of the captured images. Because surgical procedures may require imaging guidance, or imaging procedures may require surgery to access the body area to be imaged, codes for procedures may include image guidance. See for example the cardiovascular surgical code 33990, *Insertion of ventricular assist device, percutaneous including radiological supervision and interpretation; arterial access only*. Alternatively, section notes may state that imaging is included with the procedure or diagnostic study, as in this example from the Cardiovascular Surgery subsection:

> Radiological supervision and interpretation related to the pacemaker or implantable defibrillator procedure is included in 33206-33249, 33262, 33263, 33264, 33270, 33271, 33272, 33273 0387T, 0388T.

In these instances, a radiology code that describes the imaging is not reported. However, if the CPT® code description does not include radiologic supervision and interpretation, and there are no guidelines to indicate that imaging is included with the procedure, it is acceptable to assign a separate code to report the imaging service.

EXAMPLE 18.5

A patient with a mass in her left breast underwent a ductography. During the procedure, the physician injected dye into the duct. The dye created a sharper image of the breast ducts. An x-ray image was created of multiple duct glands. The physician then evaluated the image and created a written report of his findings. The physician fully reports the procedure, supervision, and interpretation with the following codes:

77054 *Mammary ductogram or galactogram, multiple ducts, radiological supervision and interpretation*

19030 *Injection procedure only for mammary ductogram or galactogram*

Modifiers are not required to report codes 77054 and 19030 together. If the physician did not perform the injection, but he supervised the procedure and interpreted the image, he would report only code 77054.

Administration of Contrast Material(s)

Contrast materials are substances used to enhance the images of internal body structures and fluids produced by x-ray imaging, computed tomography, magnetic resonance imaging, and ultrasound. Enhanced images assist the physician in identifying organ or tissue abnormalities.

The type of contrast material chosen is determined by the equipment used to capture the image and the anatomical site of the imaging. Barium sulfate and iodine-based substances (that contain iodine as the primary substance) are commonly used contrast materials. Because iodine-based contrast agents are water soluble and appropriate for many different areas of the body, these solutions have many routes of administration, with the intravenous route being the most typical. Contrast materials are commonly referred to as *dyes*, but technically they do not stain or color organs or blood vessels. Rather, they are substances with different opacities from surrounding tissues; the substances eventually absorb into the body to be eliminated through urine or bowel movements. **Opacification** causes the targeted body area to appear more opaque (not transparent) or cloudy. For example, barium sulfate agents enhance mucosal imaging details by making targeted body areas appear more opaque. Barium sulfate agents are commonly used to enhance images of the gastrointestinal tract. Figure 18.1 shows an image of the large intestine enhanced by barium sulfate. Barium sulfate may be administered orally or rectally.

Coders should review the diagnostic order (request for a test) and test report prior to code selection. When a contrast material is used in a diagnostic study, the phrase "with contrast" is written by the physician in the test order and in the diagnostic report. Coders will select the diagnostic test code that has "with contrast" in the code description. American Medical Association (AMA) and the Centers for Medicare and Medicaid Services (CMS) reporting guidelines state that if only oral and/or rectal

Figure 18.1 Image of Colonoscopy Enhanced by Use of Barium Sulfate

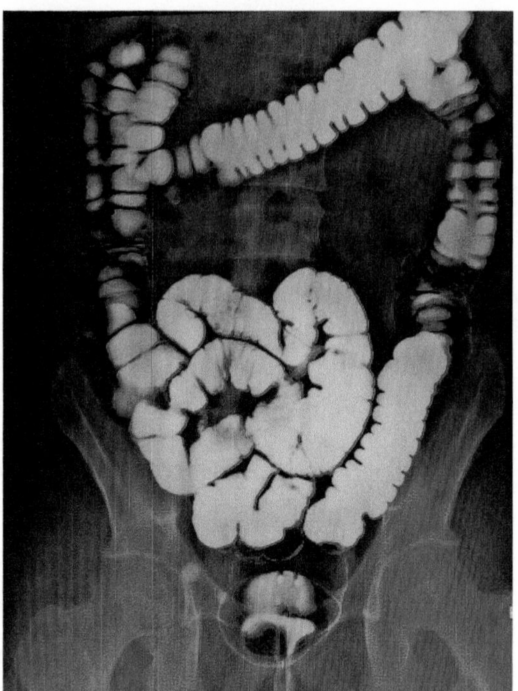

contrast are administered, select the appropriate code that states "without contrast." Contrast materials may be given by the following routes of administration:

- orally (by mouth);
- rectally (via the rectum);
- intravascularly (in a vein or artery);
- intra-articularly (in a joint);
- intrathecally (within or into the space around the brain or spinal cord).

Conditions such as pelvic pain may warrant the physician to order a study to be performed without contrast, followed by a study with contrast. The 2 images may be compared to each other for a more accurate assessment of the patient's condition. Report the CPT® code that states in the description, "without followed by contrast." This is the only code needed to report both imaging procedures.

When reporting diagnostic studies "with contrast," it is important to read the parenthetic notes under the code, which will identify if an additional code is needed to report the injection procedure used to administer the contrast or the contrast material. When used, contrast materials are reported separately from the radiology code. Contrast material codes are located in the HCPCS Level II codebook.

CONCEPTS CHECKPOINT **18.3**

Using information from the previous section, indicate if each of the following statements is true or false.

1. _____ Barium sulfate and iodine-based substances are commonly used contrast materials.
2. _____ Contrast material codes are located in the HCPCS Level II codebook.
3. _____ Contrast materials are dyes that stain organs or blood vessels.
4. _____ If only oral and/or rectal contrast is administered, the code that states "without contrast" is appropriate to select.
5. _____ When a contrast material is used in a diagnostic study, the phrase "with contrast" is written by the physician in the test order for the diagnostic study and in the diagnostic report.

Written Report(s)

A **written report** documents in detail the imaging examination and the medical findings prepared by the physician who supervised and interpreted the diagnostic procedure. The type of radiology study will determine the length of the written report. Most insurance payers do not require written reports to be submitted with insurance claims; however, if there is a report, coders must review it to verify that the documentation supports the CPT® code. The coder may find that the documentation detail indicates the reporting of a more or less extensive imaging study, necessitating a different code or modifier. In addition to the documentation, the coder should verify that the interpreting provider has signed the written report.

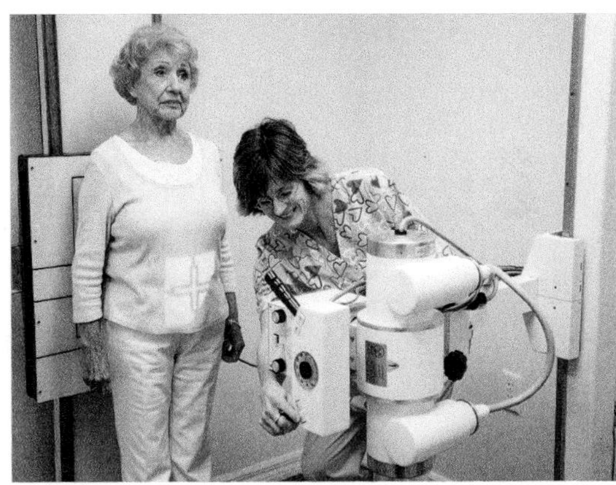

A written report documents the details of the procedure. An x-ray written report includes the number of views and the anatomical site that was imaged.

The written report will include the type of radiology service, the anatomical site, and the details of the procedure. Depending on the type of radiology service, the procedural detail will include the number of views, the status of the study as complete or limited, and the use of contrast. Figure 18.2 provides an illustration of a written report. A **complete diagnostic study** is one that includes the maximum possible images of an organ or anatomical site. A **limited diagnostic study** is one that does not include the maximum possible images of an organ or anatomical structures related to the specific body part examined.

Figure 18.2 Radiology Diagnostic Report for an Abdominal and Pelvic CT Scan With Contrast

PROCEDURE: CT abdomen pelvis with contrast

REASON FOR EXAM: Generalized abdominal pain with swelling at the site of the ileostomy

TECHNIQUE: Axial CT images of the abdomen and pelvis were obtained utilizing 100 mL of Isovue-300.

CT ABDOMEN: The liver, spleen, pancreas, adrenal glands, and kidneys are unremarkable. Punctate calcifications in the gallbladder lumen likely represent a gallstone.

CT PELVIS: Postsurgical changes of a left lower quadrant ileostomy are again seen. There is no evidence for an obstruction. A partial colectomy and diverting ileostomy is seen within the right lower quadrant. The previously seen 3.4-cm subcutaneous fluid collection has resolved. Within the left lower quadrant, a 3.4-cm x 2.5-cm loculated fluid collection has not significantly changed. This is adjacent to the anastomosis site, and a pelvic abscess cannot be excluded. No obstruction is seen. The appendix is not clearly visualized. The urinary bladder is unremarkable.

IMPRESSION:

1. Resolution of the previously seen subcutaneous fluid collection
2. Left pelvic 3.4-cm fluid collection has not significantly changed in size or appearance. These findings may be due to a pelvic abscess.
3. Right lower quadrant ileostomy has not significantly changed
4. Cholelithiasis

Diagnostic Radiology (Codes 70010-76499)

The Diagnostic Radiology subsection is divided by anatomical site. Codes for the anatomical sites in the Radiology section are sequenced by head and neck, chest, spine and pelvis, upper extremities, lower extremities, abdomen, gastrointestinal tract, urinary tract, gynecologic and obstetric, heart, and vascular procedures. Radiology procedures in the Diagnostic Radiology subsection include the following modalities:

- radiologic examinations;
- computed tomography (CT);
- magnetic resonance imaging (MRI);
- angiography and magnetic resonance angiography;
- computed tomographic angiography (CTA);
- fluoroscopy.

Radiologic Examinations

Radiologic examinations use invisible waves of energy produced by an energy source, such as an x-ray machine, to diagnose a patient's internal medical conditions. X-rays are passed through the targeted body area and are absorbed in various degrees by bones and tissues. Radiography is the process by which radiographs (x-rays) are made.

Radiologic examination codes specify the exact number of views or indicate that a complete x-ray examination was performed. A **complete radiology examination** refers to the highest number of views required to completely evaluate the patient's condition. The code for a complete study may also identify the number of views. For example, CPT® code 73564, *Radiologic examination, knee; complete, 4 or more views*, specifies both "complete" and the minimum number of views required. Do not mistake the number of views with the number of films used to capture the image. **Views** refers to the number of images taken of a body part in different positions. When the best available code describes more views than were taken, modifier 52, *Reduced services*, is appended to the CPT® code to notify the insurance payer of the decrease in services. A physician may order an x-ray procedure to diagnose a bone injury, heart problems, and digestive conditions, among many other conditions. Figure 18.3 illustrates an x-ray image of 2 views of the forearm, the radius (left) and the ulna (right).

Figure 18.3 Two X-ray Views of the Forearm

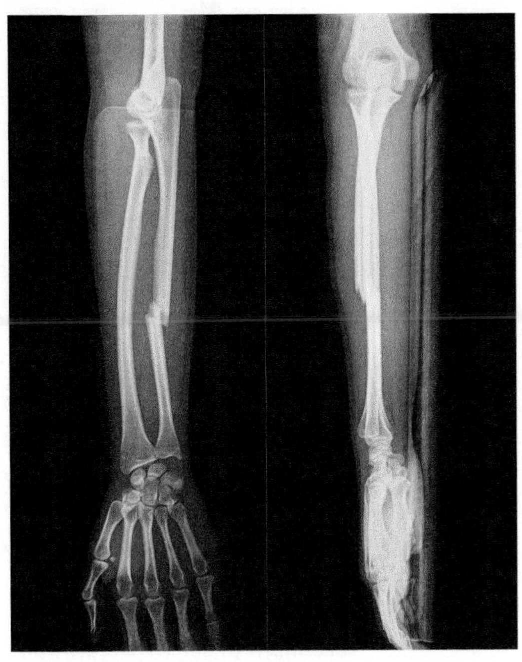

Coding for CMS

Modifier CT is appended to computed tomography services furnished using equipment that does not meet each of the standard attributes of the National Electrical Manufacturers Association (NEMA). If coding for a diagnostic facility, coders must identify the status of the CT equipment prior to appending modifier CT. Omitting modifier CT when coding for a CT scan that was performed on non-NEMA CT equipment will result in overpayment and may be considered fraud or abuse.

Computed Tomography Scan

A computed tomography (CT) scan, sometimes referred to as a *CAT scan*, is an imaging technique that uses multiple x-ray images to produce a cross-section image of soft tissues and bones. The radiographic images are captured from many different angles and then are processed by a computer to produce an image that appears to be a slice of the organ. If desired, the computer can produce a 3-D image by combining the cross-section images. Contrast materials may be used to improve the visualization of the body part.

Documentation in the written report must identify the type of contrast and route of administration when contrast material is used. Providers may order a CT scan for diagnosis of bone or muscle disorders, determination of the exact location of infections, or guidance during surgical procedures. Figure 18.4 illustrates a CT scan of a patient's brain.

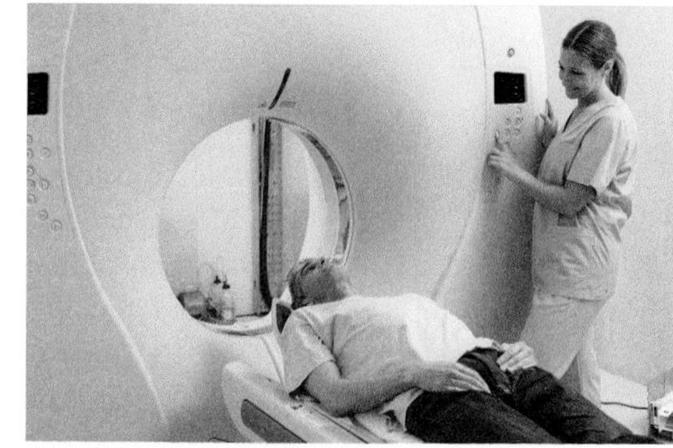

CT scans use multiple x-ray images to produce a cross-section image.

Figure 18.4 Computed Tomographic Imaging of a Patient's Brain

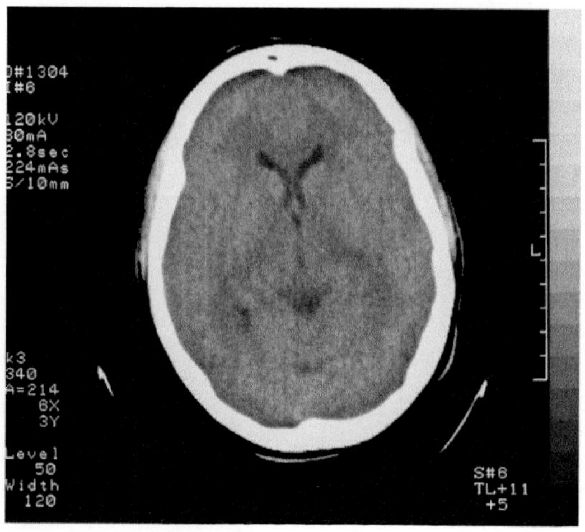

Magnetic Resonance Imaging

Magnetic resonance imaging (MRI) uses electromagnetic fields and radio waves to produce images of body parts, organs, and tissues. An MRI machine is a very large tubular structure with a moveable examination table in the center on which the patient lies flat. Activation of an electromagnetic field or of radio waves causes the body's water molecules to line up, and deactivation causes the molecules to relax. The lineup of the water molecules makes for a sharper image, and structures that contain more water allow a very sharp image to be captured. Tissues that contain very little water, such as bones, are not imaged well by MRI. Soft tissues such as the brain are the most commonly imaged by MRI and create very crisp images. Figure 18.5 shows an MRI of a patient's brain. As you can see, it is a clearer image than the brain shown in the CT scan in Figure 18.4. Contrast materials may be used to enhance the image. Documentation must support the use of contrast and its route of administration.

Figure 18.5 Magnetic Resonance Imaging of a Patient's Brain

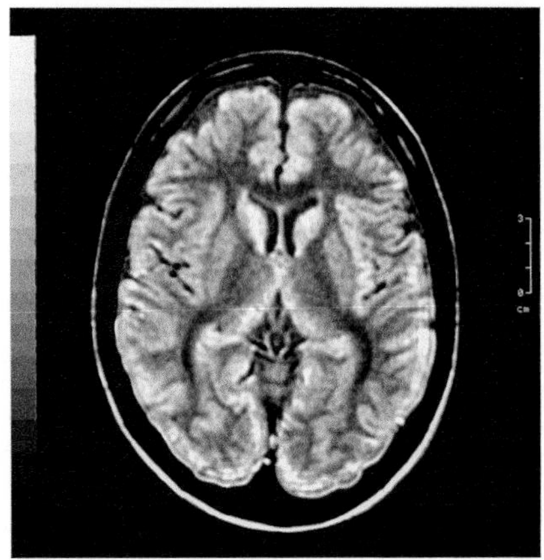

Angiography

Angiography is radiographic imaging of the inside of blood vessels. To visualize the lumen (the inside layer of a blood vessel), a catheter is inserted into the femoral artery, brachial artery, or vein. A tiny camera is used to guide the catheter to the area being studied. Contrast material (a dye) is then injected into the catheter to enable vessels, veins, and arteries to be seen on digital x-ray images or film. Angiograms may be used to identify abnormalities such as a blockage in the heart, lungs, brain, arms, legs, back, and abdomen.

When MRI technology is used instead of radiography, the procedure is called **magnetic resonance angiography (MRA)**. Not all MRAs require the use of contrast materials. Coders should review the written report to verify the use of dyes. CT scans may also be used to capture images of blood vessels, a process called **computed tomographic angiography (CTA).** All CTA tests require the use of contrast material. Figure 18.6 shows an MRA study of the carotid arteries.

Figure 18.6 Example of a Magnetic Resonance Angiography Study

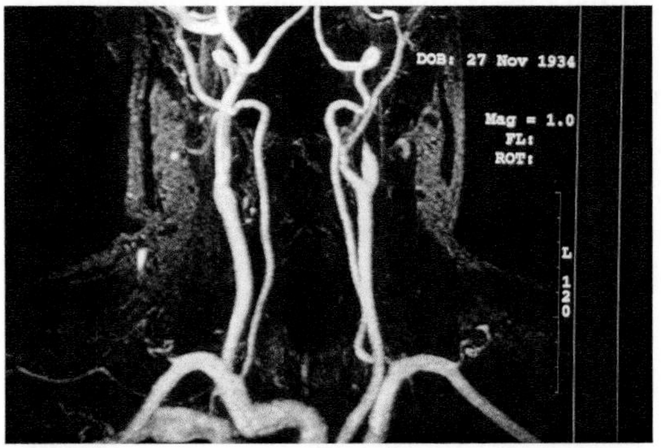

Some angiography codes are combination codes that include more than 1 anatomical site, such as code 75635, shown in Figure 18.7.

Figure 18.7 Example of an Angiography Combination Code

75635	Computed tomographic angiography, abdominal aorta and bilateral iliofemoral lower extremity runoff, with contrast material(s), including noncontrast images, if performed, and image postprocessing

The code description for code 73635 includes both the abdominal aorta and bilateral iliofemoral lower extremities. Angiography runoff studies evaluate the aorta and its branches as it flows down through the body. Prior to assigning the CPT® code, coders should carefully read the code description and any parenthetic notes.

LET'S TRY ONE **18.1**

Use the information you learned in the previous section and the report below to select the correct code for the radiologic procedure.

MRI SCAN OF THE PELVIS

CLINICAL HISTORY: Reported fullness, status post-hysterectomy and right-side oophorectomy

There are no previous films available for review. Images through the pelvis were obtained utilizing axial, sagittal, and coronal projections. Pre- and post-contrast images were obtained. Sagittal images appear normal with fluid-filled bladder. There is a linear-type low signal structure interspersed between what appears to be the rectum and bladder. This appears to be a continuation of the vaginal cuff and scar tissue from previous procedures. This does not show any specific enhancement. I do not believe this represents any bowel abnormalities. The remainder of the pelvis is otherwise unremarkable without findings of any free fluid or unusual adnexal masses. The osseous structures are unremarkable to include the iliac bones in both hips.

IMPRESSION: Linear shelflike low weakening signal scattered between the fluid-filled cystic bladder and rectum. I am unclear as to the exact significance of this finding. This may represent a component of fibrosis or scarring. This does not show any enhancement with contrast. I do not believe this represents any bowel loop. My recommendation for further evaluation would be CT scan of the pelvis with intravenous contrast to opacify the bladder and also rectal contrast to delineate the boundaries of the rectum. No clear indication of any contained mass or obvious free fluid.

Which is the appropriate code for this radiologic procedure?

a. 72195 b. 72196 c. 72197 d. 72198

CONCEPTS CHECKPOINT **18.4**

Match the medical term in the first column with the correct definition in the second column.

1. _____ angiography
2. _____ complete study
3. _____ computed tomography
4. _____ magnetic resonance imaging

a. An imaging technique that uses x-rays to capture cross-section images of soft tissues and bones
b. An imaging technique that uses electromagnetic fields and radio waves to produce images of body parts, organs, and tissues
c. X-ray imaging of the inside of blood vessels
d. The maximum number of views required to completely evaluate the patient's condition

Diagnostic Ultrasound (Codes 76506-76999)

Ultrasound, also referred to as *ultrasonography*, is an imaging procedure that uses high-frequency sound waves to capture images with measurement or real-time video of internal organs. To capture the image, the sonographer (ultrasound technician) or physician places a thin layer of gel over the skin in the area of the internal organ to be visualized. Then an instrument called a **transducer** (or probe) that transmits sound waves is placed or rolled over the gelled area. Organs are distinguished by echoes created from sound waves bouncing off tissue. The ultrasonic echoes are recorded as images, called **sonograms**.

Ultrasound codes may be differentiated by the mode or scan used. Ultrasound **modes** and **scans** identify the type of image captured during the procedure. Ultrasound modes are as follows:

- **A-mode**—Amplitude of sound (echo) creates a 1-dimensional display;
- **B-scan**—Brightness mode displays a 2-dimensional gray-scale video;
- **M-mode**—Motion mode displays a 1-dimensional video;
- **Real-time scan**—2-dimensional display of organ structure and movement in real time.

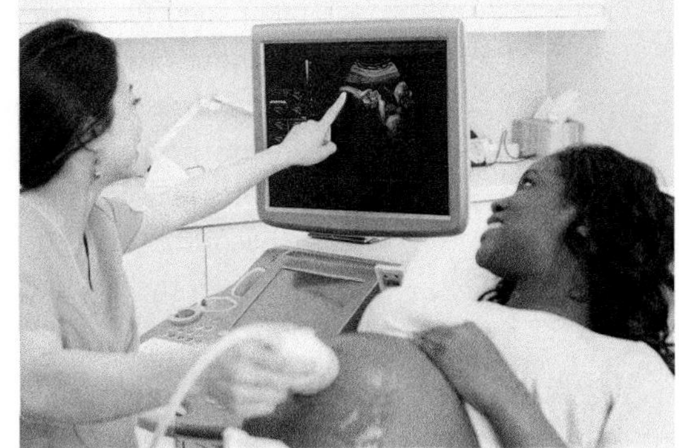

Ultrasound uses high-frequency sound waves to capture images. There are many uses of ultrasounds, including obstetric.

Many ultrasound codes include the terms "with or without Doppler" in the code description. **Doppler ultrasound** uses a special frequency that can penetrate solid or liquid to record blood flow velocity (speed). This type of ultrasound technology is primarily used to detect obstructions in blood vessels that can lead to a stroke.

Images from a Doppler ultrasound may be black and white or in full color. A **spectral Doppler scan** presents blood flow measurements plotted graphically on a grid showing flow velocities recorded over time.

A **color flow Doppler scan** shows the different levels of fluid concentration within a targeted area; it is used when the physician wants to examine movement within a structure, such as flowing blood. When documentation and images indicate a color flow Doppler scan, select the CPT® code that includes "color flow Doppler" in the description. When a color flow Doppler scan is performed in conjunction with a real-time ultrasound for identifying organ structure, the color flow Doppler scan is not reported as a separate code. Color flow Doppler echocardiography uses multiple transducers or a rotating transducer to produce 2-dimensional images of the heart. Color flow echocardiography examinations are reported with codes from the Medicine Section.

> **RED FLAG**
>
> A "complete" real-time scan of the abdomen coded with 76700 includes the liver, gallbladder, common bile duct, pancreas, spleen, kidneys, the upper abdominal aorta, and the inferior vena cava. If any of these structures are not documented in the written report as visualized during the procedure, the coder should select code 76705 that describes a "limited" procedure.

The **duplex Doppler scan** combines B-mode, spectral, and color flow Doppler imaging to produce real-time images of the pattern and direction of blood flow.

Many ultrasound codes describe the imaging of body regions with terms such as "abdominal" or "retroperitoneal." Body regions contain multiple organs and internal structures. Instructional notes to these codebook categories list the organs and/or structures included in codes that use the term "complete." When selecting an ultrasound code that describes specific organs or structures in a region, the documentation in the written report must include details of each organ and/or structure imaged. If documentation does not identify the organ(s) and/or structure(s) described by the code, the coder must report the "limited" procedure. A modifier is not required to indicate that a reduced procedure was performed.

Pelvic Ultrasound

Pelvic ultrasound codes are subdivided into obstetric and nonobstetric types of procedures. **Obstetric pelvic ultrasound** scans are taken of a pregnant uterus or of a fetus to identify the age, sex, and the number of fetuses, or to identify complications in the pregnancy. Obstetric ultrasound codes define the gestational age and the anatomical structure viewed, as seen in Figure 18.8. Coders must review the written report of the pelvic ultrasound in order to select the most accurate code. The written report should document the findings of each visualized element or the reason why a specific organ was not viewed. The approach used to capture the image must also be documented. Pelvic ultrasounds may be **transabdominal** (through the abdomen) or **transvaginal** (through the vagina). The transabdominal approach uses a transducer placed on the skin of the abdomen to capture the image. The transvaginal approach uses a probe that is inserted into the vagina. Transvaginal ultrasounds may be obstetric or nonobstetric, providing images of female reproductive organs.

Nonobstetric pelvic ultrasound may be performed on male or female patients and is used to define organs and anatomical structures viewed. When limited pelvic ultrasound is performed to view 1 or more organs or structures, or is repeated due to a previously identified abnormality, report code 76857, *Ultrasound, pelvic (nonobstetric), real time with image documentation; limited or follow-up (eg, for follicles)*. For example, if the urinary bladder alone (ie, not including the kidneys) is imaged, code 76857 should be reported rather than 76770, *Ultrasound, retroperitoneal (eg, renal, aorta, nodes), real time with image documentation; complete.*

Figure 18.8 Obstetric Pelvic Ultrasound Examination at 16 Weeks of Gestation

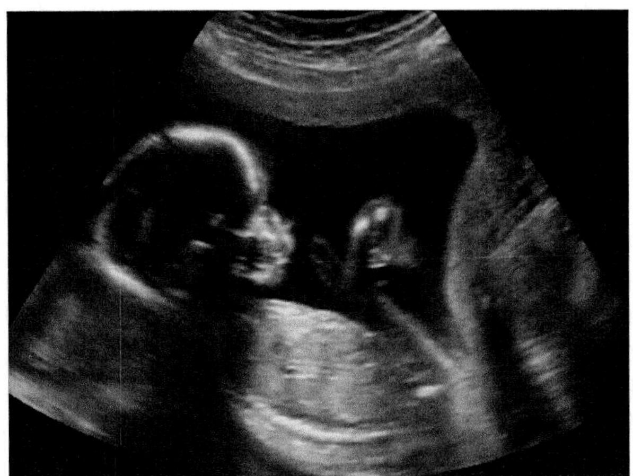

RED FLAG

An ultrasound guidance code may not be reported with a diagnostic ultrasound code.

Ultrasound may be used to guide the physician when inserting a medical device or catheter or during surgery or diagnostic procedures. When an ultrasound is used for guidance during a surgical procedure, the ultrasound code is selected based on the type of procedure performed. Be sure to read the description and notes of the surgical procedure prior to assigning an ultrasound code separate from the procedure code. An ultrasound guidance code may not be reported with a diagnostic ultrasound code. Referring to the Medicare NCCI edits and encoder systems will assist you when selecting ultrasound guidance codes.

LET'S TRY ONE **18.2**

A physician performed a transoral flexible esophagogastroduodenoscopy. During the procedure, the physician performed a transmural fine needle biopsy under ultrasound guidance. The coder locates the following 3 possible codes:

43235	*Esophagogastroduodenoscopy, flexible, transoral; diagnostic, including collection of specimen(s) by brushing or washing, when performed (separate procedure)*
43242	*Esophagogastroduodenoscopy, flexible, transoral; with transendoscopic ultrasound-guided intramural or transmural fine needle aspiration/biopsy(s) (includes endoscopic ultrasound examination of the esophagus, stomach, and either the duodenum or a surgically altered stomach where the jejunum is examined distal to the anastomosis)*
76942	*Ultrasonic guidance for needle placement (eg, biopsy, aspiration, injection, localization device), imaging supervision and interpretation*

The coder finally decides to report only code 43242. Review the code descriptions above and then select the statement below that is not applicable to the coder's selection of code 43242. _____

a. Codes 43242 and 76942 may be reported together, which better describes the procedures.
b. Codes 43235 and 76942 together do not fully describe the procedure.
c. Codes 43242 and 76942 may not be reported together because the code 43242 description includes an ultrasound exam.
d. Code 43242 fully describes the procedures, both the ultrasound and the biopsy.

A DEXA machine projects x-rays to the targeted body area. The DEXA software calculates and displays the bone density measurements on a computer monitor. Figure 18.11 illustrates a typical screen generated from a DEXA machine. Bone density studies may be recommended for postmenopausal women, men with clinical conditions with bone loss, and men and women with prolonged use of medications known to cause bone loss. DEXA procedures are coded based on the anatomical site being scanned.

Figure 18.11 DEXA Scanner Screen

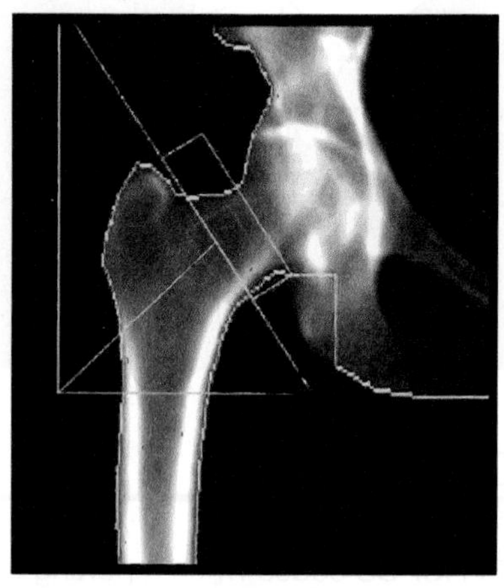

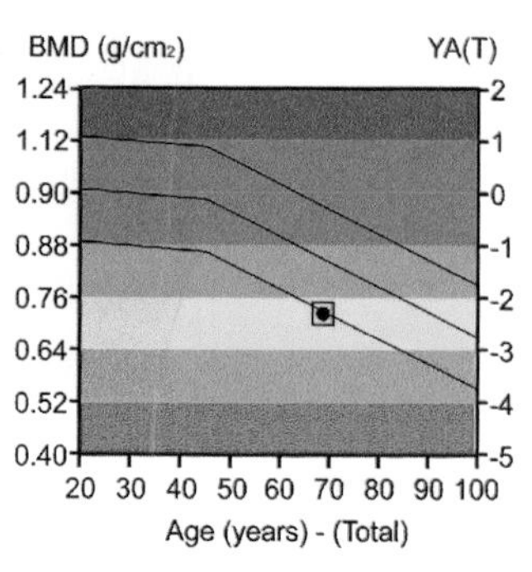

ADAM.

CONCEPTS CHECKPOINT **18.6**

Use information from the previous sections to select the correct answer to the following questions.

1. A preventive service performed on patients without signs or symptoms of breast disease is a
   a. diagnostic mammogram.
   b. galactogram.
   c. screening mammogram.
   d. ductogram.
2. All screening mammograms are
   a. unilateral.
   b. bilateral.
   c. performed only on the affected breast.
   d. None of the answers are correct.
3. Which of the following is a criterion for selecting an osseous survey code?
   a. the location of the examination
   b. whether the survey is local
   c. the specific anatomical site
   d. whether the survey is limited and complete
4. Which of the following is an acronym for bone densitometry?
   a. DEXA
   b. CT
   c. XRA
   d. MRI

LET'S TRY ONE **18.4**

A patient with a lumbar fracture underwent a bone density study. The study indicated that the bone density assessment was fair with T scores of –1.06 in the lumbar spine and almost in the middle of the normal range for the femoral neck. What code should be reported? _____

Radiation Oncology (Codes 77261-77799)

Radiation oncology is a medical specialty that uses high-energy ionizing radiation to treat malignant and benign tumors. Table 18.4 presents some of the technical terminology you are likely to encounter when using the radiation oncology codes.

Table 18.4 Radiation Oncology Terminology

Term	Definition
compensator (tissue)	Also known as a *radiation filter,* used to create variation in the amount of radiation distributed
fractions	Total number of radiotherapy sessions
IGRT	Image-guided radiation therapy
IMRT	Intensity modulated radiation therapy
isodose	Points or zones in a medium that receive equal doses of radiation
linear accelerator based	A type of radiation treatment that intensifies x-rays
megavoltage	Greater than or equal to 1 MeV
MeV	1 million electron volts
MLC	Multileaf collimator
multi-source Cobalt 60 based	A type of stereotactic radiation treatment used for cranial applications
SBRT	Stereotactic body radiation therapy
SRS	Stereotactic radiosurgery
TDF	Time/dose/fractionation
teletherapy	A variety of radiation techniques that uses a source outside the body to treat cancer
TLD	Thermoluminescent dosimeter

There are many different therapeutic methods used in radiation oncology. As we explore the subdivisions of radiation oncology, we will discuss the treatment methods described in the CPT® codebook.

The Radiation Oncology codes are subdivided into groups under the following headings:

- Consultation: Clinical Management;
- Clinical Treatment Planning;
- Medical Radiation Physics, Dosimetry, Treatment Devices, and Special Services;
- Stereotactic Radiation Treatment Delivery;
- Radiation Treatment Delivery;
- Neutron Beam Treatment Delivery;
- Radiation Treatment Management;

- Proton Beam Treatment Delivery;
- Hyperthermia;
- Clinical Intracavitary Hyperthermia;
- Clinical Brachytherapy.

The sequence roughly follows the radiation oncology process of care. First, the patient consults with a provider about the health issue. Next, clinical planning takes place, leading to the simulation and dosimetry stages to specify treatment modalities. After clinical treatment planning, treatment is administered under the management of the provider. This chapter will discuss each stage of the process.

Consultation: Clinical Management

Prior to radiation treatment, a provider evaluates a patient to determine if radiation therapy will be beneficial. This preliminary visit is reported with the appropriate evaluation and management code. When the preliminary consultation is provided by a therapeutic radiologist, the appropriate code from the medicine or surgery sections may be assigned.

Clinical Treatment Planning

After the clinical management consultation confirms that radiation therapy will be beneficial, the patient and provider will focus on developing a therapeutic radiology treatment plan and therapeutic radiology simulation.

Therapeutic Radiology Treatment Plan

The clinical treatment planning session will develop the treatment plan that will best benefit the patient. Depending on the patient's condition, the treatment plan will include the following components:

- interpretation of special testing;
- tumor localization;
- treatment volume determination;
- treatment time/dosage determination;
- choice of treatment modality;
- determination of number and size of treatment ports;
- selection of appropriate treatment devices.

Part of the planning includes determining the number and size of treatment ports. A **port** is the location where the treatment beam will enter the skin to reach the internal malignant area(s). This area is typically marked on the skin by a tattoo. Blocks are also used during treatment. **Blocks** are pieces of lead designed to shield healthy tissue from receiving radiation. The custom-designed blocks allow the targeting of radiation to focus solely on the tumor.

Treatment planning codes are selected according to the complexity of the treatment plan—simple, intermediate, or complex—predominantly based on the number of malignant areas, ports, and blocks. Table 18.5 presents the codes with the criteria that define their levels of complexity.

Table 18.5 Radiation Planning Codes: Definitions and Documentation Requirements

Radiation Planning Code	Treatment Planning Complexity	Treatment Plan Criteria
77261	Simple	• A single area of treatment • A single port or contrasting ports parallel to each other • Basic or no blocking
77262	Intermediate	• 2 separate areas of treatment • 3 or more converging ports • Multiple-blocks, or time or dosage considerations
77263	Complex	• 3 or more separate areas of treatment • Tangential ports, wedges, or compensators • Complex blocking • A combination of 2 or more methods of treatment or rotating or other beam considerations

Codes 77261 through 77263 are always reported as a complete global service and do not have technical and professional components. When radiation planning includes radiation physics consultation, simulation-aided field setting, medical radiation physics, treatment delivery, and treatment management, these services or procedures may be reported separately, in addition to the appropriate treatment planning code. The following section discusses these separate procedures in detail.

Therapeutic Radiology Simulation

During the planning process, the provider and patient will go through therapeutic radiology simulation. **Therapeutic radiology simulation** is the process of determining the targeted anatomy and collecting data and images necessary to develop the ideal radiation treatment process for the patient. Therapeutic radiology simulation codes are selected based on the complexity of the simulation process. Table 18.6 details the criteria for selecting the appropriate code.

Typical radiation therapy will require 1 to 3 simulations. However, no more than 1 simulation code may be reported on the same date of service.

Table 18.6 Simulation Codes: Definitions and Documentation Requirements

Simulation Code	Simulation-Aided Field Setting Complexity	Simulation Criteria
77280	Simple	• A single treatment area
77285	Intermediate	• 2 separate treatment areas
77290	Complex	Involvement of any of the following: • 3 or more treatment areas • Particle, rotation, or arc therapy • Complex blocking • Custom shielding blocks • Brachytherapy simulation • Hyperthermia probe verification • Any use of contrast materials

CONCEPTS CHECKPOINT **18.7**

Use information from the previous sections to select the correct answer to the following questions.

1. Preliminary clinical management consultations for radiation oncology services provided by a physician are reported with
   a. clinical management codes.
   b. radiation oncology codes.
   c. evaluation and management codes.
   d. codes from the Medicine section.
2. Treatment planning codes are based on
   a. associated oncology services.
   b. the type of cancer.
   c. the anatomic site of the cancer.
   d. the complexity of the treatment plan.
3. Complex radiation planning includes all except
   a. 3 or more separate areas of treatment.
   b. tangential ports, wedges, or compensators.
   c. a combination of 5 or more methods of treatment, or rotating or other beam considerations.
   d. complex blocking.
4. Therapeutic radiology simulation codes
   a. are selected based on the complexity of the simulation process.
   b. are selected based on the location of the port.
   c. are selected based on the number of ports.
   d. None of the answers are correct.

Medical Radiation Physics, Dosimetry, Treatment Devices, and Special Services

Information collected through the therapeutic radiology simulation is sent to medical radiation physicists and dosimetrists. Radiation physics and dosimetry are used to design specialized blocks and calculate radiation dosage. A **medical radiation physicist** works with the radiation oncologist to design a treatment schedule that will kill cancer cells. Dosimetry is the calculation of radiation dosage. The **medical radiation dosimetrist**, in conjunction with the medical radiation physicist, uses computer and mathematical calculations to design a treatment plan that includes the technique to deliver the prescribed radiation dose.

Coders must carefully read code descriptions and instructional notes prior to assigning codes from this section. There is an add-on code in the Clinical Treatment Planning group that is specified for use with codes 77295 and 77301. Report code 77293, *Respiratory motion management simulation (List separately in addition to code for primary procedure)*, in conjunction with 77295, *3-dimensional radiotherapy plan, including dose-volume histograms*, or 77301 *Intensity modulated radiotherapy plan, including dose-volume histograms for target and critical structure partial tolerance specification.*

Radiation Treatment Delivery

After the medical radiation dosimetry has been calculated, the medical physicist and radiation oncologist choose the treatment delivery method. These include stereotactic radiosurgery and external radiation, including megavoltage treatments. Megavoltage is defined as greater than or equal to 1 **megaelectron** (1 million electronvolts or 1 MeV) unit of energy. The CPT® codebook provides codes for the following methods:

- x-ray (photon) beams, which include conventional and intensity modulated radiation therapy (IMRT) beams;
- electron beams;
- neutron beams;
- proton beams.

Radiation treatment delivery codes represent technical-only services and are reported by the facility, not by the physician office. The codes are selected based on the level of complexity as indicated by the number of treatment areas; the use of ports, blocks, and wedges; the use of tissue compensators; and megavoltage (MeV). Code 77401 describes superficial radiation delivery. Table 18.7 shows the code criteria for selection of megavoltage radiation treatments.

IMRT codes are differentiated by 2 levels of complexity:

- simple: relevant to procedures on the prostate, breast, and all sites using physical compensator based IMRT;
- complex: relevant to all other sites if not using physical compensator based IMRT.

Some treatment methods require image guidance. The codebook resource "Radiation Management and Treatment Table" correlates codes with image-guided radiation therapy (IGRT). The table also indicates whether the code is reported as a technical or professional component.

Table 18.7 Code Criteria for Megavoltage Radiation Treatment Delivery

Radiation Treatment Delivery Code	Radiation Treatment Level of Complexity	Code Criteria
77402	Simple	All criteria are met: • Single treatment area • 1 or 2 ports • Up to 2 simple blocks
77407	Intermediate	Any of these criteria are met: • 2 separate treatment areas • 3 or more ports on a single treatment area • 3 or more blocks
77412	Complex	Any of these criteria are met: • 3 or more separate treatment areas • Tangential ports • Custom blocks, wedges • Rotational beam, field-in-field, or other tissue compensation that does not meet IMRT guidelines • Electron beam

Stereotactic Radiation Treatment Delivery

RED FLAG

Codes 77424 and 77425 are out of numerical sequence.

Stereotactic radiosurgery (SRS) is a radiation therapy technique used to deliver large amounts of radiation to distinct tumor sites in the brain. The principle of cranial SRS as applied to treatment of body tumors is known as **stereotactic body radiation therapy (SBRT)**. The technique is designed to minimize damage to healthy tissue while maximizing delivery of radiation to the tumor. Radiation from multiple directions is targeted on 1 or more tumors. During the procedure, the patient is fitted with a plastic mold or cast to keep the body area still so that radiation is precisely delivered. SRS codes 77371 and 77372 are reported per session and selected based on radiation source. SBRT code 77373 has parenthetic instructions that it is not reported in conjunction with certain Radiation Treatment Delivery codes. Guidance for localization of target volume is a professional component reported by a physician with code 77387.

Neutron Beam Treatment Delivery

Unlike conventional radiation therapy, neutron radiotherapy works in the absence of oxygen, a condition that enables the treatment of larger tumors. Neutron beam treatment is very effective in the treatment of inoperable (not surgically treatable) salivary gland tumors, bone cancers, and specific types of pancreas, bladder, lung, prostate, and uterine cancers.

CPT® code 77423 is the only code available to report neutron beam treatment. Code 77423 is used to report treatment of 1 or more isocenters (beam intersection points) with coplanar (linear lines) or noncoplanar geometry with blocking and/or wedge, and/or compensator(s). Coders must review the written report to verify the numbers of ports and blocks used in the procedure.

Proton Beam Treatment Delivery

Proton beam therapy uses protons rather than x-rays to treat cancer. A proton is a positively charged particle that is part of an atom. Protons are very effective in treating cancer with minimal damage to healthy cells. It is a particularly effective treatment of intraocular melanomas (cancer within the eyeball) and pituitary adenomas (cancer of the pituitary gland). Stereotactic radiosurgery is sometimes used with proton beam therapy.

Proton beam treatment delivery codes are selected based on the complexity of the treatment, categorized as simple, intermediate, or complex. Table 18.8 shows the criteria for selecting the appropriate proton beam treatment code.

Table 18.8 Criteria for Proton Beam Treatment Codes

Proton Treatment Delivery Code	Proton Treatment Level of Complexity	Code Criteria
77520	Simple, without compensation	• Single treatment area • Single nontangential/oblique port • Custom blocking without compensation
77522	Simple, with compensation	• Single treatment area • Single nontangential/oblique port • Custom blocking with compensation (custom-made devices attached to the treatment unit for manipulating the radiation dose)
77523	Intermediate	• 1 or more treatment areas • 2 or more ports or 1 or more tangential/oblique ports • Custom blocks and compensators
77525	Complex	• 1 or more treatment areas • 2 or more ports per treatment area • Matching or patching fields and/or multiple isocenters • Custom blocks and compensators

LET'S TRY ONE **18.5**

Use your CPT® codebook or encoder to select the correct code from the Radiation Oncology section.

1. Clinical treatment planning for a single area of malignancy with a single port or opposing ports parallel to each other and basic or no blocking
   a. 77261, *Therapeutic radiology treatment planning; simple*
   b. 77262, *Therapeutic radiology treatment planning; intermediate*
   c. 77263, *Therapeutic radiology treatment planning; complex*
2. Clinical treatment planning simulation of 3 or more areas of malignancy with tangential ports and complex blocking that may require customized shielding blocks, rotation or arc therapy, brachytherapy source and hyperthermia probe verification, and use of contrast materials
   a. 77280, *Therapeutic radiology simulation-aided field setting; simple*
   b. 77285, *Therapeutic radiology simulation-aided field setting; intermediate*
   c. 77290, *Therapeutic radiology simulation-aided field setting; complex*
3. Medical radiation treatment devices, design and construction, multiple blocks, stents, bite blocks, special bolus
   a. 77332, *Treatment devices, design and construction; simple*
   b. 77333, *Treatment devices, design and construction; intermediate*
   c. 77334, *Treatment devices, design and construction; complex*
4. Radiation treatment delivery 4 ports on a single treatment area
   a. 77407, *Radiation treatment delivery, >=1 MeV; intermediate*
   b. 77402, *Radiation treatment delivery, >=1 MeV; simple*
   c. 77412, *Radiation treatment delivery, >=1 MeV; complex*
5. High energy neutron radiation treatment delivery; 2 isocenters with coplanar geometry
   a. 77499, *Unlisted procedure, therapeutic radiology treatment management*
   b. 77423, *High energy neutron radiation treatment delivery; 1 or more isocenter(s) with coplanar or non-coplanar geometry with blocking and/or wedge, and/or compensator(s)*
   c. 77522, *Proton treatment delivery; simple, with compensation*

Radiation Treatment Management

Radiation treatment management is reported by the physician with codes from the Radiation Treatment Management subsection. The codes represent only the professional component of radiation delivery. The physician is required to examine the patient at least once for medical evaluation and management. The evaluation includes coordination of care; assessment of the patient's response to treatment; and the review of dose delivery, dosimetry, lab tests, patient treatment set-up, port film, treatment parameters, and x-rays. The exception to the examination requirement is code 77469 for intraoperative session management.

Radiation treatment management codes are reported in units of 5 fractions or treatment sessions. Code 77427, *Radiation treatment management, 5 treatments*, is reported at the completion of each 5 sessions. There is an exception if the patient's course of treatment is completed in 3 or more sessions. Do not report code 77427 for less than 2 sessions. When more than 1 session is performed on the same date of service, the additional session is also counted toward the 5 sessions only if documentation supports a distinct break between treatment sessions.

EXAMPLE 18.7

A patient with stage II rectal cancer had a consultation with the oncologist on Monday, June 28, about beginning her radiation therapy. She told the physician that she had a family emergency that required her to be out of town beginning Wednesday, June 30, for an indefinite time. This unexpected trip would allow her to be in town for her next round of radiation therapy; however, she did not know when she would be able to return for the fifth and final treatment. The oncologist and patient agreed to perform a lower-than-normal dose of radiation therapy at 6 a.m. the morning of Tuesday, June 29, and then a second treatment at 6 p.m. later that day to complete the fifth round. On Tuesday at 6 a.m., the patient successfully completed her fourth dose of radiation therapy. When she returned for her fifth and final round of treatment that evening, the patient received lab work and a brief examination. The physician cleared the patient for the additional dose of radiation therapy.

Although the 2 final sessions took place on the same date of service, the physician may count both radiation treatment management services toward the 5 sessions because there was a distinct break between treatment sessions. Because the second treatment on June 29 completes the fifth session, the provider may report code 77427.

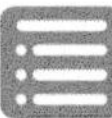

Index Insider

The radiation oncology codes are indexed under the main entry *Radiation Therapy* and organized by stage of the process (eg, *Consultation*, *Treatment Management*) or by method of delivery (eg, *Radiosurgery*, *Proton Beam*).

Radiation Therapy

Treatment Management	
1 or 2 Fractions Only	77431
Intraoperative	77469
Stereotactic	
Body	77435
Cerebral	77432
Unlisted Services and Procedures	77499
Weekly	77427

Hyperthermia and Clinical Intracavitary Hyperthermia

Localized **hyperthermia** for treatment of cancer uses heat to make tumors more susceptible to cancer therapy methods. Heat is generated by sources such as microwave, ultrasound, and radio frequency conduction. Hyperthermia codes are selected based on the mode of entry: superficial, deep, interstitial (within tissue), or intracavitary (inside the body). Superficial and deep hyperthermia are considered external procedures. Interstitial and intracavitary procedures use a probe to heat internal areas of the body.

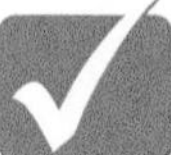

CONCEPTS CHECKPOINT 18.8

Use information from the previous section to indicate if each of the following statements is true or false.

1. _____ Radiation Treatment Management subsection codes represent only the professional component of radiation delivery.
2. _____ Radiation Treatment Management codes are reported in units of 5 fractions or treatment sessions.
3. _____ When more than 1 session is performed on the same date of service, the additional session is also counted toward the 5 sessions only if documentation supports a distinct break between treatment sessions.
4. _____ Hyperthermia codes are selected based on the mode of entry: superficial, deep, interstitial, or intracavitary.

Clinical Brachytherapy

Brachytherapy is a type of radiation therapy that uses natural or fabricated radioactive materials instilled (insertion of liquid) or implanted close to or into the tumor or treatment site. Radiation is delivered by radioactive sources in the form of wires, needles, capsules, or small seeds. These radioactive sources may be temporarily or permanently implanted. Brachytherapy is beneficial for the treatment of many different types of tumors, including cranial, breast, prostate, and esophageal tumors. Figure 18.12 illustrates brachytherapy performed in the lung.

There are currently 4 basic types of clinical brachytherapies: interstitial, intracavitary, and remote afterloading intraluminal therapy. **Interstitial brachytherapy** sources are implanted directly into the tumor. **Intracavitary brachytherapy** uses a special applicator implanted inside a body cavity, such as the vagina, for treatment of cervical cancer. **Intraluminal brachytherapy** also uses special applicators to implant radioactive sources inside a body passage, such as the esophagus for treatment of esophageal cancers. **Remote afterloading brachytherapy** uses a special mechanical-electronic machine that places extremely thin tubes or needles containing a single, high-intensity radioactive material around the tumor.

Clinical brachytherapy codes are selected based on the type of brachytherapy and the complexity of the procedure. The complexity is described in the codes as simple, intermediate, or complex, defined by the number of sources or ribbons (media carrying the therapeutic substance) used.

Figure 18.12 Brachytherapy in the Lung

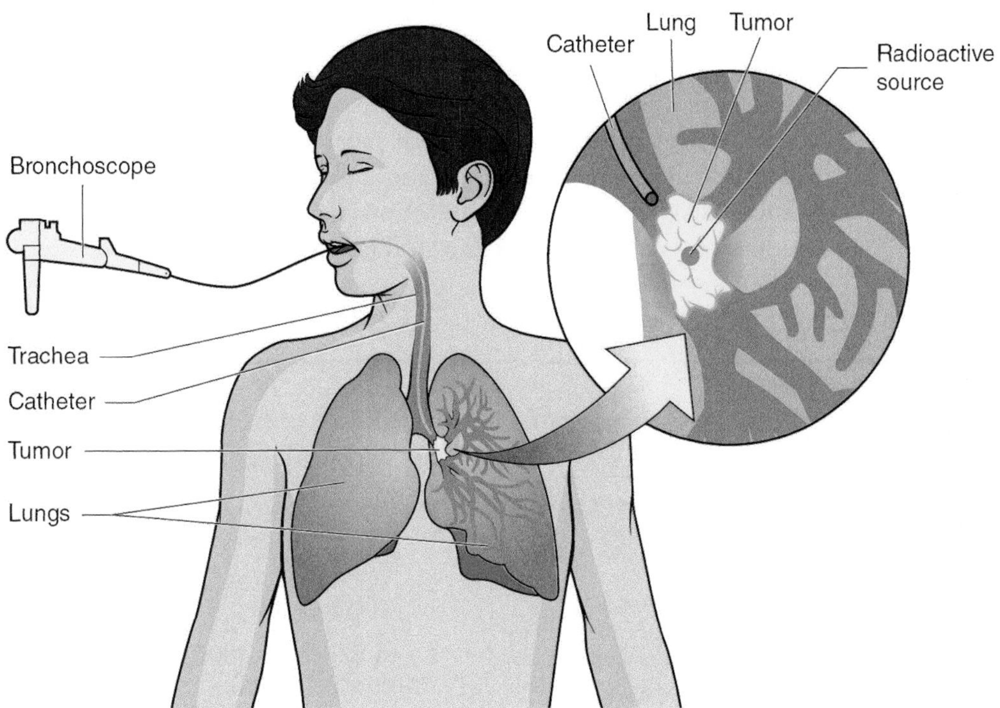

Nuclear Medicine (Codes 78012-79999)

Nuclear medicine is the clinical discipline that uses radioactive substances to diagnose and treat disease by use of radiopharmaceuticals. **Radiopharmaceuticals** (radiotracers) are a combination of chemical or pharmaceutical compounds with radioactive substances. Use of radiopharmaceuticals in diagnostic procedures allows for the enhancement of tissue or cell imaging. As a therapeutic treatment, nuclear medicine is similar to pharmacology. Specialized radiopharmaceuticals are created to treat specific types of abnormalities. The absorption of a radiopharmaceutical into the diseased tissue is called **uptake**. Therapeutic nuclear medicine can be used to treat a variety of conditions such as hyperthyroidism, thyroid cancer, and blood disorders.

Diagnostic nuclear medicine focuses on identifying abnormalities in the physiologic processes within the body, such as rates of metabolism. Single photon emission computed tomography and positron emission tomography are 2 types of radiation detecting techniques used in nuclear medicine diagnostic studies. **Single photon emission computed tomography (SPECT)** uses a gamma ray camera to capture an image of the radiation emitted from the radiopharmaceutical, creating a 3-D image with multiple planes. **Positron emission tomography (PET)** uses a machine that looks similar to an MRI or CT machine. However, a PET scan does not emit x-rays but rather detects radiation to create an image.

Nuclear medicine codes are divided into 2 sections, diagnostic and therapeutic. The diagnostic section is subdivided according to body system. Therapeutic codes are selected based on route of administration: oral, intravenous, intracavitary, interstitial, and intra-arterial. Nuclear medicine codes do not include the radiopharmaceutical or drug used, which may be reported separately. When the route of administration is intracavitary, interstitial, or intra-arterial, report an additional code for the administration of the radiopharmaceutical. It is also appropriate to report an additional procedure code for radiologic supervision and interpretation when radiologic guidance or imaging is performed. Parenthetic notes provide directions on additional code selection.

LET'S TRY ONE **18.6**

Using your codebook, select the correct code for each of the following procedures.

1. Bone marrow imaging of the entire body
   a. 78102, *Bone marrow imaging; limited area*
   b. 78104, *Bone marrow imaging; whole body*
   c. 78103, *Bone marrow imaging; multiple areas*
   d. 78120, *Red cell volume determination (separate procedure); single sampling*
2. Venous thrombosis imaging, venogram on the left and right leg
   a. 78456, *Acute venous thrombosis imaging, peptide*
   b. 78457, *Venous thrombosis imaging, venogram; unilateral*
   c. 78458, *Venous thrombosis imaging, venogram; bilateral*
   d. 78466, *Myocardial imaging, infarct avid, planar; qualitative or quantitative*
3. Bone and/or joint imaging; multiple areas
   a. 78320, *Bone and/or joint imaging; tomographic (SPECT)*
   b. 78300, *Bone and/or joint imaging; limited area*
   c. 78305, *Bone and/or joint imaging; multiple areas*
   d. 78306, *Bone and/or joint imaging; whole body*
4. Single photon emission computed tomography of liver with vascular flow
   a. 78202, *Liver imaging; with vascular flow*
   b. 78205, *Liver imaging (SPECT)*
   c. 78206, *Liver imaging (SPECT); with vascular flow*
   d. 78215, *Liver and spleen imaging; static only*

Instructions for Reporting Radiology Codes

To assign radiology codes, coders must be familiar with the Radiology section guidelines. The steps to locating radiology codes are listed below.

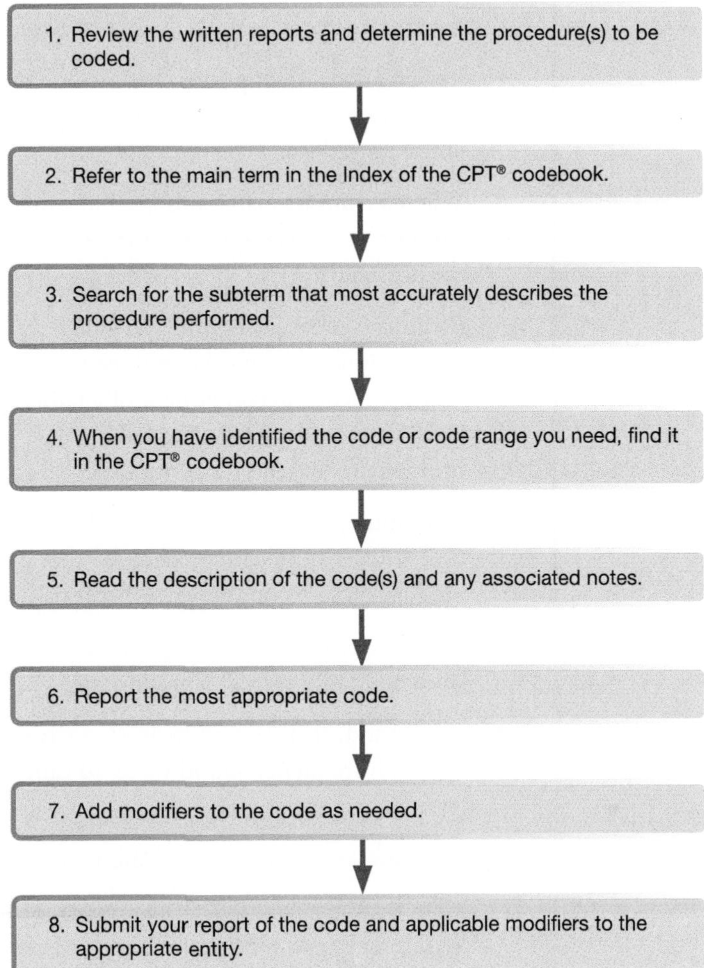

1. Review the written reports and determine the procedure(s) to be coded.
2. Refer to the main term in the Index of the CPT® codebook.
3. Search for the subterm that most accurately describes the procedure performed.
4. When you have identified the code or code range you need, find it in the CPT® codebook.
5. Read the description of the code(s) and any associated notes.
6. Report the most appropriate code.
7. Add modifiers to the code as needed.
8. Submit your report of the code and applicable modifiers to the appropriate entity.

Chapter Summary

- Radiology is the branch of medicine that uses radiation (such as x-rays) and other forms of imaging to treat and diagnose diseases. A radiologist is a medical doctor who specializes in the study of radiologic services.
- Imaging code descriptions that include the designation "separate procedure" should not be reported independently when carried out as an integral part of the procedure.
- When a contrast material is used in a diagnostic study, the phrase "with contrast" is included in the order for the study and in the written details of the procedure.
- Radiology codes are considered global services, which means that the services include a technical component and a professional component. When only the technical component of a radiology service is performed, append HCPCS modifier TC to the CPT® code. To report only the professional component, append CPT® modifier 26 to the CPT® code.
- A computed tomography scan (CT scan), sometimes referred to as a *CAT scan*, is an imaging technique that processes multiple x-rays to produce cross-section images of soft tissues and bones.
- Magnetic resonance imaging (MRI) is a technique that uses electromagnetic fields and radio waves to produce images of body parts, organs, and tissue.
- Ultrasound, also referred to as *ultrasonography*, is an imaging procedure that uses high-frequency sound waves to capture images or real-time video of internal organs.
- A fluoroscopy is an x-ray technique that captures continuous images in real time.
- Mammograms can be performed for screening or diagnostic purposes.
- Bone and joint studies identify abnormalities of bones and joints.
- Radiation oncology is a medical specialty that uses high-energy ionizing radiation to treat malignant and benign tumors.
- Nuclear medicine is the clinical discipline that uses radioactive substances to diagnose and treat diseases with chemical or pharmaceutical compounds.

Navigator

Access interactive chapter review exercises, practice activities, flash cards, and study games.

Chapter 19

Pathology and Laboratory Coding

Fast Facts

- Most cancer is diagnosed through pathology tests.
- The rate of positive pre-employment drug testing rose 5.7% in 2011. However, only 2% of the 3.4 million urine tests analyzed tested positive for marijuana.
- Approximately half of US companies perform drug testing of new hires.
- In the United States in 1970, autopsies were performed in 40% to 60% of all hospital deaths. The rate has steadily declined to approximately 5% today.

Sources: http://cancerconnect.com, http://drugwarfacts.org, http://medscape.com

Crack the Code

Review the sample autopsy report to find the correct pathology and laboratory code. You may need to return to this exercise after reading the chapter content.

EXTERNAL EXAMINATION: The body is that of a well-developed and well-nourished 54-year-old white male measuring 177 cm in length and estimated to weigh 80 kg.

RESPIRATORY SYSTEM: The right lung weighs 630 gm and the left lung 590 gm. The lungs are well inflated, and the visceral pleural surfaces are smooth and glistening. The mucous membrane is not infected.

LIVER, GALLBLADDER, AND PANCREAS: The 1900-gm liver has a smooth, intact capsule. On section, the parenchyma is variegated and yellowish green, and the central vein area is sharply demarcated and dark purple. The gallbladder contains approximately 15 cc of dark green viscid bile without stones. The bile ducts are unremarkable.

answer: 88045

Learning Objectives

19.1 Discuss the types of pathology and laboratory services reported with CPT® codes.

19.2 Locate pathology and laboratory codes in the CPT® codebook Index.

19.3 Apply symbols, guidelines, and instructional notes when coding pathology and laboratory services.

19.4 Identify the modifiers most commonly used in pathology and laboratory coding.

19.5 Describe the use of the chargemaster to code and bill for laboratory services.

19.6 Differentiate between the terms *quantitative* and *qualitative* in relation to laboratory codes.

19.7 Demonstrate the ability to assign appropriate pathology and laboratory codes.

19.8 Describe the different types of drug assays and the proper application of drug assay codes.

19.9 Describe different types of tests performed on urine samples and assign urinalysis codes.

19.10 Describe the creation of molecular pathology codes and differentiate between Tier 1 and Tier 2 molecular pathology services.

19.11 Assign codes for genomic sequencing procedures and other molecular multianalyte assays.

19.12 Describe what types of tests the chemistry section of a laboratory performs and how chemistry codes are assigned.

19.13 Define the common types of hematology and coagulation services, *complete blood count*, and *prothrombin time*.

19.14 Assign codes for different microbiology tests.

19.15 Differentiate between *presumptive identification* and *definitive identification*.

19.16 Describe the evaluation of specimens found in the surgical pathology codes. Define the 6 levels of examination.

Chapter Outline

I. Introduction to Pathology and Laboratory Services

II. Organization of the Pathology and Laboratory Section

- **A.** Pathology and Laboratory Section Conventions, Symbols, and Special Notes

III. Guidelines for Reporting Pathology and Laboratory Codes

- **A.** Modifiers Used in Pathology and Laboratory Coding

IV. Subsections of the Pathology and Laboratory Section

V. Organ or Disease-Oriented Panels (Codes 80047-80076)

VI. Drug Assay (Codes 80305-80377)

- **A.** Presumptive Drug Class Screening
- **B.** Definitive Drug Testing

VII. Therapeutic Drug Assays (Codes 80150-80299)

VIII. Evocative/Suppression Testing (Codes 80400-80439)

IX. Consultations (Clinical Pathology) (Codes 80500-80502)

X. Urinalysis (Codes 81000-81099)

XI. Molecular Pathology (Codes 81105-81479)

XII. Genomic Sequencing Procedures and Other Molecular Multianalyte Assays (Codes 81410-81471)

XIII. Multianalyte Assays With Algorithmic Analyses (Codes 81490-81599)

XIV. Chemistry (Codes 82009-84999)

XV. Hematology and Coagulation (Codes 85002-85999)

XVI. Immunology (Codes 86000-86849)

XVII. Transfusion Medicine (Codes 86850-86999)

XVIII. Microbiology (Codes 87003-87999)

XIX. Anatomic Pathology (Codes 88000-88099)

XX. Cytopathology (Codes 88104-88199)

XXI. Cytogenetic Studies (Codes 88230-88299)

XXII. Surgical Pathology (Codes 88300-88399)

XXIII. Reproductive Medicine Procedures (Codes 89250-89398)

XXIV. Instructions for Reporting Pathology and Laboratory Codes

XXV. Proprietary Laboratory Analyses (Codes 0001U-0017U)

XXVI. Chapter Summary

Introduction to Pathology and Laboratory Services

Pathology is the study of disease. Physicians known as **pathologists** examine the causes and effects of various conditions by studying samples of cells, tissues, and other bodily materials in a **laboratory**. Laboratories are usually divided into 2 sections: anatomical pathology and clinical pathology. The **anatomical pathology** section examines tissue samples and specimens from surgery, under the direction of the surgical pathologist. The **clinical pathology** section consists of microbiology, chemistry, immunology, parasitology, hematology, and other specialty units that pertain to the diagnosis of disease. In the clinical pathology section of the laboratory, technicians perform diagnostic tests to analyze blood, urine, and other material. The **analyte** is the substance or chemical constituent that is of interest in an analytical procedure. The **specimen** is the material being analyzed, a sample that represents the whole.

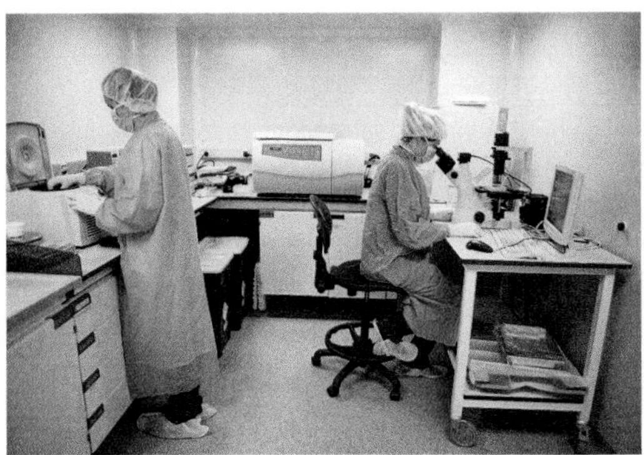

Large facilities may have separate departments for each type of lab test, while smaller facilities may cross-train their lab techs to work in several different areas.

The organization of a laboratory depends on the size: in larger facilities, there may be separate departments for each type of test; in smaller facilities, there may not be separate departmental designations, and lab techs may be cross-trained to work in several areas. The different disciplines reflected in typical laboratory departments are the following:

- **Hematology** is the study of blood. In the hematology department, routine screening to test for blood abnormalities is performed. Most of the hematology tests are done with automated instruments, but some parts of blood counts may require microscopic examination by a lab technician. **Coagulation tests,** such as prothrombin time, assess bleeding and clotting problems.
- **Urinalysis** is the analysis of urine and is used to detect disease in the urinary tract. Urinalysis can constitute a separate laboratory department.
- The **chemistry department** performs quantitative analysis on body fluids. Chemistry tests can be performed for several hundred analytes.
- The **immunology and serology department** performs testing for antigen-antibody reactions. The detection of antibodies in a patient's blood can confirm the presence of an infectious disease.
- The **microbiology department** performs identification of microorganisms that cause disease.
- **Molecular pathology** is the identification of the risk of developing a particular disease by analyzing specific genes. The data and results obtained in the laboratory from these tests help physicians and other healthcare providers evaluate and treat patients. Pathology and laboratory codes include tests and procedures performed by a physician or by laboratory technicians working under the supervision of a physician.

It is important for a coder to be familiar with laboratory technical terms to correctly report codes from the CPT® codebook Pathology and Laboratory section. Table 19.1 provides some basic terms and their definitions.

Table 19.1 Pathology and Laboratory Terminology

Term	Definition
assay	A laboratory procedure performed to obtain data about a certain drug or substance in a specimen
autopsy/necropsy	An exam performed postmortem to discover information regarding the cause of death or extent of disease
DNA/RNA	A nucleic acid that carries genetic information in cells and some viruses
gene	A unit consisting of a sequence of DNA that contains genetic information and can influence the phenotype of an organism
genome	An organism's genetic material
genomic sequencing	The process of figuring out the order of DNA nucleotides in a genome that make up an organism's DNA
immunology	The branch of science/medicine that deals with the immune system
massively parallel sequencing (MPS)	Any of several high-throughput approaches to DNA sequencing; also known as *next-generation sequencing (NGS)*
molecular	Relating to molecules
screen	A test
serology	The examination of blood serum, particularly with regard to the response of the immune system to pathogens or substances

Organization of the Pathology and Laboratory Section

Pathology and laboratory codes are located in the fifth section of the CPT® codebook (following Radiology and preceding Medicine), and the code numbers range from 80047 through 89398. A special subsection of codes for Proprietary Laboratory Analyses appear at the end of the Pathology and Laboratory section. These codes are alphanumeric and range from 0001U to 0017U. The codes in the Pathology and Laboratory section are arranged into subsections according to the type of study. Pathology and laboratory codes can easily be identified by the first digit in the code because no other codes in the CPT® code book start with the digit *8*. While not all of the pathology and laboratory codes will be explained in detail in this chapter, some of the more common and more challenging codes you may be required to report are discussed in the upcoming sections. Table 19.2 presents a list of the subsections within the Pathology and Laboratory section and the corresponding code ranges.

Pathology and Laboratory Section Conventions, Symbols, and Special Notes

The CPT® codebook Pathology and Laboratory section begins with 2 resources that provide helpful information—the table of contents and the Molecular Pathology Gene Table. The table of contents lists in sequence all the subsections and headings with the

Table 19.2 Subsections Within the Pathology and Laboratory Section of the CPT® Codebook

Subsection	Code Range
Organ or Disease-Oriented Panels	80047-80081 (out of numeric sequence)
Drug Assay	80305-80377 (out of numeric sequence)
Therapeutic Drug Assays	80150-80299 (out of numeric sequence)
Evocative/Suppression Testing	80400-80439
Consultations (Clinical Pathology)	80500-80502
Urinalysis	81000-81099
Molecular Pathology	81105-81479 (out of numeric sequence)
Genomic Sequencing Procedures (GSPs) and Other Molecular Multianalyte Assays	81410-81471
Multianalyte Assays with Algorithmic Analyses	81490-81599
Chemistry	82009-84999
Hematology and Coagulation	85002-85999
Immunology	86000-86849
Transfusion Medicine	86850-86999
Microbiology	87003-87999
Anatomic Pathology	88000-88099
Cytopathology	88104-88199
Cytogenetic Studies	88230-88299
Surgical Pathology	88300-88399
In Vivo (eg, Transcutaneous) Laboratory Procedures	88720-88749
Other Procedures	89049-89240
Reproductive Medicine Procedures	89250-89398
Proprietary Laboratory Analyses	0001U-0017U

codes associated with them. Those with an asterisk symbol (*) have special instructions unique to those codes. The Molecular Pathology Gene Table relates to codes under the Molecular Pathology heading and is discussed in this chapter.

Guidelines for Reporting Pathology and Laboratory Codes

Assignment of codes from the Pathology and Laboratory section to procedures and services is often automated, hardcoded into a facility or provider's **chargemaster** (the list of codes and associated charges) rather than manually assigned by coding staff prior to claim submission. For work performed at a hospital or facility with a lab, such as an outpatient surgery center or a rehabilitation facility, codes from the chargemaster are entered into the patient's financial record by the laboratory technicians upon completion of a test or service. Automated laboratory systems that interface with electronic health record (EHR) systems may also upload codes and charge information directly to a patient's account for billing purposes.

Therapeutic Drug Assays (Codes 80150-80299)

Therapeutic drug assays are quantitative studies, meaning that they are performed to determine the amount of a known drug present in the patient's whole blood, serum, plasma, or cerebrospinal fluid. The results are used to monitor the patient's response to a prescribed medication and correct the dosage if indicated. Therapeutic drug assay codes are listed in alphabetical order by the parent drug name.

LET'S TRY ONE **19.2**

A physician ordered a quantitative theophylline level for a 51-year-old patient with emphysema taking 400 mg of theophylline daily. The patient reported to the laboratory, where a blood sample was taken and the therapeutic drug assay was performed. What code is reported for this test? ____

Evocative/Suppression Testing (Codes 80400-80439)

The Evocative/Suppression Testing subsection provides codes for panels of tests to measure the effects of administering evocative or suppressive agents. Typically, these panels start with a chemistry test to measure the level of the analyte(s) in the blood as a baseline. The patient is then given an agent appropriate to the protocol (such as human growth hormone or insulin) by intravenous infusion. Subsequent blood samples are taken at specific intervals, such as 30, 60, and 120 minutes. Those samples are then tested to determine the levels of the analyte(s) and look for variations, which may aid in diagnosing certain conditions.

Consultations (Clinical Pathology) (Codes 80500-80502)

Under certain circumstances, a physician may request a consultation from a pathologist regarding the interpretation of test results. Pathology consultations may be ordered to interpret many types of laboratory test results, including chemistry, immunology, microbiology, and others. In response to this request, the pathologist provides a written consultation report. In this report, the pathologist does not examine or evaluate the patient but simply provides a medical interpretation of the test results. A limited clinical pathology consultation is reported with code 80500, *Clinical pathology consultation; limited, without review of patient's history and medical records.* A more in-depth consultation is reported with code 80502, *Clinical pathology consultation; comprehensive, for a complex diagnostic problem, with review of patient's history and medical records.*

EXAMPLE 19.3

A 58-year-old male with arthritic symptoms affecting his left knee underwent an arthrocentesis. The specimen of synovial fluid was submitted for crystal identification because the physician suspected chondrocalcinosis. Because crystals are found in the synovial fluid of approximately 90% of patients with inflamed joints, the attending physician requested a pathology consultation to review the results of a synovial fluid crystal identification. The pathologist reviewed the test results and provided a consultation report to the attending physician. For this service, the pathologist reports 80500, *Clinical pathology consultation; limited, without review of patient's history and medical records*.

Urinalysis (Codes 81000-81099)

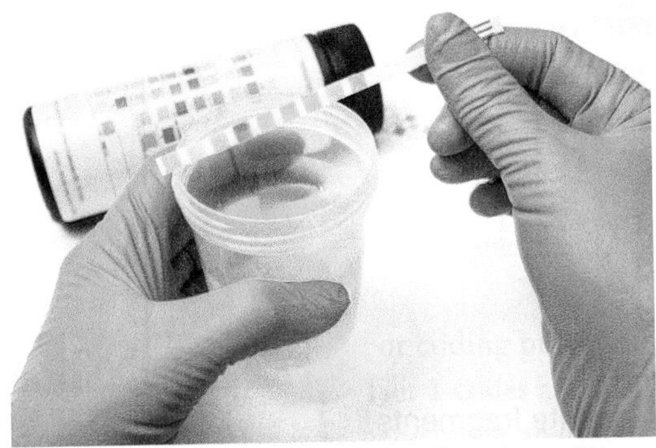
Urinalysis helps diagnose many different conditions.

The term *urinalysis* refers to tests performed on a urine sample. Urinalysis is used to help diagnose urinary tract diseases and conditions such as infection, proteinuria, or glucosuria.

Several criteria determine the appropriate code for a urinalysis procedure: the specific analyte and the methodology of testing, qualitative or quantitative, and automated or nonautomated. In most cases, laboratory technicians will enter the appropriate code from the chargemaster after test completion. The documentation in the health record will contain a urinalysis report, which the coder should review to determine the correct code. Figure 19.5 shows a sample urinalysis report.

Codes 81000 through 81003 describe specific analytes tested by dipstick or tablet reagent, with automated and nonautomated methods of interpreting results, with or without microscopy. In these types of tests, 1 or more plastic strips impregnated with chemicals that react with urine are dipped into a urine sample. Once dipped into the urine, the color of the strip changes, and the strip is then compared against a standardized color chart to interpret results. One strip will test for multiple analytes such as bilirubin, glucose, and hemoglobin, as well as for pH and specific gravity. Tablets work in much the same way, except that a drop from the urine sample is placed on the tablet rather than the tablet being placed in the sample. The chemical reaction causes a color change on the tablet, which is then compared against a standardized color chart. Tablets are usually used to measure only 1 analyte. An automated urinalysis uses an instrument to read the color changes on the strip. **Microscopy** is the examination of urine specimens under a microscope for biological abnormalities such as bacteria and chemical abnormalities such as crystals. Code 81001 is reported for an automated urinalysis with microscopy, code 81002 is reported for a nonautomated urinalysis without microscopy, and code 81003 is reported for an automated urinalysis without microscopy.

Genomic Sequencing Procedures and Other Molecular Multianalyte Assays (Codes 81410-81471)

Advances in DNA sequencing technology, next-generation sequencing (NGS), or massively parallel sequencing (MPS) required new procedure codes to report these tests. New in 2015, disorder-specific multigene assays can now be reported with codes 81410 through 81471. These codes include multianalyte assays where 1 method can simultaneously test multiple genes or genetic regions. Codes are listed in alphabetical order by the name of the disease being tested for (such as "hereditary colon cancer syndromes") or the target of the genomic sequence.

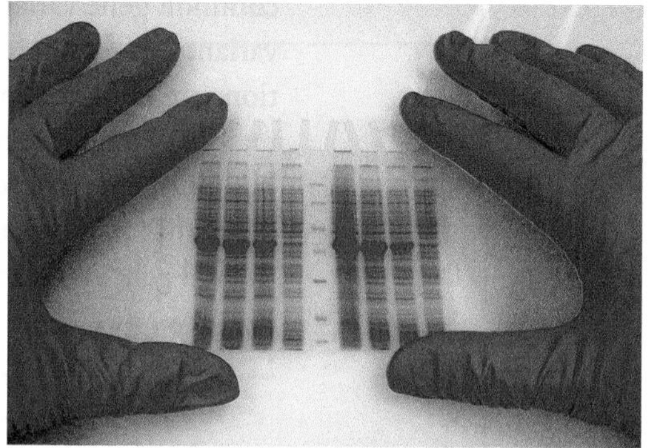

Advances in DNA sequencing technology have required codes for these new multianalyte assays.

Multianalyte Assays With Algorithmic Analyses (Codes 81490-81599)

Multianalyte assays with algorithmic analyses (MAAA) use algorithmic analysis to report a score or probability of a disease from results of the assay. MAAA procedures are proprietary and unique to a single clinical laboratory or manufacturer. Refer to Appendix O to cross-reference the proprietary names and clinical laboratory or manufacturer for these procedures with their correlated codes. MAAAs not listed in Appendix O may be reported with code 81599, *Unlisted multianalyte assay with algorithmic analysis.*

Chemistry (Codes 82009-84999)

The chemistry section of a laboratory performs tests for drugs, chemicals, and other substances. Chemistry tests can be performed on many types of specimens, including blood, urine, and cerebrospinal fluid. An example of a chemistry test that a physician may request is measuring the level of cholesterol in a patient's blood to help determine the risk for heart disease. Another example is monitoring ketone bodies in a diabetic patient's urine.

The chemistry codes are arranged in alphabetical order according to the name of the analyte (the substance or constituent being tested for). To appropriately assign codes from the Chemistry subsection, in addition to the analyte, you may need to identify the type of specimen and the specific test that was performed. The same chemistry codes are used for any type of specimen, unless the source of the specimen is specifically noted in the code description, such as in code 82757, *Fructose; semen.* When an analyte is measured multiple times from multiple specimens, each test is reported separately. These tests are quantitative unless otherwise specified in the code description, such as in code 82355, *Calculus; qualitative analysis.*

EXAMPLE **19.5**

A physician ordered a total testosterone level for a male patient who was experiencing symptoms of fatigue and reduced libido. The patient presented to the clinic for blood draw. The blood was collected and sent to the chemistry department of the laboratory. The test was performed and reported with code 84403, *Testosterone; total*.

LET'S TRY ONE **19.3**

A physician ordered a quantitative selenium level for a patient who has been taking a daily, high-dose selenium supplement. The patient presented to the clinic for blood draw. The blood was collected and sent to the chemistry department of the laboratory where the test was performed. What code should be reported for this laboratory test? _____

Hematology and Coagulation (Codes 85002-85999)

Hematology tests analyze the amount and/or function of blood cells. A physician may order a **complete blood count (CBC)** to determine how many cells of different types are present. A CBC measures red blood cells (RBC), white blood cells (WBC), hematocrit, hemoglobin, and platelets. A CBC is often used as a screening test to help the physician determine the patient's overall health status. Another common hematology test is the **prothrombin time (PT)**, which measures how long it takes blood to clot. A PT is often required for patients on the drug warfarin, which is a blood thinner taken to prevent blood clots. The hematology codes are arranged in alphabetical order according to the name of the test or the analyte being tested. As with assigning codes for other laboratory tests, you must identify the specific test, whether the test was automated or nonautomated (manual), and the methodology of testing.

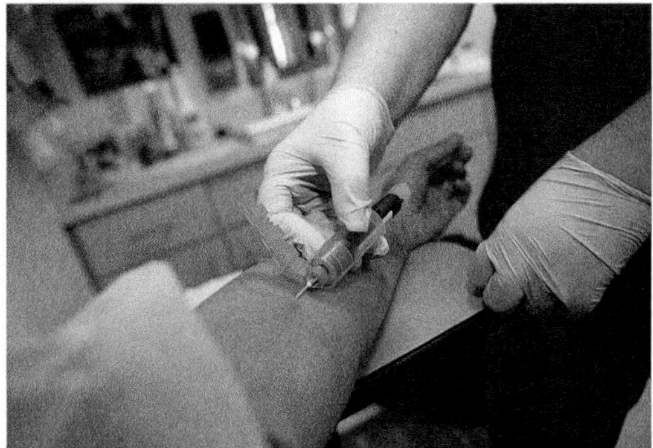

Hematology tests analyze the amount and/or function of blood cells.

Immunology (Codes 86000-86849)

Immunology is the study of the immune system. Immunology tests identify the presence of antigens and antibodies in a patient's body to help determine whether his or her immune system is functioning normally. Codes 86000 through 86593 are arranged in alphabetic order according to the name of the analyte (eg, allergen, antibody, antigen) for which a specimen is being tested or a type of test (eg, immunoelectrophoresis); codes 86602 through 86804 are arranged in alphabetic order by specific antibodies to be identified. The Tissue Typing category of codes (86805 through 86849) involves procedures to determine donor-recipient compatibility for transplantations.

Note that modifier 92, *Alternative laboratory platform testing*, is mentioned in the tabular after the codes for HIV testing (86701 through 86703). This modifier indicates that the test is performed using a kit or transportable instrument that has a single-use or disposable analytic chamber. These tests can be performed anywhere and do not require a dedicated lab space. The location of the test does not affect the use of the modifier.

EXAMPLE **19.6**

An HIV-1 and HIV-2 single-result test was performed at a walk-in clinic held in a church basement. This test would be reported with code 86703 - 92, *HIV-1 and HIV-2, single result - Alternative laboratory platform testing*.

Transfusion Medicine (Codes 86850-86999)

Codes in the transfusion medicine subsection (86850-86999) describe tests used to detect antibodies in whole blood, serologic blood typing, Rh typing, and collecting and preparing blood for transfusion.

Microbiology (Codes 87003-87999)

Microbiology tests are performed to determine the presence of bacteria, fungi, parasites, or viruses that can cause infection. Sources of microorganism specimens include blood, urine, sputum, wounds, and feces. An example of a microbiology test is a urine culture performed to identify the organism causing a urinary tract infection. Determining the cause of the infection helps the physician decide what treatment will be best for the patient.

Codes in the Microbiology codebook subsection are assigned according to the method of the test, the source of the specimen, and/or the organism being tested for. Multiple specimens may be reported with the same procedure code by appending modifier 59, *Distinct procedural service*.

When working with codes in the Microbiology subsection, you will encounter the terms *presumptive identification* and *definitive identification*. These terms refer to the depth of results that the tests provide. When a test includes **presumptive identification**, it means that a sample has been cultured or put into media to grow the microorganisms it may contain into a colony. The colony has characteristics called its *morphology*. Colony morphology is used to determine whether the sample contains pathogens or microorganisms. When a test includes **definitive identification**, it means a microorganism present in the sample has been identified down to the genus or species level. Some presumptive identification tests are followed by parenthetic instructions that refer the coder to specific tests performed for definitive identification, as the 1 that follows code 87073:

> *Culture, bacterial; quantitative, anaerobic with isolation and presumptive identification of isolates, any source except urine, blood or stool:*
>
> *(For definitive identification of isolates, use 87076 or 87077. For typing of isolates see 87140-87158).*

Culture typing procedures are performed to provide a more specific identification of a cultured pathogenic organism so that the physician can determine the best treatment. Each antibiotic drug has a range of efficacy in killing certain bacteria or pathogens and keeping them from reproducing. A culture can identify which pathogen is causing an infection so the physician can determine which antibiotic is the most appropriate treatment. A **quantitative colony count** is a measurement of individual colonies of bacteria in a urine sample that has been cultured for 24 to 48 hours. Quantitative urine cultures are necessary to differentiate a real infection from contamination of the specimen. Urine cultures are reported by colony-forming units per milliliter (CFU/mL) of urine. The result of 100,000 CFU/mL and above indicates a urinary tract infection. A lower number of colonies present can indicate contamination of the specimen, while a high colony count of a single type of pathogen can indicate infection.

Another type of microbiology test is macroscopic (visual) identification of arthropods and parasites, covered by codes 87168 through 87169. A related test is a pinworm exam, reported using code 87172. In this test, cellophane tape is briefly applied to the patient's perianal area. Once removed, the tape is sent to the laboratory on a clean slide. A microscopic examination is then performed to confirm or dismiss the presence of these tiny parasitic worms.

Identification of infectious agents, such as enterovirus or influenza B virus, is reported with codes 87260 through 87905. These codes are grouped by the technique (immunofluorescence, immunoassay, and nucleic acid) and alphabetized by infectious agent within each technique grouping. The **immunofluorescent** technique involves mixing the antigen with a fluorescent compound, then adding that to a sample of the patient's blood. If the antibody is present, the mixture will fluoresce under ultraviolet light. An **immunoassay** is any assay that measures an antigen-antibody reaction, with methods such as fluorescence, enzyme, or radioisotope markers. Another type of assay is detection by nucleic acid. **Nucleic acid (DNA** or **RNA)** is detected in the patient source specimen, which identifies the presence of an infectious agent, such as hepatitis B or chlamydia.

When separate results are reported for different species or strains of organisms, a CPT® code is assigned for each separate result. When separate results are reported for different species or strains reported with the same code, modifier 59, *Distinct procedural service*, should be applied. Molecular pathology codes (81161, 81200 through 81408) cannot be used with the microbiology codes for infectious agent antigen detection (87470 through 87801) as instructed in the notes following code 87255.

EXAMPLE **19.7**

A urine culture was performed using a quantitative colony count. This test was reported with code 87086, *Culture, bacterial; quantitative colony count, urine*. A colony count of more than 100,000 organisms per milliliter of urine was found, indicating there was a clinically significant urinary tract infection. Additional aerobic (grows in the presence of oxygen) biochemical testing was done on the bacteria found in the urine. The additional test is reported with code 87077, *Culture, bacterial; aerobic isolate, additional methods required for definitive identification, each isolate*.

LET'S TRY ONE **19.4**

A 21-year-old female presented to the physician's office after learning that her boyfriend has chlamydia. The physician ordered a chlamydia culture. The patient's vagina was swabbed, and the specimen was sent to the lab. The lab performed a culture for chlamydia. How is this test reported? _____

Anatomic Pathology (Codes 88000-88099)

The Anatomic Pathology subsection codes are reported for postmortem examinations, also known as *autopsies* or *necropsies*. A **gross examination** includes dissection of the body with examination of the organs and tissues. A **microscopic examination** involves examining organ samples under a microscope. Both gross and microscopic examinations require an examination of the body and organs, and a description of the examination and findings must be provided. Anatomic Pathology codes are assigned based on the scope of the autopsy: a gross examination only (88000 through 88016), both gross and microscopic examinations (88020 through 88029), or a limited autopsy on a single organ or on specific organs or tissues within a region of the body (88036 through 88037). These codes represent physician services only, so the use of modifier 26, *Professional component*, is not allowed.

EXAMPLE **19.8**

A pathologist was requested to perform a necropsy of the body of a 59-year-old male with a clinical diagnosis of Alzheimer's disease. The pathologist completed a gross and microscopic examination of the brain and described the findings. This is reported with code 88037, *Necropsy (autopsy) limited, gross and/or microscopic; single organ*.

RED FLAG

A necropsy (autopsy) forensic examination reported with code 88040 includes both gross and microscopic examination.

Coding Clicks

To view a short National Geographic video that highlights the work of a medical examiner, visit http://Coding.ParadigmEducation.com/MedicalExaminer. Note that the video briefly shows the autopsy procedure, which may be disturbing to some viewers.

Autopsies done for legal purposes to gather and preserve evidence are reported with code 88040, which includes both gross and microscopic examination. A **coroner** is a public official who investigates deaths that appear to be from unnatural causes. Coroners may also be required to sign death certificates for people who die while not under the care of a physician. Since only 4 states require coroners to be physicians, a coroner may request a postmortem examination to be performed by a medical examiner/physician. The physician makes an onsite gross examination and arranges for a more thorough examination under laboratory conditions. Code 88045 is reported when a gross examination is performed by the physician onsite at the request of a coroner.

Cytopathology (Codes 88104-88199)

Cytopathology is the study of disease on the cellular level. Codes describing cytopathology procedures include many for the evaluation of cervical and vaginal specimens, as well as cytopathological evaluation of fine needle aspiration specimens. Obtaining the specimen for analysis is separately reportable in most cases. Pap smears (cervical or vaginal) that are examined using the Bethesda system are reported with codes 88164 through 88167. The **Bethesda system** of reporting uses standard diagnostic terminology that includes a statement of the specimen adequacy (eg, satisfactory for evaluation), a general categorization (eg, within normal limits), and a descriptive diagnosis (eg, epithelial cell abnormalities).

Cytogenetic Studies (Codes 88230-88299)

Cytogenetics is the study of cell structure and function as it relates to genetics (heredity), distinguished from molecular pathology tests that identify inherited disorders. Codes describing cytogenetic studies include tissue cultures for neoplastic and non-neoplastic disorders and for chromosome analysis. White blood cells are the most commonly used specimen for chromosome analysis. For example, white blood cells, specifically T-lymphocytes, are stimulated and grown in tissue culture for evaluation of nonneoplastic disorders. This is reported with code 88230, *Tissue culture for non-neoplastic disorders; lymphocyte.*

Surgical Pathology (Codes 88300-88399)

Surgical pathology codes describe the evaluation of specimens for pathologic diagnosis. The coder should identify the source of the specimen and the reason for the surgical procedure to determine the level of surgical pathology examination. Surgical pathology codes are divided into 6 levels, as shown in Table 19.3. Codes 88300 through 88309 include accession of specimens, examination, and reporting.

Table 19.3 Levels of Surgical Pathology Codes

Surgical Pathology Examination Level	CPT® Code	Description
Level I	88300	Gross examination only Specimens that do not need to be examined under a microscope for diagnosis (eg, foreign body, tooth)
Level II	88302	Gross and microscopic examination Specimens usually considered normal, removed for a reason other than malignancy or disease (eg, vas deferens from a vasectomy)
Level III	88304	Gross and microscopic examination Specimens with a low probability of malignancy (eg, gallbladder with inflammation from chronic disease)
Level IV	88305	Gross and microscopic examination Specimens with a higher probability of malignancy (eg, biopsy of stomach)
Level V	88307	Gross and microscopic examination More complex pathology examinations (eg, examination of breast tissue from partial mastectomy)
Level VI	88309	Gross and microscopic examination Complex examination of neoplastic tissue or very involved specimens (eg, total lung resection)

Within each CPT® code, different anatomical specimens are listed. Each tissue submitted to pathology that requires individual examination and pathological diagnosis is considered a specimen. A separate code is reported for each specimen. Multiple surgical pathology codes may be assigned if multiple specimens are submitted and require individual and separate attention. The surgical pathology codes are arranged in ascending order of physician work. Code 88300 is reported for specimens that can be identified by the pathologist without microscopic examination. Code 88302 is used to report gross and microscopic exam to confirm identification and the absence of disease. Codes 88304 through 88309 describe higher levels of physician work and are assigned by the specimen examined. The pathologist determines the level of work involved.

Pathologists are often called to surgery to perform an intraoperative pathological examination. During the course of the operation, the surgeon requests a pathology consultation. A gross exam of tissue is performed by the pathologist. After the gross exam, consultations often involve a microscopic exam called a **frozen section** in which the specimen removed by the surgeon is immediately frozen to facilitate cutting a thin section to be placed under the microscope. The pathologist then examines the specimen and gives an opinion about the presence or absence of disease in the tissue. Surgeons use the pathological diagnosis to determine the course of the surgery. Pathology consultations during surgery are reported with codes 88329 through 88334, based on the type of examination performed.

EXAMPLE 19.9

A 24-year-old male was brought to the emergency department (ED) after being involved in a bar fight. He had an open wound of the cheek where he claimed his assailant bit him. The ED physician removed a foreign body from the open wound, which appeared to be a crowned tooth. The physician submitted the foreign body as a single specimen to the pathology department. The pathologist performed a gross examination of the specimen and confirmed that the foreign body was a tooth. This surgical pathology examination is reported with 88300, *Level I Surgical pathology, gross examination only*.

Codes 88311 through 88399 describe additional pathology services not included in the Levels I through VI codes. Unlike those tissue pathology codes, the specimen submitted for special studies may be tissue or any body fluid or blood. These codes describe the use of special stains or procedures. Some of these codes may be used alone, while others are reported in addition to the code(s) reported for the primary surgical pathology procedures.

CONCEPTS CHECKPOINT 19.3

Answer true or false to each of the following statements.

1. _____ A pathologist performs a gross examination using the microscope.
2. _____ Multiple pathology codes may be reported if multiple specimens were examined.
3. _____ A pathologist is never allowed into the surgery suite if the patient is still alive.
4. _____ A specimen requiring a very complex examination would be considered level VI.
5. _____ A specimen requiring verification of absence of disease would be considered level II.

LET'S TRY ONE 19.5

The pathologist performed a surgical pathology examination (gross and microscopic) of a kidney biopsy. What code would be reported for this examination? _____

Reproductive Medicine Procedures (Codes 89250-89398)

Codes contained in the reproductive medicine subsection (89250 through 89398) describe procedures relating to sperm and egg viability as well as the storage of sperm, eggs, and embryos. Codes 89342 through 89346 are reported by storage facilities for the long-term maintenance of preserved embryos (89342), sperm/semen (89343), testicular or ovarian tissue (89344), and oocytes (eggs) (89346). These codes are reported once per year of storage.

Coding Clicks

Medicare will use private payor prices to set payment rates for clinical diagnostic laboratory tests in 2018, as a final rule of the Protecting Access to Medicare Act of 2014. Visit http://Coding.ParadigmEducation.com/PrivatePayorPrices for more information.

Proprietary Laboratory Analyses (Codes 0001U-0017U)

Proprietary Laboratory Analyses (Codes 0001U-0017U) are a special category of tests that are provided by a single laboratory or licensed to multiple laboratories that have been cleared or approved by the FDA to provide these specific advanced diagnostic laboratory tests. These tests are an analysis of RNA, DNA, or proteins and include a unique algorithm. Codes 0001U through 0017U include multianalyte assays with algorithmic analyses (MAAA) and genomic sequencing procedures. The results of these advanced diagnostic laboratory tests predict the probability that a patient will develop a certain condition or respond to a certain therapy. The codes are very specific to the disease or drug compound to be analyzed and are requested by the laboratory or manufacturer that offers the test. These proprietary laboratory analyses codes take precedence over similar laboratory codes such as those for MAAAs in the 81490 through 81599 range.

Instructions for Reporting Pathology and Laboratory Codes

Though most laboratory procedure codes will be automatically assigned through the chargemaster, a coding specialist should be able to locate the appropriate code in the CPT® codebook. The steps to locating pathology and laboratory procedure codes are listed below.

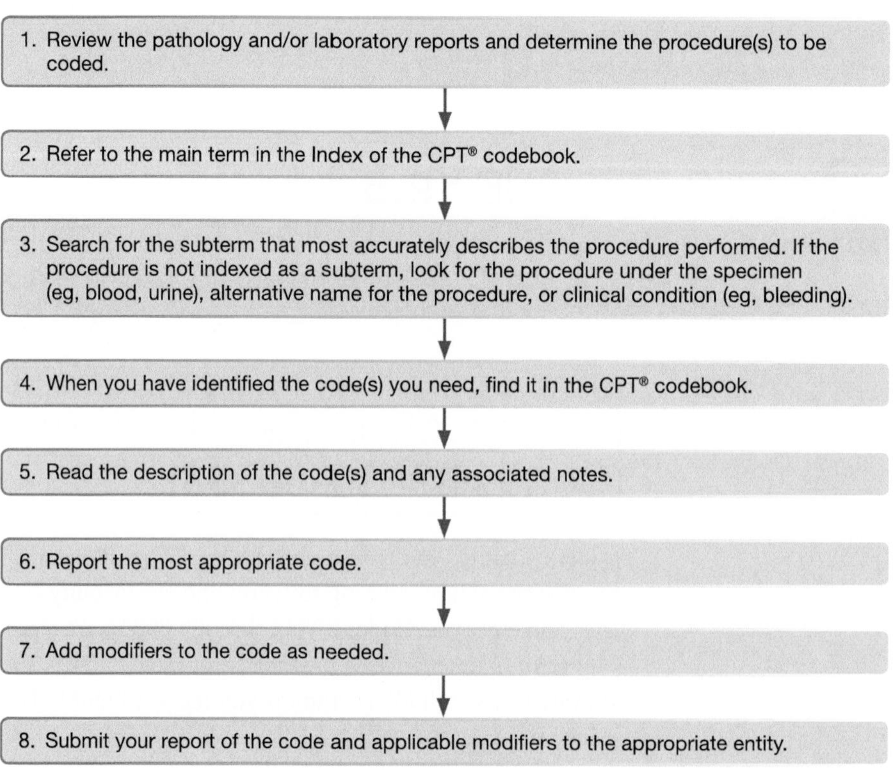

1. Review the pathology and/or laboratory reports and determine the procedure(s) to be coded.
2. Refer to the main term in the Index of the CPT® codebook.
3. Search for the subterm that most accurately describes the procedure performed. If the procedure is not indexed as a subterm, look for the procedure under the specimen (eg, blood, urine), alternative name for the procedure, or clinical condition (eg, bleeding).
4. When you have identified the code(s) you need, find it in the CPT® codebook.
5. Read the description of the code(s) and any associated notes.
6. Report the most appropriate code.
7. Add modifiers to the code as needed.
8. Submit your report of the code and applicable modifiers to the appropriate entity.

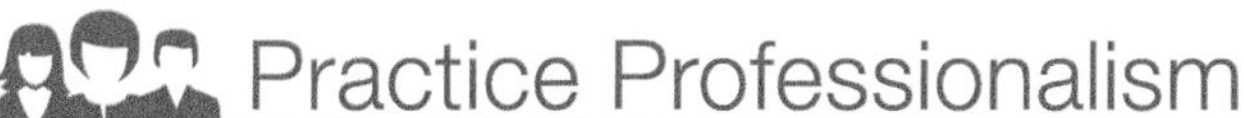

Practice Professionalism

Imagine that you are a coding specialist at a busy acute care hospital. The director of your hospital's laboratory has requested your help in updating the lab department's chargemaster for the new fiscal year. To determine if there are revised or new CPT® codes for the lab, what resources will you need?

Chapter Summary

- Pathology and laboratory codes include tests and procedures performed by a physician or by laboratory technologists working under the supervision of a physician.
- Modifier 90, *Reference (outside) laboratory*, is reported when a physician's office sends specimens to an outside laboratory (for testing and interpretation) where the tests are purchased by the physician's office.
- Modifier 91, *Repeat clinical diagnostic laboratory test*, is reported when a lab test is intentionally repeated on the same date of service to obtain subsequent results.
- All the tests listed in an organ or disease-oriented panel must be performed for that code to be reported.
- Qualitative tests determine whether a drug or substance is present or not present in the sample being evaluated but not how much is present if the results are positive. Drug testing may be both qualitative and quantitative on the same patient on the same day.
- Therapeutic drug assays (80150 through 80299) or chemistry tests (82009 through 84999) are quantitative studies that determine the amount of the substance present in the sample.
- Urinalysis tests are performed from a urine sample. The coder must identify the specific analyte, whether the test was automated or nonautomated (manual), and the methodology of testing before an appropriate code can be assigned.
- Molecular pathology tests are related to procedures that identify variants in genes associated with disorders and diseases. The molecular pathology services are placed into a 2-tiered system for coding purposes. Tier 1 codes are unique and analyte specific. Codes are based on the specific genes that are being analyzed. These analyses are qualitative. Tier 2 codes are categories of molecular pathology services grouped by the complexity and resources required for the service.
- To appropriately assign codes from the chemistry subsection, the coder must identify the specimen and the specific test that was performed. Chemistry codes are used for any type of specimen unless the source of the specimen is specifically noted in the code description.

- Hematology tests analyze the amount and/or function of blood cells. The coder must identify the specific test, whether the test was automated or nonautomated (manual), and the methodology of testing before an appropriate code can be assigned.
- Immunology tests identify conditions of the immune system caused by the actions of antibodies. These tests can determine if a patient's immune system is functioning normally.
- Microbiology tests are performed to determine the presence of bacteria, fungi, parasites, or viruses that cause infection. Microbiology tests can be performed from many types of specimens, including blood, urine, sputum, and feces.
- The Anatomic Pathology subsection of codes are reported for postmortem examinations, also known as *autopsies* or *necropsies*. Anatomic pathology codes represent physician services only, and the use of modifier 26, *Professional component*, is not allowed.
- Surgical pathology codes describe the evaluation of specimens for pathologic diagnosis. Tissue submitted to pathology that requires individual examination and pathological diagnosis is considered a specimen. A separate code is reported for each specimen.

Navigator

Access interactive chapter review exercises, practice activities, flash cards, and study games.

Chapter 20

Medicine Coding

Fast Facts

- Approximately 4 in 10 adults in the United States are using some form of alternative or complementary medicine.
- Acupuncture is a form of complementary and alternative medicine that involves inserting needles in various places on the body to alleviate pain and stimulate healing.
- Acupuncture is 1 of the oldest treatments at over 5,000 years old.
- According to the National Institutes of Health, more than half of Americans have at least 1 allergy. Allergies to shellfish, nuts, fish, milk, eggs, and other foods cause approximately 150-200 deaths per year in the United States.

Sources: http://seedswellness.com, http://www.nih.gov

Crack the Code

Review the sample operative report to find the correct medicine code. You may need to return to this exercise after reading the chapter content.

DESCRIPTION: This is an 84-hour continuous video EEG monitoring study.

TECHNICAL SUMMARY: The 22-year-old female patient was recorded from noon on 11/07/19 through midnight on 11/11/19. Patient was recorded digitally using the 10-20 system of electrode placement. Additional temporal electrodes and single channels of EOG and ECG were also used.

The occipital dominant rhythm was 10 to 10.5 Hz and well regulated. Low voltage 18 to 22 Hz activity was present in the anterior regions bilaterally.

INDUCED EVENT: The patient was informed that we would be performing prolonged photic stimulation and hyperventilation, which may induce a seizure. At 10:28 a.m. on 11/10/19, the patient was instructed to begin hyperventilation. Two minutes later we initiated photic stimulation using flickering light of random frequencies. Approximately 6 minutes into the procedure, the patient became unresponsive. Approximately 1 minute later, she began to exhibit asynchronous shaking of her extremities and her eyes were closed. Thirty seconds later, she became slowly responsive. She said she had been asleep and did not remember the event.

IMPRESSION: This patient's 84-hour continuous video EEG monitoring shows findings within the range of normal variation. No epileptiform activity present. There was 1 induced clinical event.

answer: 95951 and 95954

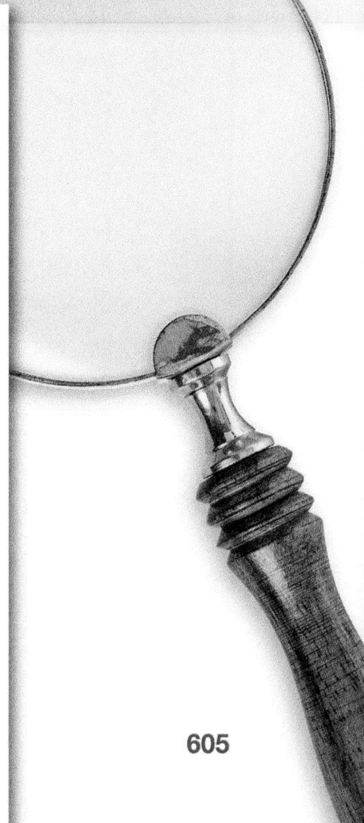

Learning Objectives

20.1 Describe the contents and structure of the Medicine section of the CPT® codebook.

20.2 Identify guidelines specific to the immunization codebook subsection.

20.3 Describe the use of therapeutic or diagnostic infusion and injection codes.

20.4 Describe the use of psychiatry codes.

20.5 Identify the elements used in assigning dialysis codes.

20.6 Describe the use of ophthalmology codes and the services that are included.

20.7 Describe the codes in the cardiovascular subsection, including cardiac catheterization and defibrillation.

20.8 Discuss the chemotherapy administration codes and circumstances in which additional codes may be reported.

20.9 Identify guidelines for allergy and clinical immunology codes and describe professional services for allergen immunotherapy

20.10 Discuss the codes included in the physical medicine and rehabilitation, osteopathic, and chiropractic manipulation codebook subsections.

20.11 Discuss the contents and limitations of codes in the special services and reports codebook subsection.

Chapter Outline

- **I.** Introduction to the Medicine Section
- **II.** Medicine Section Terminology
- **III.** Organization of the Medicine Section
  - **A.** Immunizations: Immune Globulin, Vaccine, and Toxoid Products and Their Administration (Codes 90281-90749)
  - **B.** Psychiatry (Codes 90785-90899)
  - **C.** Dialysis (Codes 90935-90999)
  - **D.** Gastroenterology (Codes 91010-91299)
  - **E.** Ophthalmology (Codes 92002-92499)
    - **i.** General Ophthalmological Services
    - **ii.** Special Ophthalmological Services
    - **iii.** Contact Lens Services
    - **iv.** Spectacles Services
  - **F.** Special Otorhinolaryngologic Services (Codes 92502-92700)
  - **G.** Cardiovascular (Codes 92920-93799)
    - **i.** Therapeutic Services and Procedures
    - **ii.** Cardiography and Cardiovascular Monitoring Services
    - **iii.** Implantable and Wearable Cardiac Device Evaluations
    - **iv.** Echocardiography
    - **v.** Cardiac Catheterization
    - **vi.** Additional Cardiovascular Procedures
  - **H.** Noninvasive Vascular Diagnostic Studies (Codes 93880-93998)
  - **I.** Pulmonary (Codes 94002-94799)
  - **J.** Allergy and Clinical Immunology (Codes 95004-95199)
  - **K.** Neurology and Neuromuscular Procedures (Codes 95782-96020)
  - **L.** Central Nervous System Assessments/Tests (Codes 96101-96127)
  - **M.** Health and Behavior Assessment/Intervention (Codes 96150-96161)
  - **N.** Hydration, Therapeutic, Prophylactic, Diagnostic Injections and Infusions, and Chemotherapy and Other Highly Complex Drug or Highly Complex Biologic Agent Administration (Codes 96360-96549)
    - **i.** Hydration
    - **ii.** Therapeutic, Diagnostic, and Prophylactic Injections and Infusions

Introduction to the Medicine Section

The Medicine section of the CPT® codebook is 1 of the more difficult sections to navigate due to the wide range of medical specialties and procedures it covers. However, there are some commonalities among the codes. The diagnostic and therapeutic services are in general noninvasive or minimally invasive. Noninvasive procedures do not enter a body cavity. Minimally invasive procedures involve skin penetration for injections, infusions, or catheterizations. These procedures are also typically performed in physician offices, clinics, or ancillary departments of hospitals.

The Medicine section contains a variety of services, such as chemotherapy administration, psychiatric therapy, and chiropractic manipulation. The codes for qualifying circumstances for anesthesia and the moderate (conscious) sedation codes are also contained in the Medicine section. Codes in this section may not include the supplies used in performing these services, and additional HCPCS codes may be reported if applicable.

Medicine Section Terminology

It is important for a coder to be familiar with a variety of diagnostic and therapeutic terms to correctly report codes from the CPT® codebook Medicine section. Table 20.1 provides an overview of some of the more commonly used terms.

Table 20.1 Medicine Terminology

Term or Phrase	Definition
administration of drugs and other substances, techniques	Introduction of a medicinal substance or nutrient material by one of the following: • injection: introduction of a medicinal substance or nutrient material into a canal or cavity of the body that lasts 15 minutes or less and may have one of several routes of administration, such as intravenous (push), intramuscular, subcutaneous, and intra-arterial • infusion: continuous intravenous administrations over time increments of 31 minutes to an hour • push: an injection in which the administering individual is continuously present to administer the injection and observe the patient, or an infusion of 15 minutes or less.
administration, routes of	Methods of giving medicine; routes can be • epidural—into the dura mater (outer protective membrane of brain and spinal cord); • intradermal (IM)—under the epidermis (skin); • intramuscular—into a muscle; • intranasal—sprayed into the nose; • intrathecal—into the space around the spinal cord; • intravenous (IV)—within a vein; • intraventricular—within a ventricle of the brain or heart; • oral—by mouth; • subcutaneous—beneath the skin.
angiography	Radiography of blood vessels after injection of contrast material
angioplasty	Reconstruction of a blood vessel
atherectomy	Invasive removal of an atheroma or plaque from an artery
endoscopy	A surgical procedure during which a surgeon uses an endoscope (a small tube with a light source) to examine or manipulate body structures
valence of vaccines	The number of antigens (substance that induces an immune response) a vaccine contains: • 1—monovalent • 2—bivalent • 3—trivalent • 4—quadrivalent • 5—pentavalent • 9—nonavalent • multi-valent—contains several different antigens • [#] valent—the digit indicates the number of antigens

Organization of the Medicine Section

Medicine codes are located in the final section of the CPT® codebook, and the codes range from 90281 through 99607. The Medicine section has 34 subsections, as shown in Table 20.2.

The Medicine section is divided into subsections, some of which are used by many providers, and some of which are specific to specialists (eg, chiropractors). In the Medicine section table of contents, subsections, categories, and subcategories of codes are marked with an asterisk (*) to indicate they have special instructions unique to the codes. This chapter does not cover every code in the Medicine section but will cover guidelines in the discussions of most subsections.

Table 20.2 Subsections Within the Medicine Section of the CPT® Codebook

Subsection	Code(s)
Immune Globulins, Serum or Recombinant Products	90281-90399
Immunization Administration for Vaccines/Toxoids	90460-90474
Vaccines,Toxoids	90476-90749
Psychiatry	90785-90899
Biofeedback	90901-90911
Dialysis	90935-90999
Gastroenterology	91010-91299
Ophthalmology	92002-92499
Special Otorhinolaryngologic Services	92502-92700
Cardiovascular	92920-93799
Noninvasive Vascular Diagnostic Studies	93880-93998
Pulmonary	94002-94799
Allergy and Clinical Immunology	95004-95199
Endocrinology	95249-95251
Neurology and Neuromuscular Procedures	95782-96020
Medical Genetics and Genetic Counseling Services	96040
Central Nervous System Assessments/Tests	96101-96127
Health and Behavior Assessment/Intervention	96150-96161
Hydration, Therapeutic, Prophylactic, Diagnostic Injections and Infusions, and Chemotherapy and Other Highly Complex Drug or Highly Complex Biologic Agent Administration	96360-96549
Photodynamic Therapy	96567-96574
Special Dermatologic Procedures	96900-96999
Physical Medicine and Rehabilitation	97001-97799
Medical Nutrition Therapy	97802-97804
Acupuncture	97810-97814
Osteopathic Manipulative Treatment	98925-98929
Chiropractic Manipulative Treatment	98940-98943
Education and Training for Patient Self-Management	98960-98962
Non-Face-to-Face Nonphysician Services	98966-98969
Special Services, Procedures, and Reports	99000-99091
Qualifying Circumstances for Anesthesia	99100-99140
Moderate (Conscious) Sedation	99151-99157
Other Services and Procedures	99170-99199
Home Health Procedures/Services	99500-99602
Medication Therapy Management Services	99605-99607

Immunizations: Immune Globulin, Vaccine, and Toxoid Products and Their Administration (Codes 90281-90749)

Immunization is the process in which an individual is made immune or resistant to an infectious disease by the administration of an agent that stimulates and strengthens a protective immune response. CPT® codes provide for the administration of 3 agents: immune globulins, vaccines, and toxoids. An **immune globulin** is a protein extracted from donated human plasma, which contains antibodies that protect from certain diseases. Specific types of immune globulins protect against specific diseases, like measles or chicken pox. **Serum globulins** are made from human blood. **Recombinant immune globulins** are made from human or animal proteins and created in a laboratory through genetic modification. The recipient of an immune globulin is immune to the disease for a short time while the immune globulin circulates through the body. The recipient's immune system does not produce its own antibodies but is able to use the donated antibodies. In contrast, a **vaccine** causes the body to create antibodies against the specific microorganism or virus that was given. A vaccine contains an agent that resembles the disease-causing organism and is often made from weakened or dead forms of the microbe. **Toxoids** or **toxoid vaccines** are inactivated toxic compounds such as tetanus. Toxoids teach the body to fight the microbe's real toxins.

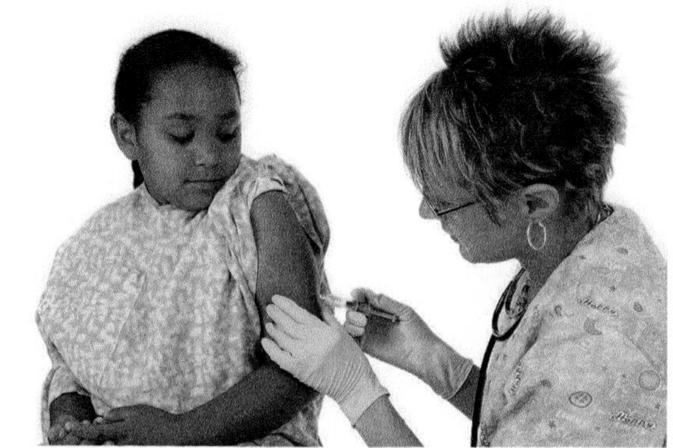

Reporting a vaccine requires at least 2 codes.

Index Insider

Immune globulin products are indexed under the main entry *Immune Globulins* and their administration under *Injection or Infusion*. There is no specific Index entry for administration of immune globulins. Vaccine and toxoid products are indexed under *Vaccines* and their administration under *Administration, Immunization*.

</> Coding for CMS

Medicare reporting for administration of immunizations may require use of HCPCS G codes. For more information, visit the Medicare Learning Network website at http://Coding.ParadigmEducation.com/MLNImmunization.

The immunization codes are differentiated by the routes of administration for both product and procedures of administration. Reporting the administration of an immune globulin, vaccine, or toxoid requires a code for the product and another code for the service of administering the product, as shown in Table 20.3.

The coding specialist should be aware of products that are bundled together. For example, code 90697 is reported for a single product that vaccinates against 6 diseases: diphtheria, tetanus, acellular pertussis, poliomyelitis, Haemophilus influenza, and hepatitis B. Reporting any of these vaccines separately when the 1 combination product is given is fraudulent.

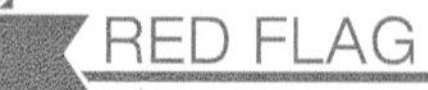

RED FLAG

Some third-party payers will require modifier 25 on the E/M code.

Immunizations are often given in conjunction with another medical service. A separate evaluation and management (E/M) code may be assigned only if a significant and separately identifiable E/M service was performed for a purpose other than the immunization. Patient visits for the sole purpose of receiving immunizations are reported with codes from the Medicine CPT® codebook section (90281 through 90749).

Table 20.3 Immunization Product and Administration Codes

Immunization Type	Product Codes	Administration Codes
Immune globulins	90281-90399	96365-96368, 96372, 96374, 96375
Vaccines/Toxoids	90476-90749	90460-90461, 90471-90474

EXAMPLE **20.1**

A new patient, an 11-year-old male, visited the physician's office for complaints of recurrent headaches. An expanded problem-focused history and physical was performed, with straightforward medical decision-making (MDM). The patient was given an IM injection of Tdap (tetanus, diphtheria, and acellular pertussis). This visit is reported with the following codes:

*99202, *Office or other outpatient visit for the evaluation and management of a new patient*;

*90471, *Immunization administration...; 1 vaccine (single or combination vaccine or toxoid)*;

*90715 *Tdap when administered to individuals 7 years or older for intramuscular use*.

EXAMPLE **20.2**

A parent brought a child into the office for a poliomyelitis vaccine. The nurse injected IPV (inactivated poliovirus vaccine). This visit is reported with the following codes:

*90471 *Immunization administration*;

*90713 *Poliovirus vaccine, inactivated (IPV) for subcutaneous or intramuscular use*.

LET'S TRY ONE **20.1**

A 54-year-old established patient came to the physician's office for a flu shot. The nurse administered the trivalent split influenza virus vaccine via an IM injection into the patient's left arm. The vaccination was the only service provided at this visit. How is this visit reported? _____

Psychiatry (Codes 90785-90899)

Psychiatry is the medical specialty that diagnoses, treats, and prevents mental illness and behavioral disorders. Codes exist for psychiatric services such as psychotherapy, pharmacological management, and diagnostic services, with add-on codes to indicate the time and complexity of the service provided. Psychiatry codes are not differentiated by setting and are reported without distinction between inpatients and outpatients.

The first code appearing in the psychiatry subsection is add-on code 90785, *Interactive complexity*. Interactive complexity is reported when there are specific factors present that make it more difficult to communicate with the patient or when third parties are involved in the services provided to the patient. Code 90785 is reported in addition to other psychiatric codes and may not be reported alone. The CPT® codebook includes extensive instructional notes regarding the use of code 90785, specifying the codes with which it can be used and the circumstances in which it is appropriate. Psychiatric procedures that may be reported with the interactive complexity code added require at least 1 of the following factors:

- Poor communication skills among participants complicates the delivery of care and requires management.
- Emotions and/or behavior from the caregiver interfere with the caregiver's ability to understand and implement the care plan.
- Evidence or disclosure of a sentinel event mandates reporting to a third party. A sentinel event is an unexpected occurrence resulting in significant psychological trauma, which requires discussion of the event and/or initiation of the report of the event with the patient and others at the visit.
- A patient is not fluent in the same language as the physician, cannot express or explain his or her symptoms and response to treatment, or lacks the receptive communication skills to understand the physician; therapy may require the use of play equipment, other physical devices, an interpreter, or a translator to communicate with the patient.

Coding Clicks

The Joint Commission created a policy on sentinel events to help hospitals investigate, analyze, and learn from them. For more information, visit http://Coding.ParadigmEducation.com/SentinelEvent.

Code 90785 cannot be reported with the codes for psychotherapy for crisis (codes 90839 and 90840).

Psychiatric diagnostic evaluations are reported with code 90791 or 90792, depending on whether a medical assessment and physical examination were performed. Codes 90791 and 90792 may be reported more than once per day if separate diagnostic evaluations are performed with the patient and other informants but may not be reported on the same day as another E/M service for the patient by the same provider.

Psychotherapy, also known as the *talking cure*, is the treatment of mental illness and behavioral disturbances through talking with a psychiatrist or other qualified health professional about thoughts and behaviors. The therapist encourages the patient to develop and change patterns of behavior to alleviate symptoms of emotional distress. This form of therapy is distinguished from psychoanalysis (code 90845), a form of psychotherapy that accesses the patient's unconscious mental processes. Psychotherapy is reported based on the time spent with the patient and/or family members in face-to-face communication. The Psychotherapy category notes augment the code descriptors with guidelines for choosing a code to report time, as shown in Table 20.4. In addition to the time element, codes are separated into those with or without E/M services.

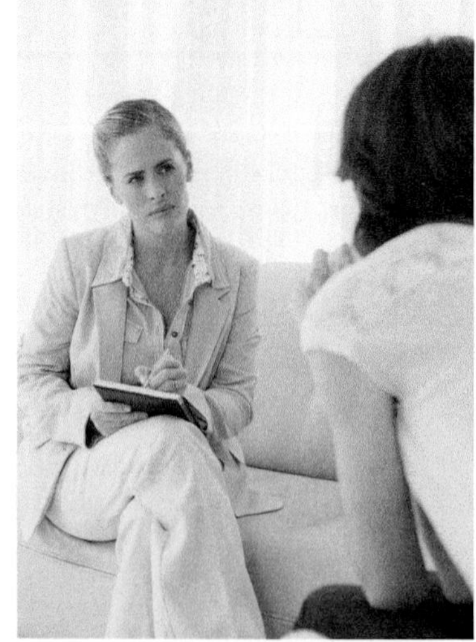

Psychotherapy is the treatment of mental illness and behavioral disturbances through talking with a qualified professional. Psychotherapy is reported based on the time spent with the patient.

Table 20.4 Psychotherapy Time Element Guidelines

Psychotherapy Time	Code for Therapy Only	Code for Therapy With an E/M Service
Less than 16 minutes	Not reported	Not reported
16-37 minutes	90832	90833
38-52 minutes	90834	90836
53 minutes or more	90837	90838

The patient must be present for some of the service for these psychotherapy service codes (90832 through 90838). The E/M Prolonged Services codes (99354 through 99360) may not be reported in addition to the psychotherapy codes with E/M services (90833, 90836, and 90838).

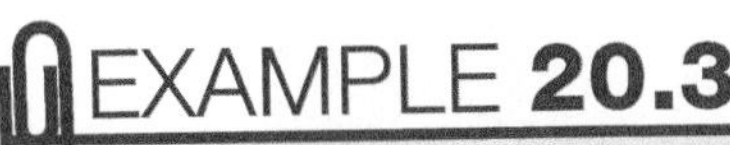

EXAMPLE **20.3**

A psychiatrist provided psychotherapy for 35 minutes to a 17-year-old male whose behavior at school was inappropriate. This service was reported with code 90832, *Psychotherapy, 30 minutes with patient and/or family member*.

LET'S TRY ONE **20.2**

A 23-year-old female with a history of obsessive-compulsive disorder (OCD) received 40 minutes of psychotherapy with her psychiatrist. Her mother then spoke to the psychiatrist for an additional 5 minutes. How would this service be reported? _____

Crisis psychotherapy codes are used when a presenting problem is complex or life threatening and requires immediate attention to a patient who is highly distressed. Services include an assessment, a history, a mental status exam, and psychotherapy or other interventions to diffuse a critical situation without injury to the patient. Psychotherapy for patients in crisis is reported with codes 90839 and 90840 depending on the face-to-face time spent with the patient and/or family, with 30 to 74 minutes reported with code 90839 and additional 30-minute increments with add-on code 90840; less than 30 minutes is reported with the psychotherapy codes 90832 or 90833. Crisis psychotherapy is reported for the time spent on any given date even if the time spent is not continuous. Code 90839 may be reported only once on a given calendar date.

Psychiatric evaluation of hospital records, psychiatric reports, and other data used to make an appropriate diagnosis and treatment plan are separately reportable with code 90885. Time spent to prepare a report of a patient's psychiatric history and treatment for individuals, agencies, or insurance carriers (other than for legal or consultative purposes) is reported with code 90889. Other psychotherapy and psychiatric services codes (90845 through 90899) include group psychotherapy, pharmacological management, narcosynthesis, transcranial magnetic stimulation (TMS), electroconvulsive therapy, biofeedback training, and hypnotherapy.

Dialysis (Codes 90935-90999)

Dialysis codes are separated into 4 categories: hemodialysis (90935 through 90940), miscellaneous dialysis procedures (90945 through 90947), end-stage renal disease services (90951 through 90970), and other dialysis procedures (90989 through 90999). **Dialysis** is the use of a machine to filter the blood when the kidneys are no longer able to function well enough to do this naturally. There are 2 types of dialysis: hemodialysis and peritoneal dialysis. In **hemodialysis**, the patient's blood is pumped out of the patient's body into a dialysis machine, filtered and washed, and returned to the body. In **peritoneal dialysis,** the peritoneum acts as a natural filter. Peritoneal dialysis requires the instillation of a sterile cleansing fluid into the patient's abdomen (through a catheter), as shown in Figure 20.1, which is then later drained and discarded.

Figure 20.1 Peritoneal Dialysis

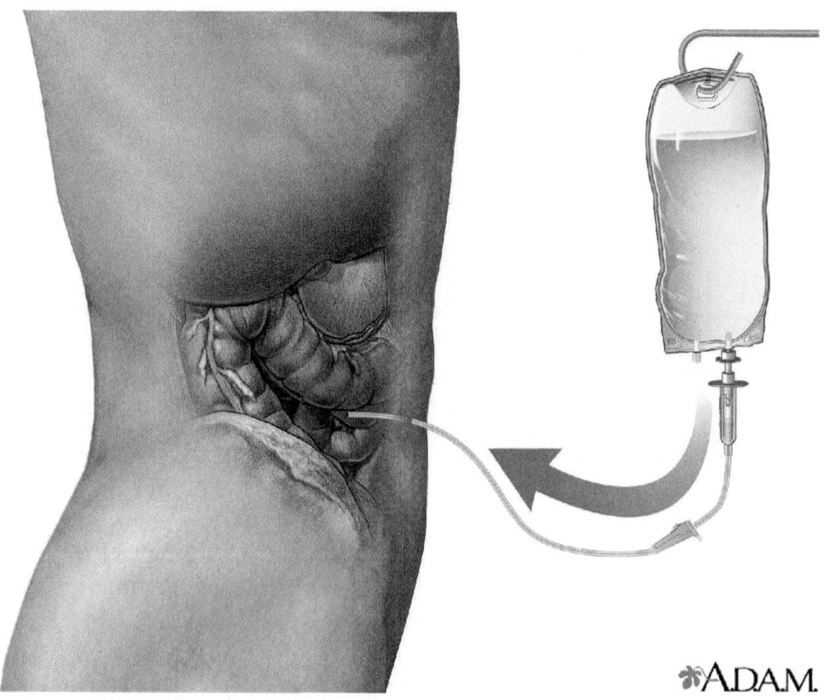

Hemodialysis codes include all evaluation and management (E/M) services that are related to the patient's renal disease on the day of hemodialysis. E/M services that are unrelated to the patient's renal disease should be reported with the appropriate E/M code and modifier 25 (for a significant, separately identifiable E/M service). A hemodialysis procedure with a single evaluation by the physician is reported with code 90935, and a hemodialysis procedure requiring repeated evaluations is reported with code 90937. A hemodialysis access flow study includes the measurement of BUN (blood urea nitrogen), a standard technique to determine blood recirculation, and is reported with code 90940.

Like hemodialysis codes, peritoneal dialysis codes (90945 and 90947) also include all evaluation and management services that are related to the patient's renal disease on the day of dialysis and follow the same guidelines for E/M reporting.

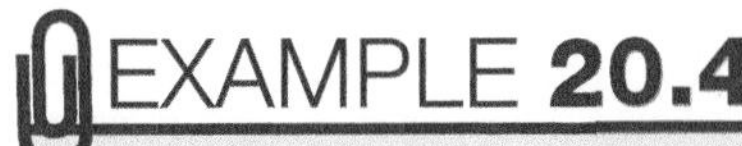

EXAMPLE 20.4

A patient in acute renal failure underwent hemodialysis. The physician responsible for the hemodialysis evaluated the patient 1 time. This is reported with code 90935, *Hemodialysis procedure with single evaluation by a physician or other qualified health care professional*.

End-stage renal disease (ESRD), also known as *chronic renal failure*, is a condition in which the kidneys are no longer able to function and dialysis or a renal transplant is needed to prolong life. Services provided for patients with ESRD are age specific and determined by the number of visits per month. ESRD services (codes 90951 through 90962) include outpatient evaluation and management of the dialysis visits, establishing a dialysis treatment cycle, telephone calls, and management. Codes are reported once per month, and in the instances in which a complete assessment was done but a full month of services was not provided, codes would be based on the number of visits. Codes 90963 through 90965 are reported for monitoring patients on home dialysis and are also differentiated by the age of the patient. Patients receiving ESRD services without a complete assessment and less than a full month of services are reported per day with codes 90967 through 90970. Each month is considered to be 30 days long. The CPT® codebook contains instructional notes and examples for reporting ESRD-related services.

EXAMPLE 20.5

A 10-year-old male patient received a full month of ESRD services with 4 physician visits. This is reported with code 90954, *End-stage renal disease related services monthly, for patients 2-11 years of age to include monitoring for the adequacy of nutrition, assessment of growth and development, and counseling of parents; with 4 or more face-to-face visits by a physician or other qualified health care professional per month*.

LET'S TRY ONE 20.3

A 14-year-old female patient received a full month of ESRD-related services. She was visited by the physician 3 times during this 30-day period. What is the appropriate code for these physician services? _____

CONCEPTS CHECKPOINT 20.1

Answer the following questions based on the information presented above.

1. In what way is hemodialysis different from peritoneal dialysis? ______________
2. Describe when E/M services may be coded in addition to dialysis services. ______________
3. What services are included in the ESRD services codes? ______________

Gastroenterology (Codes 91010-91299)

Gastroenterology is the medical specialty concerned with the structure, function, and diseases of the digestive tract. Codes in the Gastroenterology subsection describe diagnostic procedures such as the Bernstein (acid perfusion) test for esophagitis and tests of colon motility and liver elastography. Several codes for imaging studies are included. Endoscopic gastrointestinal (GI) tract imaging, also known as *capsule endoscopy*, is reported with code 91110 for a study of the esophagus through the ileum and 91111 for a study of the esophagus only. In capsule endoscopy, the patient swallows a capsule that contains a miniature camera, which then sends video images from the intestinal tract to sensors worn around the patient's waist. The capsule passes painlessly through the intestinal tract, and after 8 hours, the patient returns the equipment for processing. The images are then reviewed and interpreted for diagnostic purposes.

Ophthalmology (Codes 92002-92499)

Ophthalmology is the study of the eye, its anatomy, physiology, and diseases. The Medicine Ophthalmology codes are organized under 4 headings:

- General Ophthalmological Services (92002 through 92014);
- Special Ophthalmological Services (92015 through 92287);
- Contact Lens Services (92310 through 92326);
- Spectacles Services (92340 through 92371).

General Ophthalmological Services

General ophthalmology services are divided into new or established patients, following the E/M definitions. The codes further differentiate intermediate or comprehensive services. An **intermediate ophthalmological service** includes the evaluation of a new problem (or for an established patient, an existing condition complicated with a new diagnosis or management problem); the performance of history, external ocular, and adnexal examinations; and the use of mydriasis (dilation of the pupil) for ophthalmoscopy. An intermediate ophthalmological service for new patients is coded with 92002 and for established patients with 92012. A **comprehensive ophthalmological service** includes a general evaluation of the complete visual system. A comprehensive service includes all the elements of an intermediate service, an external and an ophthalmoscopic exam, gross visual fields, and a basic sensorimotor exam. Biomicroscopy, an exam with cycloplegia (using eye drops that paralyze eye muscle); mydriasis; and tonometry (measuring pressure in the eye) may also be included. A comprehensive service always includes diagnosis and treatment initiation. A comprehensive ophthalmological service for new patients is coded with 92004 and for established patients with 92014. A comprehensive service need not be performed all on 1 date of service; code 92014 is reported for 1 or more visits.

Special Ophthalmological Services

Special ophthalmological services codes (92015 through 92287) are for those procedures that are above and beyond the services included in general ophthalmology services or for those procedures that require special treatment. Special services include gonioscopy (testing for glaucoma by placing a special mirrored lens on the cornea), contact lens fitting for keratoconus, biometry, ophthalmoscopy, and other services. These special services may be reported in addition to the general ophthalmological service codes (92002 through 92014).

EXAMPLE **20.6**

A 48-year-old female new patient received a comprehensive ophthalmological service. In addition, she underwent provocative tests for glaucoma.
These services would be reported with code 92004 for comprehensive ophthalmological services for a new patient and code 92140, *Provocative tests for glaucoma, with interpretation and report, without tonography*.

Contact Lens Services

Contact lens services are reported with codes 92310 through 92326. The prescription and fitting of contact lenses are not a part of the general ophthalmological service and should be reported separately. The follow-up of a patient who was successfully fitted with extended-wear contact lenses is included in the general ophthalmological service codes.

Spectacles Services

Spectacles services codes (92340 through 92371) are reported when the fitting of spectacles, or eyeglasses, is a separate service. The prescription of lenses for eyeglasses is coded with 92015, *Determination of refractive state*. The fitting of spectacles includes measuring the facial characteristics of the patient, writing the laboratory specifications, and the final adjustment. A physician or other qualified healthcare professional does not need to be present for this service. Supply of materials should be reported separately. Aphakia is a condition in which the eye does not have a lens, whether due to a congenital abnormality, cataract surgery, or injury. The treatment involves the fitting of high-power lenses. There are specific codes for this service.

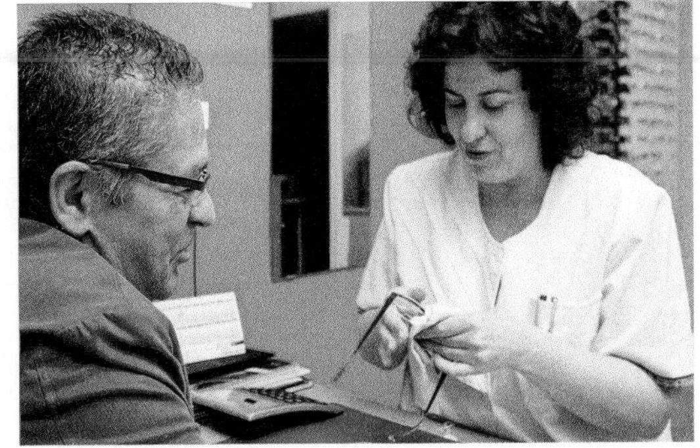

Spectacles services codes are reported when the fitting of spectacles is a separate service.

Coding for CMS

CMS does not provide benefits for spectacles. HCPCS codes (S0504 through S0510, S0516 through S0518, and S0595) may be reported for supplies related to spectacles to other third-party payers, including Medicaid, Blue Cross Blue Shield, and payers belonging to the America's Health Insurance Plans (AHIP) organization.

LET'S TRY ONE **20.4**

A 24-year-old male patient visited his ophthalmologist for an evaluation. He was last seen 2 years prior. He received a comprehensive ophthalmological service as well as a new prescription and fitting of contact lenses. (The patient does not have aphakia.) How are these services coded? _____

Special Otorhinolaryngologic Services (Codes 92502-92700)

Otorhinolaryngology is the study of diseases of the ear, nose, and throat. Special otorhinolaryngologic services codes are used to report diagnostic and treatment services not included in E/M codes. Procedures in this subsection include function studies of the nose, facial nerve, and larynx; individual and group treatment for communication disorders; and treatment of swallowing dysfunction. Vestibular function tests, audiologic tests, and diagnostic analysis of cochlear implants are also in this subsection.

EXAMPLE **20.7**

A 5-year-old patient who was unable to cooperate with an otolaryngologic exam was placed under general anesthesia. While the patient was under anesthesia, a thorough examination of the ear using otoscopy was completed successfully, and the nose and larynx were also inspected. This is reported with code 92502, *Otolaryngologic examination under general anesthesia*.

Cardiovascular (Codes 92920-93799)

Unlike other Medicine subsections, the cardiovascular subsection contains many codes for invasive procedures such as cardiac catheterizations, atherectomy, and stent placement. Diagnostic procedures such as echocardiography and electrocardiography are also in this subsection. The cardiovascular subsection is organized under 10 headings, as listed in Table 20.5.

Most of the categories have special instructions unique to that section included in the tabular. Some of the coding tips not included in the CPT® codebook will be discussed in the following paragraphs.

Table 20.5 Cardiovascular Codebook Subsection Headings and Codes

Heading	Code(s)
Therapeutic Services and Procedures	92920-92998
Cardiography	93000-93042
Cardiovascular Monitoring Services	93224-93278
Implantable and Wearable Cardiac Device Evaluations	93279-93299
Echocardiography	93303-93355
Cardiac Catheterization	93451-93583
Intracardiac Electrophysiological Procedures/Studies	93600-93662
Peripheral Arterial Disease Rehabilitation	93668
Noninvasive Physiologic Studies and Procedures	93701-93790
Other Procedures	93797-93799

Therapeutic Services and Procedures

The codebook heading Therapeutic Services and Procedures contains 2 categories of codes, and coders should note that blocks of code numbers are out of sequence:

- Other Therapeutic Services and Procedures (92950 through 92971 and 92986 through 92998);
- Coronary Therapeutic Services and Procedures (92920 through 92944 and 92973 through 92979).

Other Therapeutic Services and Procedures The first code description in the Cardiovascular subsection is 92950, *Cardiopulmonary resuscitation (eg, in cardiac arrest).* **Cardiopulmonary resuscitation (CPR)** includes assessing the patient, opening the airway, restoring breathing by mouth-to-mouth assisted breathing or "bagging" (use of a manual resuscitator or self-inflating bag), and restoring circulation (eg, by chest compressions). It is not required that the physician personally perform the chest compressions or breathing restoration to report code 92950. The code for CPR may be reported even if the physician only manages the service. CPR may be reported separately from critical care services codes (99291, 99292), but the first 30 minutes of time spent on CPR should not be included in the time counted for the critical care code.

Elective cardioversion is the use of electric shock to restore the heart back to normal sinus rhythm. Elective cardioversion is used to treat patients with atrial fibrillation and atrial flutter if the administration of antiarrhythmic drugs is unsuccessful. Code 92960, *Cardioversion, elective, electrical conversion or arrhythmia; external,* is used to report cardioversion that is performed as a separate procedure in a non-emergency situation. Code 92960 should not be reported when it is an integral part of another procedure such as coronary artery bypass graft or if provided during critical care services.

Defibrillation is the delivery of an electric impulse to the heart, performed to stop abnormal rhythms by interrupting the heart's electrical conduction (stopping the beat). The heart resumes a normal sinus rhythm if defibrillation is successful. Defibrillation may be performed during CPR, open heart surgery, cardiac catheterization, and other procedures. There is no CPT® code for defibrillation as a separate procedure; therefore, defibrillation is not reportable as a separate service.

Coronary Therapeutic Services and Procedures Coronary therapeutic services and procedures codes include percutaneous transluminal coronary angioplasty, atherectomy, and stent placement. These percutaneous coronary intervention (PCI) codes have a hierarchical structure, with less intensive services included in the more intensive services codes. An example is shown in Figure 20.2. Code 92920 is reported for angioplasty if performed alone, 92924 for angioplasty with atherectomy, and 92933 for angioplasty, atherectomy, and stent insertion.

PCI procedures are reported with a primary code for the initial major coronary artery or branch and add-on codes for each additional branch of a major coronary artery that is treated. Add-on code 92973, *Percutaneous transluminal coronary thrombectomy mechanical,* is reported when a thrombus is removed from within a vessel using a

Figure 20.2 Hierarchy of Percutaneous Transluminal Coronary Procedures

92920	Percutaneous transluminal coronary angioplasty; single major coronary artery or branch
92924	Percutaneous transluminal coronary arthrectomy, with coronary angioplasty when performed; single major coronary artery or branch
92933	Percutaneous transluminal coronary atherectomy, with intracoronary stent, with coronary angioplasty when performed; single major coronary artery or branch

motorized mechanical device such as the brand-name AngioJet. According to the *CPT® Assistant* citation under the code, AngioJet is the only device that meets the requirement of code 92973. AngioJet uses a motor that generates suction to fragment and remove clots from the coronary artery. Code 92973 is reported in addition to other PCI codes.

Cardiography and Cardiovascular Monitoring Services

Cardiography is the graphic recording of a physical or functional aspect of the heart. Procedures grouped under the Cardiography heading (codes 93000 through 93042) include routine electrocardiograms (ECGs), stress tests, and rhythm ECGs ordered in response to an event. A complete cardiography includes the tracing (the graph that is created), interpretation, and report. Portions of a complete cardiography, such as tracings only, can be reported separately if that is the only service provided (see code 93041).

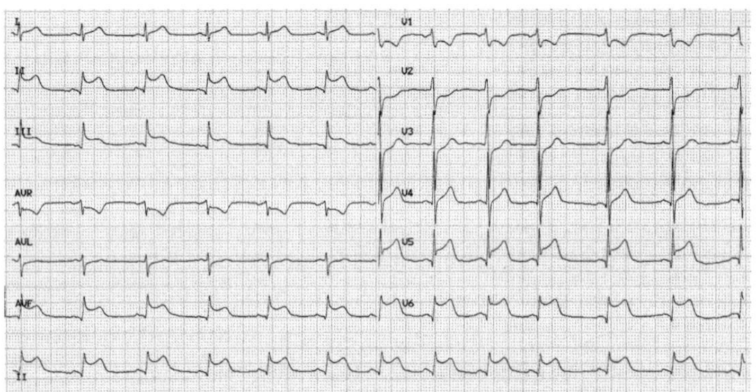

An electrocardiogram (ECG) produces a tracing of the heart's rhythm.

Cardiovascular monitoring services (codes 93224 through 93278) assess cardiovascular rhythm and include the use of Holter, mobile cardiac telemetry, and event monitors. Holter monitors can continuously monitor for up to 48 hours, and event monitors record segments of ECG recordings triggered by the patient.

Implantable and Wearable Cardiac Device Evaluations

Implantable and wearable cardiac devices are described in Chapter 12. The device evaluation codes (93279 through 93299) include procedures that use technology to access data from a pacemaker, implantable defibrillator, implantable cardiovascular monitor, or implantable loop recorder. Extensive instructional notes in the CPT® codebook describe the different devices. Some codes in this subsection may be reported once per procedure, while other codes may be reported only once every 30 or 90 days. Coders should follow the instructional notes in the tabular portion of the codebook.

Echocardiography

Echocardiography is the use of ultrasound imaging of the heart and great vessels to produce a 2-dimensional display of the size, structure, and motion of the heart. Different types of echocardiography are described in the extensive instructional notes found in the CPT® codebook. An echocardiography procedure (codes 93303 through 93355) includes the images obtained, an interpretation of the data, and documentation of all findings and measurements. If an interpretation of the information obtained during the echocardiography is performed separately, modifier 26, *Professional services*, is reported with the appropriate echocardiography code.

Cardiac Catheterization

Cardiac catheterization is a diagnostic procedure in which a catheter is threaded through a vein and into the heart to look for abnormalities. An illustration of a cardiac catheterization is shown in Figure 20.3.

Figure 20.3 Cardiac Catheterization

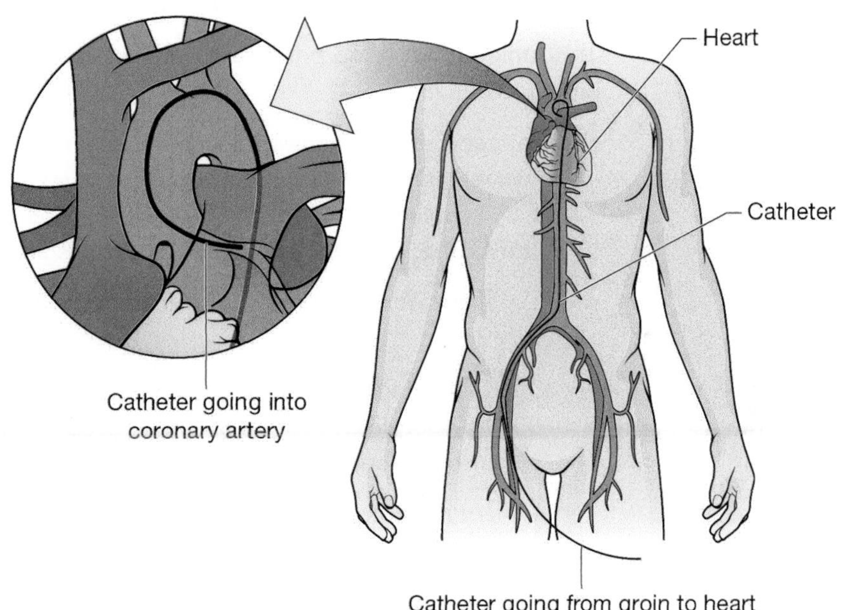

The codebook describes the division of cardiac catheterization procedures into 2 code families, for congenital heart disease or anomalies (93530 through 93533) and all other conditions (93451 through 93464). The primary criteria of code assignment are right heart and left heart. Right-heart catheterization directs the catheter into the right atrium, right ventricle, and pulmonary artery. Left-heart catheterization directs the catheter into the left atrium and left ventricle and includes injections for angiography and image supervision and interpretation. Combination codes exist that describe the performance of both right- and left-heart catheterizations (93453, 93460, 93461, and 93531 through 93533). Right-heart catheterization codes do not include angiography or contrast injections so these may be reported separately if performed. The AMA *CPT® Professional Edition* contains the table "Cardiac Catheterization Codes," which organizes the codes by catheter placement type and add-on procedures (which include transseptal and transapical punctures, studies, and injection procedures). Coders should refer to this table to determine which codes may be reported separately.

Inside the OR

For the left-heart catheterization procedure described in code 93452, the patient is placed under sedation, and a physician inserts a needle into a peripheral artery. A flexible guidewire is passed through the needle. A sheath that serves as a passageway for the catheter is introduced, and the catheter is advanced over the wire through the sheath under fluoroscopic guidance. The catheter is threaded into the heart (through the aortic valve and into the left ventricle). Intracardiac and intravascular pressures are recorded. Left-ventricular injection is performed for left ventriculography. The catheter and sheath are removed. Hemostasis is achieved by applying pressure to the wound or other means by the physician or the technician under the physician's supervision.

Additional Cardiovascular Procedures

The cardiovascular subsection also includes codes for a variety of studies and rehabilitation procedures:

- Intracardiac Electrophysiological Procedures /Studies (codes 93600 through 93662)—for diagnostic procedures used to evaluate patients with arrhythmia. The CPT® codebook contains definitions and guidelines for the procedures under the Intracardiac Electrophysiological Procedures/Studies heading;
- Peripheral Arterial Disease Rehabilitation (code 93668)—for rehabilitative physical exercise;
- Noninvasive Physiologic Studies and Procedures (codes 93701 through 93790)—for determination of venous pressure, temperature gradient studies, and ambulatory blood pressure monitoring;
- Other Procedures (codes 93797 through 93799)—for outpatient cardiac rehabilitation.

EXAMPLE **20.8**

Temperature gradient studies evaluate heart and circulatory function by taking temperatures of certain coronary vessels through an IV catheter and comparing and contrasting the results. Variations may indicate the presence of unstable coronary plaque within the artery. This is reported with code 93740, *Temperature gradient studies*.

CONCEPTS CHECKPOINT **20.2**

Answer true or false to each of the following statements.

1. _____ The code for elective cardioversion (92960) may be used to report cardioversion performed in an emergency situation.
2. _____ Defibrillation is not reportable as a separate service.
3. _____ The codes for right-heart catheterization include angiography and contrast injections.
4. _____ CPR may be reported in addition to critical care service codes.
5. _____ Right-heart catheterization when performed with left-heart catheterization always requires reporting 2 separate codes.

Noninvasive Vascular Diagnostic Studies (Codes 93880-93998)

The CPT® codebook contains definitions and guidelines for noninvasive vascular diagnostic studies at the beginning of the subsection. The codes are organized under 6 headings for anatomical sites: cerebrovascular arterial studies, extremity arterial studies, extremity venous studies, visceral and penile vascular studies, extremity arterial-venous studies, and other noninvasive vascular diagnostic studies. The codes for vascular studies include performance of the study, interpretation of the results, and documentation and analysis of all data. Arterial studies of the extremities (codes 93922 through 93923) are considered to be bilateral. If the study is performed on only 1 arm or leg, modifier 52, *Reduced services*, is reported unless 3 or more levels or provocative functional maneuvers were performed. When both the arms and legs are evaluated, code 93922 or 93923 may be reported twice, adding modifier 59, *Distinct procedural service*, to the second code.

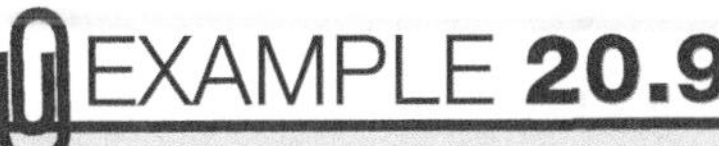

EXAMPLE **20.9**

A physician performed plethysmography of the right leg at 2 levels for a patient with an above-the-knee amputation of the left leg. This would be reported with 93922 - 52, *Limited bilateral noninvasive physiologic studies of upper or lower extremities - reduced service.*

Pulmonary (Codes 94002-94799)

Codes in the Pulmonary subsection include ventilator management and pulmonary diagnostic testing and therapies. Reporting criteria are place and type of service for ventilator management codes, and type of procedure and patient age for pulmonary diagnostic testing and therapies codes.

Patients who cannot breathe on their own due to trauma or illness may require a mechanical ventilator to help get oxygen into the lungs and carbon dioxide out. A ventilator can help the patient breathe for a short term until he or she recovers, or a patient may remain on a ventilator for a longer period of time. Figure 20.4 shows a patient receiving mechanical ventilation. Ventilator management codes (94002 through 94004) are reported per day for each day that ventilation assist and management is provided. Code 94002 is reported for the initial day of ventilation in the hospital inpatient or observation setting, while code 94003 is reported for each subsequent day. Ventilator assist and management in nursing facilities is reported with code 94004. Code 94005 for services provided to a patient on a ventilator at home (either a private residence, domiciliary, or rest home) is reported for 30 minutes or more of care plan oversight in a month's time. The ventilator care plan oversight is reported separately from home or domiciliary services.

Figure 20.4 Patient on Mechanical Ventilation

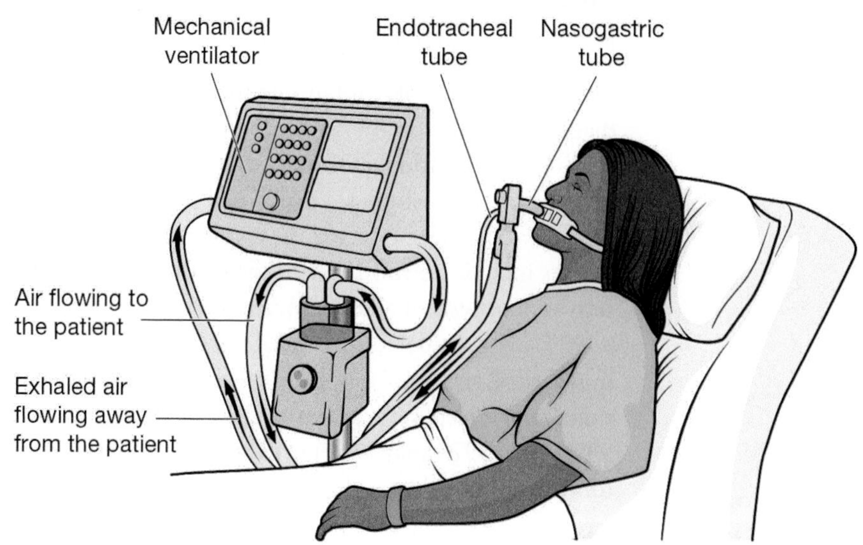

Codes for pulmonary diagnostic testing and therapies (94010 through 94799) are used to report procedures such as spirometry, breathing response, pulse oximetry, and testing for airway integrity in neonates. Codes for pulmonary diagnostic testing and therapies include both the laboratory procedures and the interpretation of test results. E/M services may be reported with codes for pulmonary diagnostic testing and therapies if the E/M services are separately identifiable.

LET'S TRY ONE **20.5**

The physician visited a hospital inpatient in the ICU to manage the ventilator on the second day of mechanical ventilation. What is the appropriate code for this physician service? _____

Allergy and Clinical Immunology (Codes 95004-95199)

Allergy and clinical immunology codes are organized under 3 headings: Allergy Testing, Ingestion Challenge Testing, and Allergen Immunotherapy.

Allergy testing involves the administration of substances to determine a patient's sensitivity to the substance. Codes are differentiated by the substance being tested (the allergen, such as venom, drugs or biologicals, and airborne allergens) and the technique for testing (such as percutaneous, patch, and mucous membrane tests).

Ingestion challenge testing, also known as an *oral food challenge*, is a way to diagnose an allergy to a specific food, drug, or other substance by observing the patient after ingestion of the suspected allergen. The patient is given a very small amount of a substance. If there is no reaction after a specified time (usually 20 minutes) then a slightly larger portion of the suspected allergen is given. This process is repeated until either the patient experiences symptoms or the predetermined amount of the suspected allergen has been ingested. Ingestion challenge testing is reported with code 95076 for the initial 120 minutes of testing, with add-on code 95079 reported for each additional 60 minutes of testing.

Allergen immunotherapy, also known as *allergy vaccine therapy*, involves giving the patient a series of injections of specific allergens in increasing doses to reduce the response to allergic triggers. The patient is observed after the administration of the allergen for a period of time, usually 20 to 30 minutes. Allergen immunotherapy requires the availability of qualified healthcare providers to administer treatment if an anaphylactic (severe or life-threatening allergic response) reaction should occur. Allergen immunotherapy codes (95115 through 95199) are reported according to the number of injections and the provision of the allergenic extract. E/M codes may be reported with codes 95115 through 95199 if separately identifiable E/M services were provided.

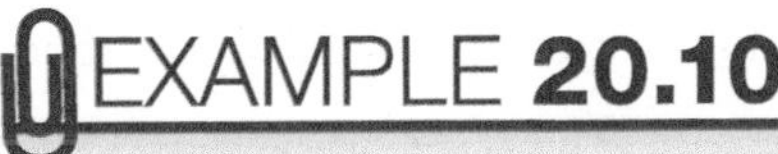

EXAMPLE **20.10**

A physician performed professional services for 3 separate injections of allergenic extracts. The extract was provided by the patient. This is reported with code 95117, *Professional services for allergen immunotherapy not including provision of allergenic extract; 2 or more injections*.

LET'S TRY ONE **20.6**

A physician performed professional services for allergen immunotherapy in the office for 2 injections of allergenic extract. The allergen extracts were provided by the office. How is this service coded? _____

Neurology and Neuromuscular Procedures (Codes 95782-96020)

The Neurology and Neuromuscular Procedures subsection contains many codes for diagnostic testing such as electroencephalography (EEG), electromyography (EMG), and other neurophysiologic studies. The codes are organized under the 14 headings listed in Table 20.6.

Table 20.6 Neurology and Neuromuscular Procedures Codebook Headings and Codes

Heading	Code(s)
Sleep Medicine Testing	95782-95811
Routine Electroencephalography (EEG)	95812-95830
Muscle and Range of Motion Testing	95831-95857
Electromyography	95860-95872, 95885-95887 (out of numerical sequence)
Ischemic Muscle Testing and Guidance for Chemodenervation	95873-95875 (out of numerical sequence)
Nerve Conduction Tests	95905-95913
Intraoperative Neurophysiology	95940-95941
Autonomic Function Tests	95921-95924, 95943 (out of numerical sequence)
Evoked Potentials and Reflex Tests	95925-95939 (out of numerical sequence)
Special EEG Tests	95950-95967
Neurostimulators, Analysis-Programming	95970-95982
Other Procedures	95990-95999
Motion Analysis	96000-96004
Functional Brain Mapping	96020

Under most of the headings, special instructions unique to its codes are provided. Some of the coding tips not included in the CPT® codebook will be discussed in the following paragraphs.

Sleep medicine studies are procedures used by physicians in the diagnosis of patients with suspected sleep disorders. Sleep studies may include monitoring heart rate, respiratory airflow, and oxygen saturation. Sleep medicine testing services are reported with codes 95800 through 95811, and all codes include recording, interpretation of data recorded during the testing, and report. Sleep studies may be attended by a technician or be unattended and performed using a portable device. Both methods require a physician to interpret the data and provide a report. Code 95807 is reported for an attended sleep study, which requires the monitoring of a patient asleep in the lab for at least 6 hours. Modifier 52, *Reduced services*, should be applied if less than 6 hours of recording takes place.

Polysomnography measures sleep staging with an electroencephalogram, an electro-oculogram, and a submental electromyogram. An electroencephalogram is a recording of the electrical activity of the brain. An electro-oculogram uses electrodes to measure eye movements. A submental electromyogram measures the electrical activity of muscle

RED FLAG

As with many other procedures performed by technicians under the supervision of physicians, polysomnography codes have both a technical and a professional component. To report only the technical component, HCPCS Level II modifier TC, *Technical component*, should be added. To report only the professional component, CPT® modifier 26, *Professional component*, should be added. To report both the technical and professional components, no modifier is required.

movements. Polysomnography codes (95808 through 95811 and 95782 through 95783) are differentiated by the age of the patient (6 years or older, or younger than 6) and the initiation of ventilation assistance. All polysomnography is attended by a technologist. Modifier 52, *Reduced services*, should be applied if total recording time is less than 6 hours.

Nerve conduction studies are diagnostic tests to assess muscle or nerve damage. After placing electrodes and then applying electrical stimulation, the provider measures the latency, amplitude, and conduction velocity of the stimulation. There are 3 types of nerve conduction studies represented by codes 95905 through 95913. For the purposes of coding these studies, a single conduction study is a sensory conduction test, a motor conduction test with or without an F wave test, or an H-reflex test. A **sensory nerve conduction study** is done by stimulating a nerve at 1 point and measuring the action potential at another point on the nerve. A **motor nerve conduction study** is done by stimulating motor nerves and measuring the compound muscle action. An **F wave test** is done by stimulating the distal end of a nerve so that the impulse travels toward the muscle fiber and back to the motor neurons of the spinal cord. The **H-reflex test** measures the Achilles muscle stretch reflex by stimulation of the tibial nerve. Code selection is determined by the number of nerve conduction tests. Each type of test is counted to determine which code to report. Each nerve constitutes 1 unit of service even if multiple sites on the same nerve are stimulated.

The CPT® codebook Appendix J correlates each sensory, motor, and mixed nerve to its appropriate nerve conduction study code. Table 1 found in Appendix J lists the type of study and the maximum number of studies that can be reported for each indication listed. Fewer studies may be performed for each indicated condition, depending on the patient's clinical presentation.

EXAMPLE **20.11**

A 54-year-old female with L5 radiculopathy complained of shooting pain from the leg to the great toe. She underwent nerve conduction studies. The following tests were performed: unilateral sural sensory nerve, unilateral peroneal motor nerve recording from extensor digitorum brevis with F wave, and unilateral tibial motor nerve with F wave. This is reported with code 95908, *Nerve conduction studies; 3-4 studies*, as a total of 3 nerve conduction studies were performed.

Central Nervous System Assessments/Tests (Codes 96101-96127)

Central nervous system assessments and tests involve the testing of cognitive function. These services include assessments of emotionality, intellectual ability, developmental milestones, cognitive performance, and other neuropsychological capacities. For example, code 96127 reports a brief emotional or behavioral assessment, such as a depression inventory or an attention deficit hyperactivity disorder (ADHD) scale. Codes comprise scoring and documentation of the standardized instruments. Time criteria are included in the codes, both for face-to-face interaction with the patient as well as for interpretation of test results and preparation of reports.

Health and Behavior Assessment/Intervention (Codes 96150-96161)

Health and behavioral assessments do not focus on mental health issues but rather on the behaviors, social factors, and cognition important to improving the patient's health. The assessment may focus on an acute or chronic illness like hepatitis, or the focus may be on the prevention of a physical illness or disability, such as ensuring that a diabetic patient follows the physician's instructions regarding foot care to avoid potential amputation. Health and behavior assessment services are provided to the individual patient, a group of patients, or the patient and family member(s). The codes (96150 through 96155) should not be reported on the same day as psychiatric services (90785 through 90899). The administration and scoring of health risk assessment instruments are reported with codes 99160 and 99161. Nonphysician clinical staff may administer the health risk assessment. The interpretation and discussion of results provided by the physician are reported with an evaluation and management code.

Hydration, Therapeutic, Prophylactic, Diagnostic Injections and Infusions, and Chemotherapy and Other Highly Complex Drug or Highly Complex Biologic Agent Administration (Codes 96360-96549)

Injection and infusion codes are divided into 3 categories: hydration (96360 through 96361); therapeutic, prophylactic, and diagnostic (96365 through 96379); and chemotherapy and other highly complex drug or biologic agents (96401 through 96549). The CPT® codebook contains detailed instructional notes regarding injection and infusion services. In the facility setting, the physician's or other qualified health professional's role is to monitor the treatment plan and provide supervision of staff. Codes in this subsection that may not be reported by the physician in a facility setting are the following:

- hydration codes 96360 and 96361;
- therapeutic, prophylactic, and diagnostic injection and infusions codes 96365 through 96379;
- chemotherapy administration codes 96401, 96402, and 96409 through 96425;
- device maintenance codes 96521 through 96523.

The services that are performed to facilitate infusion or injection are a package composed of the following components that may not be reported separately:

- use of local anesthesia;
- initial IV start;
- access to indwelling IV or subcutaneous catheter or port;
- IV flush at end of infusion;
- standard supplies.

E/M codes may be reported separately (with modifier 25) if a separately identifiable E/M service was provided in addition to the administration service.

Many drug treatments require specific administration routes for the drug to be effective, and these criteria are reflected in the code descriptors. **Intramuscular injections** are given directly into a muscle. **Subcutaneous injections** are given into the fatty tissue under the dermal layer of the skin. **Intravenous** administration infuses a drug into a vein where the drug enters the blood stream and has a systemic effect. The codes describe 3 techniques of administration, infusion, push, and injection. An infusion and a push are both delivered intravenously. Infusions are continuous administrations over time increments of 31 minutes to an hour, with add-on codes to report additional time. An intravenous or intra-arterial push has specific characteristics, being either (a) an injection in which the administering individual is continuously present to administer the injection and observe the patient, or (b) an infusion of 15 minutes or less. An injection lasts 15 minutes or less and may have 1 of several routes of administration: intravenous (push), intramuscular, subcutaneous, and intra-arterial.

Figure 20.5 Hierarchy for Facility Reporting

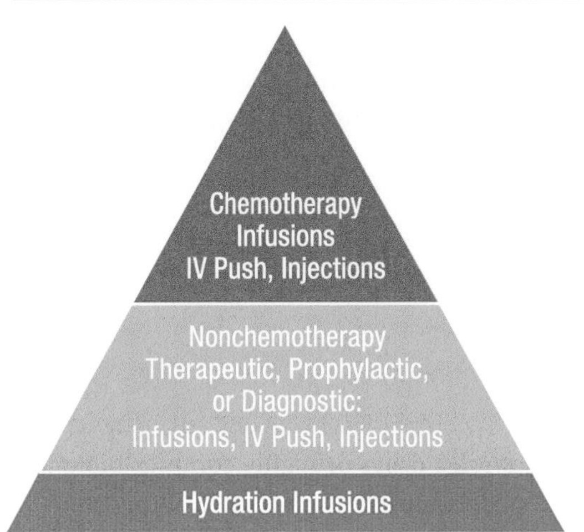

When multiple infusions/injections are administered, CPT® has developed a hierarchy for facility reporting, as illustrated in Figure 20.5. The hierarchy for reporting codes for facilities is as follows: priority is given to chemotherapy as the initial code, followed by therapeutic, prophylactic, and diagnostic infusions, and lastly by hydration services. IV infusions are reported first, followed by IV pushes, with injections reported last.

Hydration

Patients who cannot or should not get fluids through eating and drinking are often given fluids containing sugar, carbohydrates, and electrolytes through an IV line. IV hydration does not typically require special handling or disposal, and staff is not required to have advanced training to monitor patients receiving IV hydration. Hydration codes 96360 and 96361 are used to report IV infusion of fluids and electrolytes and should not be reported for administration of drugs or other substances. A minimum time of 30 minutes of infusion is required to report hydration codes. Code 96360 is reported for the initial hydration time of 31 to 60 minutes; 96361 is reported for each additional hour. Code 96361 is also reported for each interval greater than 30 minutes beyond 1-hour increments.

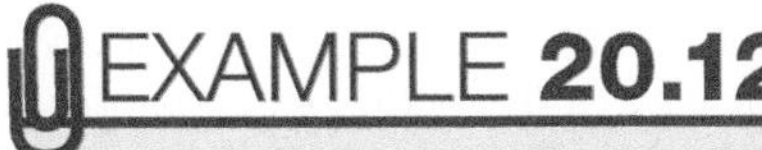

EXAMPLE 20.12

A patient received IV hydration of normal saline for a total of 2 hours and 40 minutes. Code 96360 would be reported for the first hour, 96361 for the second hour, and another 96361 for the 40 minutes beyond the second hour.

Therapeutic, Prophylactic, and Diagnostic Injections and Infusions

Therapeutic, prophylactic, and diagnostic injections and infusions codes 96365 through 96379 are reported for the administration of drugs and substances other than hydration, chemotherapy, and other highly complex drug or biologic administration. These codes (96365 through 96379) would include infusions of drugs such as antibiotics, analgesics, and narcotics. Services include direct supervision of staff since these drugs and substances typically require special handling. Staff must be trained to administer these substances and monitor the patient during infusion. Codes are differentiated by 2 criteria: the route of administration as intravenous infusion, subcutaneous infusion, or injection; and the status of the administration as initial, concurrent, or sequential.

EXAMPLE **20.13**

A patient received an IV infusion of antibiotic for 1 hour. This would be reported with code 96365, *Intravenous infusion for therapy, prophylaxis, or diagnosis; initial, up to one hour*.

Chemotherapy and Other Highly Complex Drug or Highly Complex Biologic Agents

The term **chemotherapy** is defined as the treatment of disease by chemical substances. The chemotherapy in codes 96401 through 96549 includes antineoplastic drugs as well as other highly complex drugs or highly complex biologic agents. The infusion of chemotherapy and other highly complex drugs requires advanced training for staff because of the great risk to the patient of adverse reaction to the drug. Physicians and other staff must follow special procedures for the preparation, dosage, and disposal of these potentially toxic substances. Codes are differentiated by route of administration—subcutaneous, intramuscular, intralesional, intravenous push, intravenous infusion, intra-arterial infusion, administration into a body cavity (eg, pleural, peritoneal)—and whether the administration was initial or sequential. Infusion codes are time based and reported for each hour of administration.

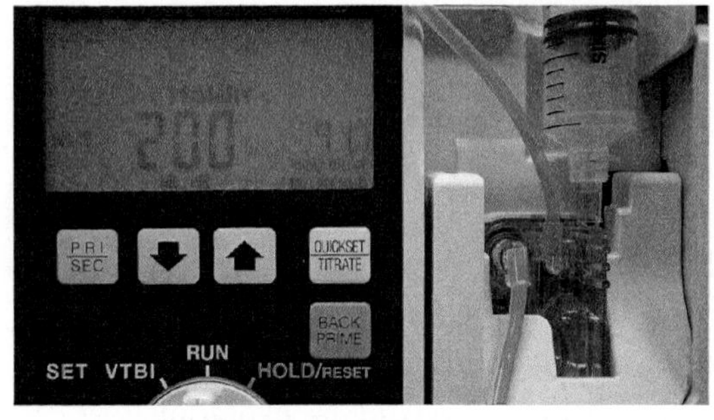

Codes for chemotherapy are differentiated by route of administration. This chemotherapy is being administered through intravenous infusion.

EXAMPLE **20.14**

A patient received a single chemotherapy drug via the IV infusion technique for a total of 6 hours. The first hour would be reported with code 96413, *Chemotherapy administration, intravenous infusion technique; up to 1 hour, single or initial substance/drug*. The remaining 5 hours would be reported with 96415 x 5 units, *Chemotherapy administration, intravenous infusion technique; each additional hour*, once for each additional hour of infusion.

LET'S TRY ONE **20.7**

A patient received a single chemotherapy drug administered by IV push over 10 minutes' time. How would this service be reported? _____

Coding Clicks

Read more about photodynamic therapy at http://Coding.ParadigmEducation.com/PhotodynamicTherapy.

Photodynamic Therapy (Codes 96567-96574)

Photodynamic therapy combines a drug that is preferentially absorbed by certain kinds of cells and a special light source. When used together, the photosensitizer and the light destroy the targeted cells. Photodynamic therapy by external application of light to destroy premalignant skin lesions, or lesions of the mucosa, is reported with code 96567 for each phototherapy exposure session. Code 96567 is reported when the physician or other qualified health professional is not directly involved with the therapy session. When photodynamic therapy is used endoscopically, such as with a bronchoscopy or GI endoscopy, the code for the appropriate endoscopic procedure is reported along with add-on code 96570 for the first 30 minutes of photodynamic therapy and 96571 for each additional 15 minutes of therapy. Code 96573 is reported when the photodynamic therapy session is provided by the physician or other qualified health professional. Code 96574 is reported for debridement of lesion(s) followed by photodynamic therapy. As noted in the CPT manual, code 96567 cannot be reported with either 96573 or 96574 for the same anatomical area.

CONCEPTS CHECKPOINT **20.3**

Answer true or false to each of the following statements.

1. _____ Physicians in facility settings should not report chemotherapy IV infusion codes.
2. _____ If a patient received multiple drug administrations, the codes for IV infusions should be reported before codes for IV pushes.
3. _____ An IV hydration infusion code should not be reported for infusions lasting less than 30 minutes.

Special Dermatological Procedures (Codes 96900-96999)

Dermatological therapies and services not included in evaluation and management services are found in the Special Dermatological Procedures subsection. Procedures include laser treatment for inflammatory skin diseases such as psoriasis, and actinotherapy using ultraviolet light.

Physical Medicine and Rehabilitation (Codes 97001-97799)

Physical medicine, also known as *physiatry* or *physical therapy*, is the medical specialty that treats disease by physical means such as manipulation, heat, electricity, or radiation, rather than by medication or surgery.

Physical medicine and rehabilitation codes are organized under 7 headings, as shown in Table 20.7.

A code from the Physical Medicine and Rehabilitation subsection is used to report each type of physical medicine service performed. Multiple codes are to be expected when treating a patient with physical medicine, so codes 97001 through 97755 should not be used with modifier 51, *Multiple procedures*.

Table 20.7 Physical Medicine and Rehabilitation Codebook Headings and Codes

Heading	Code(s)
Physical Therapy Evaluations	97161-97172 out of numeric sequence
Modalities	97010-97039
Therapeutic Procedures	97110-97546
Active Wound Care Management	97597-97610
Tests and Measurements	97750-97755
Orthotic Management and Prosthetic Management	97760-97762
Other Procedures	97799

Evaluation

Evaluations performed for physical therapy, occupational therapy, and athletic training are reported using codes based on the complexity of the evaluation. A low complexity physical therapy evaluation is reported with code 97161, moderate complexity with 97162, and high complexity with 97163. A re-evaluation of an established plan of care is reported with code 97164.The codes for occupational therapy evaluations (97165 through 97168) and athletic training evaluations (97169 through 97172) follow a similar structure. Evaluations include a history, exam of body systems, and tests such as range of motion and motor function. Documentation must include the patient's prognosis and the planned physical medicine interventions.

Modalities

Modalities are defined as physical agents applied to produce therapeutic changes to biologic tissue and include the use of hot or cold packs, electrical stimulation, whirlpool treatment, and paraffin bath treatment. Codes are categorized as either "supervised" or "constant attendance." Supervised modalities do not require one-on-one patient contact. Each modality of treatment is reported separately with codes 97010 through 97028. Electrical stimulation that is performed in conjunction with acupuncture is reported with codes 97813 and 97814 found under the acupuncture heading. Modalities that require constant attendance (direct one-on-one patient contact) include iontophoresis (a low electrical current used to deliver a drug through skin), ultrasound, and Hubbard tank (hydrotherapy) reported with codes 97032 through 97039. Modalities that require constant attendance are reported in 15-minute increments.

EXAMPLE **20.15**

A 52-year-old female patient received 15 minutes of ultrasound therapy for tendinitis in the right arm. The therapist was in constant attendance for the entire 15 minutes of ultrasound delivery. The patient then received an application of a hot pack to the elbow region for 15 minutes while the therapist was not in attendance. These services would be reported with 97035, *Application of a modality to 1 or more areas; ultrasound, each 15 minutes*; and 97010, *Application of a modality to 1 or more areas; hot or cold packs*.

Therapeutic Procedures

Therapeutic Procedures services require direct patient contact from the therapist or physician. Therapeutic procedures reported with codes 97110 through 97546 are performed to improve function and include gait training, massage, and mobilization.

Gait training is a type of physical therapy to help a patient improve the ability to stand and walk. Patients who are recovering from an illness or injury may need gait training to help them build endurance. One of the goals of gait training is to prevent falls that may lead to further injury. Patients who have suffered a stroke, are recovering from major surgery, or had a traumatic injury may require gait training. Gait training may involve the use of adaptive devices, such as teaching the patient how to use a walker correctly.

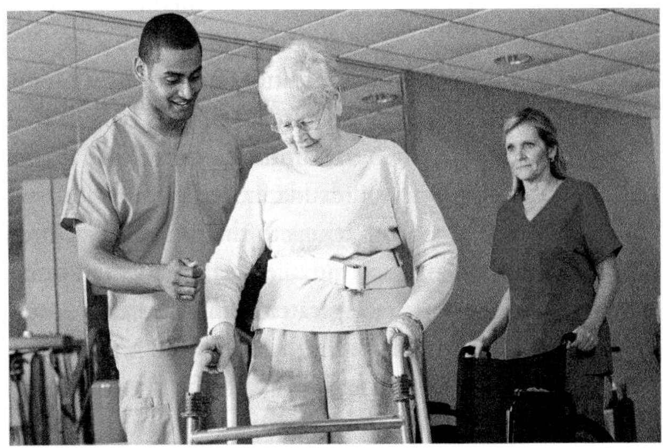

Gait training may involve adaptive devices, such as teaching a patient how to use a walker correctly.

Mobilization is a manual therapy technique in which the therapist manipulates the joint by manually applying therapeutic movements within or at the end of the range of motion. Mobilization is intended to relieve pain and muscle spasms and improve flexibility.

Work hardening is a program specifically designed to build strength and endurance for work tasks so the patient can return to work after an injury. Work hardening is reported with 97545 for the first 2 hours, with add-on code 97546 for each additional hour. Therapeutic procedures are reported individually for each 15 minutes of therapy.

EXAMPLE **20.16**

An 81-year-old female recovering from abdominal surgery was being discharged from the hospital with a walker to aid her in ambulation at home. The therapist spent 15 minutes instructing the patient. This is reported with code 97116, *Therapeutic procedure, 1 or more areas, each 15 minutes; gait training (includes stair climbing)*.

LET'S TRY ONE **20.8**

A 54-year-old male patient received 30 minutes of aquatic therapy with therapeutic exercises. How is this service reported? _____

management and training should not be reported with gait training (code 97116) for the same extremity. Code 97762 is reported for follow-up of an established patient, which includes an assessment of the patient's response and tolerance to wearing the orthotic or prosthetic device. If further training is needed for an established patient, code 97760 should be reported.

CONCEPTS CHECKPOINT **20.4**

Choose the word(s) that completes the sentence correctly.

1. Diagnostic/Therapeutic procedures are performed to improve function and include gait training, massage, and mobilization.
2. Orthotics/Prosthetics are devices that replace missing body parts.
3. All physical medicine modalities require/do not require one-on-one attendance by the therapist.
4. Codes 97001 through 97755 should/should not be used with modifier 51, *Multiple procedures*.
5. Active wound care management codes can/cannot be reported with the surgical debridement codes.

Acupuncture (Codes 97810-97814)

</> Coding for CMS

CMS does not provide benefits for acupuncture.

Acupuncture is the practice of inserting small needles into the patient in specific areas to relieve pain. Acupuncture was originally an ancient Chinese therapy but is now widely accepted in Western medicine. The needles are twirled or manipulated by hand to provide therapeutic stimulation, or the needles may be energized by electrical stimulation, as shown in Figure 20.7. Acupuncture codes 97810 through 97813 are differentiated by the use of electrical stimulation and reported in 15-minute increments. Personal one-on-one contact with the patient is required.

Figure 20.7 Acupuncture with Electrical Stimulation on Patient's Back

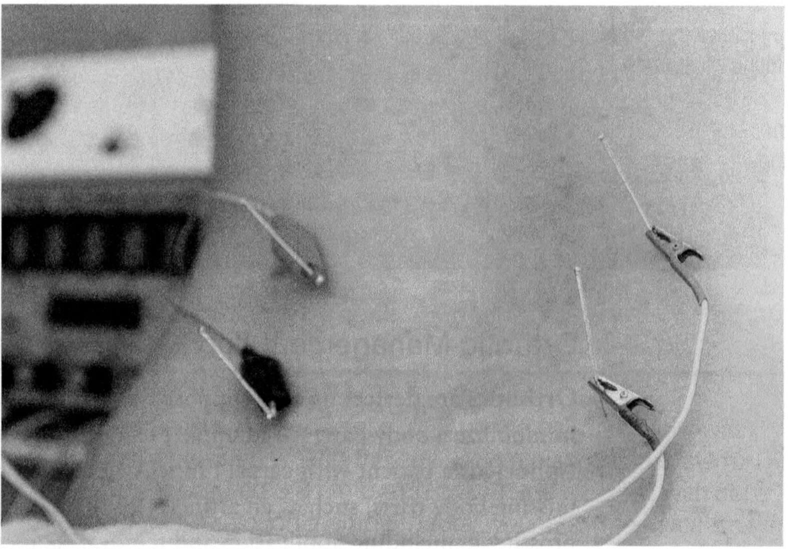

Osteopathic Manipulative Treatment (Codes 98925-98929)

Osteopathic manipulation treatment (OMT) is the use of hands to treat and prevent illness and injury by manipulation of the body using stretching, pressure, and resistance. Osteopathic manipulation treatment codes 98925 through 98929 are based on the number of body regions treated. The body regions are:

- head;
- cervical;
- thoracic;
- lumbar;
- sacral;
- pelvic;
- lower extremities;
- upper extremities;
- rib cage;
- abdomen and viscera.

The codes range from 98925 for the manipulation of 1 to 2 regions to 98929 for 9 to 10 body regions. E/M services may be reported in addition to osteopathic manipulation codes if a separately identifiable E/M service was performed. Different diagnoses are not required for reporting E/M and OMT codes on the same date of service.

Chiropractic Manipulative Treatment (Codes 98940-98943)

Chiropractic manipulation treatment (CMT), like OMT, is a manual treatment to influence joint and neurophysiologic function by using controlled force to manipulate the body, especially the spine. CMT codes 98940 through 98943 include patient assessment prior to manipulation. CMT codes are based on the number of spinal and extraspinal regions treated. The 5 spinal regions are:

- cervical (includes atlanto-occipital joint);
- thoracic (includes costovertebral and costotransverse joint);
- lumbar;
- sacral;
- pelvic (sacroiliac joint).

The 5 extraspinal regions are:

- head (including temporomandibular joint);
- lower extremities;
- upper extremities;
- rib cage;
- abdomen.

CMT codes are differentiated by the number of regions treated and whether the regions were spinal or extraspinal, as shown in Figure 20.8.

Coding for CMS

CMS does provide benefits for chiropractic services under Part B of Medicare. For more information on the services covered, visit http://Coding.ParadigmEducation.com/CMSChiropractic.

Figure 20.8 Chiropractic Manipulation Codes

98940	Chiropractic manipulative treatment (CMT); spinal, 1-2 regions
98941	spinal, 3-4 regions
98942	spinal, 5 regions
98943	extraspinal, 1 or more regions

Like OMT codes, E/M services may be reported in addition to chiropractic manipulation codes if a separately identifiable E/M service was performed. Different diagnoses are not required for reporting E/M and CMT codes on the same date of service.

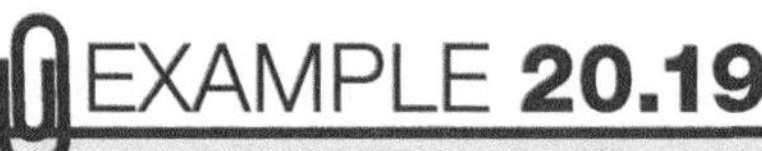

EXAMPLE 20.19

An osteopathic physician provided manipulative treatment to the pelvic and lower extremity regions. This service is reported with code 98925, *Osteopathic manipulative treatment (OMT); 1-2 body regions involved*.

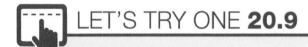

LET'S TRY ONE 20.9

An osteopathic physician provided manipulative treatment to the head, cervical, thoracic, and upper extremity regions. How is this service reported? _____

Education and Training for Patient Self-Management (Codes 98960-98962)

Codes 98960 through 98962 are used to report educational and training services for patient self-management ordered by a physician or other qualified healthcare professional and performed by a nonphysician healthcare professional using a standardized curriculum. Code 98960 reports education for individuals, 98961 for groups of 2 to 4 patients, and 98962 for groups of 5 to 8 patients.

Non-Face-to-Face Nonphysician Services (Codes 98966-98969)

Non-face-to-face Nonphysician Services codes are used to report telephone and Internet-based assessment and management services performed by nonphysicians for established patients. If the telephone or online discussion ends with a decision to see the patient in person within 24 hours or at the next available urgent visit appointment, this service is not reported. Telephone calls or electronic communications within a postoperative period or relating to any service performed within the past 7 days are not reported separately.

EXAMPLE **20.20**

A child with asthma was taught to recognize symptoms and use the nebulizer appropriately by the nurse in the physician's office. The educational service performed by the nurse is reported with code 98960, *Education and training for patient self-management by a qualified, nonphysician health care professional using a standardized curriculum, face-to-face with the patient (could include caregiver/family) each 30 minutes*.

Special Services, Procedures, and Reports (Codes 99000-99091)

The Special Services, Procedures, and Reports subsection of codes allows the physician or other provider to report miscellaneous procedures such as transport of a specimen to a laboratory, medical testimony for legal purposes, and services provided in the office on an emergency basis. The codes are reported in addition to other services rendered. Each special circumstance is reported separately, but typically only 1 special service code is reported per patient encounter. Codes for services provided in the office with special circumstances, 99050 through 99060, are reported in addition to the basic service (such as an E/M visit) and should not be reported with the use of modifier 51, *Multiple procedures*.

EXAMPLE **20.21**

A urologist is called away from his office to provide consultative services to an emergency department (ED) patient who may have kidney stones. The urologist must reschedule the office patients to accommodate this request. In addition to the consultation code (99243), the urologist reports code 99060, *Service(s) provided on an emergency basis, out of the office, which disrupts other scheduled office services, in addition to basic service*.

LET'S TRY ONE **20.10**

A physician gave medical testimony at a trial for a patient who was injured in an accident. How is this service reported? _____

Qualifying Circumstances for Anesthesia (Codes 99100-99140)

The 4 add-on codes describing qualifying circumstances for anesthesia listed in the Medicine section are the same as those listed in the Anesthesia section. The explanation of these services is included in the Anesthesia Guidelines section of the CPT® codebook and discussed in Chapter 7.

Moderate (Conscious) Sedation (Codes 99151-99157)

The codes for moderate (conscious) sedation are listed in the Medicine section, preceded by detailed instructional notes describing the services included in the codes. The Anesthesia Guidelines section of the CPT® codebook provides principles for reporting these codes. These principles and the codes are discussed in Chapter 7.

Other Services and Procedures (Codes 99170-99199)

Other services and procedures codes describe a collection of unrelated services, such as hyperbaric oxygen therapy attendance, ipecac administration, and therapeutic phlebotomy.

Home Health Procedures/Services (Codes 99500-99602)

The codes in the Home Health Procedures/Services subsection are for certain services provided by nonphysician healthcare professionals in a patient's residence, including assisted living apartments, group homes, custodial care facilities, or schools. Services such as stoma care, catheter care, newborn care, and home infusions are included in this subsection. E/M home visit codes (99341 through 99350) may be reported in addition to the home health codes (99500 through 99600) if the patient's condition required a significant separately identifiable E/M service above and beyond the home health service.

EXAMPLE **20.22**

A 45-year-old female with colon carcinoma recently underwent surgery; she was discharged to her home with a colostomy. A home health aide visited the patient to provide colostomy care. This is reported with code 99505, *Home visit for stoma care and maintenance including colostomy and cystostomy*.

LET'S TRY ONE **20.11**

A 91-year-old male with a history of incontinence has an indwelling urinary catheter. A home health aide visited the patient to provide catheter care and maintenance. How is this service reported? _____

Medication Therapy Management Services (Codes 99605-99607)

The last subsection of codes in the Medicine section describes medication management services provided by a pharmacist. The pharmacist must document a review of the patient history, a medication profile including nonprescription drugs, and recommendations for improving health outcomes and treatment compliance. Medication therapy management services are reported in 15-minute increments for face-to-face time spent with the patient.

Instructions for Reporting Medicine Codes

Though the Medicine section may seem complicated because many different services and procedures are grouped together, you can employ a step-by-step process to find the right code. The steps to locating medicine procedure codes are listed below.

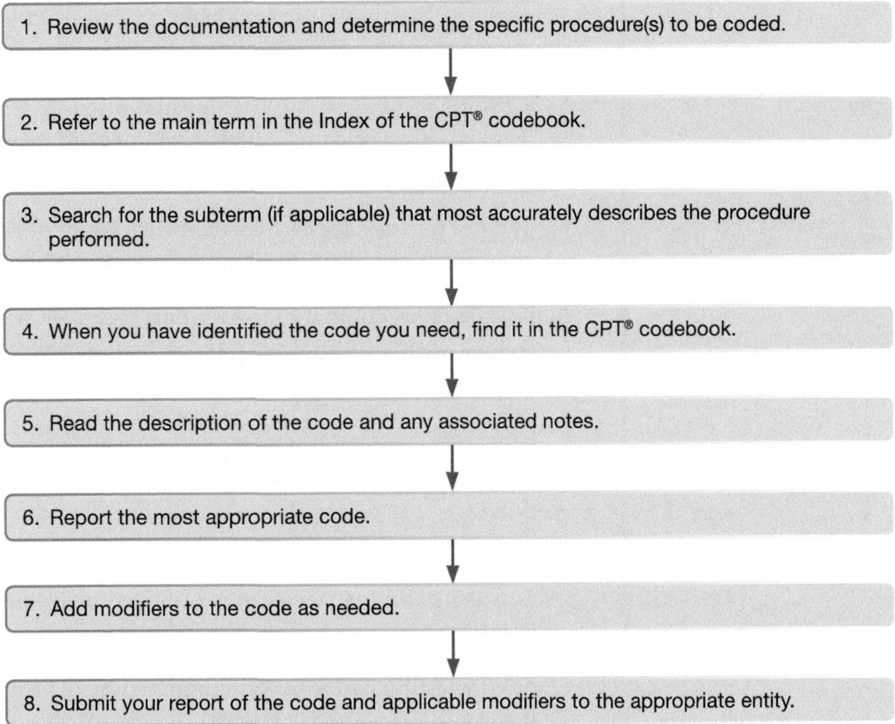

1. Review the documentation and determine the specific procedure(s) to be coded.
2. Refer to the main term in the Index of the CPT® codebook.
3. Search for the subterm (if applicable) that most accurately describes the procedure performed.
4. When you have identified the code you need, find it in the CPT® codebook.
5. Read the description of the code and any associated notes.
6. Report the most appropriate code.
7. Add modifiers to the code as needed.
8. Submit your report of the code and applicable modifiers to the appropriate entity.

Chapter Summary

- Reporting the administration of an immune globulin or vaccine requires at least 2 codes: a code for the product given and a code for the administration of the product.
- Psychiatry codes are not differentiated by setting and are reported without distinction between inpatients and outpatients.
- Psychotherapy is reported based on the time spent with the patient and/or family members in face-to-face communication.
- Psychotherapy for crisis codes are used when a presenting problem is complex or life threatening and the patient is highly distressed.
- Hemodialysis and peritoneal dialysis codes include all E/M services that are related to the patient's renal disease on the day of dialysis.

- Services provided to patients with ESRD are age specific and determined by the number of visits per month.
- General ophthalmology services are divided into new and established patients, following the E/M guidelines. Spectacle services are reported only when the fitting of eyeglasses is a separate service. A physician or other qualified healthcare professional does not need to be present for the fitting of spectacles.
- Cardiopulmonary resuscitation is reported by the physician for management of this service. The physician does not need to personally perform the chest compressions or breathing restoration to report this service.
- There is no code for cardiac defibrillation performed as a separate procedure; therefore, defibrillation is not reportable as a separate service.
- Percutaneous coronary intervention codes are structured in progressive hierarchies, with less intensive services included in the more intensive services codes.
- Codes for cardiac catheterizations are categorized into 2 code families, those for congenital heart disease or anomaly and those for all other heart conditions.
- Ventilator management codes are reported per day for each day that ventilation assist and management is provided in an inpatient hospital or nursing home setting.
- Allergy testing codes are differentiated by the substance being tested for and the technique for testing.
- Allergen immunotherapy requires the availability of qualified healthcare providers to administer treatment if an anaphylactic reaction occurs. Allergen immunotherapy codes are reported according to the number of injections and the provision of the allergenic extract.
- Sleep medicine studies may be attended or unattended, but either method requires a physician to interpret the data and provide a report.
- Injection and infusion codes are divided into categories for hydration; therapeutic, prophylactic and diagnostic; or chemotherapy and other highly complex drugs or biologicals. With multiple services, the hierarchy for facility reporting is chemotherapy codes first; therapeutic, prophylactic and diagnostic codes second; and hydration codes last. The hierarchy for facility reporting of administration routes is IV infusions, followed by IV push, with injections reported last.
- Infusion codes are differentiated by the substance administered and reported for each hour of administration.
- Physicians in the facility setting should not report chemotherapy IV infusion codes.

- Each physical medicine modality of treatment is reported separately, so modifier 51 should not be used with those codes.
- Therapeutic physical medicine services require direct patient contact from the therapist or physician.
- Active wound care management codes cannot be reported with codes for surgical debridement for treatment of the same wound.
- Many physical medicine codes are reported in 15-minute increments, including orthotic and prosthetic management codes.
- Osteopathic and chiropractic manipulation treatments are reported according to the number of regions treated.
- Codes for special services, procedures, and reports are reported in addition to codes for basic services and should not be reported with modifier 51.
- Home health procedures/services codes are reported for nonphysician healthcare professional services performed in a patient's private residence or residential facility, such as an assisted living facility or a group home.
- Medication therapy management services are performed by a pharmacist and reported in 15-minute increments for face-to-face time spent with the patient.

Navigator

Access interactive chapter review exercises, practice activities, flash cards, and study games.

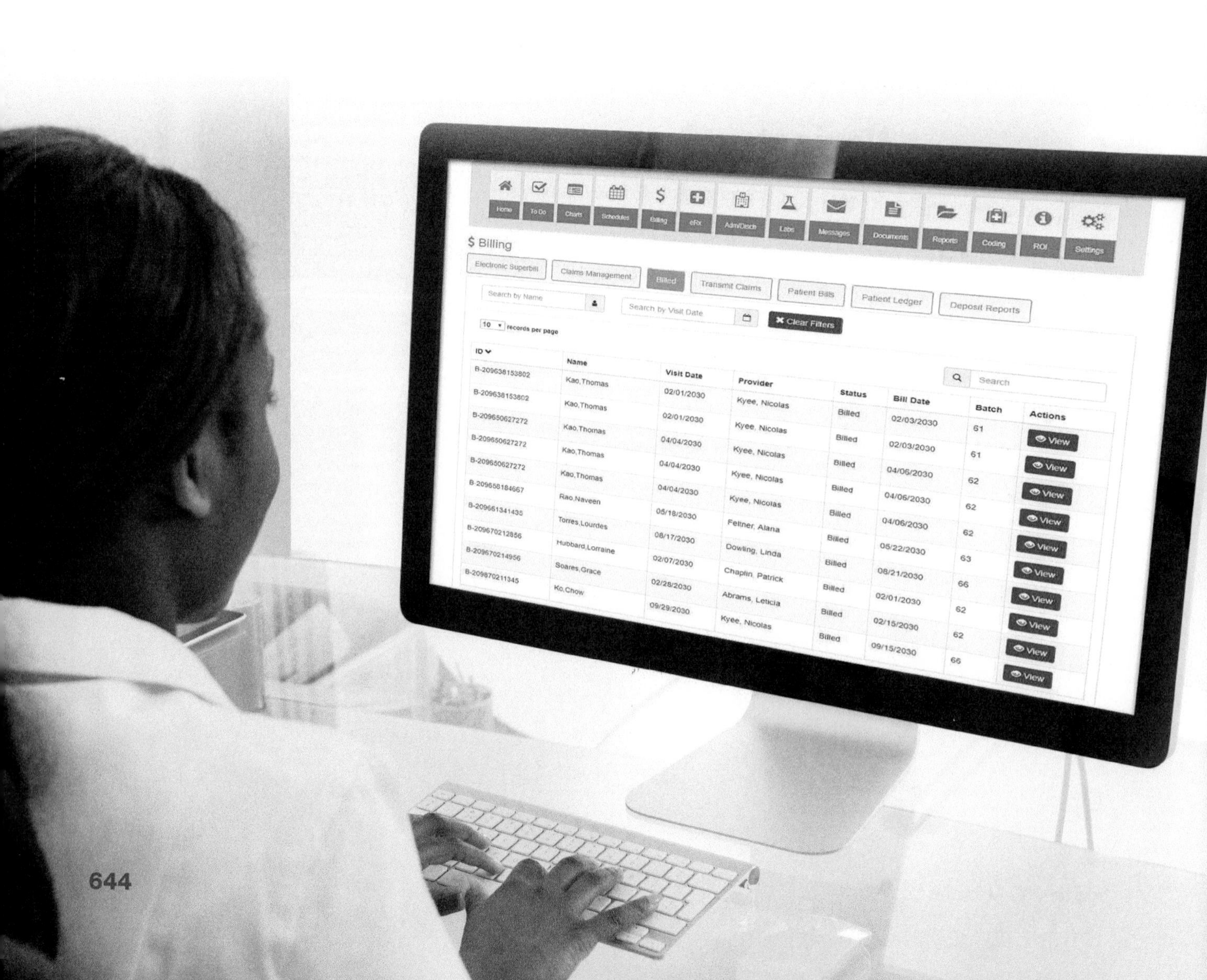
Home
To Do
Charts
Schedules
Billing
eRx
Adm/Disch
Labs
Messages
Documents
Reports
Coding
ROI
Settings
$ Billing
Electronic Superbill
Claims Management
Billed
Transmit Claims
Patient Bills
Patient Ledger
Deposit Reports
Search by Name
Search by Visit Date
Clear Filters
10 records per page
Search
ID
Name
Visit Date
Provider
Status
Bill Date
Batch
Actions
B-209638153802 Kao,Thomas 02/01/2030 Kyee, Nicolas Billed 02/03/2030 61 View
B-209638153802 Kao,Thomas 02/01/2030 Kyee, Nicolas Billed 02/03/2030 61 View
B-209650627272 Kao,Thomas 04/04/2030 Kyee, Nicolas Billed 04/06/2030 62 View
B-209650627272 Kao,Thomas 04/04/2030 Kyee, Nicolas Billed 04/06/2030 62 View
B-209650627272 Kao,Thomas 04/04/2030 Kyee, Nicolas Billed 04/06/2030 62 View
B-209658184667 Rao,Naveen 05/18/2030 Feltner, Alana Billed 05/22/2030 63 View
B-209661341435 Torres,Lourdes 08/17/2030 Dowling, Linda Billed 08/21/2030 66 View
B-209670212856 Hubbard,Lorraine 02/07/2030 Chaplin, Patrick Billed 02/01/2030 62 View
B-209670214956 Soares,Grace 02/28/2030 Abrams, Leticia Billed 02/15/2030 62 View
B-209870211345 Ko,Chow 09/29/2030 Kyee, Nicolas Billed 09/15/2030 66 View

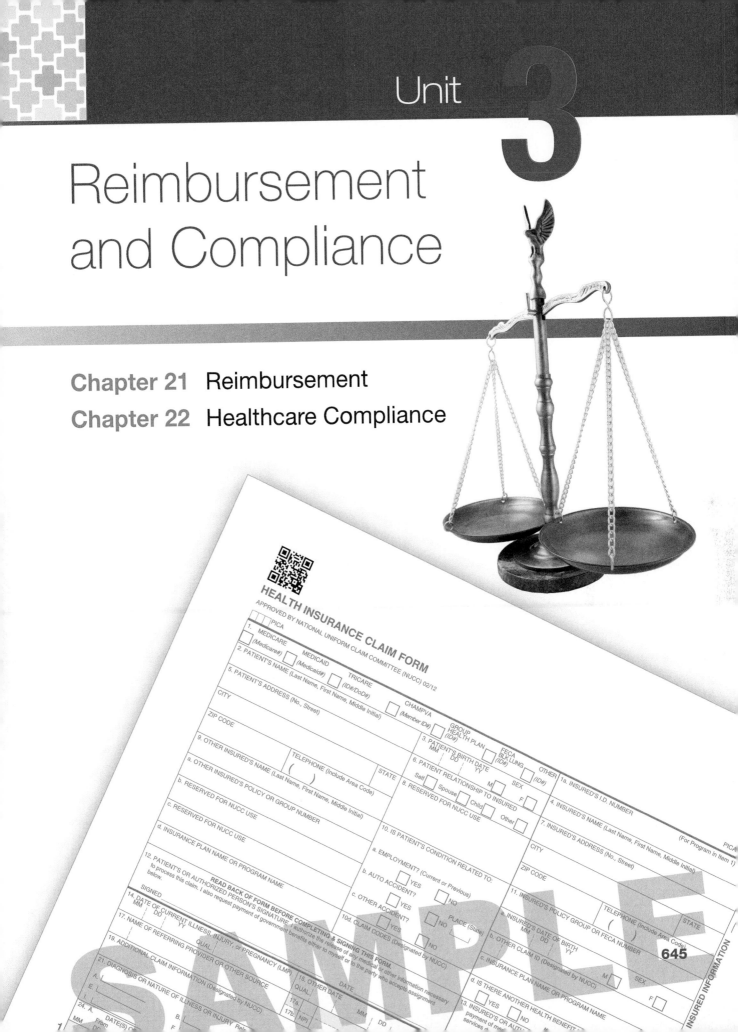

Unit 3

Reimbursement and Compliance

Chapter 21

Reimbursement

Fast Facts

- In 2014, 33.4 million people received physician services under Medicare.
- In 2012, 42.8 million Medicaid beneficiaries received physician services.
- An estimated 71.1 million people are enrolled in Medicaid in the 2016 fiscal year.
- Ranked by specialty, nonphysican practitioners and primary care providers are the largest providers of health care to Medicare patients.

Sources: http://cms.gov/fastfacts

Crack the Code

Review the sample CMS 1500 form and identify the errors. You may need to return to this exercise after reading the chapter content.

DATE OF SERVICE: 07/23/2019

DIAGNOSIS CODE: S73.012A *Posterior subluxation of left hip, initial encounter*

PROCEDURE CODE: 27252, *Closed treatment of hip dislocation, traumatic; requiring anesthesia - Modifier 53, Discontinued services*

21. DIAGNOSIS OR NATURE OF ILLNESS OR INJURY Relate A-L to service line below (24E) ICD Ind. 10

A. S73.012A	B.	C.	D.
E.	F.	G.	H.
I.	J.	K.	L.

22. RESUBMISSION CODE | ORIGINAL REF. NO.

23. PRIOR AUTHORIZATION NUMBER

24. A. DATE(S) OF SERVICE From MM	DD	YY	To MM	DD	YY	B. PLACE OF SERVICE	C. EMG	D. PROCEDURES, SERVICES, OR SUPPLIES (Explain Unusual Circumstances) CPT/HCPCS	MODIFIER				E. DIAGNOSIS POINTER	F. $ CHARGES		G. DAYS OR UNITS	H. EPSDT Family Plan	I. ID. QUAL.	J. RENDERING PROVIDER ID. #
07	23	18	07	25	18	21		27252	53				1	1710	10	1		NPI	1234567890
																		NPI	

answer: Section 21A: There should not be a decimal in the code. 24E: Should be A.

RED FLAG

Medical offices have policies and procedures regarding guarantors of children's financial accounts. These policies typically place payment responsibility on the custodial parent, requiring the custodial parent to reconcile medical expenses of the child directly with the other parent.

Patients may subcontract with a third party, either a government program or commercial health insurance, to help pay for their medical services. **Commercial health insurance**, also known as *private health insurance*, is insurance provided by a private company. Patients who have commercial health insurance purchased directly from insurance companies or subsidized by their employers are referred to as **private patients**. A private patient has an expressed physician-patient contract that places the patient responsible for payment for all services or procedures rendered, either through an insurance company or by direct payment. If an insurance policy does not cover a specific service or treatment, the patient is ultimately responsible for paying the medical bill. The insurance policy will state when the patient may not be billed for services or treatment rendered.

Other Types of Physician Contracts

Physicians may enter into other types of contracts to provide their services. Two of the more familiar agreements are managed care organizations and workers' compensation.

Managed Care Organization Contracts

A **managed care organization (MCO)** is a system of health care in which patients agree to receive care from selected doctors and hospitals. **Managed care patients** are individuals who have been assigned to or have selected physicians of a specific MCO. Managed care patients still have a physician-patient contract for treatment; however, the physician also has a contract with the MCO. The physician agrees to provide medical care to the assigned members at a discounted rate. The patient is also in a contract with the managed care plan. The patient's contract with the MCO states the patient's financial obligation to the physician. The patient and medical provider must abide by the managed care contract for the medical bills to be reimbursed.

Workers' Compensation Contracts

Workers' compensation patients seek treatment for illnesses or injuries acquired while at work. In workers' compensation cases, the contract is between the physician and the workers' compensation insurance carrier. Although the agreement is between the physician and insurance carrier, the patient is typically asked to sign a financial agreement that transfers financial responsibility from the insurance company to the patient if it is determined that the patient's condition is not work related.

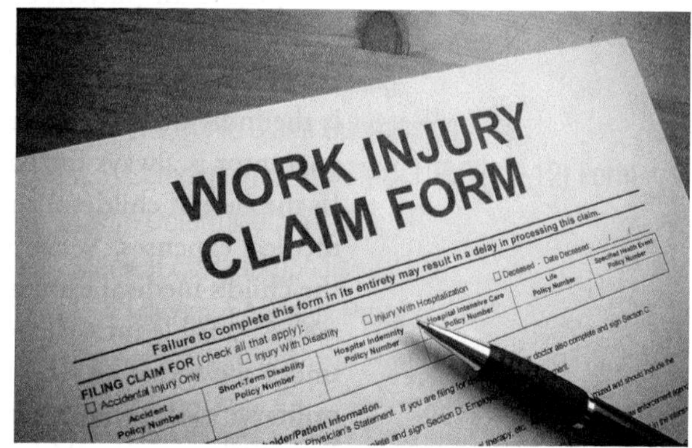

Workers' compensation is for the treatment of illnesses or injuries acquired while at work.

CONCEPTS CHECKPOINT **21.1**

Match the terms in the first column with their correct definitions in the second column.

1. _____ expressed contract
2. _____ first party
3. _____ managed care patients
4. _____ second party
5. _____ third party

a. The medical provider
b. The patient
c. Clearly states the terms of the agreement into which 2 parties enter
d. The insurance payer, other than the patient
e. Individuals who have been assigned to or have selected physicians of a specific MCO

Health Insurance

Insurance is a contract in which a private company or government agency (the insurer) agrees to compensate an individual or business (the insured) for a specified loss, damage, illness, or death in return for premiums. **Premiums** are the fees paid to the insurer by the insured for a specified length of time. **Health insurance**, also referred to as *health coverage*, is a type of insurance that pays healthcare providers for services rendered to patients or reimburses the insured (the owner of the insurance policy) for out-of-pocket medical expenses. Most patients have health insurance that reimburses (pays) the healthcare provider for medical services and surgical procedures. The purpose of health insurance is to offset the cost of medical expenses to patients. Individuals have a variety of choices when it comes to selecting health insurance. Health insurance payers determine how an insurance plan is structured and what payment methods are associated with the plan. This chapter will discuss the reimbursement (payment) process as it relates to physician and hospital outpatient services.

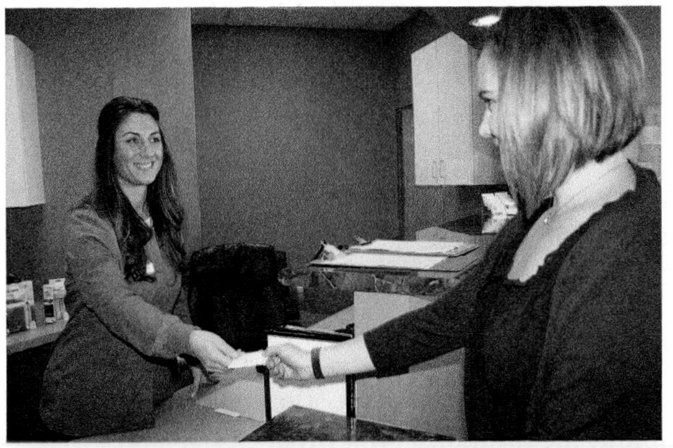

Most patients have health insurance that reimburses the healthcare provider for medical services and surgical procedures. There are a variety of health insurance options to choose from.

The History of Health Insurance

The concept of health insurance began in the 1850s, with a type of nonfatal accident coverage offered by the Franklin Assurance Company of Massachusetts. The original policies covered only passengers of steamboats and rail cars. By the early 1900s, other insurance companies adapted the original concept to also cover personal illness and injuries. These are considered the first health insurance plans.

In 1911, Montgomery Ward and Company offered its employees the option to purchase illness and injury insurance as part of its employee benefits. This was the first time individuals could purchase illness and injury coverage through their employers, and thus the concept of group plans was born. Many large employers began to offer group health plans to recruit and retain employees. In the 1940s, Kaiser Industries offered a flat-rate, prepaid plan that included hospitalization, surgeries, preventive screening, and other physician services. The model resembled some of the current managed care plans offered today. By the 1960s, commercial health insurance plans offered additional options to include hospital care, surgical fees, and physician services.

Today's health insurance plans offer a variety of coverage options and can be purchased through an employer or directly from the insurance company, or acquired through government programs or health insurance exchanges (organizations set up to facilitate the purchasing of health insurance). Government health plans use the same health insurance coverage models as commercial insurance; however, beneficiaries of government plans must meet specific eligibility criteria to enroll in the plans. The **Patient Protection and Affordable Care Act of 2010**, known as the Affordable Care Act (ACA), is a federal law that regulates American healthcare policies. The ACA is meant to improve the quality of health care and increase the number of insured Americans. One of the many provisions of the act requires that all Americans have health insurance or pay a fine. Details of specific insurance plans and provisions of the ACA are discussed later in the chapter.

The Health Insurance Policy

A **health insurance policy** is a legal contract between the holder of the policy and the insurer for reimbursement of a portion of the medical expense incurred for receiving medical treatment. The **policyholder** is the owner of the policy, and the health insurance policy covers the policyholder and eligible family members. As previously noted, the first party of the contract is the patient, and the second party is the medical provider. The **third-party payer** is an entity contracted to pay the medical provider on behalf the policyholder. Health insurance policies vary in what they cover. For example, some plans cover hospitalization only.

Policy Limitations

Health insurance policies do not cover all medical expenses. The **statement of limitations** or exclusions is a section in the insurance policy that clearly states what services, procedures, and circumstances are not reimbursed by the health insurance company. The statement of limitations also lists requirements for specific services or procedures to be covered. For example, some policies may require a physician to obtain authorization prior to performing magnetic resonance imaging (MRI). If the preauthorization procedures are not followed, the insurance policy will not reimburse for the MRI.

Coordination of Benefits

When a patient has more than 1 insurance policy (dual coverage), the contract states which policy is primary (billed first) and which is secondary (billed second). Determination of which insurance plan is primary or secondary is referred to as **coordination of benefits**. The coordination of benefits prevents overpayment.

The coordination of benefits also determines the financial responsibility of the patient. Many health insurance plans require patients to share the cost of health care by paying a portion of the medical expense. The payment may be in the form of a copay, deductible, or coinsurance. A **copay** (or **copayment**) is a fixed amount paid prior to the provision of health services. A **deductible** is the set amount the insured must pay for healthcare services before the health insurance begins to pay. **Coinsurance** is a set percentage the member pays after the deductible is met (paid). Because deductibles and coinsurance payments are based on the total fees for services provided, they are collected after services are rendered.

Medicare is the federal health insurance program for people who are 65 or older, certain younger people with disabilities, and people with end-stage renal disease (permanent kidney failure requiring dialysis or a transplant, sometimes called *ESRD*). **Medicare secondary payer (MSP)** provisions coordinate benefits to ensure that Medicare does not pay for services and items that the beneficiary's other health insurance is responsible for paying. The most common situations in which Medicare is not the primary payer involve Medicare beneficiaries in the following circumstances:

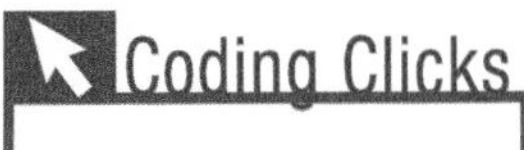

To learn more about Medicare Secondary Payer provisions, visit http://Coding.ParadigmEducation.com/MedicareSecondaryPayer.

- age 65 or older covered by a group health plan through current employment, a spouse's current employment, or self-employment, and the employer has 20 or more employees;
- disabled and covered by a group health plan through his or her own current employment, and the employer has 100 or more employees;
- ESRD patients during the 30-month coordination period;
- an accident or another situation in which no-fault or liability insurance is involved.

CONCEPTS CHECKPOINT **21.2**

Match the insurance term in the first column with the correct definition in the second column.

1. _____ coordination of benefits
2. _____ coinsurance
3. _____ deductible
4. _____ copay
5. _____ Medicare secondary payer

a. A set amount the insured must pay for healthcare services before the health insurance begins to pay
b. Determination of which insurance plan is primary or secondary
c. A fixed amount paid prior to health services being rendered
d. A set percentage the member pays after the deductible is met
e. Provision that determines when Medicare is not the primary payer

Types of Health Insurance

The current provisions of the ACA stipulate that Americans who can afford to purchase health insurance but choose not to will be subject to a fee based on income adjusted for inflation. For example, the penalty in 2017 was set at a flat fee of $695 per adult and $347.50 per child under 18, or 2.5% of the family income, whichever is greater.

There are several different healthcare plans that offer a variety of coverage options. Different plans have different eligibility requirements. The following section provides a brief overview of the basic types of health insurance plans offered in the United States.

Managed Care Insurance Plans

The managed care organization (MCO) insurance plan is a system in which patients agree to receive care only from selected doctors and hospitals. MCOs control healthcare costs by negotiating fees and monitoring treatment. The following is a list of different types of MCO plans:

- **competitive medical plan**—MCOs that meet the Centers for Medicare & Medicaid Services (CMS) criteria for enrolling Medicare beneficiaries into their managed care plans; for example, Humana is an MCO that offers several different types of plans, 1 of which is offered only to Medicare beneficiaries;
- **exclusive provider organization (EPO)**—a network of individual medical care providers, or groups of medical care providers, who have entered into a contract with an insurer to provide health insurance to members;
- **health maintenance organization (HMO)**—the most restrictive MCO; HMOs require members to select an in-network primary care physician (PCP) and request referral or preauthorization prior to receiving certain healthcare services;
- **preferred provider organization (PPO)**—the least restrictive MCO; PPOs allow members to visit any in-network physician or healthcare provider they choose without first obtaining a referral from a primary care physician;
- **point-of-service (POS) plan**—a hybrid of HMO and PPO plans; like an HMO, members select an in-network primary care provider, but like a PPO, patients may seek treatment outside of the provider network for healthcare services.

Independent/Individual Practice Association Insurance Plans

In an **independent** or **individual practice association (IPA) insurance plan**, a group or organization of private practice physicians negotiates contracts with insurance companies on their own behalf.

Government Health Insurance Plans

Federal and state programs exist to subsidize health care for people who cannot afford to purchase health insurance. The best-known programs are described in Table 21.1.

Table 21.1 Government Health Insurance Plans

Program	Government Level (Federal or State)	Description
Maternal and Child Health Program	Joint federal and state	Provides funds to agencies to address the healthcare needs of mothers, women, children, and youth, including those with special healthcare needs, and their families
Medicaid	Joint federal and state	Helps individuals with disabilities or low-income individuals or families pay for healthcare expenses; although mostly funded by the federal government, Medicaid is run by the state, where coverage may vary from state to state
Medicare	Federal	For people who are 65 or older, individuals with disabilities, and people with end-stage renal disease; Medicare gives beneficiaries 4 choices of coverage: • **Part A (hospital insurance)**—covers inpatient hospital stays, care in a skilled nursing facility, hospice care, and some home health care; • **Part B (medical insurance)**—covers certain doctors' services, outpatient care, medical supplies, and preventive services; • **Part C (Medicare Advantage plans)**—a type of Medicare health plan offered by a private company that contracts with Medicare to provide all Part A and Part B benefits. Most Medicare Advantage plans offer prescription drug coverage; • **Part D (prescription drug coverage)**—prescription drug insurance coverage provided by private companies.
Medicare/Medicaid, often referred to as Medi/Medi	Joint federal and state	Individuals who are enrolled in both Medicare and Medicaid programs
TRICARE	Federal	Healthcare program for active duty members of the military and their families, as well as activated National Guard and Reserve personnel, retired military personnel, and surviving family members of deceased veterans
CHAMPVA (Civilian Health and Medical Program of the Department of Veterans Affairs)	Federal	Healthcare program provided by the US Department of Veterans Affairs for the families of veterans permanently disabled or killed in the line of duty who are not eligible for TRICARE; CHAMPVA for Life (CFL) is an extension of CHAMPVA benefits to those 65 years and older

Coding Clicks

Find the MAC for your jurisdiction using the interactive CMS map at http://Coding.ParadigmEducation.com/CMSMap.

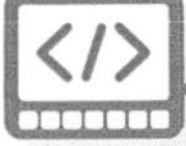

Coding for CMS

Medicare uses a network of contractors called Medicare Administrative Contractors (MACs) to process Medicare claims, enroll healthcare providers in the Medicare program, and educate providers on Medicare billing requirements. Contractors designated as "A/B MACs" process Medicare Part A and Part B claims for defined geographic areas called *jurisdictions*. As Medicare sets national coverage standards on specific services, procedures, supplies, and diagnoses, MACs are tasked with applying these national coverage determinations (NCDs) to their local jurisdictions. These local rules are called *local coverage determinations (LCDs)*. An LCD may be more restrictive than an NCD. Coders must become familiar with the LCD that applies to the jurisdiction of the patient's Medicare plan. Documentation that does not meet the LCD requirements will affect coverage of services.

CONCEPTS CHECKPOINT **21.3**

Use information from the previous section to answer true or false to each of the following statements.

1. _____ A health maintenance organization (HMO) requires members to select an in-network primary care physician (PCP) and request referral or preauthorization prior to receiving certain healthcare services.
2. _____ Preferred provider organizations (PPOs) allow members to visit any in-network physician or healthcare provider they choose without first obtaining a referral from a primary care physician.
3. _____ Medicaid is a federal program that helps low-income individuals or families pay for healthcare expenses.
4. _____ Medicare Part A covers inpatient hospital stays, care in a skilled nursing facility, hospice care, and some home health care.
5. _____ Medicare Part B covers certain doctors' services, outpatient care, medical supplies, and preventive services.
6. _____ Provisions of the Patient Protection and Affordable Care Act of 2010 required most Americans to purchase a healthcare insurance policy or be subject to a penalty.

Reimbursement Methodology

Reimbursement is the act of compensating a person for services rendered. In the healthcare industry, medical providers treat patients prior to receiving payment. Fees may not be collected prior to the patient receiving treatment because the necessary treatment is not yet known. There are many different reimbursement methods within health care. The following section reviews the most common methods.

Fee-for-Service Reimbursement

Fee for service is a reimbursement method that requests payment for each service or procedure. Each service or procedure has a set fee or charge. Providers are reimbursed only the allowed amount as listed on the third-party payer fee schedule. The **allowed amount** is the average or maximum amount that may be reimbursed per service, procedure, or item to the provider from the insurance payer.

Fee Schedules

A **fee schedule** is a price list of services and procedures. Each payer has its own customized fee schedule. However, many healthcare providers base their fees on the CMS **Medicare Physician Fee Schedule (MPFS)**. Medicare uses the **resource-based relative value scale (RBRVS)** to create the MPFS. The RBRVS sets fees for CPT® and HCPCS codes. To calculate the value of a service or procedure, the RBRVS uses 3 factors:

1. **Relative value units (RVU)** calculated by using the formula Work RVU + Practice Expense RVU + Malpractice RVU = Total RVU. The 3 components are described below:
    - work RVU—the amount of work needed to render the treatment;
    - practice expense RVU—the expense of the practice to facilitate the treatment;

- malpractice RVU—the risk of malpractice associated with the treatment.

2. **Geographic practice cost indices (GPCI)**: adjustments applied to the RVU values to account for variations in the costs of practicing medicine in specific geographic regions.
3. **Conversion factor (CF)**: a fiscal-year monetary amount arrived at by a formula set by Congress to convert the GPCI into a dollar amount that reflects several elements: the category of services (medical, surgical, or nonsurgical), the percentage of changes to the Medicare Economic Index, physician expenditures, access to health care, and quality of health care. The conversion factor is adjusted annually.

Examples of the calculations are provided in Tables 21.2 and 21.3.

The national RVU provides the base value for CPT® and HCPCS codes. Table 21.2 shows the use of the RVU formula for code 49540, *Repair lumbar hernia.* The 3 RVU components—work, practice expense, and malpractice—are given set values. The values are added together to determine the **national (standard) RVU** for the procedure: 10.74 + 6.20 + 2.48 = 19.42.

RED FLAG

When coders assign multiple codes to report surgeries that involved more than 1 procedure, they must know which code has the highest RVU. The procedure with the highest RVU is the primary procedure and is reported first. Knowing which codes have the highest RVU will also determine modifier placement for multiple procedures.

Table 21.2 Example of a National (Standard) RVU Calculation

CPT®/HCPCS Code	RVU Component			Total RVU
	Work	Practice Expense	Malpractice	
49540	10.74	6.20	2.48	19.42

However, a procedure performed in a major metropolitan city such as Los Angeles, California, will have higher work, practice expense, and malpractice costs than the same procedure in a smaller city such as Red Banks, Mississippi. The RVU is geographically adjusted by the GPCI (informally referred to as the *gypsy*). Table 21.3 compares the RVUs for the 2 cities for code 49540, calculated as:

Los Angeles = 11.24 + 7.30 + 1.72 = 20.25
Red Banks = 10.32 + 5.39 + 0.92 = 16.63

Table 21.3 Calculation of RVUs for Los Angeles, California, and Red Banks, Mississippi, Using GPCI

City	CPT®/HCPCS Code	RVU Component GPCI Value			Total RVU Value
		Work	Expense	Malpractice	
Los Angeles, CA	49540	11.24	7.30	1.72	20.25
Red Banks, MS	49540	10.32	5.39	0.91	16.63

To convert the GPCI into a dollar amount, the total RVU is multiplied by a monetary CF. CFs differ based on the category of services (medical, surgical, or nonsurgical). Using a CF of 35.99960 and the values in Table 21.3, the fees for code 49540 in Los Angeles and Red Banks are calculated by multiplying their respective GPCI-adjusted, total RVUs by the CF:

Los Angeles = 20.25 × 35.99960 = 729.08
Red Banks = 16.63 × 35.99960 = 598.77

> **Coding Clicks**
>
> The Medicare Physician Fee Schedule Look-Up Tool allows coders to search for fees by CPT® or HCPCS code. Access the tool at http://Coding.ParadigmEducation.com/FeeSchedule.

Rounding the results to the nearest penny shows that the procedure has a Medicare monetary value of $729.11 in Los Angeles and $598.77 in Red Banks.

The MPFS lists RVUs on the CMS website. The MPFS is updated on April 15 of each year. The formulas used to establish RVUs and GPCIs are published in the ***Federal Register***, the US government's daily publication of final and administrative regulations for federal agencies. Coders reference the *Federal Register* to stay current on changes that affect healthcare regulations and Medicare.

Health insurance companies base their fees on the MPFS. Physician offices may also use the MPFS to establish a fixed fee schedule for the office, which lists all services and procedures offered at that practice. However, the fees set by the practice do not determine reimbursement amounts from third-party payers. Hospitals compile all procedures, services, supplies, and drugs that are billed to insurance payers into a computer database called a **hospital chargemaster**. Most hospital chargemasters include several thousand line items that are reviewed and updated annually by a medical coder who has the title of chargemaster.

Physician offices incorporate their most common procedure and diagnosis codes into the **encounter form**, also known as a *superbill* or *charge slip*. The encounter form also includes patient information, the insurance payer, and current financial account information. Figure 21.1 shows an example of an encounter form that may be used in an orthopedic office. The master encounter form includes the set fee schedule for the physician office. These fees are typically slightly higher than the highest payer fee schedule.

EXAMPLE **21.1**

Let's look at code 20610, *Arthrocentesis, aspiration and/or injection, major joint or bursa (eg, shoulder, hip, knee, subacromial bursa); without ultrasound guidance*. Code 20610 may be reported for the removal of fluid from a major joint or bursa. It may also be reported for the injection of drugs into a major joint or bursa. Physician offices typically accept patients with Medicare, Medicaid, and commercial insurance. The physician, who is contracted with the payers, has access to the fee schedules for each payer. The following is a list of the payers' fees for code 20610 as well as the office fee:

Payers Fee Schedule for Code 20610:

Medicare	$61.73
Medicaid	$58.12
Commercial payer	$78.28

Physician Office Fee Schedule:

Code 20610	$85.00

The fee schedule shows that each payer has a different allowable fee for code 20610. The commercial payer fee represents a single amount despite the range of fees set by the many different commercial payers who all have their own fee schedules. Rather than looking up the exact fee for each payer, billing is expedited if the physician's office has 1 set fee for code 20610, typically set a few dollars above the highest listed fee on the commercial payers' fee schedules. If the fee is set lower than what is listed on the fee schedule, and the reimbursement is approved, the payer will pay only the amount requested. In our example, the physician office sets a fee of $85.00 for code 20610.

Figure 21.1 Encounter Form

Patient Identification	
Date:	
Name:	
Student ID #:	
DOB:	Gender:
Confidential visit today? ❑ Yes ❑ No	SHQ needed today? ❑ Yes ❑ No

Insurance Identification
COMPANY NAME:
Insurance #:
Provider name/NPI:
Provider signature:

OFFICE VISIT

	ESTAB		NEW	
	99211			Minimal eval.
	99212		99201	Problem focused
	99213		99202	Expanded problem focused
	99214		99203	Detailed
			99204	Comprehensive, mod. complexity, 45 min.
	99215		99205	Comprehensive, high complexity
	99354		99354	***Add-on code to 99215 or 99205*** Prolonged service; with patient contact; beyond 30-74 min.

EPSDT WELL CHILD EXAM / PREVENTIVE MEDICINE

	ESTAB		NEW	Consider use of Modifier 25 (write in +25 after code)
	99391		99381	Infant
	99392		99382	1-4 years
	99393		99383	5-11 years
	99394		99384	12-17 years
	99395		99385	18+ years

NUTRITION

	97802			Medical nutritional therapy, initial assessment and intervention, individual, each 15 min
	97803			Medical nutritional therapy, re-assessment and intervention, individual, each 15 min.

PSYCHIATRIC THERAPEUTIC PROCEDURES

	90832	Psychotherapy, 30 minutes with patient and/or family member
	90833	Psychotherapy, 30 minutes with patient and/or family member when performed with an evaluation and management service - add-on code
	90834	Psychotherapy, 45 minutes with patient and/or family member
	90836	Psychotherapy, 45 minutes with patient and/or family member when performed with an evaluation and management service - add-on code
	90837	Psychotherapy, 60 minutes with patient and/or family member
	90838	Psychotherapy, 60 minutes with patient and/or family member when performed with an evaluation and management service - add-on code

MEDICATIONS, SUPPLIES, AND DURABLE MEDICAL EQUIPMENT

	J0170	Adrenaline, epinephrine up to 1 ml	J7603	Albuterol, unit dose form, 1 mg
	J0560	Penicillin G, up to 600,000 units	A4614	Peak flow meter, hand-held
	J0570	Penicillin G, up to 1,200,000 units	A4266	Diaphragm device
	J0580	Penicillin G, up to 2,400,000 units	A4261	Cervical cap for contraceptive use
	J0696	Ceftriaxone 250 mg. IM per vial	A4267	Condom, male
	J1055	Depo Provera 150 mg. IM	A4268	Condom, female
	J1056	Medroxyprogesterone	A4269	Spermicidal agent
	J2550	Promethazine HCl, injection up to 50 mg	J8499 **U1**	Plan B or similar emergency contraception
	J7300	Intrauterine copper contraceptive	J7307	Etenogestrel contraceptive implant system
	J7302	Levonorgesterel-releasing intrauterine (Mirena)	S4989	IUD other than above (Progestacert)
	J7303	Hormone-containing vaginal ring (Nuvaring	S4993	Contraceptive pills for birth control
	J7304	Hormone-containing patch (OrthoEvra)	Q0144	Azithromycin oral powder 1 gm **Man. care only**
	J7602	Albuterol, concentrated form, 1 mg		

IMMUNIZATIONS

IMMUNIZATION ADMINISTRATION

	90471	One immunization **Managed care only**	90472	Each additional vaccine **Managed care only**

VACCINATIONS

	90633	Hep A	90702	DT
	90645	HIB(HbOC) [HibTITER]	90707	Measles, Mumps, Rubella
	90646	HIB(PRP-D) [ProHIBIT]	90712	Poliovirus
	90647	HIB(PRP-OMP) [PedvaxHIB]	90713	IPV (polio)
	90648	HIB(PRP-T) ActHIB or Omni HIB]	90715	Tdap
	90649 **HB**	HPV females 9-10 and 19-26	90716	Varicella SQ
	90649	HPV females 11-18	90718	Tetanus and Diphtheria (Td)
	90657	Influenza (split virus 6-35 mo.)	90732	Pneumococcal polyvalent, SQ or IM
	90658	Influenza (split virus 3 yrs+)	907033	Meningococcal (polysaccharide, SQ)
	90669	Pneumococcal conjugate, IM <5 yrs	90734	Meningococcal conjugate vaccine, sero-groups A, C, Y, and W-135 (tetravalent)
	90700	DTaP		
	90701	DT	90744	Hep B 3 dose IM
	90660	Influenza virus vaccine, live, for intranasal use	90748	Heb B/Hib Combination IM

FOLLOW-UP	REFERRAL
Return to EMC (follow-up date): To provider:	To:

DIAGNOSIS (ICD-10)

	Code # and name

ON-SITE LAB TESTS

X	CPT	DESCRIPTION
		No labs given
	80061	Lipid panel
	81000	Urinalysis – dip stick
	81001	Urinalysis, auto. – microscopy
	81002	Urinalysis, non-auto. – no microscopy
	81003	Urinalysis, auto – no microscopy
	81015	Urine – microscopic only
	81025	Urine pregnancy test-by visual color
	82270	Guiac, occult blood
	82465	Cholesterol, total
	82947	Glucose; quantitative; blood
	82948	Glucose fingerstick
	82962	Glucose monitoring device
	84703	hCG preg. test (urine) – qualitative
	85013	Hematocrit
	85018	Hemoglobin
	86308	Mono-spot screen
	86677	H. pylori antibody
	87210	Wet mount (e.g., saline) for infectious agents
	87430	Streptococcus, group A (culture nonbillable)
	87491	Urine CT/GC – amplified probe nonbillable
	87880	Streptococcus, group A (rapid strep test)
	Q0091	PAP smear, obtaining/preparation **Man. care only**
	Q0111	Web prep, obtaining/preparation
	92567	Tympanometry – impedance testing

PROCEDURES

10060	I&D simple
10120	I&D of foreign body, subcutaneous (simple)
11730	Nail avulsion
11740	Evacuation of subungual hematoma
11750	Excision of nail and nail maxtix, partial or complete, for permanent removal
12001	Suturing – specify body part:
12031	Layer closure of wounds of scalp, axillae, trunk, and/or extremities (excluding hands and feet) 2.5 cm
16000	Initial tx – first-degree burn (local), doc. % coverage and depth
17110	Wart removal
26641	Closed tx of carpometacarpal (thumb) dislocation
28190	Removal of foreign body, foot, subcutaneous
29130	Application of finger splint (static)
30300	Removal of foreign body, intranasal
36415	Venipuncture
54050	Destruction of lesion(s), penis
56501	Destruction of lesion(s), vulva
57170	Diaphragm fitting
58300	IUD insertion
58301	IUD removal
69200	Removal foreign body from external auditory canal
69210	Removal impacted cerumen (one or both ears)
87220	KOH for skin/hair/nails
94640	Nebulizer treatment
94010	Spirometry

TELEHEALTH SERVICE

Q3014	Telehealth originating site facility fee

EMC Medical Center

CONCEPTS CHECKPOINT **21.4**

Use information from the previous section to select the correct answer to the following multiple-choice questions.

1. The average or maximum amount that may be reimbursed per service, procedure, or item to the provider from the insurance payer is called the
   a. allowed amount.
   b. fee for service.
   c. Medicare Physician Fee Schedule.
   d. reimbursement.
2. The set value given to a service or procedure is the
   a. geographic practice cost index (GPCI).
   b. monetary conversion factor (CF).
   c. relative value unit (RVU).
   d. resource-based relative value scale (RBRVS).
3. The value set by Congress that is used to convert RVUs into dollars is the
   a. geographic practice cost indices (GPCI).
   b. *Federal Register*.
   c. monetary conversion factor (CF).
   d. resource-based relative value scale (RBRVS).
4. The US government's daily publication of final and administrative regulations for federal agencies is called the
   a. *Federal Register*.
   b. hospital chargemaster.
   c. resource-based relative value scale.
   d. None of the answers are correct.
5. A form that lists the most common procedure and diagnosis codes reported in a physician office is the
   a. superbill.
   b. encounter form.
   c. charge slip.
   d. All of the answers are correct.

Self-Pay Method

Self-pay is a fee-for-service reimbursement method by which the patient or the guarantor pays for each service or procedure rendered. Patients without health insurance may be required to pay the entire cost of the treatment on the same day of the medical service. However, most medical facilities will make payment arrangements or apply a hardship discount for patients without health insurance.

Retrospective Payment Method

Retrospective payment is a fee-for-service reimbursement method in which each service or procedure rendered is reimbursed by the insurance payer. Retrospective payment is the most common method of fee-for-service reimbursement. Most retrospective payment methods require patients to share the cost of their care through a copay, deductible, or other shared-cost payment. A copay is always collected prior to the rendering of services. The portion of the fee that is part of a patient's policy deductible and other shared costs is collected from the patient at the end of the visit. Medical practices may have office policies and procedures that collect the deductible and shared costs after the insurance payer has determined the patient responsibility.

Episode-of-Care Payment Method

The term *episode of care* refers to all services provided to a patient for a medical problem within a specific period of time across a continuum of care in an integrated healthcare system. The **episode-of-care** payment method reimburses the provider in a single lump sum for all services during a specified, continuous period of time, for a specific condition. The method controls medical costs associated with a single health condition known to require multiple services to treat. For example, home health services are reimbursed using the episode-of-care payment method. All home care services provided to a patient during a 60-day period are reimbursed with a predetermined lump-sum payment.

Capitation Payment Method

The **capitation payment method** reimburses providers a fixed amount for each assigned managed care organization member in a single lump-sum payment once a month, which is similar to an episode-of-care payment. The frequency with which a patient seeks medical services has no bearing on the amount of the reimbursement. The provider is paid the same fixed rate per assigned member, regardless of whether the patient seeks treatment several times in a month or not at all. The fixed rate is not adjustable, even when treatment requires a high complexity of care or high expenses to the medical practice. The greatest advantage of a capitated payment is the certainty of the amount of the monthly reimbursement. Disadvantages are the unpredictability of providers' time and cost commitments owing to the number of patients seeking care and the complexity of the treatment needed.

Global Payment Method

The **global payment method** is a single lump-sum payment to a medical facility that covers all services and procedures needed to treat a group of patients. The payment is the same regardless of the number of patients in the group, the complexity of the treatment, or the number of medical providers who treat the patients. The global payment method allows the provider to allocate funds to the services he or she believes will best treat the patient group. Payment is received from a single insurance payer or government agency. For example, Medicare reimburses home health services using the global payment method. The home health facility receives a lump-sum payment to provide a variety of services to homebound patients. The home health service provider must allocate funds appropriately to provide care to all patients.

Prospective Payment System

A **prospective payment system (PPS)** is a Medicare reimbursement method in which payment is made based on a predetermined, fixed amount. The payment amount for a specific service is based on the resources needed for the average patient for a set period or given set of conditions or diseases. Medicare uses PPS to reimburse hospital inpatient and outpatient facilities.

Inpatient Prospective Payment System

The **inpatient prospective payment system (IPPS)** is a payment method that determines reimbursement for Medicare Part A (hospital coverage) inpatient services based on **diagnosis-related groups (DRGs)**. DRG is a classification system that uses medical data collected from previous patients to create groups based on diagnosis, treatment plan, and length of stay. Each DRG is weighted by the average resources used to treat Medicare patients in that DRG. The payment weight is determined by the hospital location, teaching status, ratio of low-income patients, and the financial expense associated with a specific case.

DRGs are assigned based on the patient's diagnosis as reported with ICD-10-CM codes. The more severe the principal diagnosis, the higher the reimbursement. Reimbursement is increased when a patient has a comorbidity. A **comorbidity** is a preexisting condition that affects the treatment of the principal diagnosis. Inpatient coders review patients' records to assign admitting diagnoses and comorbidity. It is vital that inpatient coders have an extensive knowledge of disease severity and diagnosis codes.

Outpatient Prospective Payment System

The **outpatient prospective payment system (OPPS)** reimburses medical facilities for outpatient services provided, such as diagnostic tests, to Medicare Part B (physician coverage) beneficiaries in an acute care hospital. Reimbursement amounts are based on the **ambulatory payment classification (APC)**, which groups similar services to determine reimbursement rates. An APC group is based on diagnoses, procedures, patient age, and patient gender. APC uses ICD-10-CM, CPT®, and HCPCS code sets to identify diagnoses and procedures. Each APC group has a fixed payment amount. The fixed rate is the median cost associated with the procedure and the facility's expense. An adjustment may be made to the APC rate based on the **hospital wage index**, which reflects the levels of hospital wages in the geographic area of the hospital compared with the national average. The hospital wage index is set by the secretary of the US Department of Health and Human Services (HHS). The APC is updated twice a year in the *Federal Register*.

In the APC system, several different procedures may be bundled within a single group. Most bundled procedures may not be reported separately. **APC payment status indicators** are letters assigned to each CPT® and HCPCS code to identify how a code is reimbursed in the OPPS system.

It is possible for more than 1 APC to be billed for in 1 visit. CPT® modifiers may be reported with hospital outpatient procedures. Some encoder programs have APC features that allow coders to enter the CPT® code to locate the associated APC group code. Encoder programs also provide assistance in determining if a procedure may be reported separately from the associated APC. Figure 21.2 illustrates how APC indicators and price groups are associated with codes by using pacemaker codes as an example.

Coding Clicks

Review a Medicare Learning Network article that provides guidance regarding OPPS reimbursement at http://Coding.ParadigmEducation.com/OPPS.

Figure 21.2 Hospital Outpatient Billing and Payment and Associated Ambulatory Payment Classification Groups

+ signifies add-on code		*PHYSICIAN[2]			ASC[3]	HOSPITAL OUTPATIENT[4]		HOSPITAL INPATIENT[5]		
CPT® Code[1]	CPT® Descriptions	In-Hospital (-26)	In-Office (Global)	*Work RVU* Total RVU8	ASC Payment[3]	APC Category	APC Payment[4]	Possible ICD-10-CM Codes	Possible MS-DRG Assignment	MS-DRG Payment[6]
	Cardiac Rhythm Management Device Implant Procedures									
33206	Insertion of new or replacement of permanent pacemaker with transvenous electrode(s); atria	$472	N/A	*7.39* 13.17	**$7,575**	APC 89	$8,790	I44.0 I44.1 I44.2 I44.30 I44.39 I44.4 I44.5	Permanent cardiac pacemaker implant MS-DRG 244 without CC/MCC MS-DRG 243 with CC MS-DRG 242 with MCC	 $12,532 $15,494 $21,743
33207	Insertion of new or replacement of permanent pacemaker with transvenous electrode(s); ventricular	$503		*8.05* 14.04				I44.39 I44.4 I44.5 I44.60 I44.69 I44.7 I45.0		
33208	Insertion of new or replacement of permanent pacemaker with transvenous electrode(s); atrial and ventricular	$545		*8.77* 15.20	**$9,286**	APC 655	$10,588	I44.30 I44.39 I44.4 I44.5 I44.60		
33212	Insertion of pacemaker pulse generator only; with existing single lead	$341		*5.26* 9.52	**$6,269**	APC 90	$7,353	I45.6 I45.81 I45.9 I47.1 I48.0	Cardiac pacemaker replacement MS-DRG 259 without MCC MS-DRG 258 with MCC	 $11,287 $15,792

CONCEPTS CHECKPOINT **21.5**

Match the payment method in the first column with its description in the second column.

1. _____ capitation
2. _____ episode of care
3. _____ global payment method
4. _____ retrospective payment
5. _____ self-pay

a. The patient or the guarantor pays for each service rendered

b. Each service or procedure rendered is reimbursed by the insurance payer

c. Reimburses the provider 1 lump sum for all services during a specified continuous period of time for a specific condition

d. Reimburses providers a fixed amount for each assigned member in a single lump-sum payment once a month

e. A single lump-sum payment to a medical facility that covers all services and procedures needed to treat a group of patients

The Revenue Cycle

The process of requesting reimbursement from third-party payers is part of the revenue cycle, also known as the *billing cycle.* The revenue cycle begins when a patient presents to the medical office for a healthcare appointment and ends when all charges associated with that specific date of service are reimbursed or deemed uncollectable. See

Figure 21.3. A patient's financial account may have multiple revenue cycles in progress at any given time. A single billing cycle may take a few days or several months. This section discusses the revenue cycle up to the completion of the insurance claim.

Figure 21.3 The Medical Office Revenue Cycle

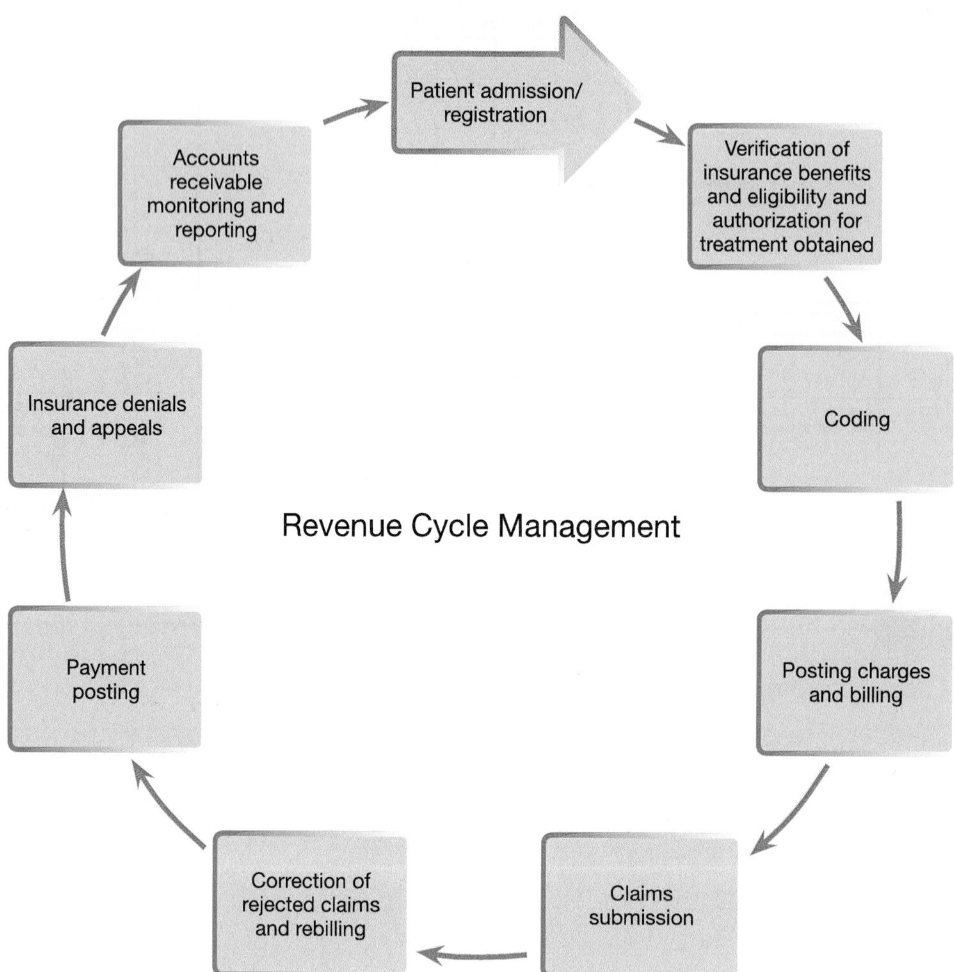

The **practice management system (PMS)** is the computer program that manages the daily operation of the medical office. The PMS organizes patient demographic information, appointments, insurance payer data, and medical codes. The PMS also performs each phase of the billing cycle and can generate reports.

Patient Registration

Prior to receiving services from a medical office, the patient must be entered into the PMS. Collection and entry of a patient's personal information such as guarantor and insurance coverage is referred to as **patient registration**. It is during the registration phase that a patient is assigned an account number in the PMS. The account number allows the PMS to store and organize all data associated with the patient for retrieval to make future appointments and track the reimbursement process. Some PMS programs allow patients to self-register using a kiosk or mobile device provided in the medical office. Registration is the beginning of the billing process, and data entered into the PMS must be accurate and complete to prevent delays in reimbursement. During the registration phase, the patient is apprised of and acknowledges office policies and procedures related to reimbursement and patient privacy practices.

Medicare requires a patient to give permission to the provider to bill for the services. Most patient registration forms include a statement that gives the medical provider permission to file a medical claim on behalf of the patient and have the payment sent directly to the medical provider. When the patient signs the statement, the Medicare patient signature requirement is met, as long as the signature remains on file.

Insurance Verification

Insurance verification is the process of verifying the patient's active health insurance benefits. Insurance companies supply patients with insurance cards that contain basic information regarding the patient's coverage. The front of the insurance card lists general coverage information, such as the member name, member ID number, and group number. The insurance card also lists insurance contact information and any special instructions regarding the insurance policy, often on the back of the card. Figure 21.4 shows an example of a healthcare insurance card. Health information management (HIM) professionals use information on the insurance card to access patient healthcare benefits by telephone or **electronic data interchange (EDI)**, the exchange of information from computer to computer. EDI healthcare eligibility websites are web-based programs that allow subscribers to verify healthcare benefits for different healthcare providers. Verifying that a patient has health insurance and the services covered under the insurance policy does not guarantee payment from the third-party payer.

Figure 21.4 Health Insurance Card

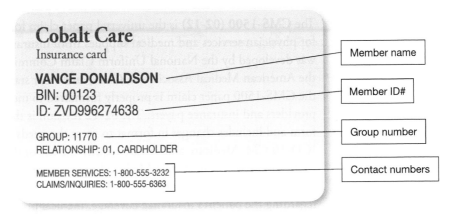

After verifying insurance, the HIM professional will update the PMS and follow the medical office policy in collection of the patient's shared cost. Patients who have a copay make the copayment prior to receiving services. Deductibles and coinsurance payments are collected after services have been rendered. Some offices calculate the amount prior to the patient leaving, and others request payment from the insurance payer first and then bill the patient.

Figure 21.6 CMS-1450 Universal Billing Form for Institutional Providers

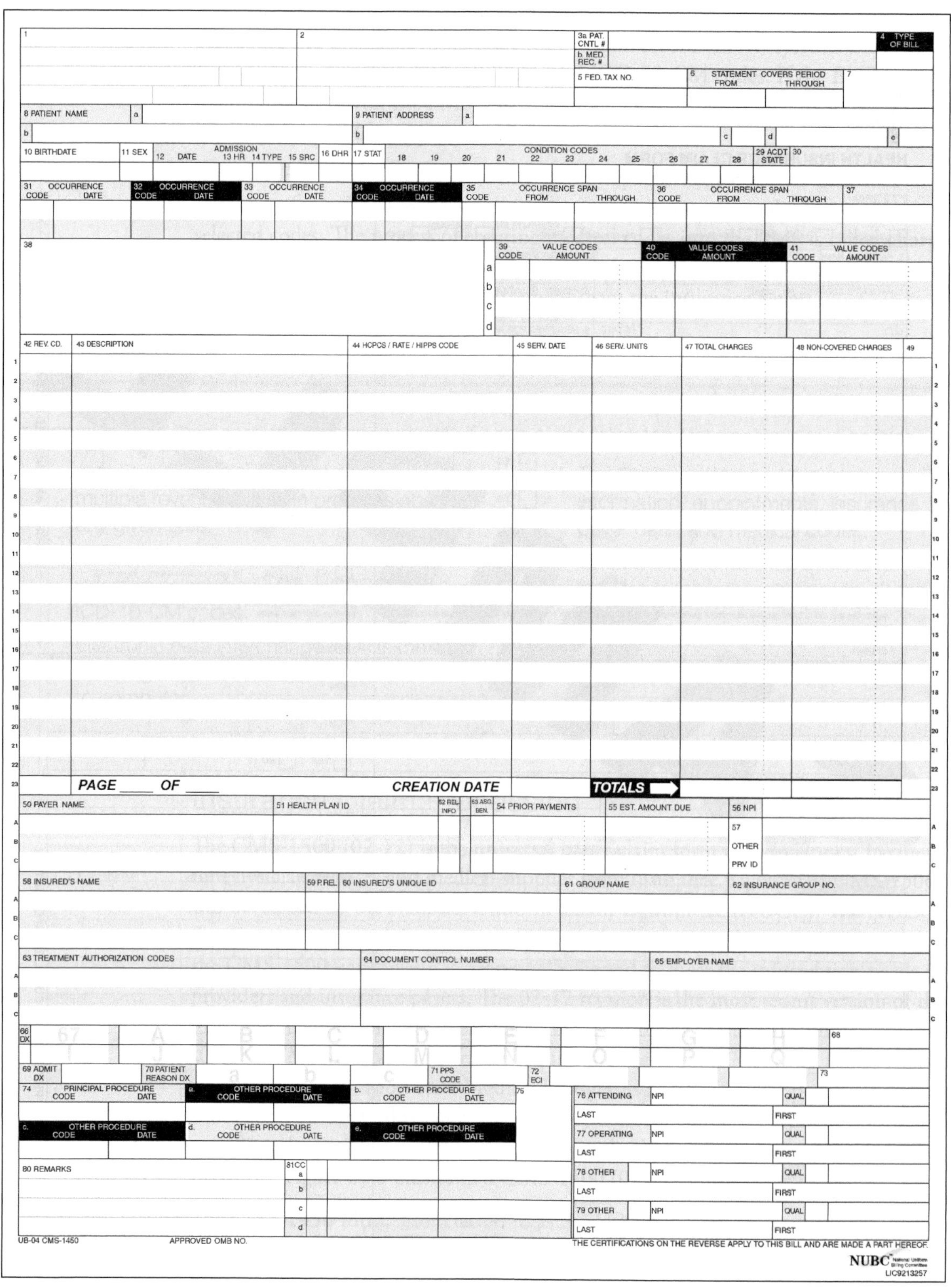

1
2
3a PAT. CNTL #
b. MED. REC. #
4 TYPE OF BILL
5 FED. TAX NO.
6 STATEMENT COVERS PERIOD FROM THROUGH
7
8 PATIENT NAME a
b
9 PATIENT ADDRESS a
b c d e
10 BIRTHDATE
11 SEX
ADMISSION 12 DATE 13 HR 14 TYPE 15 SRC
16 DHR
17 STAT
CONDITION CODES 18 19 20 21 22 23 24 25 26 27 28
29 ACDT STATE
30
31 OCCURRENCE CODE DATE
32 OCCURRENCE CODE DATE
33 OCCURRENCE CODE DATE
34 OCCURRENCE CODE DATE
35 CODE OCCURRENCE SPAN FROM THROUGH
36 CODE OCCURRENCE SPAN FROM THROUGH
37
38
39 CODE VALUE CODES AMOUNT
40 CODE VALUE CODES AMOUNT
41 CODE VALUE CODES AMOUNT
a b c d

42 REV. CD. | 43 DESCRIPTION | 44 HCPCS / RATE / HIPPS CODE | 45 SERV. DATE | 46 SERV. UNITS | 47 TOTAL CHARGES | 48 NON-COVERED CHARGES | 49

1 2 3 4 5 6 7 8 9 10 11 12 13 14 15 16 17 18 19 20 21 22 23

PAGE ____ OF ____
CREATION DATE
TOTALS

50 PAYER NAME
51 HEALTH PLAN ID
52 REL. INFO
53 ASG. BEN.
54 PRIOR PAYMENTS
55 EST. AMOUNT DUE
56 NPI
57 OTHER PRV ID
A B C
58 INSURED'S NAME
59 P. REL.
60 INSURED'S UNIQUE ID
61 GROUP NAME
62 INSURANCE GROUP NO.
A B C
63 TREATMENT AUTHORIZATION CODES
64 DOCUMENT CONTROL NUMBER
65 EMPLOYER NAME
A B C
66 DX
67 A B C D E F G H
I J K L M N O P Q
68
69 ADMIT DX
70 PATIENT REASON DX a b c
71 PPS CODE
72 ECI
73
74 PRINCIPAL PROCEDURE CODE DATE
a. OTHER PROCEDURE CODE DATE
b. OTHER PROCEDURE CODE DATE
75
76 ATTENDING NPI QUAL
LAST FIRST
c. OTHER PROCEDURE CODE DATE
d. OTHER PROCEDURE CODE DATE
e. OTHER PROCEDURE CODE DATE
77 OPERATING NPI QUAL
LAST FIRST
80 REMARKS
81CC a b c d
78 OTHER NPI QUAL
LAST FIRST
79 OTHER NPI QUAL
LAST FIRST
UB-04 CMS-1450
APPROVED OMB NO.
THE CERTIFICATIONS ON THE REVERSE APPLY TO THIS BILL AND ARE MADE A PART HEREOF.
NUBC National Uniform Billing Committee
LIC9213257

Electronic Claim Submission

As technology has evolved, insurance payers and providers prefer to submit insurance claims electronically. To ensure the security of patient information during electronic transactions, in 2002 the Administrative Simplification Compliance Act (ASCA) required the HHS to adopt standards for electronic transactions involving healthcare data. EDI facilitates the exchange of business documents from computer to computer in a standard electronic format. The requirement to adopt a single EDI format reduced the hundreds of different formats used by insurance companies and patient management systems to 1 standard format. The CMS-1500 and CMS-1450 have unique EDI formats that allow for the electronic submission of both forms. Submitting claims in a timely manner is essential to the reimbursement process. **Timely filing** is the period of time that the provider has to submit the first insurance claim to the payer. Claims not received within the timely filing period are denied. Medicare and most third-party payers' timely filing period is 12 months (1 calendar year) from the date of service.

The ASCA also required that all claims sent to the Medicare program be submitted electronically, starting October 16, 2003. There are exceptions to the ASCA that allow submission of paper claims. Because of this, health information management (HIM) professionals must have knowledge of how to complete the CMS-1500 (02-12) claim form, discussed in the following section.

Completion of the CMS-1500 (02-12) Form

Coding Clicks

The NUCC *1500 Health Insurance Claim Form Reference Instruction Manual for Form Version 02/12* can be found at http://Coding.ParadigmEducation.com/1500.

The CMS-1500 form may be completed electronically or by hand. A complete guide is available on the NUCC website. In an electronic application, the PMS populates patient data collected during the medical visit to the CMS-1500. The top half of the CMS-1500 form includes the patient and the insured information. The second half of the form includes the physician or supplier information. Coders are most concerned with the second half of the form. Medical codes are entered on the CMS-1500 form in Items 21 and 24.

Form CMS-1500 Item 21 The patient's diagnosis or nature of illness or injury is reported in Item 21 by inputting ICD-9-CM codes or ICD-10-CM codes. ICD codes report the medical condition of the patient and justify the medical service or procedure provided to the patient. Figure 21.7 shows Item 21 populated with ICD-9-CM codes, and a figure callout shows where to indicate whether ICD-9 or ICD-10 codes are used.

Form CMS-1500 Item 24 CPT® codes, HCPCS codes, and modifiers are reported in Item 24. Information associated with the services is provided in the 10 fields shown in Figure 21.8. Figure 21.9 shows brief field-by-field detail on the information needed for Item 24.

CONCEPTS CHECKPOINT **21.7**

Using information from the previous section, identify the correct fields on the CMS-1500 form for the following information.

1. _____ Date(s) of Service
2. _____ Procedures, Services, or Supplies
3. _____ Place of Service
4. _____ Units
5. _____ Rendering Provider ID

Figure 21.7 Item 21 of Form CMS-1500 (02-12)

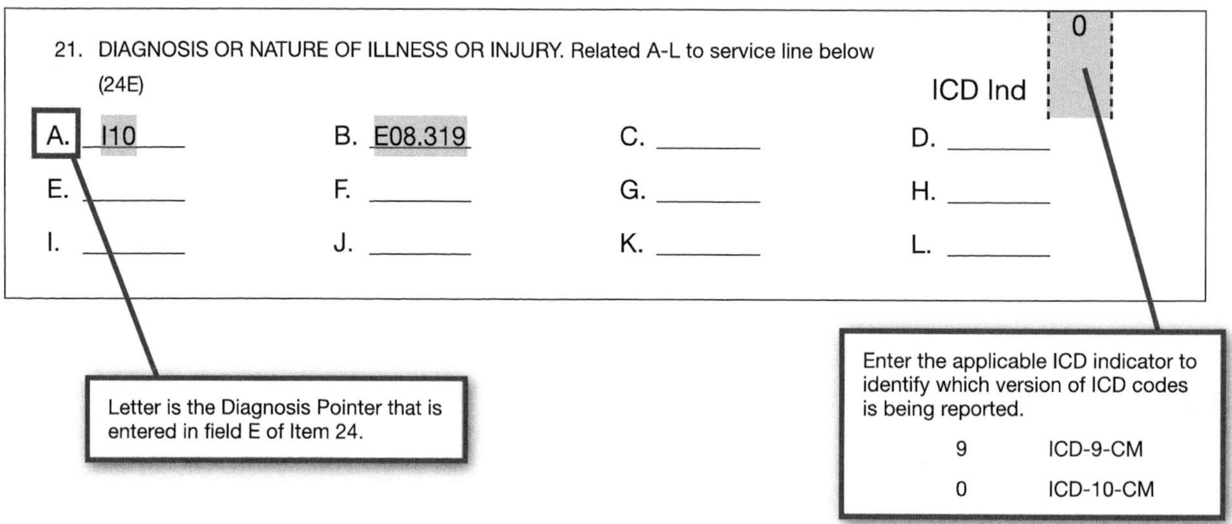

21. DIAGNOSIS OR NATURE OF ILLNESS OR INJURY. Related A-L to service line below (24E)

ICD Ind 0

A. I10	B. E08.319	C. ____	D. ____
E. ____	F. ____	G. ____	H. ____
I. ____	J. ____	K. ____	L. ____

Figure 21.8 Item 24 of the CMS-1500 Form

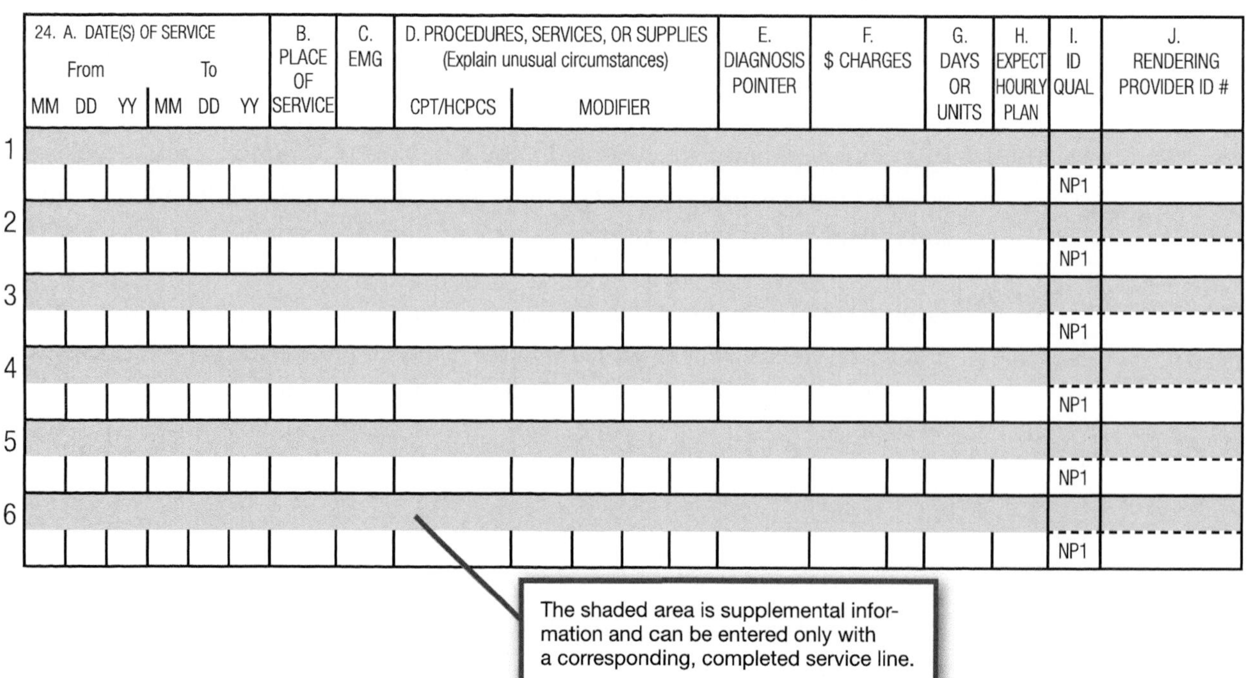

	24. A. DATE(S) OF SERVICE From MM DD YY	To MM DD YY	B. PLACE OF SERVICE	C. EMG	D. PROCEDURES, SERVICES, OR SUPPLIES (Explain unusual circumstances) CPT/HCPCS	MODIFIER	E. DIAGNOSIS POINTER	F. $ CHARGES	G. DAYS OR UNITS	H. EXPECT HOURLY PLAN	I. ID QUAL	J. RENDERING PROVIDER ID #
1											NP1	
2											NP1	
3											NP1	
4											NP1	
5											NP1	
6											NP1	

Figure 21.9 Information for Item 24 in Form CMS-1500

	A. DATE(S) OF SERVICE						B.	C.	D. PROCEDURES, SERVICES, OR SUPPLIES (Explain Unusual Circumstances)					E.	F.		G.	H.	I.	J.
	From			To			PLACE OF SERVICE	EMG	CPT/HCPCS	MODIFIER				DIAGNOSIS POINTER	$ CHARGES		DAYS OR UNITS	EPSDT Family Plan	ID. QUAL.	RENDERING PROVIDER ID. #
	MM	DD	YY	MM	DD	YY														
1																				20%, $500
	03	13	19	03	13	19	11	Y	99214					AB	69	00	1			[NPI #]
2																				0
	03	13	19	03	13	19	11	Y	71010	TC				A	77	00	1			[NPI #]

Fields designated A through J have the following characteristics:

A	Date(s) of Service	Enter the beginning and ending service dates. The date of service was March 13, 2019.
B	Place of Service	Enter the 2-digit code that describes the place of service. Place of service codes are typically listed on the inside cover of the CPT® codebook. The place of service was the office.
C	EMG	Emergency Indicator: Mark this box with a "✓," an "X," or a "Y" if the service was an emergency service, regardless of where it was provided.
D	Procedures, Services, or Supplies Required	Enter the CPT® or HCPCS procedure code that identifies the service provided. If the same procedure is provided multiple times on the *same date of service*, check with insurance payer for modifier requirements. The established patient was seen in the office for a moderate complexity evaluation and management. A single-view, frontal x-ray study was done of the patient's chest.
E	Diagnosis Pointer	Link the service provided to the diagnosis code(s) listed in Field 21 by entering the letter of the appropriate diagnosis. See Figure 21.7 for Field 21. Do not enter the diagnosis code. Only enter the reference letter(s) from Field 21 (A - L). A maximum of 4 letters may be entered in this space. Place letters in order of importance.
F	$ Charges	Enter the total charges for each procedure. If more than 1 unit of service was provided, multiply the charge by the number of units and then enter the total charges for all units.
G	Days or Units	Enter the units (number of services or procedures) on the date(s) in Field A. Bill all units of service provided on a given date on 1 line.
H	EPSDT/Family Planning	Early Periodic Screening, Diagnosis, and Treatment (EPSDT) is a Medicaid program for minors. If preventive services were performed to a Medicaid beneficiary who is a minor, mark this box with a "✓," an "X," or a "Y" in Box H. The patient was an adult, so the field was left blank.
I	ID Qualifier	Enter in the shaded area 1 of 5 qualifier ID numbers if the provider does not have a National Provider Identification (NPI) number: 0B State License Number 1G Provider UPIN Number G2 Provider Commercial Number LU Location Number ZZ Provider Taxonomy
J	Rendering Provider ID	(SHADED AREA) – Use for coordination of benefit information and to report Medicare and/or other insurance information. For Medicare, enter the coinsurance and deductible amounts. If the member has Medicare coverage but the service is not covered by Medicare or the provider has received no reimbursement from Medicare, the provider should "zero fill" (enter zeroes). *Leaving this field blank will cause the claim to be denied.* (NONSHADED AREA) – Use for the Rendering Provider's NPI, which is required for all providers who are mandated to maintain an NPI number.

Figure 21.14 Patient Statement

PATIENT STATEMENT

EMC Medical Center
222 Oak Drive
Boston, MA 79699

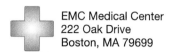

DATE
2/11/2019

FOR SERVICES RENDERED TO:
CATHY HERNANDEZ 1234 MAIN ST. BOSTON, MA 79567 PAT#10000

AMOUNT DUE	AMOUNT ENCLOSED
$75.00	

DATE	TRANSACTION	AMOUNT	BALANCE
12/31/2019	Balance forward		0.00
1/1/2019	99212 SUBSEQUENT OFFICE VISIT	45.00	45.00
1/3/2019	99212 SUBSEQUENT OFFICE VISIT	45.00	90.00
1/4/2019	99212 SUBSEQUENT OFFICE VISIT	45.00	135.00
1/4/2019	PMT – Insurance Check	60.00	75.00

0-30 DAYS	31-60 DAYS PAST	61-90 DAYS PAST	OVER 90 DAYS	AMOUNT DUE
				75.00

Collections

Collections is the term used to describe the process of collecting unpaid balances. The collection process of unpaid balances begins once the insurance payer has reviewed the insurance claim and determines the reimbursement amount and the financial responsibility of the insured. A patient's outstanding balance for a specific date of services or the entire account may become uncollectable if the guarantor refuses to pay, the insurance payer determines services or procedures are not reimbursable, and the insurance payer determines that the patient is not financially responsible. Uncollectable balances are also referred to as *bad debt.* When a patient's balance is uncollectable, the healthcare provider may decide do a write-off or use a collection agency to collect the bad debt. A **write-off** is the process of canceling out the uncollectable balance. A **contractual write-off** is the process of canceling the balance after the allowed amount has been paid and the balance is not the responsibility of the patient. Medical offices have policies and procedures for write-offs of uncollectable balances.

A **collection agency** is a business that pursues payments on debts owed by individuals or businesses. The Federal Trade Commission and the Bureau of Consumer Financial Protection are the federal agencies that oversee collection practices. The **Fair Debt Collection Practices Act** is the federal law that governs collection practices of all kinds, including collection agencies and collection departments within a business. Some of the prohibited practices stated in the Fair Debt Collection Practices Act are:

- contacting consumers by telephone outside of the hours of 8 a.m. to 9 p.m.;
- knowingly contacting a consumer at his or her place of employment;
- use of deception to misrepresent the debt;
- falsely stating that the collection actions are represented by an attorney or a law enforcement officer.

In addition to the federal agencies and regulations, many states have regulations that require collection agencies to be licensed and bonded (insured). Collection agencies that specialize in medical debt typically employ medical coders and billers to review unpaid claims.

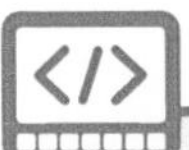

Coding for CMS

Medicare requires the medical facility to make a reasonable effort to collect deductibles and coinsurance from beneficiaries. An example of a reasonable effort is the issuance of a patient statement within 90 days of the healthcare provider receiving the EOB/ERA and the use of a collection agency. If a payment is not received by 120 days of the issuance of the first patient statement, the balance may be deemed uncollectable. Arbitrarily writing off Medicare beneficiaries' balances may be considered a violation of the False Claims Act (FCA). The FCA is discussed in Chapter 22.

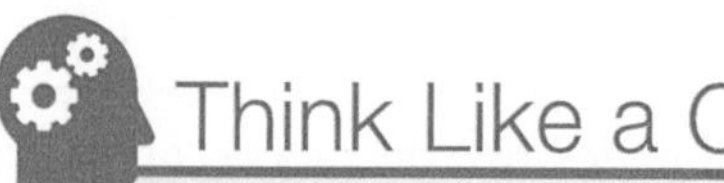

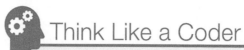

Think Like a Coder

Zion is a registered health information technician (RHIT) who is the appeals department manager. His team is responsible for compiling information and reviewing medical documentation prior to filing an appeal. During the past 3 months, Zion has identified many common errors that have led to the denial of multiple claims. Zion determines that these claims do not meet the criteria for filing an appeal. Discuss actions that can be taken to decrease the following common errors that lead to the denial of claims:

- terminated coverage;
- exclusions or noncovered services;
- invalid CPT® or HCPCS codes.

Chapter Summary

- The physician-patient contract gives permission to the physician to provide medical care to the patient. The physician-patient contract may be implied or expressed.
- A health insurance policy is a legal contract to reimburse the policyholder for a portion of the medical expense incurred for receiving medical treatment.
- A copay is a fixed amount paid prior to health services being rendered. A deductible is the set amount the insured must pay for healthcare services before the health insurance begins to pay.
- Coinsurance is a set percentage the member pays after the deductible is met (paid).
- Medicare gives beneficiaries 4 choices of coverage: Part A (hospital insurance), Part B (medical insurance), Part C (Medicare Advantage Plans), and Part D (prescription drug coverage).
- Fee for service is a reimbursement method that requests payment for each service or procedure.
- The resource-based relative value scale (RBRVS) is the method used by Medicare to create the Medicare Physician Fee Schedule (MPFS).
- The prospective payment system (PPS) is a Medicare reimbursement method in which payment is made based on a predetermined, fixed amount.
- The inpatient prospective payment system (IPPS) is a payment method that determines reimbursement for Medicare Part A (hospital insurance) inpatient services based on diagnosis-related groups (DRG).
- The outpatient prospective payment system (OPPS) reimburses medical facilities for outpatient services provided to Medicare Part B (medical insurance) beneficiaries in an acute care hospital.
- Diagnosis-related groups (DRGs) is a classification system that uses medical data collected from previous patients to create groups based on diagnosis, treatment plan, and length of stay.
- The medical billing cycle is the process followed to request reimbursement from third-party payers.
- Form CMS-1500 (02-12) is the universal paper claim form used to request payment for physician services and medical supplies from insurance payers.
- A denial of claim is the refusal of an insurance payer to reimburse the healthcare provider for medical services or procedures rendered.
- A rejected claim is one that contains a correctable error or needs additional documentation to support the claim.

- Documentation may not be added to the medical record to support the reported code after a claim has been submitted.
- A medical claim appeal is a process of requesting that a previously denied claim be reevaluated for payment.
- The Medicare appeals process consists of 5 levels and may be started after the payment determination of the first claim.
- A patient statement is a bill sent directly to the patient that requests payment for medical services, procedures, or items.
- A contractual write-off is the process of canceling the balance after the allowed amount has been paid and the balance is not the responsibility of the patient.

Navigator

Access interactive chapter review exercises, practice activities, flash cards, and study games.

Chapter 22

Healthcare Compliance

Fast Facts

- Between 2008 and 2011 there was a 75% increase in the number of individuals charged with criminal healthcare fraud.
- In 2014 Medicare made $36 billion in improper payments.
- Medicaid identified $14.4 billion in improper payments made in 2014.
- The Medicare Fraud Strike Force was established in March 2007, and as of 2015, it has recovered $1.6 billion and issued 1,808 indictments.
- In 2011, CMS began using fraud detection technology that screens all fee-for-service Medicare claims through the Fraud Prevention System. In its first year, the system generated 538 fraud investigation leads.

Sources: http://cms.gov, https://oig.hhs.gov/fraud/strike-force, http:www.stopmedicarefraud.gov

Crack the Code

Review the scenario and identify what fraud law was violated. You may need to return to this exercise after reading the chapter content.

DATE: February 24, 2019

LOCATION: Alabama Physician and Medical Practice

DESCRIPTION: The Alabama Physician and Medical Practice settles a fraud case. The group performed in-office urine drug tests of high complexity when it could have performed less-expensive, low/moderate complexity drug tests. The practice also exceeded the number of billable drug screens allowed by Medicare. In seeking reimbursement for these services, the practice reported inappropriate codes that bypassed computer programming safeguards that would have otherwise rejected such claims.

answer: False Claims Act

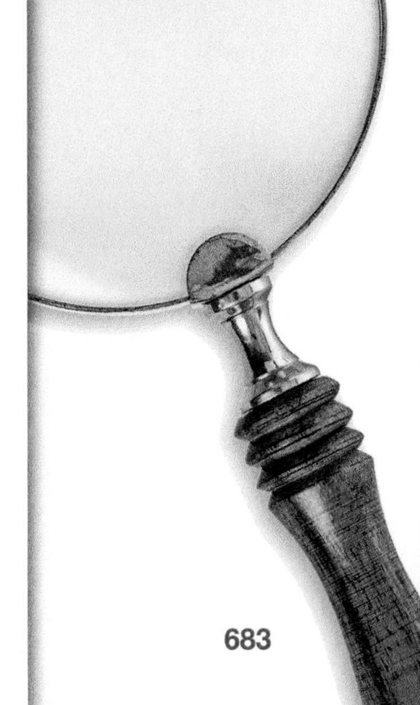

Learning Objectives

22.1 Explain the need for healthcare compliance.

22.2 Define the terms *fraud* and *abuse*.

22.3 Describe fraud and abuse laws and associated penalties.

22.4 Discuss the HIPAA Privacy Rule.

22.5 Discuss federal coding and documentation integrity programs.

22.6 Describe core elements of a medical compliance program.

22.7 Understand medical coding ethics.

Chapter Outline

The Need for Healthcare Compliance

There are many federal and state laws, regulations, and guidelines that are meant to protect the patients who receive health care paid for by federal government payers, such as Medicare and Medicaid. These federal and state laws also protect government insurers from paying for services that are considered medically unnecessary, fraudulent, or unethical. Violation of government and/or state laws and regulations may result in exclusion from participation in federal or state-funded healthcare programs, hefty monetary fines, and/or jail time.

Many of these laws and regulations govern how the business of health care is conducted. Acting in accordance with the laws and regulations that protect a specific segment of the population or a specific industry is referred to as **compliance**. Inaccurate clinical documentation and coding can place the facility at risk of violating laws and regulations. Medical coders and facilities should attempt to have a coding accuracy rate of at least 95%. A high accuracy rate will increase a facility's compliance with coding and documentation guidelines, thus decreasing the risk of legal and regulatory violations. This chapter provides coders with an in-depth look at how government agencies monitor, support, and enforce compliance to reduce the misuse of Medicare, Medicaid, and other government healthcare funds.

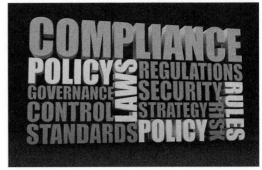

Compliance is acting in accordance with laws and regulations.

Fraud and Abuse

When fraud and abuse are associated with services rendered to Medicare and Medicaid beneficiaries, federal fraud and abuse laws apply. Many states enforce similar laws with regard to state-funded medical programs and private-pay patients. Table 22.1 lists examples of fraud and abuse and shows the distinctions between them. **Fraud** is defined by the Centers for Medicare and Medicaid Services (CMS) as making false statements or misrepresenting material facts in order to obtain some benefit or payment for which no entitlement would otherwise exist. Fraud may be committed for an

Table 22.1 Examples of Fraud and Abuse

Fraud	Abuse
Fraudulent billing practices include these scenarios: • billing for services that were not furnished and/or supplies not provided; • billing Medicare for appointments that the patient failed to keep; • altering claims forms and/or receipts in order to receive a higher payment amount; • duplicating billings to receive payment greater than allowed, such as billing both the Medicare program and the beneficiary, Medicaid, or some other insurer; • billing a person who has Medicare coverage for services provided to another person not eligible for Medicare coverage; • waiving patient financial responsibilities, such as copays, coinsurance, and deductibles. Fraudulent misuse of Medicare resources includes: • offering, paying, soliciting, or receiving bribes, kickbacks, or rebates, directly or indirectly, in cash or in kind, in order to induce referrals of patients or the purchase of goods or services that may be paid for by the Medicare program; • using another person's Medicare card to obtain medical care.	Abusive billing practices include these scenarios: • charging excessively for services or supplies; • misusing codes on a claim, such as upcoding or unbundling codes; • submitting bills to Medicare that are the responsibility of other insurers under the Medicare Secondary Payer (MSP) regulation. Abuse of Medicare resources includes: • providing medically unnecessary services or services that do not meet professionally recognized standards; • excessive referrals to other providers for unnecessary services; • violating the participating physician/supplier agreement.

Adapted from CMS, *Medicare General Information, Eligibility and Entitlement Manual*, Publication 100-01, Revision 80, 10-26-12. CMS.gov. Accessed March 24, 2015, at http://www.cms.gov/Regulations-and-Guidance/Guidance/Manuals/Downloads/ge101c01.pdf.

individual's own interest or for the benefit of another person, group, or organization. The accusing agency must prove that the act of fraud was committed intentionally, willfully, or knowingly.

Abuse is defined by CMS as practices that directly or indirectly result in unnecessary costs to the Medicare program. Improper payments are the outcome of a spectrum of improper practices from honest mistakes to intentional deception. Abuse is typically the precursor of fraud. It may begin with unintentional billing or coding errors or lack of knowledge regarding beneficiary responsibilities. Eventually abuse may escalate to fraud by intentionally and willfully ignoring CMS billing and coding guidelines. CMS uses 3 standards to determine abuse:

- Is the service or procedure medically reasonable and necessary?
- Does the service or procedure conform to professionally recognized standards?
- Are the prices for the service or procedure fair?

CONCEPTS CHECKPOINT **22.1**

Using information from Table 22.1, identify each of the following scenarios as fraud or abuse. Place an *F* to indicate Fraud and an *A* to indicate Abuse.

1. A provider repeatedly submits claims to Medicare first, even when Medicare is not the primary payer. _____
2. A provider waives deductibles for Medicare beneficiaries to increase her patient base. _____
3. A patient uses his brother's Medicare coverage to get treatment for a medical condition. _____
4. A family practice provider conducts urinalysis on all new patients. _____

Fraud and Abuse Laws

Healthcare fraud takes many forms, from fraudulent billing practices to providing medical services that are not medically reasonable or necessary. Healthcare fraud costs taxpayers billions of dollars and places patients' health at risk. Fraud and abuse laws authorize federal enforcement agencies, such as the Department of Justice, to bring criminal and/or civil actions against individuals or organizations that commit fraud and abuse in the Medicare and Medicaid programs. Violations of these laws may result in nonpayment of claims, exclusion from participation in federal healthcare programs, imprisonment, or monetary penalties.

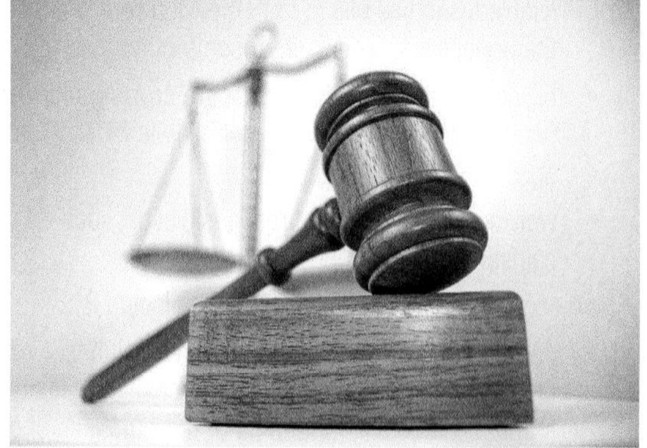

Fraud and abuse laws authorize federal enforcement agencies to bring criminal and/or civil actions against those who commit fraud and abuse.

Social Security Act Civil Monetary Penalty Provision Section 1128A of the Social Security Act provides for the levying of civil monetary penalties by the secretary of the US Department of Health and Human Services (HHS). **Civil monetary penalties (CMPs)** are substantial fines assessed against an organization, agency, or other entity (structured business) based on the type of fraud or abuse committed. The Office of Inspector General (OIG) may also impose CMPs. The type of violation committed determines the amount of the CMP. The secretary of HHS, acting through the OIG, may also exclude individuals and organizations from participation in federal healthcare programs.

False Claims Act The **False Claims Act (FCA)** is found in Title 31, Section 3729, of the United States Code. The statute prohibits individuals from knowingly submitting or causing the submission of false or fraudulent claims. FCA violations require that the person committing the act knows or should know that his or her actions will result in the submission of false information to a government healthcare program. For example, when a biller submits a claim to Medicaid for a patient whom the biller and the provider both know did not keep the appointment, the provider and the biller are both in violation of the FCA. False information on a healthcare claim may include reporting medical codes for procedures not supported by medical documentation, for services that did not take place, or for supplies not provided to a patient. **Embezzlement** is stealing money that you have been entrusted to manage. Willfully changing information on a medical claim form to divert payment to someone other than the provider of the service is a form of embezzlement and violates the FCA. An individual who attempts to cover up schemes or conceal evidence related to the willful submission of false information on a medical claim has also violated the FCA. Violations of the FCA may result in civil monetary penalties of $10,957 to $21,916 per claim and up to 3 times the amount in damages. The following actions place an individual or organization at risk of violating the FCA:

- routinely billing the same procedure or evaluation and management (E/M) code, even when documentation supports a different CPT® code;
- billing for services not provided;
- billing for services that are not medically necessary;
- billing for nonphysician providers who do not meet documentation and coding guidelines;
- submitting duplicate billings;
- retaining overpayment balances;
- incorrectly unbundling services, procedures, or products;
- reporting codes for a more extensive service than provided (**upcoding**);
- reporting lower levels of services than provided (**downcoding**).

Qui Tam Lawsuit Qui Tam (pronounced "kwee tahm") is a set of provisions that allows US citizens to sue a person or company on behalf of the US government under the False Claims Act. The term *qui tam* is derived from a Latin phrase that means "he who brings a case on behalf of the king, as well as for himself." A person who initiates the qui tam lawsuit is referred to as a *relator* or a *whistleblower*. A **whistleblower** reveals misconduct or informs the government of fraudulent acts. The initiator of the lawsuit must be represented by an attorney during the qui tam suit. The requirements to file a qui tam suit are as follows:

- The specific details must be confirmed by Medicare Integrity Contractors.
- Confirmed allegations must be referred to the Office of Inspector General.
- The whistleblower may not be currently excluded from participation in federal or state healthcare programs.
- The whistleblower may not have participated in the fraud.
- The person or group being reported is not already under investigation.
- The report leads to the recovery of at least $100 of Medicare funds.

All qui tam suits are filed under seal, which means that all records related to the suit remain secret while the Department of Justice or the local state's attorney investigates the claims. Once the government completes its investigation, it may decide to join the case as a plaintiff with the whistleblower, decline to join the case, require that the case be dismissed, or negotiate a settlement prior to the case being brought before the courts. If the case is declined by the government, the whistleblower may pursue the qui tam suit on his or her own. If the government declines to join the suit and the whistleblower wins the case, the whistleblower is entitled to a reward of 25% to 30% of the funds recovered. If the government joins the case, the whistleblower is entitled to a reward of 15% to 25% of the funds recovered. The remaining funds are returned to the agency that was violated.

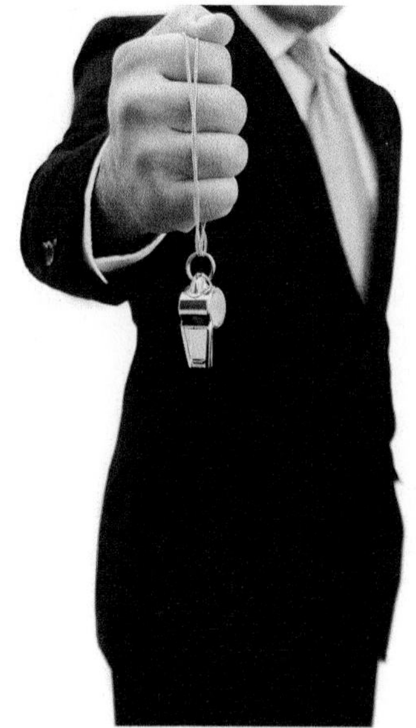

Whistleblowers reveal misconduct or inform the government of fraudulent acts.

Anti-Kickback Statute and Physician Self-Referral Law (Stark Law) Have you ever received money or a gift for referring someone to a business? Have you ever gotten a free gift for trying a new service or product? If you can answer yes to either of these scenarios, you may have been part of a kickback. A **kickback** is a payment made to someone who has aided in a transaction or appointment, especially illegally. Kickbacks are illegal in many industries. The **Anti-Kickback Statute (AKS)** prohibits knowingly and willfully offering, paying, or receiving any remuneration to induce or reward referrals for services or supplies reimbursable by Medicare or Medicaid. In health care, a kickback may influence medical decision-making by all involved parties. **Remuneration** refers to money paid for work or service. The AKS prohibits remuneration for payments made directly to the individual or indirectly, when the services are prohibited by law. The AKS seeks to protect Medicare or Medicaid beneficiaries from receiving unreasonable or unnecessary medical services or procedures due to the monetary influence. Violations of the AKS may result in criminal fines up to $10,000, civil penalties up to $50,000 for each violation, damages of up to 3 times the amount of remuneration, and possible exclusion from participation in federal healthcare programs. The OIG does not take into account whether some of the remuneration was for a legitimate purpose.

Coding Clicks

Did you ever wonder if your healthcare provider has received money from a pharmaceutical company? The Open Payments website allows you to check. Visit http://Coding.ParadigmEducation.com/OpenPayment.

Although kickbacks may be associated with any type of remuneration, the relationship between physicians and pharmaceutical companies is one that has been scrutinized for years. In 2010 the **Physician Payments Sunshine Act** was enacted to increase the public's awareness of the financial relationship between healthcare providers and pharmaceutical companies. The act requires manufacturers of drugs, medical devices, and biological and medical supplies that have relationships with government payers (Medicare, Medicaid, and the State Children's Health Insurance Program) to report to CMS all financial relationships with physicians and teaching hospitals. Information regarding these financial relationships is available to the public on the Open Payments web page on the CMS website.

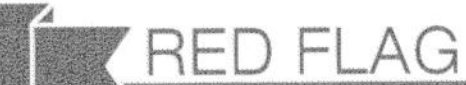

The AKS involves any type of referral. The physician self-referral law involves referrals from a physician.

The **physician self-referral law**, commonly referred to as the *Stark law*, prohibits a physician from referring patients for designated health services to an entity in which the physician or immediate family member has a financial interest. The physician self-referral law also prohibits submitting claims associated with self-referrals to Medicare. Violations of the Stark law may result in monetary penalties of up to $15,000 CMP for each service, damages of up to 3 times the amount of remuneration, and possible exclusion from participation in the Medicare or Medicaid program.

Safe Harbor Regulations Not all payments made to providers result in an AKS violation. Exceptions to the AKS are designated as safe harbors. **Safe harbors** are practices that would typically violate the AKS but are exempt from prosecution because they fit certain criteria. Examples of safe harbors are

- investments in underserved areas;
- practitioner recruitment in underserved areas;
- obstetrical malpractice insurance subsidies for underserved areas;
- sales of practices to hospitals in underserved areas;
- investments in ambulatory surgical centers;
- investments in group practices;
- referral arrangements for specialty services;
- cooperative hospital service organizations.

Coding Clicks

The Anti-Kickback Statute (AKS) and physician self-referral law (Stark law) are very similar. The OIG website provides a comparison of the laws at http://Coding.ParadigmEducation.com/AKS-Stark.

For a provider or organization to be protected by safe harbor regulations, they must meet specific criteria associated with each type of safe harbor protection. The OIG HHS website details safe harbor criteria and allows individuals to request an advisory opinion.

CONCEPTS CHECKPOINT 22.2

Read the real fraud cases below and indicate the fraud and abuse law that was violated.

1. A medical supplier in Illinois was accused by the OIG of enticing physicians and other customers to provide referrals by offering them an all-expenses-paid golf outing to the Masters Tournament. The company agreed to pay approximately $127,000 for the alleged violations. ______________

2. A Detroit-area physician admitted to conspiring with others to commit healthcare fraud by referring Medicare beneficiaries for home health care that was not medically necessary and then submitting false and fraudulent claims for the purported care to Medicare for reimbursement. He was fined $19 million for the home healthcare fraud scheme. ______________

Coding Clicks

Learn more about medical identity theft and its effect on the healthcare community at http://Coding.ParadigmEducation.com/MedicalIdentityTheft.

Medical Identity Theft **Medical identity theft** is perpetrated when a person uses someone else's name or insurance information to obtain medical treatment, acquire prescription medication, or receive payment for false claims. Depending on the actions of the thief, medical identity theft may violate the FCA, Health Insurance Portability and Accountability Act of 1996 (HIPAA) Privacy and Security Rules, and/or the Fair Credit Reporting Act (FCRA). The FCRA is violated when healthcare professionals or health information management (HIM) staff use another person's information to submit false claims to government payers. When a patient's protected health information is improperly used or shared with a medical identity thief, the HIPAA Privacy and Security Rules are violated. **Protected health information (PHI)** consists of test results, diagnoses, treatment, medications, and any other information that can be directly linked to a patient or identify the status of a patient's health. Some medical offices report unpaid debt to credit reporting agencies. The FCRA does not permit any debt associated with medical identity theft to be reported to the credit reporting companies. If medical debt associated with medical identity theft is reported, the medical facilities may be in violation of the FCRA if immediate action is not taken to correct the credit report.

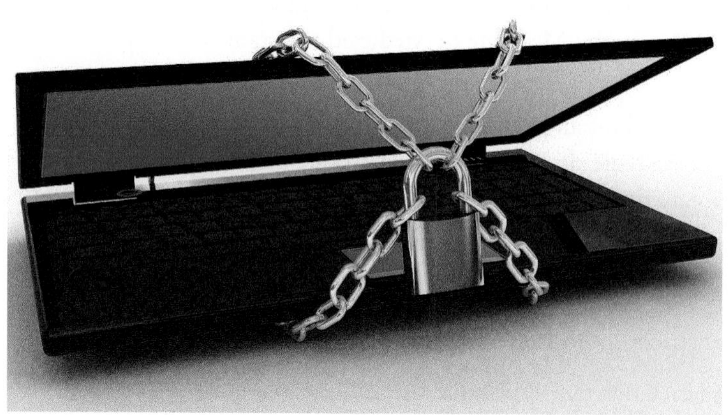

Medical identity theft may violate the FCA, HIPAA, and/or the FCRA.

The Standards for Privacy of Individually Identifiable Health Information (The Privacy Rule) The **Privacy Rule** is a set of national standards enacted to regulate the protection of health information and its selective release to improve quality of care. The Privacy Rule provides restrictions on disclosing and using individuals' PHI. The Privacy Rule was implemented by the HHS as a requirement of the HIPAA legislation. HIPAA covers only organizations that meet the criteria of a **covered entity**. HIPAA defines the following as covered entities:

- health plans, including insurance companies, health maintenance organizations (HMOs), company health plans, and government programs that pay for health care;

- healthcare clearinghouses that process health record information into standard (electronic or data) formats;
- healthcare providers who electronically transmit any health information in connection with transactions for which HHS has adopted standards.

HIPAA allows for disclosure of health information to the individual patient and for purposes of treatment, payment, and healthcare operations. Disclosures are limited to the minimum necessary when being shared within a medical facility. For example, a medical assistant may need to have access to the patient's insurance information to set up appointments with other providers. However, he or she will not need access to the payment history of the patient's account. Individuals and/or facilities may be penalized for violation of the Privacy Rule. The HHS Office for Civil Rights (OCR) is responsible for administering and enforcing compliance with the Privacy Rule. Civil monetary penalties for violations prior to February 18, 2009, were up to $100 per violation, with a cap of $25,000 per year. Violations after that date may receive CMP of $100 to $50,000 or more per violation, with a calendar year cap of $1.5 million.

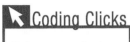

To learn more about the HIPAA Privacy Rule, visit http://Coding.ParadigmEducation.com/Privacy.

CONCEPTS CHECKPOINT **22.3**

Match the term in the first column with the correct definition in the second column.

1. _____ embezzlement
2. _____ identity theft
3. _____ remuneration
4. _____ safe harbor

a. Stealing money that has been entrusted to you to manage
b. Money paid for work or service
c. Practices exempted from prosecution under the Anti-Kickback Statute because of special criteria
d. Use of someone else's name or insurance information to obtain medical treatment, acquire prescription medication, or receive payment for false claims

Coding and Documentation Integrity Programs

It is a momentous task for the government to monitor the integrity of Medicare, Medicaid, and other government healthcare providers and suppliers. In 2015, the federal government recovered more than $2.4 billion due to self-disclosures of overpayments from Medicare and Medicaid programs as well as identification of fraud and abuse. **Self-disclosure** is the process of healthcare providers becoming aware of and reporting compliance violations to the appropriate agency or program. Self-disclosure allows the disclosing facility the opportunity to self-correct the identified violation and may minimize monetary penalties. Much of the recovery can be attributed to CMS **contracted reviewers**, who audit and review providers' documentation. They are assigned to monitor specific areas of risk in provider compliance with Medicare coverage and coding rules and to identify improper payments in the Medicare fee-for-service program. In addition to CMS, the OIG and Department of Justice have programs to prevent and combat fraud and abuse. Table 22.2 organizes some of the primary government integrity programs. The following sections discuss each program and its relevance to coders.

Table 22.2 Governmental Healthcare Integrity Programs

Program Name	Abbreviation	Agency	Purpose/Methodology
Comprehensive Error Rate Testing	CERT	CMS/HHS	Yearly audits of a random sample of claims
Medicare Administrative Contractors[a]	MACs	CMS	Provide prevention by using data collected from CERT and recovery contractors to target improper payment risks within their jurisdictions; focus on clarifying providers' use of CMS documentation and reporting guidelines in an effort to prevent improper payments
Recovery Audit Contractors	RACs	CMS	Audit data abstracted from claim submission to identify current and past improper payments
Zone Program Integrity Contractors	ZPICs	CMS	Extract data from audits and other monitoring activities to identify fraud and monitor Medicare/Medicaid data matches for 7 geographic zones
Medicaid Integrity Contractors	MICs	Medicaid	Review Medicaid provider activities, audit claims to identify overpayments and potential areas of fraud risk, and educate providers and others
Payment Error Rate Measurement	PERM	Medicaid and CHIP	Measures improper payment to produce error rates that are used to create statistical data by which audits are conducted
Health Care Fraud Prevention and Enforcement Action Team	HEAT	DOJ, OIG, HHS, CMS	Task force to improve effectiveness in combating fraud, waste, and abuse, and to provide education
List of Excluded Individuals/Entities	LEIE	OIG	Searchable database on OIG website that lists individuals and entities that are not allowed to work with Medicare, Medicaid, and other federally funded healthcare programs
Office of Inspector General (OIG) Work Plan		OIG	Presents the primary objectives of the OIG monitoring activities for the upcoming fiscal year

Abbreviations: CHIP, Children's Health Insurance Program; CMS, Centers for Medicare and Medicaid Services; DOJ, US Department of Justice; HHS, US Department of Health and Human Services; OIG, Office of Inspector General

[a]Contracted reviewers may receive a percentage of the recovered funds.

Comprehensive Error Rate Testing Contractors

The CMS implemented the **Comprehensive Error Rate Testing (CERT)** program in compliance with the **Improper Payments Elimination and Recovery Improvement Act (IPERIA)** of 2012. IPERIA required that HHS conduct annual reviews to reduce and recover improper payments. In the CERT program, a random sample of claims is selected for analysis. CERT contractors seek to identify improper payment by analyzing the medical documentation supporting a claim. A team of nurses, doctors, and certified coders review the documentation and assign the following error categories:

- no documentation;
- insufficient documentation;
- lack of medical necessity;
- incorrect coding.

If documentation review identifies that improper payments were made, CMS and CERT contractors analyze improper payment rate data and develop Error Rate Reduction Plans to reduce future improper payments. Corrective actions may include provider education, monitoring programs, recommendations to improve documentation, and updates to provider compliance programs.

Medicare Administrative Contractors

Medicare Administrative Contractors (MACs) use data collected from CERT and recovery contractors (Medicare auditors who collect overpayments) to target improper payment risks within their jurisdictions. See the jurisdictions map in Figure 22.1. MACs focus on clarifying providers' use of CMS documentation and reporting guidelines in an effort to prevent improper payments. Their efforts typically involve publishing new or revised local coverage determinations (LCDs), informative articles, and coding and documentation instructions. Coders often reference LCDs to identify documentation requirements for specific procedure code selection or to identify when a procedure is medically necessary. MACs also educate and audit providers based on the highest targeted improper payment rates.

Figure 22.1 Medicare Administrative Contractors Jurisdictions Map for Medicare Parts A and B

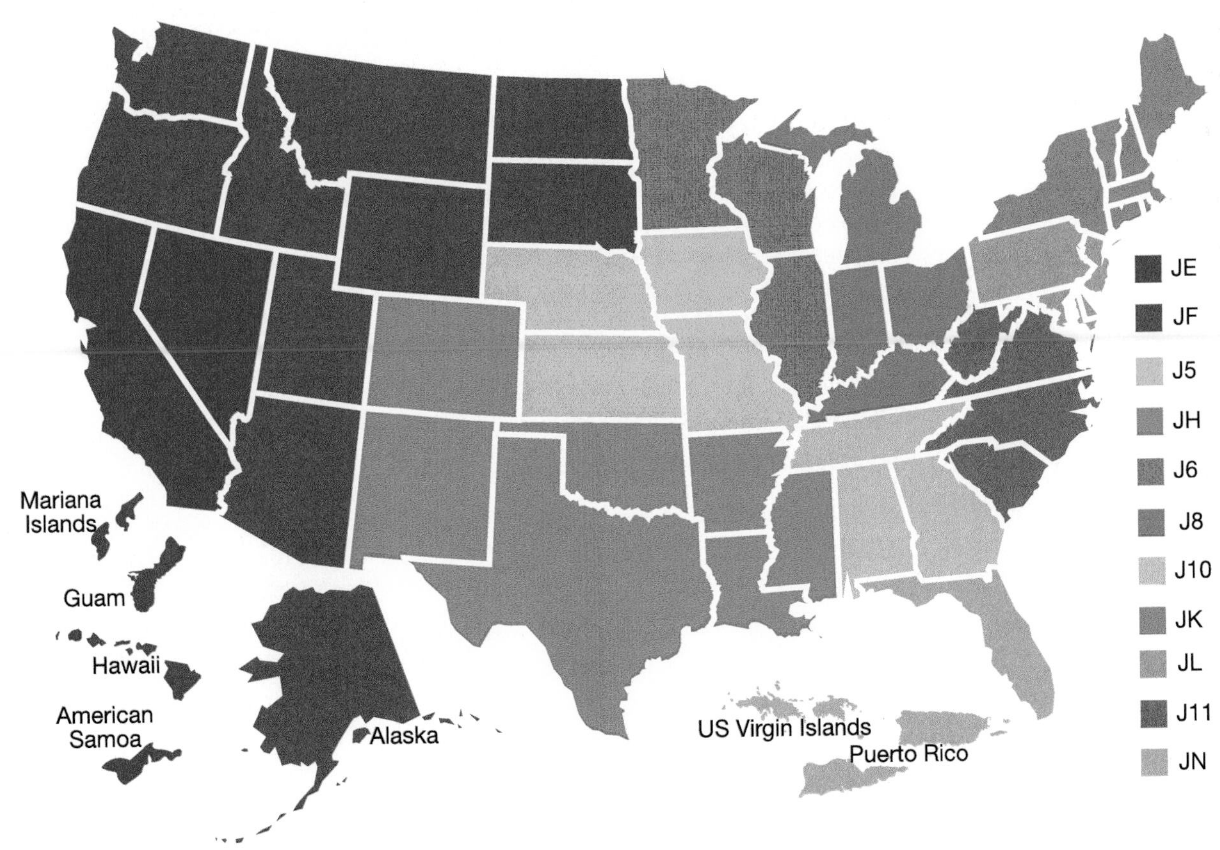

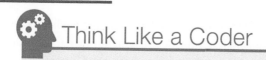

Think Like a Coder

The following is an excerpt from a CMS MAC's local coverage determination regarding the removal of benign or premalignant skin lesions. Read the LCD excerpt and then determine if the case below it can be reported for reimbursement.

Local Coverage Determination (LCD): Removal of Benign or Premalignant Skin Lesions (L27527)

Limitations

Removal of certain benign skin lesions that do not pose a threat to health or function is considered cosmetic, and as such, is not covered by the Medicare program. Lesions in sensitive anatomical locations that are not creating problems do not qualify for removal coverage on the basis of location alone. If the beneficiary wishes 1 or more of these benign asymptomatic lesions be removed for cosmetic purposes, the beneficiary becomes liable for the service rendered. The physician has the responsibility to notify the patient in advance that Medicare will not cover cosmetic dermatological surgery and that the beneficiary will be liable for the cost of the service. It is strongly advised that the beneficiary, by his or her signature, accept responsibility for payment. Charges should be clearly stated as well. Such claims billed to Medicare should append the GY - item or service is statutorily excluded or the service does not meet the definition of Medicare Benefit modifier to the CPT®/HCPCS code billed.

Scenario

Jane is a Medicare beneficiary who has a small red lesion on her arm. She tells the dermatologist that the lesion is not bothering her; however, she does not like the way it looks when she wears sleeveless shirts. The dermatologist recommends that it be removed, and the patient agrees. The dermatologist removes the lesion during the visit and sends the specimen to a pathologist to determine if it is malignant or benign. The patient is not notified of the possibility that the removal of the lesion may be denied by Medicare, and she is not asked to sign an Advance Beneficiary Notice of Noncoverage (ABN). When the report returns the following day, it is determined that the lesion is benign.

Can the service be reported?

a. Yes, all medical services performed by a licensed physician are billable.
b. Based on the LCD, the service is not billable to Medicare, but the physician may bill the patient.
c. Based on the LCD, the service is not billable to either Medicare or the patient.
d. Based on the LCD, the service is billable to Medicare but not to the patient.

Recovery Audit Contractors

Recovery Audit Contractors (RACs) analyze data abstracted from claim submissions to identify current and past improper payments. Originally, RACs monitored only Medicare Parts A and B; however, the program was expanded under the Affordable Care Act. Currently RACs review claims from Medicaid and Medicare Parts A, B, C, and D. When RACs identify likely improper payments, medical record reviews are conducted to confirm improper payment. Coders' knowledge of Medicare coding and documentation guidelines help decrease overpayment, which also helps decrease the possibility of being selected for an RAC audit. RACs are paid a percentage of the funds identified as improper payment.

Coding for CMS

As you have learned in previous chapters, Medicare has 4 parts:

- Part A—hospital insurance;
- Part B—medical insurance;
- Part C—Medicare Advantage/supplementary;
- Part D—prescription coverage.

Chapter 21 discusses Medicare coverage in detail.

Zone Program Integrity Contractors

Zone Program Integrity Contractors (ZPICs), formerly known as Program Safeguard Contractors (PSCs), are responsible for identifying fraud. The program divides the United States into 7 geographic zones, as illustrated in Figure 22.2. ZPICs extract data from audits that are reported monthly to CMS and monitor Medicare/Medicaid data matches (key links between different sets of data) for Medicare Parts A and B. In order to improve the continuity of the integrity program, CMS shares ZPIC statistics with other contracted reviewers. Coding managers may review ZPIC statistics to identify possible fraud risk areas in their practices. For example, if the ZPIC statistic identifies a high number of improper payments associated with knee replacement surgery, a coding manager will want to educate coders on documentation requirements for this procedure.

Figure 22.2 Zone Program Integrity Contractors Regional Map

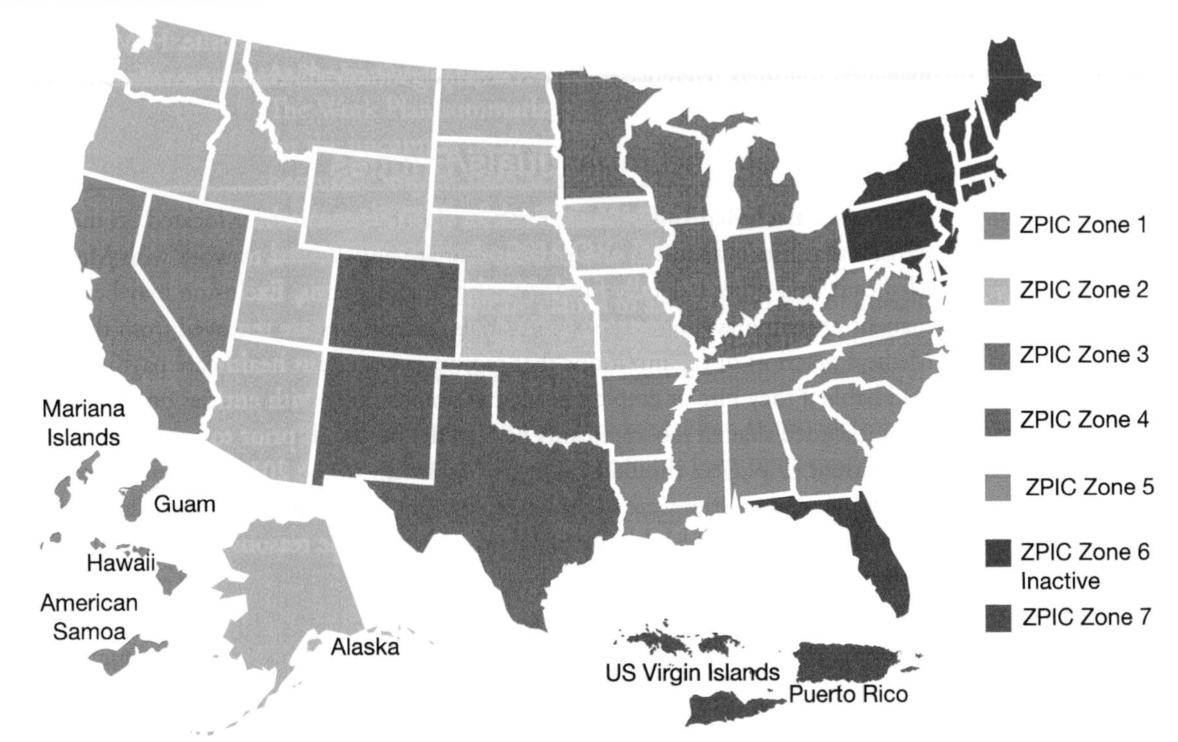

Individuals may also report fraud directly to the OIG. Claims of fraud may be reported anonymously by calling 1-800-HHS-TIPS (1-800-447-8477). Individuals who report fraud or abuse directly to the OIG or the US Office of Special Counsel (OSC) are protected from retaliation under the Whistleblower Protection Act, which states that it is illegal to take or threaten action against an employee for reporting fraud or abuse. In addition, actions may not be taken against an individual who

- files an appeal, complaint, or grievance;
- helps someone file or testifies on that person's behalf;
- cooperates with or discloses information to the OSC or OIG;
- refuses to obey an unlawful order.

If it is found that a whistleblower has suffered damages caused by retaliation, the individual may be entitled to

- job restoration;
- reversal of any suspension and other adverse actions;
- back pay;
- reasonable and foreseeable consequential damages, such as medical costs, attorney fees, and compensatory damages;
- attorney fees and expenses incurred due to retaliation.

Auditing and Monitoring

Medical facilities must have mechanisms in place to determine if a compliance program is working and to identify areas of noncompliance. Auditing and monitoring enable the facility to set standard methods of measuring the effectiveness of a compliance program and identifying risks of noncompliance. **Auditing** is a formal, unbiased review of records to check for accuracy and/or adherence to compliance policies. A compliance program may require medical record audits, human resource audits, and financial record audits. Medical record audits, also referred to as *physician documentation reviews*, are an effective means of identifying noncompliance and areas of risk associated with coding and documentation. A compliance program may require internal and external medical record audits. **Internal medical record audits** are conducted by employees of the medical practice or organization, and **external medical record audits** are conducted by outside companies. A medical record audit may be conducted when a new physician joins the practice, if a review reports possible noncompliance, after a compliance officer makes a request, or when the compliance program generates a random selection. Auditors may use audit tools or audit checklists to enhance the accuracy of the audit. Table 22.3 contains examples of questions that may appear on a medical record audit checklist.

Monitoring is the process of observing or checking the effectiveness of the compliance program over an extended period. The compliance program will determine the frequency and scope of the monitoring. This monitoring will enable a facility to remain aware of risks and ensure that all employees are following the compliance program.

Table 22.3 Example of a Medical Record Audit Checklist

Area of Compliance	Questions to Consider During Audit
Medical Necessity	❑ Are details, timing, and intensity of complaint documented? ❑ Are all diagnostic impressions documented? ❑ Did the examination include an exam of the area(s) of chief complaint? ❑ Is each diagnosis supported by the patient's chief complaint and clinical findings? ❑ Is there an appropriate diagnosis in the record to support each service provided?
Coding and Documentation	❑ Is the chief complaint clearly documented? ❑ Given the results of the diagnostic tests and other available information, is the diagnosis accurate? ❑ Does the record reflect a review of the chief complaint? ❑ If an examination was billed to the payer, is it documented in the record? ❑ If the diagnosis changed, does the healthcare record include a modified or new treatment plan? ❑ Is causation (accident, injury, and etiology) documented? ❑ Is the E/M code supported by appropriate documentation? ❑ Was the correct E/M code reported to the payer? ❑ Was the diagnosis supported by the chief complaint and objective clinical exam findings? ❑ Were all services provided and billed to the payer documented in the health record? ❑ Were services provided by a nonphysician provider? ❑ If modifiers were used, were they supported? ❑ If an Advance Beneficiary Notice form was required, was it completed in its entirety and signed by the patient?

Consistent Discipline

The facility's written policy must clearly state how compliance violations will be addressed. The written policy should address disciplinary actions associated with noncompliance, failure to detect noncompliance even when the compliance program was followed, and failure to report actual or suspected noncompliance. Discipline must be consistent, timely, and specific to the violation. The medical practice or organization should ensure that all employees know the consequences related to noncompliance. This may be accomplished by including details of disciplinary actions in new-hire orientations or during annual compliance training.

Corrective Action

When an effective compliance program exposes violations or risks of violations, steps must be taken to correct the issues. The written policy should detail what corrective actions will take place to remedy potential or actual violations. For example, if a compliance audit identifies overpayment due to inappropriate code assignment, the compliance program will detail how refunds of overpayment are handled. In addition to correcting the overpayment, the compliance program should address corrective action in relationship to the person responsible for the coding error.

CONCEPTS CHECKPOINT **22.5**

Use information from the above section to match the compliance program core elements in the first column with the correct compliance actions in the second column.

1. _____ Written policies, procedures, and standards of conduct
2. _____ Compliance program oversight
3. _____ Training and education
4. _____ Open lines of communication
5. _____ Auditing and monitoring
6. _____ Consistent discipline
7. _____ Corrective action

a. Posting the compliance hotline in the staff break room
b. Completing annual compliance training
c. Requesting medical record documentation review for a new provider
d. Terminating an employee due to verified fraud activities
e. Discussing corrective actions with human resources to ensure they are fair and consistent with labor laws
f. Contracting out compliance officers
g. Making available a complete copy of the compliance program in a binder in the coding office

Medical Coding Ethical Standards

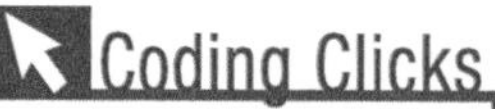

Coding Clicks

Need more guidance on coding ethics? Read the article "American Health Information Management Association Standards of Ethical Coding" in the AHIMA library at http://Coding.ParadigmEducation.com/AHIMAEthics.

In medical coding, a **code of ethics** is a compilation of standards of conduct that apply set principles by which coders may determine appropriate behavior in relationship to patients, physicians, and insurance companies. Coding ethics are not laws; however, many of the principles identified by coding ethics are based on laws. Adhering to a code of ethics will guide coders when facing ethical dilemmas that may place their integrity in jeopardy. Coding and HIM professional associations, such as the American Health Information Management Association (AHIMA) and the AAPC, have codes of ethics to which members agree to adhere when joining the organizations. Violating a professional association's code of ethics may result in loss of membership or the revocation of coding credentials. See Figure 22.3 to read the AHIMA Standards of Ethical Coding. See Figure 22.4 to read the AAPC Code of Ethics.

Figure 22.3 AHIMA Standards of Ethical Coding

Coding professionals should:

1. Apply accurate, complete, and consistent coding practices for the production of high-quality healthcare data.
2. Report all healthcare data elements (eg, diagnosis and procedure codes, present on admission indicator, discharge status) required for external reporting purposes (eg, reimbursement and other administrative uses, population health, quality and patient safety measurement, and research) completely and accurately, in accordance with regulatory and documentation standards and requirements and applicable official coding conventions, rules, and guidelines.
3. Assign and report only the codes and data that are clearly and consistently supported by health record documentation in accordance with applicable code set and abstraction conventions, rules, and guidelines.
4. Query provider (physician or other qualified healthcare practitioner) for clarification and additional documentation prior to code assignment when there is conflicting, incomplete, or ambiguous information in the health record regarding a significant reportable condition or procedure or other reportable data element dependent on health record documentation (eg, present on admission indicator).
5. Refuse to change reported codes or the narratives of codes so that meanings are misrepresented.
6. Refuse to participate in or support coding or documentation practices intended to inappropriately increase payment, qualify for insurance policy coverage, or skew data by means that do not comply with federal and state statutes, regulations, and official rules and guidelines.
7. Facilitate interdisciplinary collaboration in situations supporting proper coding practices.
8. Advance coding knowledge and practice through continuing education.
9. Refuse to participate in or conceal unethical coding or abstraction practices or procedures.
10. Protect the confidentiality of the health record at all times and refuse to access protected health information not required for coding-related activities (examples of coding-related activities include completion of code assignment, other health record data abstraction, coding audits, and educational purposes).
11. Demonstrate behavior that reflects integrity, shows a commitment to ethical and legal coding practices, and fosters trust in professional activities.

Figure 22.4 AAPC Code of Ethics

AAPC members shall:

- Maintain and enhance the dignity, status, integrity, competence, and standards of our profession.
- Respect the privacy of others and honor confidentiality.
- Strive to achieve the highest quality, effectiveness, and dignity in both the process and products of professional work.
- Advance the profession through continued professional development and education by acquiring and maintaining professional competence.
- Know and respect existing federal, state, and local laws, regulations, certifications, and licensing requirements applicable to professional work.
- Use only legal and ethical principles that reflect the profession's core values, and report activity that is perceived to violate this Code of Ethics to the AAPC Ethics Committee.
- Accurately represent the credential(s) earned and the status of AAPC membership.
- Avoid actions and circumstances that may appear to compromise good business judgment or create a conflict between personal and professional interests.

Practice Professionalism

Myla is a certified coding specialist, accredited by AHIMA, who is responsible for auditing medical records for a cardiovascular surgeon. The physician sees patients in the hospital, and the medical office bills for the inpatient E/M visits. Myla runs a billing report and randomly selects 10 inpatient E/M records to review. She requests the medical records from the medical records department. She discovers that of the 10 records requested, only 3 records exist. Myla determines that the other 7 records have been billed, but the medical records to support that a visit took place do not exist. She discusses the findings with a coworker who states, "Dr. Levy always forgets to dictate his notes. Just tell him; he will get it done for you." If Myla does what the coworker suggests, which AHIMA ethical coding standard does her actions violate? Refer to Figure 22.3 to read the AHIMA Standards of Ethical Coding. Discuss what Myla should do instead regarding the missing documentation.

Chapter Summary

- *Fraud* is defined by CMS as making false statements or misrepresenting material facts in order to obtain some benefit or payment for which no entitlement would otherwise exist.
- *Abuse* is defined by CMS as practices that, either directly or indirectly, result in unnecessary costs to the Medicare program.
- The Social Security Act enables the secretary of the US Department of Health and Human Services (HHS) to impose civil monetary penalties (CMPs), substantial fines levied against an entity (structured business) that is involved in fraud and abuse.
- The False Claims Act (FCA) prohibits individuals from knowingly submitting or causing the submission of false or fraudulent claims.
- Contracted reviewers are specialized auditors and documentation reviewers assigned to monitor specific areas of risk in provider compliance with Medicare coverage and coding rules and identify improper payments in the Medicare fee-for-service program.
- Contracted reviewers are Comprehensive Error Rate Testing (CERT) contractors, Medicare Administrative Contractors (MACs), Recovery Auditors Contractor (RACs), Zone Program Integrity Contractors (ZPICs), and Medicaid Integrity Contractors (MICs).
- The List of Excluded Individuals/Entities (LEIE) is a database on the OIG website that lists individuals and entities that are not allowed to work with Medicare, Medicaid, and other federally funded healthcare programs.
- *Compliance* refers to acting in accordance with the laws and regulations enacted to protect a specific segment of the population or a specific industry.
- A compliance program is a formal plan that outlines how an organization or medical practice will monitor, identify, correct, and disclose actions that may place the organization at risk of violating laws and regulations that affect its business. There are 7 core elements of a compliance program: (1) written policies, procedures, and standards of conduct; (2) compliance program oversight; (3) training and education; (4) open lines of communication; (5) auditing and monitoring; (6) consistent discipline; and (7) corrective action.
- Medical coding ethics are standards of conduct that apply set principles by which coders may determine appropriate behavior in relation to patients, physician, and insurance companies.

Navigator

Access interactive chapter review exercises, practice activities, flash cards, and study games.

Appendix

Answer Keys

Concepts Checkpoint Answer Key

Chapter 1

Concepts Checkpoint 1.1

1. diagnosis
2. procedure
3. supports
4. Coding
5. The health record

Concepts Checkpoint 1.2

1. g
2. e
3. b
4. d
5. c
6. f
7. a

Concepts Checkpoint 1.3

1. health information management/HIM
2. inpatient coders
3. revenue cycle
4. chargemaster
5. CPT® and HCPCS (HCPCS Level I and Level II codes)

Concepts Checkpoint 1.4

1. RHIT
2. 20 hours every 2 years
3. 20 hours every 2 years
4. 30 hours every 2 years
5. CCA, CCS, CCS-P

Concepts Checkpoint 1.5

1. the daily operations of the coding department. They may also be required to provide training to keep coders knowledgeable of coding and reporting guidelines.
2. ICD-10, CPT®, and HCPCS codes, and must have strong computer and communication skills.

Concepts Checkpoint 1.6

1. standards
2. A compliance plan
3. intentionally

Chapter 2

Concepts Checkpoint 2.1

1. October 1, 2015
2. AMA
3. Healthcare Common Procedure Coding System
4. National Codes
5. CPT® Codes

Concepts Checkpoint 2.2

1. a
2. b
3. a
4. d

Concepts Checkpoint 2.3

1. b
2. d
3. c
4. d

Concepts Checkpoint 2.4

1. d
2. c
3. a

Concepts Checkpoint 2.5

1. d
2. a
3. c
4. b

Concepts Checkpoint 2.6

1. a
2. b
3. c
4. d
5. c

Chapter 3

Concepts Checkpoint 3.1

b, c, e, f, g, h, i

Concepts Checkpoint 3.2

1. F
2. T
3. T
4. T
5. F

Concepts Checkpoint 3.3

1. e
2. c
3. d
4. b
5. a

Concepts Checkpoint 3.4

1. medical office
2. self-administered
3. administration
4. route of administration
5. integral part

Concepts Checkpoint 3.5

1. T
2. T
3. F
4. F
5. T

Chapter 4

Concepts Checkpoint 4.1

1. F
2. T
3. F
4. T

Concepts Checkpoint 4.2

1. a
2. c
3. b

Concepts Checkpoint 4.3

Answers will vary, and include 6 of the following modifiers:

24, 25, 27, 57, 58, 59, 78, 79, 91

Concepts Checkpoint 4.4

1. T
2. F
3. B
4. A

Concepts Checkpoint 4.5

1. T
2. F
3. Two services described by timed codes are performed sequentially during the same encounter.
4. A diagnostic procedure is the basis for performing a therapeutic procedure.
5. A diagnostic procedure occurs subsequent to a completed therapeutic procedure.

Chapter 5

Concepts Checkpoint 5.1

1. c
2. a
3. d
4. d
5. b

Concepts Checkpoint 5.2

1. T
2. F
3. T
4. F
5. T

Chapter 6

Concepts Checkpoint 6.1

1. social history
2. low severity
3. chief complaint
4. 3
5. family history

Concepts Checkpoint 6.2

1. problem-focused
2. comprehensive
3. 2
4. brief
5. modifying

Concepts Checkpoint 6.3

1. d
2. b
3. a
4. c

Concepts Checkpoint 6.4

1. 1. Number of diagnoses or management options;
   2. Amount and/or complexity of data to be reviewed;
   3. Risk of significant complications, morbidity, and/or mortality
2. 2
3. Two of the 3 levels must be met or exceeded to qualify for the level of MDM chosen.

Concepts Checkpoint 6.5

1. F
2. F
3. T
4. T
5. T

Concepts Checkpoint 6.6

1. 99282, *Evaluation and Management, Office and Other Outpatient*
2. 99284, *Evaluation and Management, Emergency Department*
3. No, they must be hospital-based and open 24 hours.

Chapter 7

Concepts Checkpoint 7.1

1. b
2. a
3. e
4. d
5. c

Concepts Checkpoint 7.2

1. T
2. F
3. T
4. T
5. F

Concepts Checkpoint 7.3

1. T
2. T
3. F
4. F
5. T

Concepts Checkpoint 7.4

1. F
2. T
3. F
4. T
5. F
6. F

Concepts Checkpoint 7.5

1. 00322, *Anesthesia, thyroid*
2. 01961, *Anesthesia, childbirth, cesarean delivery*
3. 00172, *Anesthesia, cleft palate, repair*
4. 01472, *Anesthesia, Achilles tendon repair*
5. 00454, *Anesthesia, clavicle*
6. 00144, *Anesthesia, corneal transplant*
7. 00864, *Anesthesia, cystectomy*
8. 00794, *Anesthesia, pancreatectomy*
9. 00921, *Anesthesia, vasectomy*
10. 00862, *Anesthesia, nephrectomy*

Chapter 8

Concepts Checkpoint 8.1

1. c
2. e
3. g

4. a
5. d
6. f
7. b
8. i
9. h
10. j

Concepts Checkpoint 8.2

1. Yes
2. No
3. No
4. Yes
5. Yes
6. No
7. Yes
8. Yes

Concepts Checkpoint 8.3

1. T
2. T
3. F
4. T
5. F

Concepts Checkpoint 8.4

1. T
2. F
3. F
4. T
5. T

Concepts Checkpoint 8.5

1. 60100, Thyroid gland, needle biopsy; Biopsy, thyroid
2. 59514, Cesarean delivery, delivery only; Pregnancy, cesarean delivery, only
3. 40720, Cleft Lip, repair, secondary; Repair, cleft lip
4. 48150, Whipple Procedure; Pancreatectomy, partial
5. 55259, Vasectomy; Vas Deferens, excision

Chapter 9

Concepts Checkpoint 9.1

1. d
2. b
3. e
4. f
5. c
6. a

Concepts Checkpoint 9.2

1. T
2. T
3. F

Concepts Checkpoint 9.3

1. F
2. T
3. F
4. T
5. T

Concepts Checkpoint 9.4

1. T
2. F
3. F
4. T

Chapter 10

Concepts Checkpoint 10.1

1. c
2. e
3. b
4. a
5. d

Concepts Checkpoint 10.2

1. T
2. T
3. F

Concepts Checkpoint 10.3

1. T
2. T
3. T

Concepts Checkpoint 10.4

1. T
2. F
3. F

Chapter 11

Concepts Checkpoint 11.1

1. e
2. d
3. c
4. a
5. b

Concepts Checkpoint 11.2

1. T
2. T
3. F

Concepts Checkpoint 11.3

1. T
2. F
3. T
4. T
5. F

Concepts Checkpoint 11.4

1. F
2. T
3. T
4. T

Concepts Checkpoint 11.5

1. is not
2. may
3. assisted
4. is

Chapter 12

Concepts Checkpoint 12.1

1. c
2. d
3. a
4. b
5. e

Concepts Checkpoint 12.2

1. d
2. b
3. d

Concepts Checkpoint 12.3

1. centrally
2. 5
3. repair
4. is
5. does

Concepts checkpoint 12.4

1. a, b

Concepts Checkpoint 12.5

1. F
2. F
3. T

Chapter 13

Concepts Checkpoint 13.1

1. digestive system
2. oral cavity
3. small
4. large

Concepts Checkpoint 13.2

1. T
2. T
3. F
4. T

Concepts Checkpoint 13.3

1. c
2. d
3. e
4. b
5. a

Concepts Checkpoint 13.4

1. T
2. T
3. T
4. T
5. T

Concepts Checkpoint 13.5

1. c
2. a
3. b
4. d
5. e

Concepts Checkpoint 13.6

1. d
2. b
3. f
4. c
5. e
6. a

Concepts Checkpoint 13.7

1. T
2. F
3. F
4. T
5. T
6. T

Chapter 14

Concepts Checkpoint 14.1

1. cystorrhaphy
2. cysto and vesico
3. surgically crushing a stone in the kidney
4. visual exam of the kidney using a scope
5. nephropexy
6. bladder
7. ureters
8. urethra

Concepts Checkpoint 14.2

1. cadaver
2. backbench
3. allotransplantation
4. allotransplantation
5. autotransplantation

Concepts Checkpoint 14.3

1. a
2. d
3. d

Concepts Checkpoint 14.4

1. F
2. T
3. T
4. F
5. F

Concepts Checkpoint 14.5

1, 5, and 6

Concepts Checkpoint 14.6

1. F
2. F
3. F
4. F
5. F

Chapter 15

Concepts Checkpoint 15.1

1. c
2. d
3. e
4. b
5. a

Concepts Checkpoint 15.2

1. F
2. F
3. T

Concepts Checkpoint 15.3

1. c
2. d
3. b
4. e
5. a

Concepts Checkpoint 15.4

1. a
2. b
3. c
4. b
5. c

Concepts Checkpoint 15.5

1. a
2. b
3. b

Chapter 16

Concepts Checkpoint 16.1

1. meninges
2. cerebellum
3. autonomic
4. central
5. ventricles

Concepts Checkpoint 16.2

1. F
2. F
3. F

Concepts Checkpoint 16.3

1. T
2. T
3. F

Concepts Checkpoint 16.4

1. F
2. T
3. F
4. T
5. T

Chapter 17

Concepts Checkpoint 17.1

1. c
2. a
3. d
4. b
5. c

Concepts Checkpoint 17.2

1. b
2. a
3. c
4. a
5. b

Concepts Checkpoint 17.3

1. b
2. a
3. c
4. c
5. b

Concepts Checkpoint 17.4

1. T
2. T
3. T
4. T
5. F

Concepts Checkpoint 17.5

1. b
2. c
3. d
4. a

Concepts Checkpoint 17.6

1. b
2. d
3. c
4. e
5. a

Chapter 18

Concepts Checkpoint 18.1

1. a
2. e
3. c
4. b
5. d

Concepts Checkpoint 18.2

1. c
2. d
3. b
4. a
5. b

Concepts Checkpoint 18.3

1. T
2. T
3. F
4. T
5. T

Concepts Checkpoint 18.4

1. c
2. d
3. a
4. b

Concepts Checkpoint 18.5

1. F
2. T
3. T
4. T
5. F

Concepts Checkpoint 18.6

1. c
2. b
3. d
4. a

Concepts Checkpoint 18.7

1. c
2. d
3. c
4. a

Concepts Checkpoint 18.8

1. T
2. T
3. T
4. T

Chapter 19

Concepts Checkpoint 19.1

1. F
2. F
3. F
4. T
5. T

Concepts Checkpoint 19.2

1. T
2. T
3. T

Concepts Checkpoint 19.3

1. F
2. T
3. F

4. T
5. T

Chapter 20

Concepts Checkpoint 20.1

1. Hemodialysis filters blood through venous access; peritoneal dialysis filters peritoneal fluid through an opening in the abdomen.
2. E/M services not related to renal disease can be coded separately.
3. ESRD services (90951-90966) include outpatient evaluation and management of the dialysis visits, establishing a dialysis treatment cycle, telephone calls, and management of the patient.

Concepts Checkpoint 20.2

1. F
2. T
3. F
4. T
5. F

Concepts Checkpoint 20.3

1. T
2. T
3. T

Concepts Checkpoint 20.4

1. Therapeutic
2. Prosthetics
3. do not require
4. should not
5. cannot

Chapter 21

Concepts Checkpoint 21.1

1. c
2. b
3. e
4. a
5. d

Concepts Checkpoint 21.2

1. b
2. d
3. a
4. c
5. e

Concepts Checkpoint 21.3

1. T
2. T
3. F
4. T
5. T
6. T

Concepts Checkpoint 21.4

1. a
2. c
3. c
4. a
5. d

Concepts Checkpoint 21.5

1. d
2. c
3. e
4. b
5. a

Concepts Checkpoint 21.6

1. T
2. F
3. T
4. T
5. T

Concepts Checkpoint 21.7

1. a
2. d
3. b
4. g
5. j

Concepts Checkpoint 21.8

1. Procedure code was invalid on the date of service.
2. The procedure is inconsistent with the patient's age.
3. This procedure or procedure/modifier combination is not compatible with another procedure or procedure/modifier combination provided on the same day according to the National Correct Coding Initiative or workers compensation state regulations/ fee schedule requirements.
4. Service not furnished directly to the patient and/ or not documented.

5. The procedure code is inconsistent with the patient's gender.

Concepts Checkpoint 21.9

1. F
2. T
3. T
4. T
5. F

Chapter 22

Concepts Checkpoint 22.1

1. A
2. F
3. F
4. A

Concepts Checkpoint 22.2

1. AKS
2. AKS and False Claims Act

Concepts Checkpoint 22.3

1. a
2. d
3. b
4. c

Concepts Checkpoint 22.4

1. b
2. c
3. d

Concepts Checkpoint 22.5

1. g
2. f
3. b
4. a
5. c
6. e
7. d

Let's Try One Answer Key

Chapter 2

Let's Try One 2.1

1. Graft, bone; mandible (includes obtaining graft)
2. Computed tomography, bone mineral density study, 1 or more sites; axial skeleton (eg, hips, pelvis, spine)
3. Aspiration and/or injection of ganglion cyst(s) any location
4. Esophagogastroduodenoscopy, flexible, transoral; with directed submucosal injection(s), any substance

Let's Try One 2.2

1. 99429, *Unlisted preventive medicine service*
2. 29799, *Unlisted procedure, casting or strapping*
3. 69979, *Unlisted procedure, temporal bone, middle fossa approach*

Let's Try One 2.3

4, 5, and 8 are not in the E/M Guidelines.

Let's Try One 2.4

1. 1050F, *Performance Measures, Melanoma, history, moles*
2. 4016F, *Performance Measures, osteoarthritis, interventions, anti-inflammatory/analgesics*
3. 6020F, *Performance Measures, Stroke & Stroke Rehabilitation, Patient Safety, NPO order*

Let's Try One 2.5

1. 00100, *Anesthesia for procedure on salivary glands*
2. 10021, *Fine needle aspiration; without imaging guidance*
3. 70010, *Myelography, posterior fossa*
4. 1000F, *Tobacco use assessed*
5. 3006F, *Chest X-ray results documented and reviewed*
6. 0019T, *Extracorporeal shock wave*

Let's Try One 2.6

1. Possible answers:
   Aspiration/Cyst
   Cyst/Ganglion
   Ganglion/Cyst
2. Possible answers:
   Esophagogastroduodenoscopy/Transoral
   Esophagogastroduodenoscopy/Biopsy
3. Possible answers:
   Arteriovenous Fistula/Repair
   Arteriovenous Fistula/Abdomen

Let's Try One 2.7

1. ⊘
2. ▲
3. +
4. #
5. ⊘
6. ▲
7. ★

Chapter 3

Let's Try One 3.1

1. P9035
2. A4580, A4590, Q4001-Q4051
3. L0180-L0200
4. L6900-L6915
5. A7003, A7005, A7006

Let's Try One 3.2

1. A4423, *Ostomy, pouches*
2. A5114, *Leg, strap, replacement*
3. A4252, *Blood, keytone test*
4. A7046, *Humidifier*

Let's Try One 3.3

1. E0157, *Walker, attachments*
2. E1003, *Wheelchair, accessories*
3. G0372, *Service, physician, for mobility device*
4. G0437, *Counseling, smoking and tobacco cessation*
5. G0177, *Training services, mental health*

Let's Try One 3.4

1. J1573, *Immune, globulin, HepaGam B*
2. J2590, *HCPCS Table of Drugs, Oxytocin, up to 10 mg.*
3. J7610, *HCPCS Table of Drugs, Albuterol, concentrated*
4. J7336, *Capsaicin patch*

Let's Try One 3.5

1. K0858, *Wheelchair*
2. L0220, *Rib belt, thoracic*
3. L1960, *Orthotic devices, ankle-foot*
4. P9047, *Albumin, human 25%*
5. Q0114, Fern test

Let's Try One 3.6

1. S0618, Evaluation, hearing
2. V2631, *Lens, intraocular*
3. T5001, *Positioning seat*
4. V2502, *Lens, contact*
5. V2624, *Prosthesis, eye*

Chapter 4

Let's Try One 4.1

1. X
2. Yes
3. No
4. No
5. Yes
6. Yes
7. Yes

Let's Try One 4.2

32

Let's Try One 4.3

1. 51
2. 55
3. 53

Let's Try One 4.4

1. 66
2. 77

Let's Try One 4.5

1. c
2. a
3. b
4. d

Chapter 5

Let's Try One 5.1

1. Drainage of generalized peritonitis, appendectomy
2. Pre-op diagnosis: Acute appendicitis
   Post-op diagnosis: ruptured appendicitis with peritonitis
3. Yes, an appendectomy was done.

Chapter 6

Let's Try One 6.1

99204, *Evaluation and Management, Office and Other Outpatient*

Let's Try One 6.2

99231, *Evaluation and Management, Hospital*

Let's Try One 6.3

99354, 99355, *Evaluation and Management, Prolonged Services*

Let's Try One 6.4

99386, *Evaluation and Management, Preventive Services*

Let's Try One 6.5

99462, *Evaluation and Management, Newborn Care*

Let's Try One 6.6

99497, 99498, *Evaluation and Management, Advanced Care Planning*

Chapter 7

Let's Try One 7.1

1. No
2. No
3. Yes

Let's Try One 7.2

1. $700.00; 4 base units + 3 time units x $100 = $700

Let's Try One 7.3

1. No, epidural catheter was used for administering anesthesia and is not separately reportable.
2. Yes
3. Yes, 01996
4. No
5. No

Let's Try One 7.4

1. General
2. Yes
3. Anesthesia, hernia repair abdomen, lower
4. Yes, under 1 year of age
5. No, procedure is specifically for a patient under 1 year of age. CPT® note under code states, "Do not report 00834 in conjunction with 99100"
6. 00834

Let's Try One 7.5

1. General
2. Yes
3. Anesthesia, tubal ligation
4. P2
5. No
6. 00851

Chapter 8

Let's Try One 8.1

50543, *laparoscopy, surgical; partial nephrectomy*

Let's Try One 8.2

11100, +11101, *skin biopsy*

Let's Try One 8.3

1. 57200, *Colporrhaphy, nonobstetrical*
2. 19318, *Mammaplasty, reduction*
3. 32555, *Thoracentesis, with imaging guidance*

Let's Try One 8.4

1. Hernia Repair
2. 49500, *Hernia Repair, inguinal, initial, child under 5 years*

Chapter 9

Let's Try One 9.1

10180, *Incision and Drainage, wound infection, skin*

Let's Try One 9.2

1. b
2. c
3. d
4. 11000, 11001, *Debridement, skin, eczematous*
5. 11004, *Debridement, skin, infected*

Let's Try One 9.3

1. 11406, *Excision, lesion, skin, benign. Simple closure is included in the excision.* (4.0 +0.5 margin + 0.5 margin= 5 cm)
2. 11643, *Excision, lesion, skin, malignant. Single layer closure is a simple closure. Simple closure is included in the excision.* (2.0 + 0.3 margin +0.3 margin =2.6cm)
3. 11644, 11603-51, *Excision, lesion, skin, malignant. Simple closure is included in the excision.*
   (Lip 2.5 +0.3+0.3 = 3.1, Chest 1.5 +0.3+ 0.3=2.1)

Let's Try One 9.4

1. 12001, *Repair, wound, simple*
2. 12042, *Repair, wound, intermediate*
3. 12051, *Repair, wound, intermediate*

Let's Try One 9.5

1. 15002, 15003, *Preparation, recipient site, skin graft* 15100, 15101 *Skin graft and flap, split graft*

2. 14040, *Adjacent tissue transfer or rearrangement, forehead, cheeks, chin, mouth, neck, axillae, genitalia, hands and/or feet; defect 10 sq cm or less*
3. 15275, *Application of skin substitute graft to face, scalp, eyelids, mouth, neck, ears, orbits, genitalia, hands, feet, and/or multiple digits, total wound surface area up to 100 sq cm; first 25 sq cm or less wound surface area* for feet, 15271, *Application of skin substitute graft to trunk, arms, legs, total wound surface area up to 100 sq cm; first 25 sq cm or less wound surface area* +15272 x2, *each additional 25 sq cm wound surface area, or part thereof*, for calf and ankle.

Let's Try One 9.6

1. 17000, 17003, 17003, Destruction, lesion, skin, premalignant
2. 17271, Destruction, lesion, skin, malignant
3. 17004, Destruction, lesion, skin, premalignant

Chapter 10

Let's Try One 10.1

1. 20550, *Injection, tendon sheath*
2. 20550, *Injection, tendon sheath*
3. 20551, *Injection, tendon origin, insertion*
4. 20550, *Injection, tendon sheath*

Let's Try One 10.2

1. 20610, *Injection, joint*
2. 20553, *Injection, trigger point, three or more muscles*
3. 20526, *Injection, carpal tunnel, therapeutic*

Let's Try One 10.3

1. 27445, *Arthroplasty, knee, hinge prosthesis (eg, Walldius type)*
2. RT

Let's Try One 10.4

1. 28292-RT, *Bunion Repair, Mayo*
2. 28292-RT, *Bunion Repair, Mayo*
3. 28291-LT, *Hallux Rigidus Correction with implant*
4. 28289-RT, *Cheilectomy, metatarsophalangeal joint release*

Let's Try One 10.5

1. 27758, *Fracture, tibia, shaft*
2. RT

Let's Try One 10.6

1. Bilateral retinacular release
2. 29873, *Arthroscopy, knee, surgical; with lateral release*
3. 50, *Bilateral procedure*

Chapter 11

Let's Try One 11.1

30400, *Rhinoplasty, primary*

Let's Try One 11.2

1. 31255, *Ethmoidectomy, endoscopic*
2. 30110, *Polypectomy, nose, simple*
3. 31256, *Antrostomy, sinus, maxillary*
4. 30430, *Rhinoplasty, secondary*
5. 30300, *Nose, removal, foreign body*

Let's Try One 11.3

1. Direct
2. Yes
3. Yes
4. 31536, *Laryngoscopy, direct, biopsy*

Let's Try One 11.4

1. Fiberoptic bronchoscopy
2. No
3. 31622, *Bronchoscopy, exploration*

Let's Try One 11.5

32554, *Thoracentesis, needle or catheter, aspiration of the pleural space; without imaging guidance*

Let's Try One 11.6

1. Biopsy lung nodule
2. VATS (thoracoscopy)
3. Answers may vary. Possible answers include: Lung, biopsy, thoracoscopy, nodule Biopsy, lung, thoracoscopy
4. 32608-RT *Thoracoscopy; with diagnostic biopsy(ies) of lung nodule(s) or mass(es), (eg. Wedge, incisional), unilateral RT (right)*

Chapter 12

Let's Try One 12.1

1. 33207, *Insertion of new or replacement of permanent pacemaker with transvenous electrode(s); ventricular*
2. 33233, *Pacemaker, removal, pulse generator only*, 33234 *Pacemaker, removal, transvenous electrode*, 33207 *Pacemaker, replacement, insertion*
3. 33214, *Pacemaker, upgrade*

Let's Try One 12.2

1. 33511, *Coronary Artery Bypass Graft, Venous Bypass*
2. 33534, *Coronary Artery Bypass Graft, Arterial Bypass*
3. 33534, *Coronary Artery Bypass Graft, Arterial Bypass*, +33517, *Coronary Artery Bypass Graft, Arterial-Venous Bypass*

Let's Try One 12.3

1. Endovascular repair of infrarenal abdominal aortic aneurysm
2. Aortic tube
3. 34800, *Aneurysm Repair, Abdominal Aorta*

Let's Try One 12.4

1. 35556, *Bypass Graft, Venous, Femoral-Popliteal*
2. 35621, *Bypass Graft, Venous, Axillary-Femoral*
3. 35583, *Bypass In-Situ, Femoral-Popliteal*

Let's Try One 12.5

1. Yes
2. Centrally inserted
3. Yes
4. Port
5. 36561, *Central venous catheter placement, insertion, central, tunneled with port*

Chapter 13

Let's Try One 13.1

40702, *Plastic repair of cleft lip/nasal deformity; primary bilateral, 1 of 2 stages*

Let's Try One 13.2

1. 2
2. 1
3. Yes
4. 40812, *Excision of lesion of mucosa and submucosa, vestibule of mouth; with simple repair*, 40812-59, *Excision of lesion of mucosa and submucosa, vestibule of mouth; with simple repair – distinct procedural service*, 40808-59, *Biopsy, vestibule of mouth – distinct procedural service*

Let's Try One 13.3

1. 40845, *Vestibuloplasty*
2. 41252, *Repair, Tongue, Laceration*

Let's Try One 13.4

1. 42107, *Excision, Uvula, Lesion*
2. 42210, Cleft Palate, Repair

Let's Try One 13.5

42507, *Salivary Duct, Diversion*

Let's Try One 13.6

1. 42831, *Adenoids, Excision*
2. 42860, *Tonsils, Excision, Tag*

Let's Try One 13.7

1. An oblique cervical incision and a horizontal upper midline abdominal incision.
2. No
3. Yes
4. Yes
5. 43108, *Total or near total esophagectomy, without thoracotomy; with colon interposition or small intestine reconstruction, including intestine mobilization, preparation and anastomosis(es)*

Let's Try One 13.8

1. 43217, *Esophagoscopy, Transoral, Removal, Tumor/Polyp*
2. 43204, *Esophagoscopy, Injection*

Let's Try One 13.9

43239, *Endoscopy, Gastrointestinal, Upper, Biopsy*

Let's Try One 13.10

1. 43275, *Cholangiopancreatography, with Removal, Stent*
2. 43260, Cholangiopancreatography

Let's Try One 13.11

43279, *Esophagomyotomy, laparoscopic*

Let's Try One 13.12

44365, *Small intestinal endoscopy, enteroscopy beyond second portion of duodenum, not including ileum; with removal of tumor(s), polyp(s), or other lesion(s) by hot biopsy forceps or bipolar cautery*

Let's Try One 13.13

44820, *Excision, lesion, mesentery*

Let's Try One 13.14

47135, Transplantation, liver

Let's Try One 13.15

47610, *Cholecystectomy, with exploration, common duct*

Let's Try One 19.5

88305, *Level IV*

Chapter 20

Let's Try One 20.1

90471, 90658, *Administration, Immunization, One vaccine/toxoid*

Let's Try One 20.2

90834, *Psychotherapy, Individual patient/family member*

Let's Try One 20.3

90958, *ESRD, End Stage Renal Disease Services*

Let's Try One 20.4

92014, *Eye Exam, Established patient*
92310, *Contact Lens Services, Fitting and Prescription*

Let's Try One 20.5

94003, *Pulmonary, therapeutic, ventilation assist*

Let's Try One 20.6

95125, *Allergen Immunotherapy, Allergenic Extracts, Injection and Provision*

Let's Try One 20.7

96409, *Chemotherapy, intravenous, push*

Let's Try One 20.8

97113 x 2, *Physical Medicine/Therapy/Occupational Therapy, Aquatic therapy*

Let's Try One 20.9

98926, *Osteopathic manipulation*

Let's Try One 20.10

99075, *Special Services, Medical testimony*

Let's Try One 20.11

99507, *Home Services, catheter care*

Glossary

\+ Add-on code.

⊘ Code exempt from use with modifier.

▲ Description has been substantially altered from the previous years.

⊙ Moderate (conscious) sedation.

● New code.

▶◀ New or revised text.

( ) Parenthetic note.

✗ Pending FDA approval.

Resequenced code.

AAPC A group that offers its members education and training programs, certifications, and networking and job opportunities. Formerly known as the *American Academy of Professional Coders.*

abdomen The area of the body between the chest and the pelvis.

abdominal hernia A protrusion of the abdominal organs or structures through the front of the abdominal wall.

ablation The removal of a body part or destruction of its function by vaporization, chipping, or other erosive processes.

abortion A spontaneous or surgically assisted termination of a pregnancy.

abscess A localized collection of pus at the site of an infection; a cavity formed by liquefactive necrosis within solid tissue.

abstract To take away.

abstracting Sifting through the data in a patient's health record to extract the pertinent information for reporting the appropriate code(s).

abuse Incidents or practices (usually considered fraudulent) that are inconsistent with accepted sound medical business or fiscal practices.

accessory sinuses A network of sinuses around the nasal cavity.

acupuncture The practice of inserting small needles into the patient in specific areas to relieve pain.

add-on code A code that describes additional procedures or services that are related to the primary procedure performed and are reported in addition to the code for the primary procedure.

adenoidectomy The surgical removal of the adenoids.

adenoids Structures located at the back of the throat. Also known as the *pharyngeal tonsils.*

adhesion Inflammatory bands that connect opposing serous surfaces resulting from trauma or inflammation.

adipose tissue Fat.

administrative data Data that include identifying information: patient's full name, address, date of birth, gender, marital status, place of employment, insured status, payment arrangements, and other personal details that the facility or provider wishes to collect. adnexa The eye's accessory structures, which include the lacrimal glands, extraocular muscles, eyelids, eyelashes, eyebrows, and the conjunctiva.

adrenal gland A gland that sits on top of the each kidney and secretes the hormones cortisol, aldosterone, epinephrine (adrenaline), and norepinephrine (noradrenaline).

adrenalectomy The removal of the adrenal glands.

Advance Beneficiary Notice of Noncoverage (ABN) A standardized notice that a healthcare provider or vendor must give to a Medicare beneficiary before providing certain services or procedures that Medicare may deem not medically necessary.

advance directive A legal document that contains the patient's wishes regarding medical treatment and life-supporting measures.

allergen immunotherapy A therapy that involves giving the patient a series of injections of specific allergens in increasing doses to reduce the response to allergic triggers. Also known as *allergy vaccine therapy.*

allergy testing A type of testing that involves the administration of substances to determine a patient's sensitivity to the substance.

allied health professional A person that provides ancillary and support services to assist in the care of patients.

allogenic An organ or tissue that comes from a donor.

allogenic transplantation A procedure that involves receiving organs or tissue from a donor. Also known as *allotransplantation.*

allotransplantation A procedure that involves receiving organs or tissue from a donor. Also known as *allogenic transplantation.*

allowed amount The average or maximum amount that may be reimbursed per service, procedure, or item to the provider from the insurance payer.

alveoloplasty The smoothing or re-contouring of the alveolar ridge or tooth sockets, usually performed prior to fitting for dentures.

ambulatory payment classification (APC) A system that groups similar services to determine reimbursement rates.

American Dental Association (ADA) An organization that maintains CDT codes.

American Health Information Management Association (AHIMA) An organization that developed a core data set for physician practices with elements for history and physicals, problem lists, and other data elements used by physicians.

American Medical Association (AMA) An organization that develops, revises, and licenses CPT® codes for publication.

American Society of Anesthesiologists (ASA) An organization that annually publishes a relative-value guide that contains the base values for anesthesia codes, physical status modifiers, and qualifying circumstances codes.

amniocentesis The removal of fluid from the sac around the baby in the uterus.

A-mode An amplitude of sound (echo) that creates a 1-dimensional display.

anal fissure A tear that may occur when muscles of the anal sphincter begin to spasm due to the passage of feces.

anal sphincterotomy The surgical incision or division of the sphincter muscle that controls the anus for defecation.

analyte The substance or chemical constituent that is of interest in an analytical procedure.

anastomosis The creation of a surgical connection between tubular structures, such as the intestines.

anatomical pathology A section that examines tissue samples and specimens from surgery, under the direction of the surgical pathologist.

anesthesia The administration of gasses or drugs that inhibit pain and sensation during procedures and surgical operations.

anesthesia base unit A number assigned to each CPT® anesthesia code that reflects the difficulty and skill required to administer that form of anesthesia.

anesthesia note A written note that documents the anesthesia drugs provided to the patient, including their doses and method of administration, the vital signs of the patient while under anesthesia, and any other services provided, such as a blood transfusion.

anesthesia time A measurement of time that starts when the anesthesiologist begins to prepare the patient to receive services and ends when the anesthesiologist is no longer in personal attendance, at which point the patient may be placed in postoperative care.

anesthesiologist A licensed physician who administers anesthesia and manages its effects on vital functions during surgery.

anesthesiology The practice of medicine dedicated to the relief of pain and the care of the surgical patient before, during, and after surgery.

aneurysm The ballooning of a weakened portion of arterial wall.

angiography The radiographic imaging of the inside of blood vessels.

angioplasty The surgical repair of a blood vessel to dilate the opening.

aniridia A disorder in which the patient does not have a visible iris.

ankyloglossia A condition in which the lingual frenum is too short, limiting the mobility of the tongue. Also known as *tongue tie.*

anomaly An abnormality.

antepartum The period of fetal gestation after confirmation of pregnancy until the beginning of labor, usually 36 weeks.

anterior The position located at the front relative to surrounding anatomical structures.

anterior chamber The fluid-filled space inside the eye between the iris and the back side of the cornea.

anterior lamellar keratoplasty A procedure that replaces the front part of the cornea.

anterior sclera The tough, white, outer coating of the eyeball in the front part of the eye.

anterior synechiae Adhesions of the iris to the cornea. anteroposterior (AP) projection The direction of an x-ray beam from the patient's front (anterior) to back (posterior).

Anti-Kickback Statute (AKS) A statute that prohibits knowingly and willfully offering, paying, or receiving any remuneration to induce or reward referrals for services or supplies reimbursable by Medicare or Medicaid.

antrotomy A procedure that involves cutting through the antrum wall to make an opening in the sinus.

antrum A cavity within a bone.

antrum The lower stomach.

aqueous humor The clear fluid that fills the space in front of the eyeball.

aorta The largest blood vessel in the body, arising from the left ventricle.

aortic aneurysm A bulge in a weakened part of the aortic wall caused by the pressure of the blood pumping.

APC payment status indicators Letters that are assigned to each CPT® and HCPCS code to identify how a code is reimbursed in the OPPS system.

appendix An organ located in the lower right abdominal quadrant, on the cecum at the cecum-ileum junction.

approach procedure The method used to reach a lesion.

arrhythmia An irregular heart rate or rhythm.

arteriovenous (AV) fistula A surgically created opening between an artery and a vein. Also known as a *fistula*

arteriovenous anastomosis A surgically created opening between an artery and a vein. Also known as a *fistula.*

artery A vessel that carries oxygenated blood away from the heart to the body.

arthrocentesis The aspiration or draining of fluid from a joint.

arthrodesis The surgical fixation or fusion of a joint.

arthrography The visualization of the inside of a joint by use of CT, MRI, or fluoroscopic imaging.

arthroplasty A procedure that involves surgically repairing a joint by replacing, reshaping, reconstructing, or remodeling it.

arthroscope An endoscope specially designed for viewing and treating the insides of joints.

arthroscopy A surgical procedure during which the surgeon makes a small incision and inserts an arthroscope.

arthrotomy A procedure performed to create an opening in a joint.

articular cartilage A smooth layer of fibrous tissue that covers the contact surfaces of joints.

arytenoid cartilages A pair of pyramid shaped structures that form part of the larynx where the vocal cords are attached.

assay A laboratory procedure performed to obtain data about a certain drug or substance in a specimen.

assessment The provider's documentation of the evaluation; includes his or her diagnosis or assessment of the situation.

assistive technology assessment An evaluation performed to determine what technology is available to maximize the patient's functional ability or environmental accessibility.

atherectomy The invasive removal of an atheroma or plaque from an artery.

atresia The absence of the external ear canal.

atrium The upper chamber of the heart.

auditing A formal, unbiased review of records to check for accuracy and/or adherence to compliance policies.

autogenic A procedure in which the patient's own kidney is moved to a new site.

autograft A skin graft taken from the patient's own skin.

autologous A graft in which the donor and recipient areas are in the same person. Also known as an *autograft.*

autonomic nervous system A system that controls involuntary automatic bodily functions such as heart rate, breathing, and digestion.

autopsy An exam performed postmortem to discover information regarding the cause of death or extent of disease.

avulsion A tearing away or forcible separation.

backbench work The preparation of a donor organ for transplant. Also known as *back table prep.*

bariatric surgeries Various open and laparoscopic gastric restriction techniques used to treat morbid obesity.

Bartholin's glands A pair of mucus-producing glands located on each side above the vaginal opening.

base procedure The most basic procedure or service of the group of codes.

benign Not harmful.

Bethesda system A system of reporting that uses standard diagnostic terminology that includes a statement of the specimen adequacy, a general categorization, and a descriptive.

bilateral Relating to both sides of a 2-sided anatomical structure.

bile A fluid that travels from the liver to the gallbladder.

biliary tract The tract that contains the gallbladder, intrahepatic bile ducts, cystic duct, and common bile duct.

bilobectomy The removal of two lobes.

biofilm A slimy film of microorganisms adhering to the surface of a structure.

biological valve A valve made of bovine (cow), porcine (pig), or human tissue.

biologicals Vaccines, prophylactics, and substances made from organic compounds used to treat patients.

biometry The analysis of biological data using mathematical and statistical methods.

biopsy A diagnostic procedure that examines excised tissue for the presence, cause, or extent of disease.

bipolar cautery A tool the same shape as tweezers that is used to remove a tumor, polyp, or other lesion.

bladder The muscular, hollow organ that temporarily stores urine.

block A piece of lead designed to shield healthy tissue from receiving radiation.

body The middle stomach.

bone age study A study to estimate the maturity of a child's skeletal system, which may be stunted due to disease or hormone abnormalities.

bone and joint study A study performed to identify abnormalities of bones and joints.

bone densitometry An x-ray technology used to measure the density of the bone. Also known as *dual-energy x-ray absorptiometry.*

bone length study A study to determine discrepancies in the length of limbs.

brachytherapy A type of radiation therapy that uses natural or fabricated radioactive materials instilled or implanted close to or into the tumor or treatment site.

bronchi Tubes that conduct air into the lungs.

bronchoscopy A visual examination of the trachea, bronchi, and lungs using a rigid or flexible endoscope.

B-scan A brightness mode scan that displays a 2-dimensional gray-scale video.

bunionectomy A repair of a bunion by removing bone, which relieves pain and realigns the joint.

burr drill A special electric drill designed to stop drilling once the skull is penetrated.

burr hole A hole created using a burr drill.

bursa A fluid-filled sac that allows for easy movement of joints.

bypass To go around.

calculus An organic or inorganic concretion formed in any part of the body.

canal of Schlemm A circular channel in the eye that collects aqueous humor in the anterior chamber. It passes through the anterior ciliary veins to the blood stream.

cancer registry A registry that keeps track of statistical information regarding cancer behaviors and characteristics and supplies this information to physicians, hospitals, and researchers.

cannula A tube-shaped portal.

cannulation The insertion of a metal tube into the body to draw off fluid or to introduce medication.

capitation payment method A method that reimburses providers a fixed amount for each assigned managed care organization member in a single lump-sum payment once a month, which is similar to an episode-of-care payment.

cardiac catheterization A surgery in which a catheter is threaded through the vein and into the heart to look for abnormalities and restore blood flow to the heart. Also known as *coronary artery bypass*.

cardiography The graphic recording of a physical or functional aspect of the heart.

cardiopulmonary Refers to the heart and lungs.

cardiopulmonary bypass A heart/lung machine used during open heart surgery so blood bypasses the heart.

cardiopulmonary resuscitation (CPR) A set of steps that includes assessing the patient, opening the airway, restoring breathing by mouth-to-mouth assisted breathing or "bagging," and restoring circulation.

cardiovascular system A body system that includes the heart and blood vessels and circulates blood throughout the body.

cardioverter-defibrillator A device that directs an electrical shock to the heart to restore normal rhythm.

care plan A plan that includes the necessary interventions for treatment and also documents any medications, tests, and medical or surgical interventions required to treat the patient's condition. Also known as *plan for care*.

carpal tunnel syndrome (CTS) An injury caused by repetitive motion of the wrist that commonly affects cashiers, office workers, and factory assembly-line workers.

case management A process of initiating and administrating a patient's required healthcare services in addition to providing direct care of the patient.

cast A dressing that is molded to the body and hardens as it dries; used to hold a broken bone in place until it heals.

cataract The clouding of the lens caused by the accumulation of protein, which results in blurry vision.

category A group that gathers the CPT® codes by a further level of specific topic related to the codes.

Category I A group of codes that is the first and largest set of codes in the CPT® codebook.

catheter A tube placed in the body to put fluid in or take fluid out.

cauliflower ear An injury that occurs primarily from trauma to the ear; cartilage is separated from the blood supply, and because of the lack of nutrients from the blood supply, fibrous tissues begin to form in the external ear, which causes the ear to swell.

cecum A section of the large intestine.

Center for Improvement in Healthcare Quality A CMS-approved organization that assures hospitals comply with Medicare conditions of participation.

Centers for Medicare & Medicaid Services (CMS) An organization that requires that facilities and providers meet their conditions of participation, which are set forth in federal regulations.

central nervous system A system made up of the brain and spinal cord.

central venous access device (VAD) A small flexible tube placed in a large vein for a patient who needs long-term intravenous therapy such as chemotherapy or antibiotics.

centrally inserted VAD A device that has an entry site of the jugular, subclavian, or femoral vein, or the inferior vena cava.

cerclage of cervix The suturing of the cervix to keep it closed during pregnancy.

cerebellum The hindbrain, located under the posterior portion of cerebrum.

cerebrospinal fluid (CSF) Clear, colorless fluid that flows through the subarachnoid space around the brain and spinal cord.

cerebrospinal fluid shunt A device implanted in patients suffering from hydrocephalus.

cerebrum The largest portion of brain, divided into right and left hemispheres.

Certificate of Medical Necessity (CMN) A form used to determine and document medical necessity for requesting specific medical equipment.

certified professional coder (CPC) An AAPC member who successfully passes the certification examination in medical coding for physician offices and is awarded a certificate.

cerumen A waxy substance found in the external ear canal that protects and lubricates the ear.

cervical The neck.

cervix A narrow passage located at the base of the corpus uteri. Also known as the *cervix uteri.*

cervix uteri A narrow passage located at the base of the corpus uteri. Also known as the *cervix.*

cesarean delivery The extraction of a fetus from the uterus via abdominal incision.

chamber The portions of the heart that include the right and left atriums and right and left ventricles.

charge entry The process of entering medical codes into the PMS.

chargemaster A comprehensive listing maintained by a hospital that contains all the services, procedures, and even medicines they provide, along with the price they charge for each one.

cheilectomy A surgery performed to correct hallux rigidus.

cheiloplasty The surgical repair of the lip for cosmetic purposes or to repair a defect or injury.

chemistry department A department that performs quantitative analysis on body fluids.

chemodenervation A procedure performed by injecting a neurotoxin such as botulinum toxin type A to paralyze dysfunctional muscle tissue by blocking the nerve signals.

chemotherapy The treatment of disease by chemical substances.

chief complaint The reason a patient is seeking care.

chiropractic manipulation treatment (CMT) A manual treatment to influence joint and neurophysiologic function by using controlled force to manipulate the body, especially the spine.

cholecystectomy The surgical removal of the gallbladder.

cholelithiasis Gallstones.

cholesteatoma A cyst that grows on the margins of the eardrum.

chordee A congenital condition in which the penis curves downward.

ciliary photocoagulation A method used to treat glaucoma.

circumcision The removal of the foreskin, a fold of skin covering the tip of the penis.

civil monetary penalty (CMP) A substantial fine assessed against an organization, agency, or other entity (structured business) based on the type of fraud or abuse committed.

classic radical mastectomy A procedure that includes the removal of the entire breast including overlying skin, pectoral muscles, and axillary lymph nodes.

classification system A system used to organize like medical conditions, procedures, or concepts into categories and assign them codes that, when deciphered, describe each item in detail.

clean claim A claim that is free of errors and contains all necessary information to pay the claim.

cleft lip A congenital defect in which the tissue that forms the upper lip does not join during fetal development.

cleft palate An opening in the hard palate or the soft palate; a congenital defect that results from the nonunion of the palate during gestation.

clinical data The collective body of documentation that contains every diagnosis and procedure related to caring for a patient.

clinical pathology A section that consists of microbiology, chemistry, immunology, parasitology, hematology, and other specialty units that pertain to the diagnosis of disease.

clitoris The highly erogenous erectile body located anterior to the urethra.

closed reduction The manipulation of the fractured bone to return it to the proper alignment by simply pushing the fracture back into place.

closed treatment A procedure in which the surgeon does not expose the bone or directly view the fracture to provide care.

CMS-1450 A form used by institutional providers to bill Medicare when a provider is eligible to submit paper claims. Also known as *UB-04.*

CMS-1500 (02-12) The universal paper claim form used to request payment for physician services and medical supplies from insurance payers.

coagulation test A test that assesses bleeding and clotting problems.

cochlea The spiral-shaped part of the inner ear that transforms sound into nerve impulses that travel to the brain.

cochlear device An electronic medical mechanism that receives sound, processes it, and sends small electric currents near the auditory nerve.

code of ethics A compilation of standards of conduct that apply set principles by which coders may determine appropriate behavior in relation to patients, physicians, and insurance companies.

codebook conventions The words, symbols, punctuation, formatting, and abbreviations that are used to help locate and assign codes.

coding ethics The standards that medical coders are expected to follow as they perform their daily tasks.

coinsurance A set percentage the member pays after the deductible is met.

cold knife A technique that uses a scalpel or other sharp instrument to cut away a tissue specimen.

colectomy The removal of the colon/large intestine.

collection agency A business that pursues payments on debts owed by individuals or businesses.

collections The process of collecting unpaid balances.

colon A section of the large intestine.

colon decompression The removal of air from the colon, reducing possible future tears.

colonoscopy An endoscopic exam, using a flexible colonoscope, of the rectum to the cecum, which may include examination of the terminal ileum.

color flow Doppler scan A scan that shows the different levels of fluid concentration within a targeted area; used when the physician wants to examine movement within a structure, such as flowing blood.

colostomy A surgical opening of the colon.

colotomy An incision of the colon.

colporrhaphy Repair by suturing.

colposcope A binocular lighted microscope.

colposcopies Endoscopies that use a colposcope to directly visualize the vagina, cervix, and other structures.

combination code A single code that includes more than one procedure.

commercial health insurance Insurance provided by a private company. Also known as *private health insurance*.

comminuted A fracture in which the bone is broken into more than 2 pieces.

Commission on Accreditation for Health Informatics and Information Management Education (CAHIIM) An organization that promotes and enforces accreditation standards for health information and health informatics education programs.

common bile duct A duct through which bile passes from the gallbladder to the duodenum.

communication skills The ability to convey information in a way that your audience can easily understand.

comorbidity A preexisting diagnosis that affects the treatment of the principal diagnosis.

compensator (tissue) A tissue used to create variation in the amount of radiation distributed. Also known as a *radiation filter*.

competitive medical plan A managed care organization that meets the Centers for Medicare & Medicaid Services criteria for enrolling Medicare beneficiaries into their managed care plans.

complete A term in radiology that indicates the maximum possible views taken.

complete blood count (CBC) A test used to determine how many cells of different types are present.

complete diagnostic study A study that includes the maximum possible images of an organ or anatomical site.

complete PFSH A comprehensive type of history that requires a review of at least 2 of the 3 areas; some E/M categories would require all 3 areas.

complete radiology examination The highest number of views required to completely evaluate the patient's condition.

complete ROS A review of systems that involves 10 or more body systems.

complex closure A procedure that may require undermining, obtaining hemostasis, or placing sutures to avoid distortion.

complex repair A procedure that involves repairing wounds with more extensive methods than just a layered closure.

compliance Acting in accordance with the laws and regulations that protect a specific segment of the population or a specific industry.

compliance committee A group of professionals with knowledge of specific areas of an organization who work together to create policy and monitor a compliance program.

compliance officer An employee who is responsible for the daily monitoring of the compliance program.

compliance plan An internal process that allows the medical facility to identify incidents that may result in the violation of federal or state regulations.

comprehensive A complete examination of a single system or a general multisystem exam of 8 or more body systems.

comprehensive A history that requires the chief complaint; an extended HPI; a review of systems related to the problem identified in the HPI, plus a review of all additional body systems; and complete past, family, and social history.

Comprehensive Error Rate Testing (CERT) A program implemented by CMS to comply with IPERIA; CERT contractors seek to identify improper payment by analyzing the medical documentation supporting a claim.

comprehensive ophthalmological service A service that includes a general evaluation of the complete visual system.

computed tomographic angiography (CTA) When CT scans are used to capture images of blood vessels.

computed tomography (CT) The computer processing of a series of x-ray views taken from many different angles to create cross-sectional images of bones and soft tissues.

computer assisted coding (CAC) A software program that analyzes text from EHR documentation and assigns codes accordingly.

concurrent care The care that occurs when a patient is seen by more than 1 provider on the same date of service.

conization A procedure that removes a cone-shaped wedge of tissue for biopsy. Also known as *cone biopsy*.

conjunctiva A thin, clear membrane that protects the anterior portion of the sclera and the inside of the eyelid.

conjunctivoplasty The surgical repair of the conjunctiva.

conscious The state of being awake; aware of physical sensations and surroundings.

conscious sedation A state in which a patient is drowsy, relaxed, and able to respond to verbal commands. Also known as *moderate sedation*.

consultation A type of E/M service provided when a physician requests the advice and opinion of another physician.

continuing education (CE) Education that typically comprises courses, webinars, workshops, and other offerings that allow professionals to stay up-to-date with changes and innovations in their field.

contracted reviewer A worker who audits and reviews providers' documentation; assigned to monitor specific areas of risk in provider compliance, coding rules, and to identify improper payments in the Medicare fee-for-service program.

contractual write-off The process of canceling the balance after the allowed amount has been paid and the balance is not the responsibility of the patient.

contrast A radiopaque substance used during an x-ray exam (or some MRI exams) to provide visual contrast in the pictures of different tissues and organs; the substance can be given orally or intravenously. Also known as *contrast material*.

contrast material A radiopaque substance used during an x-ray exam (or some MRI exams) to provide visual contrast in the pictures of different tissues and organs; the substance can be given orally or intravenously. Also known as *contrast*.

contributing components The 4 of 7 components that must be considered before selecting the level of service: counseling, coordination of care, the nature of the presenting problem, and time.

controlled hypotension A therapeutic treatment involving the intentional reduction of blood pressure to reduce blood loss.

convention An abbreviation, symbol, or note to help guide coders to the most accurate code.

conversion factor (CF) A percentage to convert the geographic practice cost indices into a dollar amount that reflects category of services, percentage of changes to the Medicare Economic Index, physician expenditures, access to health care, and quality of health care.

coordination of benefits The determination of which insurance plan is primary or secondary.

coordination of care The deliberate organization of the patient's care between the physician and another caregiver, whether it be another physician, health professional, or facility, to ensure that the patient's needs are met.

copay A fixed amount paid prior to health services being rendered. Also known as *copayment*.

copayment A fixed amount paid prior to health services being rendered. Also known as *copay*.

cordocentesis The removal of a sample of a baby's blood from the umbilical cord.

cornea A dome-shaped transparent fibrous tissue that covers the pupil and iris.

coronary artery A structure that supplies blood to the heart.

coronary artery bypass A surgery that may be performed to restore blood flow to the heart. Also known as *cardiac catheterization*.

coronary artery bypass graft (CABG) A procedure performed to reestablish blood supply to the heart and prevent permanent damage to the heart itself. 361

coroner A public official who investigates deaths that appear to be from unnatural causes.

corpectomy The removal of the body of the vertebra.

corporate integrity agreements (CIAs) The negotiated obligations between corporate entities and the OIG due to violations or self-disclosure settlements, assisted with the False Claims Act.

corpus (pl., corpora) cavernosa A column of tissue along the length of the penis that expands with blood during penile erection.

corpus uteri The large central portion of the uterus above the cervix and below the openings of the fallopian tubes.

cost sharing The amount a patient must pay, such as a co-pay, a deductible, or coinsurance.

counseling A discussion with the patient and/or family regarding the patient's care and treatment options.

covered entity Groups such as health plans, healthcare clearinghouses, or healthcare providers that electronically transmit any health information in connection with transactions for which HHS has adopted standards.

cranial suture A fibrous joint where the skull bones meet.

craniectomy A procedure in which a portion of the skull is removed but not immediately replaced.

craniosynostosis The premature closure of the sutures of the skull.

craniotomy A procedure in which a portion of the skull is temporarily removed to provide access to the brain for surgery and then replaced once the surgery has been completed.

cricoid The ring of cartilage around the trachea.

cricopharyngeal muscle The part of the pharyngeal constrictor muscle near the cricoid cartilage at the top of the esophagus.

critical thinking skills Skills that include the ability to formulate ideas, solve problems, analyze situations, and think creatively.

cross coder A book or software that links codes commonly used by anesthesiologists to corresponding CPT® surgical codes. Also known as *crosswalk*.

crosswalk A book or software that links codes commonly used by anesthesiologists to corresponding CPT® surgical codes. Also known as *cross coder*.

cryosurgery A procedure that destroys a lesion through the use of extreme cold.

cryptorchidism An undescended testicle(s).

culture typing A test that provides a more specific identification of a cultured pathogenic organism so that the physician can determine the best treatment.

curettage A scraping of the interior of a cavity.

curette A narrow, spoon-shaped instrument used to scrape the lining of the endocervical canal to obtain the specimen.

Current Dental Terminology (CDT) The common language used when describing dental procedures. Also known as the *Code on Dental Procedures and Nomenclatures*.

Current Procedural Terminology (CPT®) HCPCS Level I codes that are used to report medical services and procedures performed by outpatient providers.

cyst A fluid-filled sac.

cystocele A herniation of the bladder located against the anterior vaginal wall, causing the wall to bulge.

cystometrogram A study that can determine how much the bladder can hold, how much pressure builds up within the bladder, and how full the bladder is before the patient has the urge to urinate.

cystourethroscopy The visual examination of the bladder and urethra using a scope.

cytogenetics The study of cell structure and function as it relates to genetics.

cytopathology The study of disease on the cellular level.

da Vinci surgical system A computer system that allows a surgeon to use external controls to manipulate miniaturized instruments placed inside the patient while viewing a highly magnified 3-D image of the surgical site.

debridement The surgical excision procedure using forceps, scissors, scalpel, or dermatome to remove dead or infected tissue to promote healing and the growth of healthy tissue.

debridement depth The tissue layer of the debridement site.

debridement surface area The extent of the wound that was debrided, described in square centimeters or percentage of body surface.

declared brain dead A physician-diagnosed condition characterized by permanent, complete, irreversible cessation of brain function.

decompression A surgical operation for relief of pressure on the spinal cord and nerves.

deductible The set amount the insured must pay for healthcare services before the health insurance begins to pay.

deemed status The status granted by CMS to authorize an organization to participate in and receive payment from the Medicare and Medicaid programs.

defecation The process in which feces are eliminated from the body by moving from the small intestines to the large intestines to the anus and out of the body.

defibrillation The delivery of an electric impulse to the heart, performed to stop abnormal rhythms by interrupting the heart's electrical conduction.

definitive identification A microorganism present in the sample that has been identified down to the genus or species level.

definitive procedure The resection, excision, or other treatment of a lesion.

dehiscence The gaping or splitting of a sutured wound.

delivery The process of passing the fetus and the placenta from the womb into the external world.

denied claim The refusal of an insurance payer to reimburse the healthcare provider for medical services or procedures rendered.

dentoalveolar structures Comprise the teeth and the bone structure that hold the teeth in place.

dermis The living, functioning layer of the skin, where blood vessels and nerves are active.

destruction The ablation of lesions by any method, including electrosurgery, cryosurgery, laser treatments, and chemical treatments.

detailed An extended exam of the affected body area(s) as well as 2 to 7 other symptomatic or related organ systems.

detailed A history that requires the chief complaint, an extended HPI, problem-pertinent systems review extended to include a review of a limited number of additional body systems, and a pertinent PFSH directly related to the patient's current problems.

determination A decision made by the payer to either pay the claim in full or in part, or to deny a claim.

DEXA An x-ray technology used to measure the density of the bone.

diagnosis A statement or conclusion that describes a patient's illness, disease, or health problem.

diagnosis-related group (DRG) A classification system that uses medical data collected from previous patients to create groups based on diagnosis, treatment plan, and length of stay.

diagnostic The procedures performed to identify illness, diseases, or injuries indicated by a patient's current medical signs and/or symptoms.

***Diagnostic and Statistical Manual of Mental Disorders* (DSM)** A standard classification system developed by the American Psychiatric Association and used by mental health professionals to categorize mental illnesses.

diagnostic coronary angiography Using x-ray imaging to see the coronary vessels.

diagnostic endoscopy A procedure performed to identify abnormal conditions of the structure or organ viewed.

diagnostic mammogram A procedure performed after a lump or other symptoms of disease are detected.

diagnostic nuclear medicine A type of medicine that focuses on identifying abnormalities in the physiologic processes within the body, such as rates of metabolism.

diagnostic order A request with instructions for a diagnostic procedure.

diagnostic report A report that communicates the results from procedures such as laboratory tests and radiological exams and helps a provider make decisions about a patient's condition and treatment.

dialysis A process that artificially filters waste products from the blood.

diaphragm The muscular partition that separates the thoracic cavity from the abdominal cavity.

differential diagnosis A diagnosis that distinguishes a disease from others with similar signs or symptoms.

digest The process of breaking down food.

digestive system The body system that ingests, processes, absorbs, and eliminates food. Also known as the *gastrointestinal tract.*

direct laryngoscopy A procedure that involves visualizing the larynx with a rigid or flexible scope.

discussion The process of breaking down of abnormal lens material.

dislocation An injury in which one or more bones separates from the joint.

DNA A nucleic acid that carries genetic information in cells and some viruses.

documentation review program A program used by coding professionals to review health records.

Doppler ultrasound An imaging technique that uses a special frequency that can penetrate solid or liquid to record blood flow velocity.

downcoding The process of reporting a code that represents a lower level of service or a less extensive procedure than what is supported by the documentation. Also known as *undercoding.*

drain A medical device implanted at a surgical site to collect fluid that may build up after surgery.

dual chamber pacemaker system A system that includes a pulse generator and one electrode in the right atrium and one electrode in the right ventricle.

dual-energy x-ray absorptiometry An x-ray technology used to measure the density of the bone. Also known as *bone densitometry.*

dual leads The wires that control the pacing and sensing functions in both one atrium and one ventricle; the leads are located in two chambers of the heart.

ductography A specialized diagnostic mammogram performed to identify abnormalities of the breast ducts that produce milk.

duodenum A section of the small intestine.

duplex Doppler scan A scan that combines B-mode, spectral, and color flow Doppler imaging to produce real-time images of the pattern and direction of blood flow.

durable medical equipment (DME) The equipment provided to patients to treat a disease, increase mobility, or improve their quality of life.

Durable Medical Equipment, Prosthetics, Orthotics, and Supplies (DMEPOS) The supplier application that providers complete to apply for a DME number.

DXA An x-ray technology used to measure the density of the bone.

ear The pathway of sound reception.

echocardiography The use of ultrasound imaging of the heart and great vessels to produce a 2-dimensional display of the size, structure, and motion of the heart.

ectopic pregnancy The implantation of an embryo in a location other than the uterus such as the fallopian tubes, usually requiring termination of the pregnancy.

ectropion A condition in which the eyelid is turned outward, leaving the inside of the eyelid exposed.

education A process similar to training; however, education typically involves multiple learning sessions and provides the student with in-depth knowledge of a specific subject.

elective cardioversion The use of electric shock to restore the heart back to normal sinus rhythm.

electrocautery A procedure in which a probe heated by electricity is used to burn and/or remove tissue.

electrode A lead that transfers electricity to the atrium or ventricle.

electromyographic (EMG) A test that studies anal or urethral sphincter function by measuring the electrical signals that cause muscles to contract, allowing the physician to see if the muscle being measured is healthy.

electronic data interchange (EDI) The exchange of information from computer to computer.

electronic health record (EHR) A record that collects patient data in a computerized format designed to facilitate sharing across a continuum of healthcare entities.

electronic remittance advice (ERA) A digital explanation of benefits.

emancipated minor A person under the age of 18 who is married, divorced, or a parent; is in the military; is a college student living away from home; or is a minor who has successfully petitioned the court to sever parental relationships.

embezzlement A crime involving stealing money that you have been entrusted to manage.

embolectomy A procedure that removes blockage from vessels.

embolism A blood clot, air, or fat that moves into a blood vessel and causes a blockage.

embryo An unborn offspring in the stage of development from implantation of the zygote to the second month of pregnancy.

emesis Vomiting.

encoder An online database that allows coders to look up codes, review detailed descriptions of procedures, and review coding and reimbursement guidelines.

encounter form A form in which physician offices incorporate their most common procedure and diagnosis codes. Also known as a *superbill* or *charge slip*.

endarterectomy An incision into an artery to remove the inner lining to eliminate disease or blockage.

endocervical curettage A procedure in which the surgeon uses a narrow, spoon-shaped instrument called a curette to scrape the lining of the endocervical canal to obtain the specimen.

endocrine system A body system made up of glands located throughout the body.

endoscope A tubular instrument with a light source designed for examining and performing surgeries on hollow body organs such as the stomach.

endoscopic A surgery that provides an alternative to the traditional open technique by using an endoscope.

endoscopic retrograde cholangiopancreatography (ERCP) An examination that combines the use of a flexible endoscope with x-ray imaging to examine the biliary ducts that drain the liver, gallbladder, and pancreas to the duodenum.

endoscopic ultrasound (EUS) A procedure that allows the physician to view inside the body by use of an ultrasound device attached to the tip of the endoscope.

endoscopy A procedure that allows the physician to view inside the body by use of an endoscope.

endothelial keratoplasty A procedure that replaces the endothelial layer of the cornea.

end-stage renal disease (ESRD) A condition in which the kidneys are no longer able to function and dialysis or a renal transplant is needed to prolong life. Also known as *chronic renal failure*.

enteral nutrition therapy The process of providing a patient with nutrition via a feeding tube.

enterectomy The removal of the small intestine.

enterocele A herniation of the small intestine that protrudes into the tissues between the bladder and vagina or the rectum and the vagina.

enterostomy The creation of an artificial opening in the intestine through the abdominal wall to the outside of the body that allows fecal matter to be drained.

enterotomy An incision of the small intestine.

entropion A condition in which the eyelid turns inward.

enucleation The removal of the eye from the orbit while leaving in place all other orbital structures.

epicardially On the heart's surface.

epidermis The outermost layer of skin; consists of dead cells generated by the dermis.

epididymis The tubes where sperm are stored.

epidural The space outside the dura mater.

epidural anesthesia Anesthesia that is most commonly used for obstetric patients during labor and delivery.

epiglottis A flap of cartilage attached to the muscles of the larynx; covers the trachea while swallowing.

episiotomy An incision made between the vagina and anus to facilitate delivery.

episode-of-care A payment method that reimburses the provider in a single lump sum for all services during a specified, continuous period of time, for a specific condition.

eponym A name of a person to whom a procedure is attributed.

eschar A leathery slough resulting from a third-degree burn injury.

escharotomy A procedure in which the surgeon makes an incision through the eschar to expose the tissue below.

esophageal dilation A procedure that widens a narrowed area of the esophagus.

esophageal stent A flexible mesh tube placed into a narrowed area of the esophagus.

esophagectomy The surgical removal of part or all of the esophagus.

esophagogastroduodenoscopy (EGD) The visualization of the esophagus, stomach, and duodenum by means of an endoscope.

esophagoscopy The visualization of the esophagus by the use of an endoscope.

esophagotomy An incision into the esophagus.

esophagus A 9- to 10-inch muscular tube that connects to the stomach.

established patient Someone who is not considered a new patient.

ethics A generally accepted standard of moral conduct.

ethmoid sinuses A structure located between the nose and the eyes.

eustachian tube A narrow passage leading from the pharynx to the cavity of the middle ear.

eustachian tube dysfunction A condition that blocks the drainage of fluid and disrupts the equalization of pressure in the middle ear.

evaluation and management (E/M) The codes that describe services that a physician or other qualified healthcare professional provides to evaluate patients and manage their care.

evisceration The removal of the eyeball (globe) while leaving the sclera and extraocular muscles in place.

excision A removal of a lesion through the dermal layer of the skin.

excisional biopsy A biopsy procedure that involves the removal of the entire lesion.

exclusive provider organization (EPO) A network of individual medical care providers, or groups of medical care providers, who have entered into a contract with an insurer to provide health insurance to members.

exenteration A procedure that removes the eye, adnexa, and part of the bony orbit.

exostosis The development of new bone on the surface of an existing bone in the external auditory canal. Also known as *surfer's ear.*

expanded problem-focused A limited exam of the affected body area or organ system and other symptomatic or related organ systems.

expanded problem-focused A history that requires the chief complaint, a brief history of present illness, and a problem-pertinent systems review.

expanded problem-focused level of exam An exam that requires the chief complaint, a brief history of present illness and a problem-pertinent systems review, which pertains only to the chief complaint.

explanation of benefits (EOB) A letter or statement that details the reason a claim is accepted or denied and what the patient's financial responsibility will be.

expressed contract A contract that clearly states the terms of the agreement into which the parties enter.

extended radical mastectomy The removal of the entire breast and the axillary and internal mammary lymph nodes, including the pectoralis muscle.

extended ROS Involves the review of 1 body system that is related to the patient's current problem as well as 2 to 9 additional body systems.

external auditory canal A short tube that ends at the tympanic membrane.

external cephalic version A procedure to turn a fetus from a side-lying or breech position to a head-down position.

external fixation A procedure using skeletal pins or screws attached to a device outside the skin to realign the bone.

external hemorrhoid A swollen, inflamed vein located beneath the skin, just outside of the anus.

external medical record audit An audit conducted by an outside company.

extracapsular cataract extraction (ECCE) The removal of the natural lens from the protective capsule.

Extracorporeal Life Support (ECLS) A procedure that provides support to the heart and/or lungs, allowing patients to rest and recover from sickness or injury. Also known as *Extracorporeal Membrane Oxygenation (ECMO).*

Extracorporeal Membrane Oxygenation (ECMO) A procedure that provides support to the heart and/or lungs, allowing patients to rest and recover from sickness or injury. Also known as *Extracorporeal Life Support (ECLS).*

extracorporeal shockwave lithotripsy (ESWL) A procedure that uses sound waves to break up kidney stones.

extraoral The area outside of the mouth.

eyeball The part of the eye that has a slightly elongated globe shape and measures about 1 inch in diameter.

eyelashes The hairs that grow out of the eyelid.

eyelid The skin that covers the eye.

F wave test A test done by stimulating the distal end of a nerve so that the impulse travels toward the muscle fiber and back to the motor neurons of the spinal cord.

facet joints The bony surfaces between the vertebrae that articulate with each other.

Fair Debt Collection Practices Act The federal law that governs collection practices of all kinds, including collection agencies and collection departments within a business.

fallopian tubes The tubes that serve as a passageway for the mature oocytes or ova to move from the ovary to the uterus. Also known as *oviducts.*

False Claims Act (FCA) An act found in Title 31, Section 3729, of the United States Code; prohibits individuals from knowingly submitting or causing the submission of false or fraudulent claims.

family history The part of the history that documents the diseases of biological family members that may place the patient at risk or may be hereditary.

fascia The connective tissue that surrounds muscles, blood vessels, and nerves.

feces The materials from broken-down food that are not absorbed; solid waste.

Federal Register The US government's daily publication of final and administrative regulations for federal agencies.

fee for service A reimbursement method that requests payment for each service or procedure.

fee schedule A price list of services and procedures.

fenestrate To perforate or pierce with one or more openings.

fetus The gestational unborn child from the end of the eighth week to the moment of birth.

fifth level of appeal The level of appeal that may be requested up to 60 days after receiving notice of a Medical Appeals Council's decision; judicial review is conducted by the Federal District Court.

fimbrioplasty The repair of ovarian fimbria.

first level of appeal An appeal that may be requested up to 120 days after receiving initial determination; a Medicare Administrative Contractor will review the claim and documentation.

fissurectomy The removal of a portion of the anus that has been torn.

fistula An abnormal opening from one area to another, inside or outside the body.

fistulization The creation of a passageway.

fixation The placement of screws, rods, plates, or pins to hold a bone in place while healing.

flap A piece of tissue adjacent to the reconstruction site that remains attached to the body by a major artery or vein at the base and is rotated to the recipient site on the body.

fluorescein dye An orange organic dye injected into the eye during a slit lamp examination to improve the detection of a foreign body.

fluoroscopy An imaging technique that uses x-rays transmitted to a monitor to display real-time, moving images of the internal structures of a patient.

foramen The opening in the vertebra formed by the vertebral body and arch.

foreskin A fold of skin covering the tip of the penis.

fourth level of appeal An appeal that may be requested up to 60 days after receiving notice of an administrative law judge's decision. If the time frame expires, the Medicare Appeals Council conducts a review of the decision, and a request for oral arguments may be made.

fraction The total number of radiotherapy sessions.

fracture A break in a bone.

fragmenting The act of separately reporting services inherent in a procedure or group of procedures. Also known as *unbundling*.

fraud The act of intentionally submitting false information to benefit yourself or others.

free skin graft A graft that contains the entire epidermis and dermis layers. Also known as *full-thickness graft*.

frenotomy A procedure in which an incision is made into the lingual frenum, releasing it and allowing the tongue to move more freely.

frontal sinuses The structures located in the frontal bone located just above the eyes.

frozen section A microscopic exam in which the specimen removed by the surgeon is immediately frozen to facilitate cutting a thin section to be placed under the microscope.

full-thickness graft A graft that contains the entire epidermis and dermis layers. Also known as *free skin graft*.

fundus The upper stomach.

gait training A type of physical therapy to help a patient improve the ability to stand and walk.

galactogram A special type of mammogram used for imaging the breast ducts. Also known as *mammary ductogram*.

gallbladder An organ that stores bile from the liver for use later to help food pass through the small intestine.

gallstones Bile crystals that have slowly accumulated in the gallbladder, causing inflammation, infection, and blockage in the associated biliary ducts.

gamete A mature sex cell, sperm, or ovum.

gas-liquid chromatography A method of analysis that can identify a specific drug by measuring how fast a component of the sample being tested moves through an instrument.

gastrectomy The surgical removal of all or part of the stomach; used as treatment for morbid obesity in bariatric surgery.

gastric bypass A procedure that removes a portion of the stomach and creates a new passageway directly to the jejunum.

gastric neurostimulator A stimulating device indicated for patients with gastroparesis.

gastroenterologist A physician who diagnoses and treats conditions of the digestive system.

gastroenterology The medical specialty concerned with the structure, function, and diseases of the digestive tract.

gastrointestinal tract The system that ingests, processes, absorbs, and eliminates food. Also known as the *digestive system*.

gastrotomy A procedure involving incisions in the stomach.

gene A unit consisting of a sequence of DNA that contains genetic information and can influence the phenotype of an organism.

general anesthesia Anesthesia that affects the entire body and causes a loss of consciousness.

genome An organism's genetic material.

genomic sequencing The process of figuring out the order of DNA nucleotides in a genome that make up an organism's DNA.

geographic practice cost indices (GPCI) Adjustments applied to the relative value units to account for variations in the costs of practicing medicine in specific geographic regions.

gingivectomy The removal or trimming of overgrown gums.

gingivoplasty The surgical repair of the gums.

glaucoma A disease that results from the inability of aqueous humor to drain from the eye through the canal of Schlemm into the bloodstream.

global days The length of time over which a typical patient receives follow-up care for a surgical procedure. Also known as *global period.*

global payment method A single lump-sum payment to a medical facility that covers all services and procedures needed to treat a group of patients.

global period The length of time over which a typical patient receives follow-up care for a surgical procedure. Also known as *global days.*

global procedure A procedure that clearly defines both the technical component and the professional component used to complete the procedure.

global services Services that include both the technical and professional component of a service.

glossectomy The surgical removal of a portion or all of the tongue.

goiters An enlarged thyroid.

goniotomy A surgical procedure that lowers intraocular pressure.

grading The cell stage.

great saphenous vein The longest vein in the body: extending from the foot to the groin.

gross exam An exam conducted with the naked eye.

gross examination An exam that includes dissection of the body with examination of the organs and tissues.

grouper A program that sorts codes into groups for prospective payment system calculations.

guarantor The individual who agrees, in writing, to pay for the patient's medical care.

guide wire A thin, flexible wire that can be inserted to guide another instrument.

H reflex test A test that measures the Achilles muscle stretch reflex by stimulation of the tibial nerve.

hallux rigidus A stiffness caused by a bone spur that prevents movement in the big toe.

hallux valgus An enlargement of the base of the metatarsophalangeal joint of the big (great) toe.

HCPCS Level II The codes that are another nomenclature of procedures, services, drugs, and items. Also known as *National Codes.*

HCPCS Level II modifiers The modifiers that may be required when reporting anesthesia services to Medicare and other third-party payers.

HCPCS Level II tabular list An alphanumeric list of HCPCS codes organized by sections.

HCPCS Release and Code Sets A CMS web page that publishes HCPCS Level II procedure codes and modifiers quarterly.

heading A group in the CPT® codebook that can refer to a patient population, an anatomical site, or a type of procedure or service.

Health Care Fraud Prevention and Enforcement Action Team (HEAT) A joint effort of government agencies that work together to prevent fraud and enforce current antifraud laws.

health information management (HIM) The practice of analyzing, maintaining, and protecting traditional and digital confidential patient information.

health insurance A type of insurance that pays healthcare providers for services rendered to patients, or reimburses the insured for out-of-pocket medical expenses. Also known as *health coverage.*

health insurance policy A legal contract between the holder of the policy and the insurer for reimbursement of a portion of the medical expense incurred for receiving medical treatment.

Health Insurance Portability and Accountability Act of 1996 (HIPAA) Federal legislation enacted to provide continuing health coverage, reduce healthcare costs, and guarantee the security and privacy of health information.

health maintenance organization (HMO) The most restrictive managed care organization; requires members to select an in-network primary care physician and request referral or preauthorization prior to receiving certain healthcare services.

health record A legal document that contains descriptions of all the products and services provided to a patient. Also known as *medical record.*

Healthcare Common Procedure Coding System (HCPCS) The standards used to report medical, surgical, and diagnostic procedures as well as products and drugs.

healthcare practitioner Another name for a person who practices medicine.

healthcare provider An individual who has completed the required education and is licensed to practice medicine, provide medical care, and/or perform procedures in a medical facility.

heart An organ with four chambers: the upper chambers are the right atrium and left atrium, and the lower chambers are the right ventricle and left ventricle.

hematology The study of blood.

hematopoiesis The formation of blood cells.

hematopoietic progenitor cell A cell that is transplanted and produced in the bone marrow and able to replicate and differentiate for cellular functions.

hemic system The body system that consists of the organs and processes involved in the production of blood, including the vessels and bone marrow.

hemilaminectomy A surgery performed to remove part of the lamina. Also known as *laminotomy.*

hemodialysis A procedure in which the patient's blood is pumped out of the patient's body into a dialysis machine, filtered and washed, and returned to the body.

hemoptysis The condition of spitting up blood.

hemorrhoid ligation A treatment used to treat internal hemorrhoids.

hemorrhoid sclerotherapy A treatment used to treat internal hemorrhoids.

hemostasis The stopping of the flow of blood.

hepatectomy The surgical removal of the liver.

high severity A problem that has a high-to-extreme risk of morbidity and mortality without treatment.

histology The study of microscopic anatomy. Also known as *morphology.*

history A component of the E/M code that includes the chief complaint; the history of present illness; the review of systems; and past, family, and social histories.

history and physical (H&P) The patient's medical history and results of a physical examination.

history of present illness (HPI) The chronological description of the development of the patient's current illness.

hospital chargemaster A computer database in which hospitals compile all procedures, services, supplies, and drugs that are billed to insurance payers.

Hospital Outpatient Prospective Payment System (OPPS) A reimbursement method used by CMS to reimburse hospital services for certain medical services that take place in the outpatient department.

hospital wage index An index that reflects the levels of hospital wages in the geographic area of the hospital compared with the national average.

hot biopsy forceps A tool that produces heat in the metal portion of the forceps by an electric current that flows from the device to a grounding pad on the patient's body.

hybrid record A health record that is a combination of paper and electronic formats.

hydatidiform mole An abnormal mass of tissue that forms in the uterus at the beginning of a pregnancy.

hydrocele A collection of serous fluid.

hydrocephalus An accumulation of cerebrospinal fluid; literally translated as "water on the brain."

hymen A fold of membrane found near the opening of the vagina.

hyoid bone A U-shaped bone that is located between the base of the tongue and the larynx.

hyperthermia A procedure that uses heat to make tumors more susceptible to cancer therapy methods.

hyperthyroidism A condition of overactive thyroid.

hyphema A condition caused by blood filling the anterior chamber.

hypodermis The innermost layer of the skin. Also known as *subcutaneous tissue.*

hypospadias A congenital condition in which the opening of the urethra is on the underside of the penis instead of at the tip.

hysterectomy A procedure to remove the uterus.

ICD-10-CM A diagnosis classification system that is scheduled to replace the ICD-9 diagnosis classification system in October 2015.

ICD-10-PCS A classification system used to report procedures performed in an inpatient setting.

ICD-9 A diagnosis and procedure classification system used in the United States.

ICD-O-3 A neoplasm classification system that categorizes neoplasms by their anatomical site, histology, behavior, and grading. Its codes are also known as *morphology codes.*

IGRT An imaged guided radiation therapy.

ileostomy A surgical opening in the ileum of the small intestine.

ileum A section of the small intestine.

imaging modality A type of imaging technology such as radiographic imaging, ultrasonography, or magnetic resonance imaging.

immune globulin A protein extracted from donated human plasma, which contains antibodies that protect from certain diseases.

immunization The process in which an individual is made immune or resistant to an infectious disease by the administration of an agent.

immunoassay Any assay that measures an antigen-antibody reaction, with methods such as fluorescence, enzyme, or radioisotope markers.

immunofluorescent A technique that involves mixing the antigen with a fluorescent compound, then adding that to a sample of the patient's blood.

immunology The branch of science/medicine that deals with the immune system.

immunology and serology department The department that performs testing for antigen-antibody reactions.

implantable defibrillator A device that can use high-energy pulses to treat life-threatening arrhythmia or low-energy pulses like a pacemaker. Formerly known as a *pacing cardioverter-defibrillator*.

implantable defibrillator system A system that includes a pulse generator and electrodes.

implied contract An unwritten agreement established through actions, words, or circumstances.

Improper Payments Elimination and Recovery Improvement Act (IPERIA) An act that requires HHS to conduct annual reviews to reduce and recover improper payments.

IMRT Intensity modulated radiation therapy.

in-situ In place.

in vitro fertilization (IVF) A series of procedures used to treat fertility problems.

incarcerated hernia A hernia that is not reducible because the protruding organ or structure is stuck in the tear in the abdominal wall.

incision and drainage (I/D) Procedure that involves cutting into the skin to remove fluid.

incisional biopsy A biopsy procedure that involves cutting into a lesion to obtain a specimen.

incus A bone in the ear that transmits sound vibrations.

indented code A code listed below the parent code; refers back to the base procedure or service and supplies additions to or variations of the base procedure.

independent insurance plan A group or organization of private practice physicians that negotiates contracts with insurance companies on their own behalf. Also known as *individual practice association (IPA)*.

Index The last section of the CPT® codebook that is the starting point for locating a code for a service or procedure.

indirect laryngoscopy A procedure that visualizes the larynx with a mirror held just below the back of the patient's throat.

individual practice association (IPA) A group or organization of private practice physicians that negotiates contracts with insurance companies on their own behalf. Also known as *independent insurance plan*.

induced abortion A medically assisted termination of a pregnancy.

infarction Necrosis caused by obstruction of circulation to an area.

informational modifiers Modifiers that provide additional information; may state whether a service is reasonable and necessary, and should be used in the second, third, or fourth modifier field.

infusion The process of administering nutrients.

ingesting The process when food enters the oral cavity and digestion begins.

ingestion challenge testing A way to diagnose an allergy to a specific food, drug, or other substance by observing the patient after ingestion of the suspected allergen. Also known as an *oral food challenge*.

injection Forcing fluid into a vessel or cavity.

inpatient A patient who is formally admitted to the hospital for treatment, usually requiring at least one overnight stay.

inpatient coders Hospital coders who use ICD-10 codes to report diagnoses and procedures.

inpatient procedures Medical procedures performed in the hospital.

inpatient prospective payment system (IPPS) A payment method that determines reimbursement for Medicare Part A inpatient services based on diagnosis-related groups.

insulin A hormone that regulates the absorption of glucose and other nutrients.

insurance A contract in which a private company or government agency (the insurer) agrees to compensate an individual or business (the insured) for a specified loss, damage, illness, or death in return for premiums.

insurance verification The process of verifying the patient's active health insurance benefits.

integrity agreement An agreement that outlines the obligations that a provider or small medical group has agreed to as part of a civil settlement.

intermediate ophthalmological service A service that includes the evaluation of a new problem; the performance of a history, external ocular, and adnexal examinations; and the use of mydriasis (dilation of the pupil) for ophthalmoscopy.

intermediate repair A layered closure of one or more of the deeper layers of subcutaneous tissue and superficial fascia in addition to the skin closure.

internal hemorrhoid A small swollen vein in the wall of the anal canal that may become very large, causing the vein to expand and protrude out of the anus.

internal fixation Devices such as pins, screws, metal plates, wires, or rods that are usually placed through the use of image guidance.

internal medical record audit An audit conducted by employees of a medical practice or organization.

International Classification of Diseases (ICD) A statistical classification system maintained by the World Health Organization (WHO).

International Classification of Functioning, Disability, and Health (ICF) A classification system used to categorize the health and disability functionality of individuals and the general population.

Internet-Only Manuals (IOMs) Publications that were once printed or sent to providers annually on computer disc and are now published only on the CMS website.

internship A type of job that allows medical students to practice medicine in a medical setting under the supervision of a teaching physician.

intersex surgery An operation to change genitalia from male to female or female to male. Also known as *sex reassignment surgery*.

interstitial brachytherapy A procedure in which sources are implanted directly into the tumor.

intervertebral disk A pad of cartilage found between the vertebrae.

intracapsular cataract extraction (ICCE) A procedure in which the lens and the capsule that houses the lens are removed.

intracavitary brachytherapy A procedure that uses a special applicator implanted inside a body cavity for treatment of cervical cancer.

intraluminal brachytherapy A procedure that uses special applicators to implant radioactive sources inside a body passage, such as the esophagus for treatment of esophageal cancers.

intramuscular injection An injection given directly into a muscle.

intraoral Within the mouth.

intravenous A process that infuses a drug into a vein where the drug enters the blood stream and has a systemic effect.

Introduction The section located at the beginning of the CPT® codebook.

introitus The entrance to the vagina.

intubation The placement of a tube in the trachea.

iridectomy The removal of the iris.

iris The colored portion of the eye.

ischemia A deficient blood supply due to obstruction of a blood vessel.

island pedicle flap A flap formed near but not immediately adjacent to the recipient site.

isodose The points or zones in a medium that receive equal doses of radiation.

jejunum A section of the small intestine.

Johannsen type urethroplasty A complex procedure that is performed in 2 stages during 2 different operative episodes several months apart.

joint An area that occurs where 2 bones meet.

keratoplasty The surgical repair of the cornea.

key components Three of 7 components that must be considered before selecting the level of service: history, examination, and medical decision making.

kickback A payment made to someone who has aided in a transaction or appointment, especially illegally.

kidney calculus or stone A concretion of minerals and acid salts formed when urine becomes concentrated, allowing the minerals to crystalize.

kidneys A pair of bean-shaped organs located behind the peritoneum on each side of the vertebral column.

knowledge-based encoder An encoder that has a format similar to the codebook, meaning that the coder must have knowledge of the CPT® codebook's guidelines and Index to successfully use the encoder.

labium (pl., labia) The fold at the margin of the vulva.

laboratory A place usually divided into 2 sections: anatomical pathology and clinical pathology.

laboratory report A report that contains results from laboratory tests performed on blood, urine, and other specimens from the patient.

labyrinth The internal ear, consisting of a bony portion and a membranous portion.

labyrinthectomy The removal of the incus, stapes, and the content of the vestibule.

labyrinthotomy A surgical incision into the labyrinth of the inner ear.

lacrimal bone A bone that forms part of the medial (middle) wall of the orbit.

lamina The portion of a vertebra that covers the nerve root.

laminectomy A surgery performed to remove the lamina, thereby relieving pressure on the spinal cord and nerves.

laminotomy A surgery performed to remove the part of the lamina. Also known as *hemilaminectomy*.

laparoscope A small, flexible tube with a tiny camera on the tip.

laparoscopic A surgery that provides an alternative to the traditional open technique by using a laparoscope.

laparoscopy The viewing of the abdominal organs or female reproductive organs through a laparoscope.

large intestine An organ that contains 3 components: cecum, colon, and rectum; helps move food materials that are not needed for nutrition out of the body.

laryngectomy A removal of the larynx.

laryngopharynx The distal portion of the pharynx.

larynx A tube-shaped organ located between the pharynx and the trachea containing the vocal cords.

laser coagulation A procedure that heats the prostate tissue to a point where cells cannot survive.

laser enucleation The removal of the whole prostate organ.

laser vaporization A procedure that uses a green-light laser that emits energy that vaporizes (converts into gas) tissue.

laterality modifier A modifier used to report anatomical location, that is, the side of the body on which a procedure was performed.

layered closure A procedure that requires closure of both the skin and subcutaneous layers and is reported with the codes for intermediate wound repair.

left atrium An upper chamber of the heart.

left ventricle A lower chamber of the heart.

lens A transparent body behind the pupil.

levels of E/M services Levels that describe variations in the scope of services rendered and are the qualifying factors that distinguish codes within their respective categories and subcategories.

ligament The fibrous tissue that connects bone to bone.

ligation The tying off of veins and arteries.

limited diagnostic study A diagnostic study that does not include the maximum possible images of an organ or anatomical structures related to the specific body part examined.

linear accelerator based A type of radiation treatment that intensifies x-rays.

lingual Tongue.

lingual frenum The fold of skin that connects the tongue to the floor of the mouth.

lips The external part of the mouth, located in the lower center portion of the face.

List of Excluded Individuals/Entities (LEIE) A database on the OIG website that lists individuals and entities that are not allowed to work with Medicare, Medicaid, and other federally funded healthcare programs.

lithiasis The formation of a calculus.

liver An organ located in the upper right quadrant of the abdomen; filters blood that passes from the capillaries of the small intestine, processing nutrients, chemicals, and drugs that enter the body.

lobectomy The excision of a lobe of the lung.

local anesthesia Anesthesia that affects only a small, specific area of the body, causing loss of pain, feeling, and temperature sensation, as well as muscle relaxation.

local coverage determinations (LCDs) An online CMS resource that details how Medicare Administrative Contractors (MACs) apply national coverage determinations (NCDs) to their assigned jurisdictions (regions).

localization device A clip, metallic pellet, wire/needle, or other device inserted into tissue using image guidance to mark a biopsy site for greater accuracy.

locum tenens physician A substitute physician when a regular physician is not able to care for a patient due to extenuating circumstances.

logic-based encoder An encoder in which the coding specialist enters a main term and then answers a series of questions so that the encoder can provide the appropriate code.

longitudinal gastrectomy A procedure that removes a portion of the stomach and uses staples to create a smaller elongated, sleeve-shaped stomach. Also known as a *vertical sleeve gastrectomy.*

loop electrosurgical excision procedure (LEEP) A procedure in which a thin wire and an electrical current are used to cut away tissue from the cervix for biopsy.

low complexity A type of straightforward medical decision making.

low severity A problem that has a low risk of morbidity (disease) without treatment, little to no risk of mortality (death), and an expected full recovery without any functional impairment.

lower esophageal sphincter A muscle at the top of the stomach that contracts and relaxes, allowing food to enter the stomach and not return to the esophagus.

lumbar puncture A procedure in which a needle is inserted into the lumbar spine to obtain cerebrospinal fluid. Also known as *spinal tap* and *spinal puncture.*

Lund-Browder Classification Method A method used for estimating the total body surface area (TBSA) of burns.

lungs Two organs that bring oxygen to the blood and remove carbon dioxide from the body.

lymph A clear, colorless tissue fluid

lymph vessel A structure that transports lymph.

lymphadenectomy The removal of lymph nodes.

lymphatic system The body system that consists of lymph nodes, lymph vessels, the spleen, and the thymus gland.

macula A yellowish circle area within the retina that allows for central vision.

macular degeneration The progressive damage to the macular of the retina, causing loss of central vision.

magnetic resonance angiography (MRA) The use of magnetic resonance imaging equipment and contrast materials to better visualize blood vessels.

magnetic resonance imaging (MRI) A technique that uses a magnetic field and radio waves to create detailed images of the organs and tissues within the body.

main term The primary component of a service or procedure.

malignant Invasive, progressively worsening.

malleus A bone in the ear that transmits sound vibrations.

mammary ductogram A special type of mammogram used for imaging the breast ducts. Also known as *galactogram.*

mammography The radiographic visualization of the breast.

managed care organization (MCO) A system of healthcare in which patients agree to receive care from selected doctors and hospitals.

managed care patient An individual who has been assigned to or has selected physicians of a specific managed care organization.

manipulation The therapeutic manual adjustment of an anatomical site.

margin The area surrounding the lesion that is free from disease but is also excised to make sure all the diseased cells have been removed.

marsupialization The surgical alteration of a cyst or similar enclosed cavity by making an incision and suturing the flaps to the adjacent tissue, creating a pouch.

massively parallel sequencing (MPS) Any of several high-throughput approaches to DNA sequencing. Also known as *next-generation sequencing (NGS).*

mastectomy The removal of the breast.

masticator space An area from base of the mouth to the hyoid bone.

mastoid An air space in the temporal bone.

mastoidectomy A surgery to remove infected cells in the hollow, air-filled spaces in the skull, postauricular.

mastoiditis An inflammation of the mastoid.

mastotomy An incision into the breast.

maxillary sinuses Structures located in the maxillary bone located under the eyes.

measurement of post-voiding residual urine A test that involves using ultrasound to measure the residual urine or bladder capacity after the patient has urinated.

mechanical thrombectomy The removal of a thrombus to restore circulation, and which may be performed for a patient diagnosed with a thrombus or an embolus.

mechanical valve A valve made of metal or carbon parts that is more durable than a biological valve.

Meckel's diverticulum A pouch on the wall of the lower part of the intestine.

MEDCIN A medical nomenclature used in EHR systems that enables the system to index, store, and combine medical data.

mediastinum The space in the chest between the lungs.

Medicaid Integrity Contractors (MICs) Contracted reviewers who are assigned to review Medicaid provider activities, audit claims, identify overpayments, and educate providers and others.

medical claim appeal The process of requesting that a previously denied claim be reevaluated for payment.

medical coding The process of assigning standardized alphanumeric identifiers to the diagnoses and procedures documented in a health record.

medical compliance The process of meeting the regulations, recommendations, and expectations of federal and state agencies that pay for medical services and procedures.

medical compliance program A formal plan that outlines how an organization or medical practice will monitor, identify, correct, and disclose actions that may place the organization at risk of violating laws and regulations that affect their businesses.

medical decision making (MDM) The complexity of establishing a diagnosis and/or selecting a management strategy.

medical identity theft A crime perpetrated when a person uses someone else's name or insurance information to obtain medical treatment, acquire prescription medication, or receive payment for false claims.

medical radiation dosimetrist A person who uses computer and mathematical calculations to design a treatment plan that includes the technique to deliver the prescribed radiation dose.

medical radiation physicist A person who works with the radiation oncologist to design a treatment schedule that will kill cancer cells.

medical record A legal document that contains descriptions of all the products and services provided to a patient. Also known as a *health record.*

medical team conference A meeting of at least 3 providers from different specialties to develop and implement healthcare services for a patient.

Medically Unlikely Edits A tool used to identify codes that should never be reported together.

Medicare The federal health insurance program for people who are 65 or older, individuals with disabilities, and people with end-stage renal disease.

Medicare Administrative Contractors (MACs) People who use data collected from Comprehensive Error Rate Testing and recovery contractors to target improper payment risks within their jurisdictions.

Medicare Claims Processing Manual A manual that contains guidelines that specify what makes a specific service or procedure billable.

Medicare Learning Network (MLN) A page on the CMS website that provides educational and reference materials related to various Medicare documentation and coding guidelines.

Medicare National Coverage Determinations (NCD) Manual A manual that contains Medicare's interpretation of how a specific treatment or diagnosis is covered.

Medicare Physician Fee Schedule (MPFS) A price list of services and procedures set by CMS.

Medicare Program Integrity Manual A manual that contains guidance for CMS contactors who are responsible for reviewing provider records and reimbursements for compliance with CMS policies.

Medicare secondary payer (MSP) A provision that coordinates benefits to ensure that Medicare does not pay for services and items that the beneficiary's other health insurance is responsible for paying.

megaelectron 1 million electronvolts or 1 MeV.

megavoltage Greater than or equal to 1 MeV.

Meniere's disease The build-up of endolymph in the inner ear.

meninges The layers of membranes that cover the brain and spinal cord: dura mater, arachnoid, and pia matter.

meningitis A condition of swelling of the brain.

MeV 1 million electron volts.

microbiology laboratory A laboratory that performs identification of microorganisms that cause disease.

microscopic exam An exam conducted under a microscope.

microscopic examination A process that involves examining organ samples under a microscope.

microscopy The examination of urine specimens under a microscope for biological abnormalities such as bacteria, and chemical abnormalities such as crystals.

middle ear The tympanic cavity.

middle fossa approach A technique that involves an incision above the ear and a craniotomy over the temporal lobe of the brain.

mid-level A medical provider who has completed under-graduate studies in a specific scope of patient care. Also known as a *nonphysician practitioner (NPP).*

minimal A problem that may not require the presence of a physician to treat.

minor A problem that is transient and is not likely to alter the patient's health status permanently or has a good prognosis if the patient complies with medical treatment. Also known as *self-limited.*

MLC Multileaf collimator.

M-mode An imaging mode that displays a 1-dimensional video.

mobilization A manual therapy technique in which the therapist manipulates the joint by manually applying therapeutic movements within or at the end of the range of motion.

modality A physical agent applied to produce therapeutic changes to biologic tissue that includes the use of hot or cold packs, electrical stimulation, whirlpool treatment, and paraffin bath treatment.

mode The type of ultrasound image captured during a procedure.

moderate (conscious) sedation A state created by providing the patient with a combination of sedatives and analgesics to help him or her tolerate an uncomfortable procedure.

moderate complexity A level of medical decision making.

moderate sedation A state in which a patient is drowsy, relaxed, and able to respond to verbal commands. Also known as *conscious sedation.*

moderate severity A problem that has a moderate risk of morbidity without treatment, a moderate risk of mortality without treatment, an uncertain prognosis, or a higher risk of prolonged functional impairment.

modified radical mastectomy A procedure that involves the removal of the breast, overlying skin, and axillary lymph nodes.

modifier A 2-character code that is sometimes added to CPT® or HCPCS codes when the procedure, service, or item was altered from the code description.

modifying term A term that provides a description of a code associated with the main term.

molecular A term relating to molecules.

molecular pathology The identification of the risk of developing a particular disease by analyzing specific genes.

monitored anesthesia care (MAC) A professional service that involves both the administration of sedatives and analgesics as well as the intraoperative monitoring of a patient's vital functions during a procedure in anticipation of the need for general anesthesia.

monitoring The process of observing or checking the effectiveness of the compliance program over an extended period.

morbidity Statistics regarding illness.

morcellation A procedure in which tissue is divided and removed in small pieces.

moribund A terminal patient.

morphology The study of microscopic anatomy. Also known as *histology.*

morphology codes Codes that describe the form and structure of tumors.

mortality Statistics regarding death.

motor nerve conduction study A study done by stimulating motor nerves and measuring the compound muscle action.

multifetal reduction (MPR) A procedure used to reduce the number of fetuses carried to gestation.

multiple leads Three or four leads with pacing and sensing functions in any combination of atrium and ventricle.

multi-source Cobalt 60 based A type of stereotactic radiation treatment used for cranial applications.

SBRT Stereotactic body radiation therapy.

scan The type of ultrasound image captured during the procedure.

sclera The tough, white, outer coating of the eye.

scleral buckling A procedure that involves the physician exploring the sclera to locate the site of the retinal detachment.

sclerectomy The removal of the sclera with punch or scissors.

screen A test.

screening mammogram A preventive service performed on patients without signs or symptoms of breast disease.

scrotum A pouch of skin that holds the testes.

secondary defect The site of the tissue being transferred to repair the primary defect.

secondary rhinoplasty A revision of an original rhinoplasty to correct unfavorable results.

second level of appeal The level of appeal where a qualified independent contractor will review any evidence not previously reviewed at a lower level for a second redetermination.

second-look operation A procedure to check for recurrence of tumor(s).

section A group in the CPT® codebook of which there are six: evaluation and management, anesthesiology, surgery, radiology, pathology and laboratory, and medicine.

segmentectomy The removal of a lung segment.

self-disclosure The process of healthcare providers becoming aware of and reporting compliance violations to the appropriate agency or program.

self-limited A problem that is transient and is not likely to alter the patient's health status permanently or has a good prognosis if the patient complies with medical treatment. Also known as *minor*.

self-pay A fee-for-service reimbursement method by which the patient or the guarantor pays for each service or procedure rendered.

self-pay patients Patients who pay for the entire visit themselves.

seminal vesicles The glands that produce fluid to mix with semen.

senile macular degeneration A disease that causes vision loss in people over the age of 50. Also known as *age-related macular degeneration (AMD)*.

sensory nerve conduction study A study done by stimulating a nerve at one point and measuring the action potential at another point on the nerve.

separate procedure A procedure or service that is usually carried out as an integral component of a larger service but which may be reported separately under certain circumstances.

septal defect Any anomaly in the separating wall.

septum A thin partition that separates the nostrils.

sequential procedure When a surgery is attempted as a laparoscopic procedure but must be converted to an open procedure.

serology The examination of blood serum, particularly with regard to the response of the immune system to pathogens or substances.

serum globulin A protein made from human blood.

sex reassignment surgery An operation to change genitalia from male to female or female to male. Also known as *intersex surgery*.

shaving The removal of dermal or epidermal lesions horizontally or transversely, without full-thickness (epidermal and dermal) excision.

sialography An x-ray image of the salivary glands.

sialolithotomy An incisional treatment for a salivary duct stone.

sigmoidoscopy The endoscopic examination of the entire rectum and sigmoid colon, which may include a portion of the descending colon.

simple closure The suturing (stitching) of one layer of the skin.

simple mastectomy The removal of the entire breast for a patient with no lymph node involvement or one who may not be able to tolerate a more extensive procedure.

simple repair A closure that involves only one layer of the skin.

single chamber pacemaker system A system that includes a pulse generator and one electrode placed in either the atrium or ventricle.

single lead A pacemaker or implantable defibrillator that has pacing and sensing functions in either the atrium or the ventricle, but not both.

single photon emission computed tomography (SPECT) The radioactive tracers used in combination with a CT scan to visualize blood flow to tissue and organs.

sinus of Valsalva The aortic sinus: a dilatation in the aortic wall and valves.

sinuses The air cavities within the cranial bone that open into the nasal cavity.

skin graft A graft that uses transplanted tissue to repair a defect.

skin grafting The process of transplanting skin.

skin substitute graft A temporary wound closure used to promote healing until a permanent graft can be applied.

skull base The structure made up of the regions of the anterior, middle, and posterior cranial fossae.

sleep medicine study A procedure used by physicians in the diagnosis of patients with suspected sleep disorders.

slit lamp An instrument that produces low-intensity light beams to provide an enlarged, three-dimensional view of the front parts of the eye.

small bowel The organ that includes 3 sections: duodenum, jejunum, and ileum; contains millions of capillaries that allow nutrients to pass into the bloodstream. Also known as *small intestine.*

small intestine The organ that includes 3 sections: duodenum, jejunum, and ileum; contains millions of capillaries that allow nutrients to pass into the bloodstream. Also known as *small bowel.*

snare technique A procedure in which a wire is wrapped around a lesion, then heated, causing the lesion to be shaved off by the heated wire.

SNOMED-CT A nomenclature that is specially designed to improve the accuracy of information entered into EHR systems as well as improve communication between EHR systems, thereby improving the quality of care patients receive when they seek treatment from different medical providers. CT stands for *clinical terminology.*

SOAP note A progress note format representing the *subjective, objective, assessment,* and *plan* categories of information.

social history The history that documents the social factors that may affect the patient's health.

soft tissue The tissue that supports or surrounds other structures in the body; includes ligaments, tendons, and fascia, among others.

somatic nervous system The system that deals with voluntary movement.

sonogram An image recorded from ultrasonic echoes.

special report The documentation that provides additional information about the service or procedure to the insurance payer, such as length of time spent, the extent and effort required, equipment used, and the medical necessity of the service or procedure.

specimen The material being analyzed; a sample that represents the whole.

spectral Doppler scan A scan that presents blood flow measurements plotted graphically on a grid showing flow velocities recorded over time.

spermatic cord A cord that suspends the testes in the scrotum; contains the vas deferens, vessels, and nerves.

sphenoid sinuses The structures located behind the nasal cavity at the base of the skull.

sphincter A muscle that opens and closes access to a duct, tube, or orifice.

sphincter of Oddi A valve-like structure surrounding pancreatic and common bile ducts.

spinal anesthesia Anesthesia that is similar to epidural anesthesia in its effect on a large area of the body.

spinal cord A band of nervous tissue that connects the brain to the rest of the body.

spinal puncture A procedure in which a needle is inserted into the lumbar spine to obtain cerebrospinal fluid. Also known as *lumbar puncture* and *spinal tap.*

spinal tap A procedure in which a needle is inserted into the lumbar spine to obtain cerebrospinal fluid. Also known as *lumbar puncture* and *spinal puncture.*

spine The structure made up of a collection of small bones called vertebrae and extends from the skull to the lower back. Also known as the *vertebral column.*

splenectomy The excision of the spleen.

split-thickness graft A graft that contains the epidermis and a portion of the dermis of the donor site.

spontaneous abortion The termination of pregnancy through miscarriage before 20 weeks, 0 days.

SRS Stereotactic radiosurgery.

stab phlebectomy A procedure in which tiny stab incisions are made over a varicose vein and a phlebectomy hook is used to grab the vein.

staghorn calculus A stone that fills the renal pelvis and calyces.

stapes A bone in the ear that transmits sound vibrations.

stapled hemorrhoidopexy A procedure used for prolapsed internal hemorrhoids.

statement of limitations A section in the insurance policy that clearly states what services, procedures, and circumstances are not reimbursed by the health insurance company.

stereotactic body radiation therapy (SBRT) The principle of cranial SRS as applied to treatment of body tumors; designed to minimize damage to healthy tissue while maximizing delivery of radiation to the tumor.

stereotactic radiosurgery (SRS) A radiation therapy technique used to deliver large amounts of radiation to distinct tumor sites in the brain.

stereotaxis The use of 3-dimensional imaging to locate the site of surgery or radiation.

stoma A surgical opening.

stomach The organ that includes 3 parts: fundus, body, and antrum; the lining contains mucous membranes that secrete digestive proteins to continue the digestion process.

strabismus A condition characterized by an imbalance of extraocular muscles that control movement of the eyeball.

straightforward complexity A low level of medical decision making.

strangulated hernia An incarcerated hernia that is losing or has lost blood supply.

strapping Reinforcing and providing support for ligament structures by wrapping them with overlapping strips of adhesive plaster or tape to exert pressure and hold a structure in place.

subcutaneous injection An injection given into the fatty tissue under the dermal layer of the skin.

subcutaneous mastectomy The removal of all breast tissue, leaving the skin and nipple intact.

subcutaneous tissue The innermost layer of the skin. Also known as *hypodermis*.

subjective documentation A statement, in the patient's or family's own words, describing how the patient is feeling or why he or she is seeing the provider.

sublingual Under the tongue.

sublingual glands The salivary glands.

submandibular The salivary glands.

submandibular space The area below the mandibular/jaw bone.

submental space The area below the chin.

subsection A group in the CPT® codebook that is titled based on procedures or anatomical sites.

sunset date The date when a procedure or service is automatically removed from the CPT® codebook.

supervision and interpretation The medical provider's use of imaging equipment during a surgical procedure or diagnostic study and the medical opinion of the captured images.

supine position A patient positioned on back, face up.

surfer's ear The development of new bone on the surface of an existing bone in the external auditory canal. Also known as *exostosis*.

surgical package A package made up of the services and time involved in performing a normal, uncomplicated surgical service.

sympathetic nervous system The system that activates the "fight or flight" response that prepares the body to react to a stressful situation by increasing the heart rate and slowing digestion.

symptomatic aortic stenosis A narrowing of the valve that constricts normal blood flow. 360

system review A series of questions asked by the provider to obtain information from the patient about his or her current condition. Also known as *review of systems (ROS)*.

Systematized Nomenclature of Medicine (SNOMED) A nomenclature that contains the names of diseases, bacteria, anatomic sites, procedures, and other medical terms, as well as the corresponding medical codes.

systemic disease The condition that affects multiple organs and tissues or the whole body.

tarsorrhaphy To partially suture together to narrow an opening.

TDF Time/dose/fractionation.

technical component The component that reports the deployment of equipment for the diagnostic test by the owner of the equipment.

technical skills The knowledge and ability to work efficiently with technology.

telehealth services Services rendered via a real-time interactive audio and video telecommunications system. Reported with modifier 95. The beneficiary must be located at an eligible originating site (a Rural Health Clinic and/or a county outside of a Metropolitan Statistical Area).

teletherapy A variety of radiation techniques that uses a source outside the body to treat cancer.

temporal bone The bone located at the base of the skull underneath the temple.

temporal fossa The area on the skull just below the temporal lines.

tendon A band of fibrous tissue that connects muscle to bone.

testes The paired male reproductive organs that produce sperm and testosterone. Also known as *testis* or *testicles*.

testicles The paired male reproductive organs that produce sperm and testosterone. Also known as *testis* or *testes*.

testis The paired male reproductive organs that produce sperm and testosterone. Also known as *testes* or *testicles*.

The Joint Commission An accrediting organization that has been approved by CMS as having standards and a survey process that exceed federal requirements.

therapeutic Procedures performed to treat illness, disease, or injuries.

therapeutic drug assay A quantitative study performed to determine the amount of a known drug present in the patient's whole blood, serum, plasma, or cerebrospinal fluid.

therapeutic radiology simulation The process of determining the targeted anatomy and collecting data and images necessary to develop the ideal radiation treatment process for the patient.

third level of appeal An appeal that may be requested up to 60 days after receiving notice of a qualified independent contractor (QIC) decision or if a decision is not received from the QIC before the applicable time frame.

third-party payer An entity contracted to pay the medical provider on behalf the policyholder. 6, 686

thoracentesis The surgical puncture of the thoracic cavity to remove fluid.

thoracic The chest.

thoracoscopy The use of a lighted endoscope to view pleural spaces and thoracic cavity or perform surgical procedures.

thoracostomy A procedure to drain the space around the lungs when a disease causes pleural effusion (fluid buildup) or an injury causes blood or air to build up in the chest cavity.

thoracotomy The surgical incision into the chest cavity.

thrombosis The presence or condition of a blood clot in a vessel.

thrombosis (clotted) hemorrhoids Hemorrhoids caused by clotted blood.

thymectomy The removal of the thymus gland.

thymus gland A gland located above the heart that produces T lymphocytes during early childhood.

thyroid The largest endocrine gland, located in the neck.

thyroidectomy The removal of the thyroid.

time A factor in the description of many E/M codes.

time-based code A Category I code that may be applied based on the amount of face-to-face time the healthcare provider spends with the patient.

timely filing The period of time that the provider has to submit the first insurance claim to the payer.

tissue transfer A skin graft in which the piece of skin used for transplant is still partially attached to the donor site and is used to cover an adjacent defect.

TLD Thermoluminescent dosimeter.

tomography A radiographic technique that produces cross section images of tissue structures at a predetermined depth.

tongue tie A condition in which the lingual frenum is too short, limiting the mobility of the tongue. Also known as *ankyloglossia*.

tonsillectomy The removal of the tonsils, a viable treatment for chronic tonsillitis or for cancer of the tonsils.

total body hypothermia The therapeutic treatment involving intentional reduction of body temperature to reduce tissue metabolism.

toxoid vaccines Vaccines made up of inactivated toxic compounds. Also known as *toxoids*.

toxoids Vaccines made up of inactivated toxic compounds. Also known as *toxoid vaccines*.

trachea The airway that connects the larynx to the primary bronchi.

tracheostomy A procedure that creates an opening in the neck to the trachea.

traction The application of force to a limb for the purpose of straightening bones or relieving pressure.

training The act of teaching or reinforcing skills or applications.

transabdominal Through the abdomen.

tympanic membrane A membrane that vibrates in response to sound waves.

transcatheter aortic valve implantation (TAVI) A procedure for patients with aortic stenosis who are not candidates for open chest surgery. Also known as *transcatheter aortic valve replacement*.

transcatheter aortic valve replacement (TAVR) A procedure for patients with aortic stenosis who are not candidates for open chest surgery. Also known as *transcatheter aortic valve implantation*.

transcatheter mitral valve repair (TMVR) A procedure used to treat mitral regurgitation.

transducer An instrument that transmits sound waves.

transfer of care A process that occurs when a physician gives the responsibility of providing services to a patient to another physician who explicitly agrees to accept this responsibility.

transforaminal injection An injection given through the foramen.

transluminal A procedure performed through the lumen or opening.

transurethral resection of the prostate (TURP) A surgical procedure used to treat patients with prostate cancer.

transvaginal Through the vagina.

trephination A technique that uses a trephine to cut out circular sections of the iris and sclera.

trephine A cylindrically shaped surgical saw used to remove a circular section of the skull.

trigger point Spots of hypersensitive irritability within a band of muscle. Also known as *muscle knot*.

truncus arteriosus An arterial trunk: undivided short portion.

tunica vaginalis The serous membrane that surrounds testes.

twist drill A manually operated drill.

tympanoplasty The surgical repair of a perforated tympanic membrane.

tympanostomy The insertion of plastic or metal ventilating tubes to allow for fluid drainage; an effective treatment for conditions such as eustachian tube dysfunction and conductive hearing loss.

ultrasound A procedure that uses sound waves to create images.

unbundling The practice of using multiple codes when one code could sufficiently cover all the components of a service.

undermining Surgically separating the skin from its underlying connective tissue.

unilateral Relating to 1 side of a 2-sided anatomical structure.

unlisted code A code used to report the services or procedures that do not have a Category I or temporary code. Also referred to as a *dummy code*.

unlisted procedure code A code used when a surgeon performs a procedure or service that is not specifically listed in the CPT® codebook.

upcoding The process of reporting a service or procedure that is more extensive than what the documentation supports. Also known as *overcoding*.

uptake The absorption of a radiopharmaceutical into the diseased tissue.

ureterolithotomy The removal of calculus by making an incision into the ureter.

ureteroliths Stones that have developed in the kidney and have moved to the ureter.

ureterostomy An opening.

ureterotomy A small incision.

ureters 2 tubes (one connected to each of the kidneys) that carry the urine from the kidney to the bladder.

urethra The single tube that passes the urine from the bladder to the outside of the body.

urethrography X-ray imaging of the urethra.

urethroplasy The repair of a defect in the urethra, often performed on a patient with urethral stricture due to scarring.

urinalysis The analysis of urine; used to detect disease in the urinary tract.

urinary system The system that removes waste from the body, regulates fluid volume, and maintains electrolyte balance in the fluids within the body.

urodynamics The study of how well the bladder is holding and emptying urine.

uroflowmetry (UFR) A study that measures urine speed and volume.

uterine tubes The tubes that allow ova to move from the ovaries to the uterus. Also called *fallopian tubes* or *oviducts*.

uterus An organ involved with the functions of menstruation, pregnancy, and labor.

uvula The tissue in the back of the throat.

vaccine An injection that causes the body to create antibodies against the specific microorganism or virus that was given.

vagina The tube that connects the uterus to the outside of the body.

vaginal birth after cesarean (VBAC) A planned vaginal delivery for a patient who has previously delivered by C-section.

valve A membranous fold in a passage that prevents reflux.

varicose vein A common condition of the valves in the vein not functioning properly, allowing the vein to become filled with blood.

vas deferens The tube that transports sperm.

vasectomy The removal of vas deferens.

vasovasostomy The reversal of a vasectomy.

vein A vessel that carries deoxygenated blood from the body to the heart.

venography The radiographic visualization of a vein.

ventricle The lower chamber of the heart.

ventricles The spaces within the brain that contain cerebrospinal fluid.

vermilion The red epithelium that starts at the intraoral "moist line" and extends outward on the face. Also known as *vermilion border*.

vermilion border The red epithelium that starts at the intraoral "moist line" and extends outward on the face. Also known as *vermilion*.

vermilionectomy An excision performed on the vermilion of the lip.

vertebral body A thick segment of bone in each vertebra.

vertebral column A structure made up of a collection of small bones called vertebrae that extends from the skull to the lower back. Also known as the *spine*.

vertebral corpectomy The removal of part or all of the vertebral body and the intervertebral discs above and below the segment.

vertical sleeve gastrectomy A procedure that removes a portion of the stomach and uses staples to create a smaller elongated, sleeve-shaped stomach. Also known as a *longitudinal gastrectomy*.

vesical neck The structure that connects the urinary bladder to the urethra.

vestibule The mucous membrane–lined arch around the front and sides of the oral cavity in front of the teeth and gingiva and inside of the lips and cheeks.

vestibuloplasty A surgical modification to increase the depth and width of the vestibule of the mouth.

view A radiographic image study described by an x-ray exposure of an anatomical site.

vitrectomy The removal and replacement of vitreous.

vitreous humor The clear gel that fills the eye.

vocal cords 2 bands of muscle that form a V shape inside the larynx.

vulva The external genitalia that surrounds the vagina.

vulvectomy An excision of the vulva.

warfarin An anticoagulant (blood-thinner) drug that prevents blood clots. Also known by brand name *Coumadin*.

wet macular degeneration A disease caused by the leaking of fluids from blood vessels or blood into the macula.

Whipple procedure A procedure that removes the head of the pancreas, where tumors are most likely to occur.

whistleblower A person who reveals misconduct or informs the government of fraudulent acts.

work hardening A program specifically designed to build strength and endurance for work tasks so the patient can return to work after an injury.

workers' compensation A contract in which patients seek treatment for illnesses or injuries acquired while at work.

write-off The process of canceling out the uncollectable balance.

written report A report that documents in detail the imaging examination and the medical findings prepared by the physician who supervised and interpreted the diagnostic procedure.

x-ray High-energy electromagnetic radiation with short wavelengths that are absorbed to different degrees by different materials; popularly, an image created by use of x-ray technology.

Z-plasty An incision in which the letter Z is centered over the defect, and the two incisions at each end are equal in length to the center incision.

Zone Program Integrity Contractors (ZPICs) People who are responsible for identifying fraud in 7 geographic zones in the United States. Formerly known as *Program Safeguard Contractors (PSCs).*

zygote A cell formed by the union of the sperm and the ovum.

Index

Symbols

A

B

C

F

G

H

I

J

K

L

M

N

O

P

Q

R

S

T

U

V

Photo Credits

xxviii top © iStock.com/Maartje van Caspel; xxviii bottom © iStock.com/JLGutierrez; 1 © iStock/alexsl; 3 © RTimages/Shutterstock.com; 7 © iStock.com/seanami; 8 © Paradigm Publishing; 16 © iStock.com/PeopleImages; 21 © iStock.com/bjdlzx; 23 © Paradigm Publishing; 25 © iStock.com/Elenathewise; 26 © iStock.com/sturti; 31 © RTimages/Shutterstock.com; 33 © iStock.com/ eyenigelen, 33 © iStock.com/mattjeacock; 34 © iStock.com/ineskoleva; 38 © iStock.com/AMR Image; 45 © iStock.com/ Alina555; 65 © RTimages/Shutterstock.com; 74 © Tristanb at the English language Wikipedia; 76 © iStockphoto.com/danielzgombic; 78 © iStock.com/bowdenimages; 82 © iStock/danr13; 89 © RTimages/Shutterstock.com; 92 © Dragon Images/ Shutterstock.com; 99 © Poznyakov/Shutterstock.com; 103 © ProStockStudio/Shutterstock.com; 106 © fivepointsix/Shutterstock.com; 113 © Tyler Olson/Shutterstock.com; 115 © CandyBox Images/Shutterstock.com; 125 © RTimages/Shutterstock.com; 148 © iStock.com/ BeyzaSultanDURNA, 148 © iStock.com/sturti; 149 © iStock.com/Ratsanai; 151 © RTimages/Shutterstock.com; 155 © iStock.com/fstop123; 163 © iStock.com/michaeljung; 173 © iStock.com/asiseeit; 178 © iStock.com/ddea; 180 © iStock.com/YvanDube; 184 © iStock.com/ M_a_y_a; 185 © iStock.com/RapidEye; 193 © RTimages/Shutterstock.com; 195 © iStock.com/stoffies; 217 © RTimages/Shutterstock.com; 219 © Kotin/Shutterstock.com; 225 © iStockphoto.com/sturti; 227 © herjua/Shutterstock.com; 241 © RTimages/Shutterstock.com; 254 Reprinted with permission from DermNetNZ.org., 254 Reprinted with permission from DermNetNZ.org.; 275 © RTimages/Shutterstock.com; 294 © R.C.Hall - K.Kaplan - Medical Media / Custom Medical Stock Photo—All rights reserved.; 301 © RTimages/Shutterstock.com; 317 Reprinted with permission from Harald Krauss, Kaiser-Franz-Josef Hospital, Vienna, Austria.; 318 © Guzel Studio/Shutterstock.com; 327 © RTimages/Shutterstock.com; 361 © RTimages/Shutterstock.com; 367 © Aleksandr Markin/Shutterstock.com; 415 © RTimages/Shutterstock .com; 439 © RTimages/Shutterstock.com; 463 © iStock/Trish233; 475 © RTimages/Shutterstock.com; 503 © RTimages/Shutterstock.com; 512 © Custom Medical Stock Photo / Custom Medical Stock Photo—All rights reserved.; 539 © RTimages/Shutterstock.com; 541 © iStock.com/4774344sean; 550 © Praisaeng/Shutterstock.com; 551 © iStock.com/lisafx; 553 © ntdanai/Shutterstock.com; 554 © CristinaMuraca/Shutterstock.com, 554 © Gloszilla Studio/Shutterstock.com; 555 © IxMaster/Shutterstock.com, 555 © S. Grover/Custom Medical Stock Photo—All rights reserved.; 557 © Monkey Business Images/Shutterstock.com; 559 © CristinaMuraca/Shutterstock.com; 579 © RTimages/Shutterstock.com; 581 © iStock.com/Alija; 587 © iStock.com/CarolinaSmith; 591 © Alexander Raths/Shutterstock.com; 594 © iStock.com/elkor; 595 © iStock.com/ftwitty; 605 © RTimages/Shutterstock.com; 610 © iStock.com/PhotoEuphoria; 612 © iStock.com/4774344sean; 617 © iStock .com/Maica; 620 © J. Cavallini / Custom Medical Stock Photo—All rights reserved.; 630 © Li Wa/Shutterstock.com; 633 © iStock.com/kali9; 634 © 3660 Group / Custom Medical Stock Photo—All rights reserved.; 636 © iStock.com/seiki14; 644 © Andrey_Popov/Shutterstock.com; 645 © iStock.com/jsmith, 645 public domain; 647 © RTimages/Shutterstock.com, 647 Public domain; 649 © iStock.com/vm; 650 © iStock.com/KLH49; 651 © Paradigm Publishing; 683 © RTimages/Shutterstock.com; 685 © iStock.com/rozkmina; 686 © Junial Enterprises/Shutterstock.com; 688 © suphakit73/Shutterstock.com; 690 © iStock.com/Daniilantiq; 701 © Matej Kastelic/ Shutterstock.com.

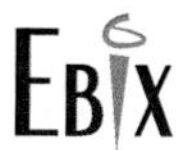

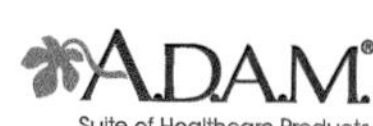

Images courtesy of A.D.A.M. a business unit of Ebix, Inc. All rights reserved. Images may not be reproduced in any manner without express written consent of A.D.A.M., a business unit of Ebix, Inc.; 1 Ebix Way, Johns Creek, GA 30097 USA

Page 1252, 291, 320, 369, 393, 489, 506, 522, 531, 535, 563, 564, 614

nucleus

Illustration Copyright © 2017 Nucleus Medical Media, All rights reserved.
www.nucleusmedicalmedia.com

Page 289, 290, 294, 340, 371, 393, 398, 399, 451, 480, 486, 500